Surgery of the Salivary Glands

AF871812

Mahmoud Sakr

Surgery of the Salivary Glands

Diagnostic and Therapeutic Strategies

Springer

Mahmoud Sakr
Faculty of Medicine, Department of Surgery
Alexandria University
Alexandria, Egypt

ISBN 978-3-031-82071-7 ISBN 978-3-031-82069-4 (eBook)
https://doi.org/10.1007/978-3-031-82069-4

© The Editor(s) (if applicable) and The Author(s), under exclusive license to Springer Nature Switzerland AG 2024

This work is subject to copyright. All rights are solely and exclusively licensed by the Publisher, whether the whole or part of the material is concerned, specifically the rights of translation, reprinting, reuse of illustrations, recitation, broadcasting, reproduction on microfilms or in any other physical way, and transmission or information storage and retrieval, electronic adaptation, computer software, or by similar or dissimilar methodology now known or hereafter developed.
The use of general descriptive names, registered names, trademarks, service marks, etc. in this publication does not imply, even in the absence of a specific statement, that such names are exempt from the relevant protective laws and regulations and therefore free for general use.
The publisher, the authors and the editors are safe to assume that the advice and information in this book are believed to be true and accurate at the date of publication. Neither the publisher nor the authors or the editors give a warranty, expressed or implied, with respect to the material contained herein or for any errors or omissions that may have been made. The publisher remains neutral with regard to jurisdictional claims in published maps and institutional affiliations.

This Springer imprint is published by the registered company Springer Nature Switzerland AG
The registered company address is: Gewerbestrasse 11, 6330 Cham, Switzerland

If disposing of this product, please recycle the paper.

To my dear students and colleagues

Preface

Management of salivary gland disorders encompasses a broad array of both benign and malignant diseases. The purpose of this authored book is to provide a comprehensive review of the current knowledge of the pathophysiology, diagnostic techniques, and therapeutic strategies of salivary gland disorders. We have endeavored to give some rein to the new developments, which are evidence-based and widely supported in the literature.

This book, in 28 chapters with 137 images, 37 tables, and 2260 references, will provide a valuable source of knowledge and reference for all specialists and trainees entrusted with the care of patients suffering from salivary gland disorders. It addresses a wide range of topics including embryological development and anomalies, histology, surgical anatomy, and applied physiology of the salivary glands. Parotid gland topics included assessment and evaluation, traumatic injuries and fistulae, calculi, sialadenosis (sialosis), sialadenitis, cysts and tumors of the parotid gland, the various techniques and potential complications of parotidectomy including Frey's syndrome, in addition to extra-temporal facial nerve reconstruction procedures. Likewise, topics of the submandibular gland included evaluation, sialolithiasis, inflammatory disorders, sialadenosis, tumors, and different techniques and complications of submandibular sialoadenectomy. In addition, this book includes two chapters discussing topics related to surgery of the sublingual gland and minor salivary glands.

The book has been structured in such a way as to facilitate quick reference and serve as a practical manual for the clinicians of many specialties who treat patients with salivary gland disorders. It is my collective hope that head and neck surgeons, maxillofacial surgeons, orthopedic surgeons, endocrinologists, oncologists, pediatricians, and clinicians of other specialties will find this book to be a useful and indispensible resource as they face the most challenging of salivary gland disorders to help provide individual patients with the best possible outcome.

Alexandria, Egypt — Mahmoud Sakr

Acknowledgments

I would like to thank all those who helped and encouraged me during the writing, editing, and revision of this book. I would like to express my appreciation and gratitude to my wife and children for their continuous support and unconditioned love.

Contents

Embryology and Developmental Disorders

1

1.1 Embryology

The salivary gland system can be divided into two distinct exocrine groups: the major salivary glands, which include the three paired parotid, submandibular, and sublingual glands, and the minor salivary glands, which are hundreds (600–1000) of small glands lining the mucosa of the upper aero-digestive tract. Together, these glands produce saliva, which contains digestive enzymes, antibodies, growth factors, and coating substances essential for eating, speaking, tasting, and oral hygiene [1, 2]. The embryological development of the salivary glands is the result of a complex interaction between two distinct tissues: the oral epithelium and the underlying mesenchyme [3, 4]. All of the salivary glands share a common embryogenesis; they all develop from growths of the oral epithelium into the underlying mesenchyme.

Embryological development of the major salivary glands consists of three main stages [5, 6]. The first stage is marked by the presence of a primordial anlage (from the German verb anlagen, to set a foundation) and the formation of branched duct buds due to repeated epithelial cleft and bud development. Ciliated epithelial cells form the luminal lining, while external surfaces are lined by ectodermal myoepithelial cells [7]. During the second stage, early appearance of lobules and duct canalization takes place, resulting in the appearance of primitive acini and distal duct regions. The third stage is marked by maturation of acini and intercalated ducts, and reduced prominence of interstitial connective tissue.

The primordial "parotid" gland is the first to appear, during the sixth gestational week, when oral ectodermal outpouchings extend into the adjacent mesoderm and serve as the site of origin for the growth of glands. After a short journey of dorsal and lateral migration, the parotid gland resides in the pre-auricular region. The facial nerve arbitrarily divides the gland into superficial and deep lobes by the 10th week of gestation. By the 12th week, the stroma, which comprises the capsule of each gland, and the septae that divide the gland into lobes and lobules develop from

© The Author(s), under exclusive license to Springer Nature Switzerland AG 2024
M. Sakr, *Surgery of the Salivary Glands*,
https://doi.org/10.1007/978-3-031-82069-4_1

cranial neural crest cells, which are cells that originate from the dorsal part of the neural tube epithelium [5, 8].

During the sixth week of embryonic life, small buds appear in the floor of the mouth lateral to the tongue and extend posteriorly around the mylohyoid muscle into the submandibular triangle. These buds eventually develop into the "submandibular glands." A capsule from the surrounding mesenchyme is fully formed around the gland by the third gestational month [6].

During the ninth embryonic month, the "sublingual gland" anlage is formed from multiple endodermal epithelial buds in the paralingual sulcus of the floor of the mouth. Absence of a capsule is due to infiltration of the glands by sublingual connective tissue. Intraglandular lymph nodes (LNs) and major ducts also do not generally develop within sublingual glands. The upper respiratory ectoderm gives rise to simple tubulo-acinar units. They develop into the "minor salivary glands" during the 12th intrauterine week [9].

The eventual development of the salivary glands does not solely depend on the coordinated development of the epithelium and the mesenchyme, but, in addition, there must be endothelial cells for vessels and neuronal cells for nerves that have to be organized and incorporated into the final complex structure of the gland [10].

1.2 Developmental Disorders

When normal salivary gland tissue develops in an "abnormal" body location, it is referred to as a choristoma, ectopic salivary gland tissue, or salivary heterotopia. When this salivary tissue has a ductal system, the tissue is now referred to as an aberrant salivary gland. The most common location for salivary heterotopia in the head and neck is in the peri-parotid and parotid lymph nodes [11]. This occurrence is likely related to the encapsulation of the salivary glands and the associated development of the cervical lymphatic system. In addition, heterotopic salivary gland tissue can rarely be found in the following anatomical areas; the middle ear [12], remnant of Rathke pouch [13], the cerebello-pontine angle [14, 15], the posterior or anterior mandible [16, 17], the palatine and lingual tonsils [18], the parathyroid and thyroid glands [19, 20], the soft tissues of the neck, and medial to the sternocleidomastoid (SCM) muscle [21]. There is even a report of such heterotopic salivary tissue in the rectum [22]. The most common site for "accessory" parotid tissue is overlying the masseter muscle, with the ductal system draining into Stensen's duct [23]. The next most common location is in the anterior triangle of the neck, followed by the posterior triangle [21, 24].

Aside from "heterotopic salivary glands," developmental disorders of these glands are rare. Reported congenital anomalies include aplasia (absence) [25–28] gland duplication [29], as well as congenitally atretic, imperforate, ectatic, and duplicated ducts [30, 31]. Agenesis may be associated with abnormalities of the lacrimal apparatus and may also be genetically transmitted [27]. Agenesis may be partial or total, unilateral or bilateral, and may involve more than one salivary gland. Association with "specific syndromes" such as Levy–Hollister syndrome, Down syndrome, or Klinefelter syndrome has been reported. The true incidence of parotid agenesis is unknown since most of the cases are asymptomatic. Symptoms may include dental caries, thirst, xerostomia, and gingival infections. Oral examination reveals the absence of the papilla of Stensen's duct. When suspected, magnetic resonance imaging (MRI) is the imaging tool of choice to demonstrate replacement of the glandular bed by fat. Congenital parotid fistula is another developmental disorder that may be encountered.

Tumor-like presentations of maldevelopment include rare hamartomas of the hard palate [32] and unusual cystic choristomas of the submandibular gland [33], which appear to be a mixture of epithelium of both ectodermal and endodermal derivation. The congenital salivary gland anlage tumor or congenital pleomorphic adenoma is thought to represent a hamartoma of minor salivary gland origin [34].

References

1. Carpenter GH. The secretion, components, and properties of saliva. Annu Rev Food Sci Technol. 2013;4:267–76.
2. Andrew DJ, Henderson KD, Seshaiah P. Salivary gland development in Drosophila melanogaster. Mech Dev. 2000;92:5–17.
3. Miletich I. Introduction to salivary glands: structure, function and embryonic development. Front Oral Biol. 2010;14:1–20.
4. Tucker AS. Salivary gland development. Semin Cell Dev Biol. 2007;18:237–4.
5. Arey LB. Developmental anatomy; a textbook and laboratory manual of embryology. Revised 7th ed. Philadelphia, PA: WB Saunders, Inc.; 1974.
6. Gibson MH. The prenatal human submandibular gland: a histological, histochemical and ultrastructural study. Anat Anz. 1983;153(1):91–105.
7. Bernfield MR, Banerjee SD, Cohn RH. Dependence of salivary epithelial morphology and branching morphogenesis upon acid mucopolysaccharide-protein (proteoglycan) at the epithelial surface. J Cell Biol. 1972;52(3):674–89.
8. Yamamoto S, Fukumoto E, Yoshizaki K, Iwamoto T, Yamada A, Tanaka K, et al. Platelet-derived growth factor receptor regulates salivary gland morphogenesis via fibroblast growth factor expression. J Biol Chem. 2008;283:23139–49.
9. Kontis TC, Johns ME. Anatomy and physiology of the salivary glands. In: Bailey BJ, editor. Head and neck surgery—otolaryngology. Philadelphia, PA: Lippincott Williams & Wilkins; 2001
10. Som PM, Miletich I. The embryology of the salivary glands: an update. Neurographics. 2015;5(4):167–77.
11. Daniel E, McGuirt WF Sr. Neck masses secondary to heterotopic salivary gland tissue: a 25-year experience. Am J Otolaryngol. 2005;26:96–100.
12. Enoz M, Suoglu Y. Salivary gland choristoma of the middle ear. Laryngoscope. 2006;116:1033–4.
13. Ranucci V, Coli A, Marrucci E, Paolo MP, Della Pepa G, Anile C, et al. Ectopic salivary gland tissue in a Rathke's cleft cyst. Int J Clin Exp Pathol. 2013;6:1437–40.
14. Rodriguez F, Scheithauer BW, Ockner DM, Giannini C. Solitary fibrous tumor of the cerebellopontine angle with salivary gland heterotopia: a unique presentation. Am J Surg Pathol. 2004;28(139–42):45.
15. Curry B, Taylor CW, Fisher AW. Salivary gland heterotopia: a unique cerebellopontine angle tumor. Arch Pathol Lab Med. 1982;106:35–8.
16. Dorman M, Pierse D. Ectopic salivary gland tissue in the anterior mandible: a case report. Br Dent J. 2002;193:571–2.

17. Miller AS, Winnick M. Salivary gland inclusion in the anterior mandible. Report of a case with a review of the literature on aberrant salivary gland tissue and neoplasms. Oral Surg Oral Med Oral Pathol. 1971;31:790–7.
18. Banerjee AR, Soames JV, Birchall JP, Reid C, Bray RJ. Ectopic salivary gland tissue in the palatine and lingual tonsil. Int J Pediatr Otorhinolaryngol. 1993;27:159–62.
19. Park JY, Kim GY, Suh YL. Intrathyroidal branchial cleft-like cyst with heterotopic salivary gland-type tissue. Pediatr Dev Pathol. 2004;7:262–7.
20. Edwards PC, Bhuiya T, Kahn LB, Fantasia JE. Salivary heterotopia of the parathyroid gland: a report of two cases and review of the literature. Oral Surg Oral Med Oral Pathol Oral Radiol Endod. 2005;99:590–3.
21. Marshall JN, Soo G, Coakley FV. Ectopic salivary gland in the posterior triangle of the neck. J Laryngol Otol. 1995;109:669–70.
22. Weitzner S. Ectopic salivary gland tissue in submucosa of rectum. Dis Colon Rectum. 1983;26:814–7.
23. Ramachar SM, Huliyappa HA. Accessory parotid gland tumors. Ann Maxillofac Surg. 2012;2:90–3.
24. Haemel A, Gnepp DR, Carlsten J, Robinson-Bostom L. Heterotopic salivary gland tissue in the neck. J Am Acad Dermatol. 2008;58:251–6.
25. Myers MA, Youngberg RA, Bauman JM. Congenital absence of the major salivary glands and impaired lacrimal secretion in a child: case report. J Am Dent Assoc. 1994;125(2):210–2.
26. Wiedemann HR. Salivary gland disorders and heredity. Am J Med Genet. 1997;68(2):222–4.
27. Kwon SY, Jung EJ, Kim SH, Kim TK. A case of major salivary gland agenesis. Acta Otolaryngol. 2006;126(2):219–22.
28. Karakoc O, Akcam T, Kocaoglu M, Yetiser S. Agenesis of the unilateral parotid gland associated with pleomorphic adenoma of the contralateral parotid gland. J Laryngol Otol. 2005;119(5):409–11.
29. Codjambopoulo P, Ender-Griepekoven I, Broy H. Bilateral duplication of the submandibular gland and the submandibular duct. Rofo. 1992;157(2):185–6.
30. Pownell PH, Brown OE, Pransky SM, Manning SC. Congenital abnormalities of the submandibular duct. Int J Pediatr Otorhinolaryngol. 1992;24(2):161–9.
31. Amin MA, Bailey BM. Congenital atresia of the orifice of the submandibular duct: a report of 2 cases and review. Br J Oral Maxillofac Surg. 2001;39(6):48048–2.
32. Harada H, Morimatsu M, Kusukawa J, Kameyama T. A hamartoma-like mass on the palate? A possible discussion regarding the components of a pigmented naevus and hyperplastic salivary gland. J Laryngol Otol. 1997;111(3):296–9.
33. Tang TT, Glicklich M, Siegesmund KA, Oechler HW, McCreadie SR. Neonatal cystic choristoma in submandibular salivary gland simulating cystic hygroma. Arch Pathol Lab Med. 1979;103(10):536–9.
34. Dehner LP, Valbuena L, Perez-Atayde A, Reddick RL, Askin FB, Rosai J. Salivary gland anlage tumor ("congenital pleomorphic adenoma"). A clinicopathologic, immunohistochemical and ultrastructural study of nine cases. Am J Surg Pathol. 1994;18(1):25–36.

2 Histology of the Salivary Glands

2.1 Histological (Microscopic) Features

All salivary glands in general are derived from epithelial cells and consist of "parenchyma" or "functional unit" (secretory unit and associated ducts), and "stroma" (surrounding connective tissue that penetrates and divides the gland into lobules). Interlobular regions include large excretory ducts and neurovascular bundles. The salivary gland secretes saliva via ducts from a flask-like, blind-ended secretory structure called the "acinus" [1]. Thus, the microanatomy of the major salivary gland includes the following: connective tissue (stroma), secretory units (acini), myoepithelial cells, and ductal units, as shown in Fig. 2.1.

2.1.1 Secretory Unit (Acinus)

Acini can be composed predominantly of serous or mucous cells or can be mixed seromucous type.

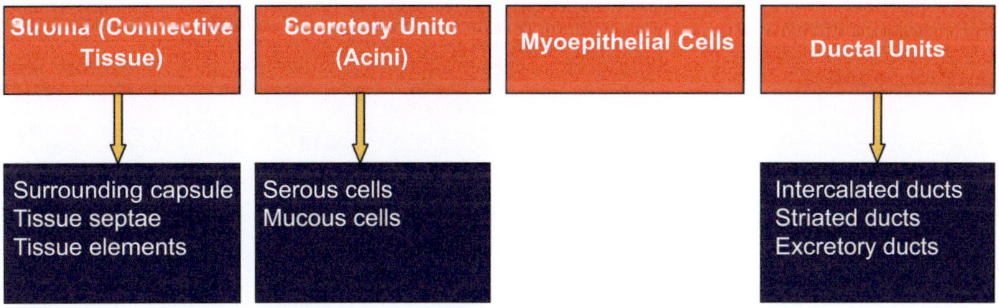

Fig. 2.1 Microanatomy of the parotid gland (stroma–acini–myoepithelial cells–ductal units)

© The Author(s), under exclusive license to Springer Nature Switzerland AG 2024
M. Sakr, *Surgery of the Salivary Glands*,
https://doi.org/10.1007/978-3-031-82069-4_2

2.1.1.1 Serous Acini

Serous acini are the dominant component in the parotid gland (Fig. 2.2) and von Ebner glands of the tongue (minor salivary glands). Cells are polygonal-shaped with dense, intracytoplasmic, basophilic (eosinophilic) zymogen enzyme-containing granules. Their nuclei are spherical in appearance. Cells are periodic acid-Schiff (PAS) reagent positive.

2.1.1.2 Mucous Acini

Mucous acini are the dominant component in the minor salivary glands of the palate and base of the tongue. Cells are round in shape, have a pale-staining, bubbly cytoplasm filled with mucin, and contain a basally located, condensed nucleus (Fig. 2.3). Cells are positive for mucicarmine, alcian blue, and PAS with diastase resistance (DPAS).

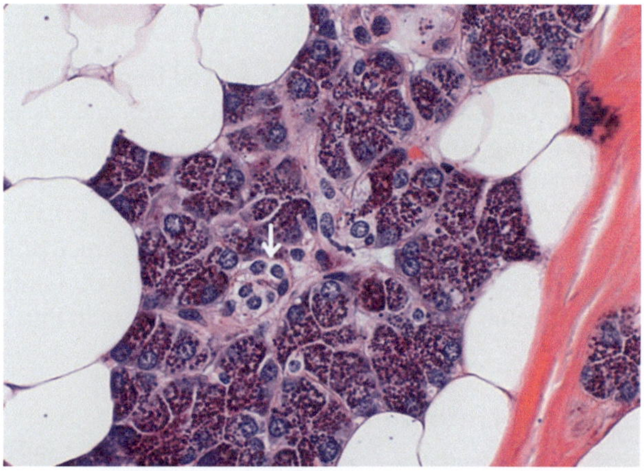

Fig. 2.2 The serous acinar cells of the parotid gland are polygonal in shape with dense, intracytoplasmic, eosinophilic zymogen granules. The intercalated duct (white arrow) is lined by a single layer of cuboidal epithelium. H&E stain

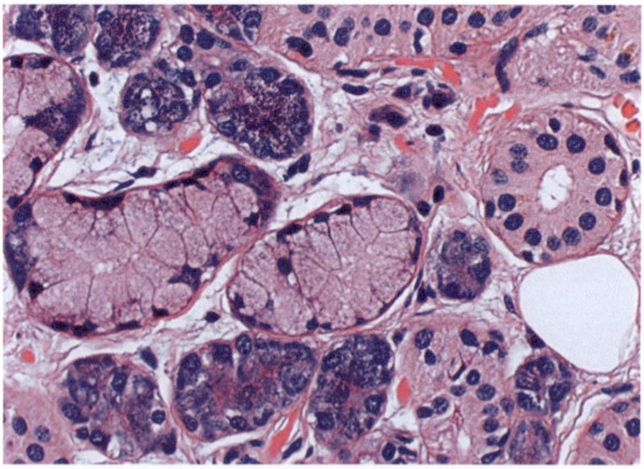

Fig. 2.3 Mucous acinar cells of the submandibular gland are round, filled with mucin, and contain a basally located, condensed nucleus. H&E stain

2.1.1.3 Mixed Seromucous Acini

The mixed seromucous acini are the dominant component in the submandibular (serous predominance) and sublingual (mucous predominance) glands (Fig. 2.4), minor salivary glands of the lip, cheek, and anterior tongue. They are mucous acini with crescent-shaped caps (demilunes) of serous cells.

This histological description results in parotid thin watery, saliva, devoid of mucins, submandibular mixed saliva, and sublingual more viscous, mucin-rich saliva [2].

2.1.2 Myoepithelial Cells

Myoepithelial cells are critical for the expulsion of saliva. They surround acini, intercalated ducts, and striated ducts. These cells are located between epithelial cells and the basement membrane, embracing the secretory unit with long cytoplasmic processes. They are stellate-shaped with blunt-ended nuclei and numerous, elongated, branching cytoplasmic processes that envelop the secretory end piece. They may be fusiform-shaped with fewer processes. These processes are filled with actin and soluble myosin. Contraction of these processes provides support to the end pieces during active secretion of saliva [3]. Recent advances also suggest that these cells provided signals to the end pieces during active secretion of saliva.

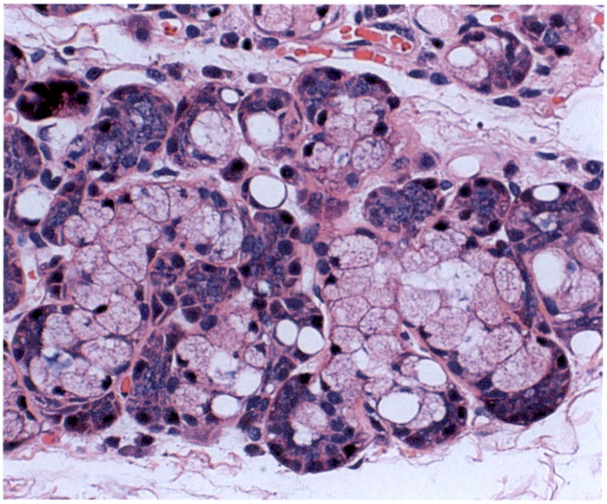

Fig. 2.4 Seromucous acinar cells of the sublingual gland. Mucous acini with crescent-shaped caps (demilunes) of serous cells. H&E stain

2.1.3 Ductal Unit

The ductal unit consists of three main types of ducts: intercalated, striated, or interlobular. The minor salivary gland duct system is simpler than that of the major salivary glands, whereas the intercalated ducts are longer and the striated ducts are either less developed or not present [2].

2.1.3.1 Intercalated Ducts

Intercalated ducts are intralobar and have the smallest caliber. They emerge from the acinar unit to drain the acini and are lined by a single irregular myoepithelial cell layer lined with squamous or low cuboidal epithelium, and in turn drain into the "striated ducts." Intercalated ducts contain reserve cells that regenerate the terminal secretory unit.

2.1.3.2 Striated Ducts

Striated ducts, which are also intralobar, proceed from the intercalated ducts. They are an intermediate caliber between intercalated and interlobular ducts, and are lined by columnar epithelium containing basal cytoplasmic striations, formed by rows of mitochondria alternating with folded cell membrane [3] (Fig. 2.5). Striated ducts contribute to the ionic composition of the saliva and drain into the interlobular ducts.

2.1.3.3 Interlobular Ducts

Interlobar ducts have the largest caliber and are located within the interlobular septa and lined by pseudo-stratified columnar epithelium (Fig. 2.6). They merge to form the major excretory duct outside the gland, lined distally by non-keratinized stratified squamous epithelium (Stensen's duct in the parotid gland, Wharton's duct in the submandibular gland, and Bartholin's duct in the sublingual gland).

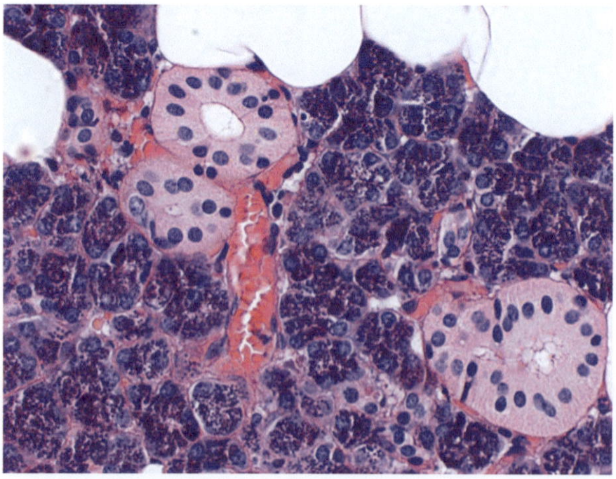

Fig. 2.5 Striated ducts (of the parotid gland) are lined by simple columnar epithelium containing densely packed mitochondria that form cytoplasmic striations. H&E stain

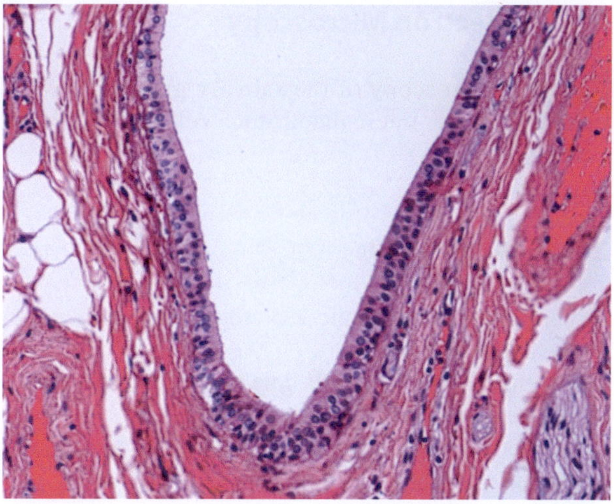

Fig. 2.6 Interlobar ducts (of the parotid gland) are located within the interlobular septa and lined by pseudo-stratified columnar epithelium. Note the adjacent neurovasculature. H&E stain

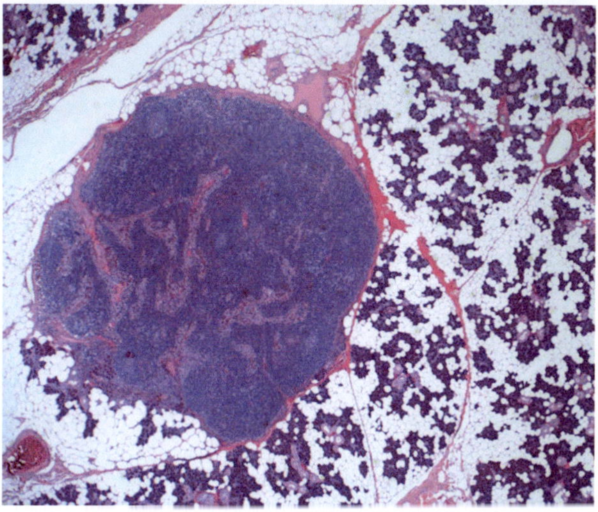

Fig. 2.7 Histopathology of the parotid gland showing an intraparenchymal lymph node. H&E stain

2.1.4 Normal Inclusions within the Salivary Glands

The presence of sebaceous glands within the parotid gland is common and is usually found to be associated with interlobular ducts or may exist as isolated cells within the wall of intercalated or striated ducts [4].

Unique to the parotid gland is the presence of intraparotid lymph nodes (LNs) (Fig. 2.7), most of which are located superficial to the facial nerve. Often, the LNs may lack a well-defined capsule and merge with the adjacent salivary gland acini. Fatty infiltration of the major salivary glands is an age-induced variation [4].

2.2 Electron Microscopy

Electron microscopy of the salivary glands can show the following description of acinar cells, intercalated duct cells, myoepithelial cells, and striated duct cells [5].

2.2.1 Acinar Cells

- Numerous cytoplasmic secretory (zymogen) granules in the apical portion of the cell.
- Extensive rough endoplasmic reticulum (ER) and Golgi.
- Numerous mitochondria.
- Numerous folds are present in the basal lamina of acinar cells that are not distended with secretory product.
- Mucous acinar cells have larger, more irregular secretory droplets that are more electron lucent than in serous acinar cells.

2.2.2 Intercalated Duct Cells

- Few special ultrastructural features.
- May have some secretory granules.
- Scant cytoplasm has basal rough ER, apical Golgi, and mitochondria.
- Lateral membranes interdigitate with neighboring cells.

2.2.3 Myoepithelial Cells

- Between basal plasma membrane of acinar and intercalated duct cells and basal lamina.
- Flattened and elongated with cytoplasmic processes extending around acinar and intercalated duct cells.
- Long/irregular nuclei.
- Desmosomes attach the myoepithelial cells to the acinar and ductal cells.

2.2.4 Striated Duct Cells

- Striations are due to basal vertical folds.
- Numerous mitochondria are present.

2.3 Effect of Aging

There is no overall change in the amount of saliva secreted with advancing age. However, aging of salivary glands shows some structural changes, which include the following [6 ,7]:

- Decrease in the volume of acinar tissue
- Increase in the fibrous tissue
- Increase in the adipose tissue
- Ductal hyperplasia and dilation

  In addition, there are also some changes in the salivary contents:
- Decrease in the concentration of secretory IgA
- Decrease in the amount of mucin

References

1. Tandler B, Pinkstaff CA, Phillips CJ. Interlobular excretory ducts of mammalian salivary glands: structural and histochemical review. Anat Rec A Discov Mol Cell Evol Biol. 2006;288(5):498–526.
2. Junqueria L, Carneiro J. Basic histology: text and atlas. 10th ed. New York, NY: McGraw-Hill; 2003.
3. Riva A, Valentino L, Lantini MS, Floris A, Riva FT. 3D-structure of cells of human salivary glands as seen by SEM. Microsc Res Tech. 1993;26:5.
4. Martinez-Madrigal F, Micheau C. Histology of the major salivary glands. Am J Surg Pathol. 1989;13(10):879–99.
5. Garcia JJ. Atlas of salivary gland pathology. 1st ed. Berlin: Springer-Verlag; 2019.
6. Vissink A, Spijkervet FK, Van Nieuw AA. Aging and saliva: a review of the literature. Spec Care Dent. 1996;16(3):95–103.
7. Kim SK, Allen ED. Structural and functional changes in salivary glands during aging. Microscop Res Tech. 1994;28(3):243–53.

Surgical Anatomy of the Salivary Glands 3

3.1 Surgical Anatomy of the Parotid Gland

The parotid gland is a paired organ, weighing about 15–30 g each, and is the largest of the major salivary glands. It consists of two lobes, superficial and deep, with regard to its relation with the facial nerve. It is wrapped around the mandibular ramus and secretes saliva through the parotid (Stensen's) duct in the oral cavity.

The parotid gland is pyramidal-shaped and is encased in robust parotid fascia, which is a continuation of deep cervical fascia as it travels superiorly. It is located in a shallow, pre-auricular compartment (the word "parotid" literally means around the ear, that is, para-otic) defined as follows:

- Superficially: the superficial musculo-aponeurotic system (SMAS) forming parotid fascia and platysma
- Inferiorly: the anteromedial margin of the sternocleidomastoid (SCM) muscle
- Medially: the para-pharyngeal space
- Antero-medially: the mandibular ramus covered by the masseter muscle
- Posteriorly: the cartilage of the ear canal and temporal bone

3.1.1 Structures Related to the Parotid Gland

Several structures run through the parotid gland: (1) the terminal segment of the external carotid artery (ECA), which gives the posterior auricular artery just before entering the gland and terminates by dividing into the superficial temporal artery and the maxillary artery; (2) retro-mandibular vein; (3) facial nerve (extracranial trunk), which soon gives two divisions (temporofacial and cervicofacial), giving off five terminal branches inside the gland radiating forward superficial to the vein and artery to supply muscles of facial expression; and (4) parotid lymph nodes (LNs).

© The Author(s), under exclusive license to Springer Nature Switzerland AG 2024
M. Sakr, *Surgery of the Salivary Glands*,
https://doi.org/10.1007/978-3-031-82069-4_3

3.1.2 Parotid Fascia

The deep cervical fascia continues superiorly to form the parotid fascia, which is split into superficial and deep layers to enclose the parotid gland. The thicker adherent, inelastic, superficial fascia extends up to be attached to the zygomatic arch while the thinner deep one is attached to the styloid process, angle, and posterior border of the ramus of the mandible and tympanic plate. A portion of the deep lamina thickens to form the stylomandibular ligament, which separates the parotid gland from the submandibular gland.

3.1.3 Parotid Duct (Stensen's Duct, Ductus Parotideus)

The parotid gland drains its serous secretions through the long (~7 cm) Stensen's duct that arises from the most anterior superficial part of the gland, travels parallel and 1 cm below the zygoma, running on the lateral surface of masseter, just deep to the skin, then finally dives at an angle of 90° at the anterior border of masseter to pierce the buccal pad of fat, buccopharyngeal fascia, then buccinator, and opens in the oral (gingivo-buccal) vestibule opposite the second maxillary molar tooth over the summit of a papilla [1, 2].

3.1.4 Accessory Parotid Gland

Accessory parotid tissue (lobe or gland) can be identified in approximately 20% of individuals, usually residing over the masseter muscle between the zygomatic arch and Stensen's duct [3]. As proved histologically, this accessory glandular tissue secretes mucous in addition to serous secretions drained through a single short duct that joins the main duct [4].

3.1.5 Surface Anatomy of the Parotid Gland

The anterior border of the gland corresponds to a line that extends from the ear tragus to the posterior border of the masseter opposite the angle of the mouth, the inferior border from there to below and behind the angle of the mandible, the posterior border from there to the mastoid process, and the superior border from the mastoid process to the ear tragus. Surface anatomy of the parotid duct corresponds to the middle third of an imaginary line that extends from the tragus of the ear to the middle portion of the upper lip.

3.1.6 Nerve Supply

The facial nerve (CN-VII) exits the skull base through the stylomastoid foramen and immediately gives off three motor branches for the posterior belly of the digastric, the stylohyoid, and the post-auricular muscles. Its main trunk then enters the posterior portion of the parotid gland. Inside the gland, it divides into two divisions: upper temporofacial and lower cervicofacial, approximately 1.3 cm from the stylomastoid foramen. The temporofacial division gives off the temporal, zygomatic, and buccal branches, while the cervicofacial gives off the marginal mandibular and cervical branches.

During parotidectomy, the facial nerve must be traced from behind forward as it emerges from the stylomastoid foramen and enters the parotid gland. The nerve is surrounded by a leash of veins called the neurovenous plexus of Patey, which must be followed with fine dissection, preferably under the microscope, to surgically divide the isthmus (between the superficial and the deep parotid lobes).

The temporal branch passes with the superficial temporal vessels over the zygoma to supply the frontal belly of occipitofrontalis, orbicularis oculi, corrugator supercilii, and anterior and superior auricular muscles. The zygomatic branch passes over the periosteum of the zygomatic arch to supply the zygomatic, orbital, and infraorbital muscles. The buccal branch travels with the Stensen's duct to supply the buccinator, upper lip, and nostril muscles. The marginal mandibular branch (also known as the marginal mandibular nerve) travels along the inferior border of the parotid gland just deep to the platysma muscle but superficial to the posterior facial and retromandibular veins, to supply the lower lip and chin muscles. Running in the same plane is the cervical branch, which supplies the platysma muscle. All the muscles supplied by the facial nerve are muscles of facial expression.

The great auricular nerve (C2,3) is a sensory branch of the cervical plexus that provides general sensation to the parotid gland, the skin of the posterior portion of the ear pinna and the ear lobule. It accompanies the external jugular vein along the lateral surface of the SCM muscle toward the tail of the parotid gland, and there it splits into anterior and posterior branches. It is often injured during parotidectomy, leaving the ear lobule senseless. Its harvesting for facial nerve grafting may be needed when the latter is injured or sacrificed.

The auriculotemporal nerve (ATN) is a branch of the mandibular division of the trigeminal nerve (CN-V). After exiting the foramen ovale, it runs parallel to the superficial temporal vessels and anterior to the external auditory canal to innervate the skin and scalp immediately anterior to the ear.

The glossopharyngeal nerve (CN-IX) provides visceral secretory innervation to the parotid gland. The nerve carries preganglionic parasympathetic fibers from the inferior salivatory nucleus in the medulla through the jugular foramen. Then, a small branch of the CN-IX (Jacobsen's nerve) re-enters the skull through the inferior tympanic canaliculus and into the middle ear to form the tympanic plexus.

The preganglionic fibers then travel as the lesser petrosal nerve into the middle cranial fossa and out through the foramen ovale to synapse in the otic ganglion. Postganglionic parasympathetic fibers exit the otic ganglion to join the ATN in the infratemporal fossa. The ATN enters the substance of the gland from its deep aspect along the neck of the mandible and emerges from the gland just inferior to the root of the zygomatic arch. The ATN so carries fibers that innervate the parotid gland for the secretion of saliva. Thus, parasympathetic syndromes cause salivation.

Postganglionic sympathetic fibers innervate the salivary glands, sweat glands, and cutaneous blood vessels, mediating vasoconstriction, through the external carotid plexus from the superior cervical ganglion. Sympathetic syndromes cause dry mouth. Acetylcholine serves as the neurotransmitter for both postganglionic sympathetic and parasympathetic fibers. This physiological coincidence allows for the occasional development of "gustatory sweating" (also known as "Frey's syndrome") following parotidectomy [5].

3.1.7 Arterial Supply

The external carotid artery (ECA) arrives at the posteromedial surface of the parotid gland, dividing into two terminal branches, the superficial temporal artery and maxillary artery, which exit from superior and anteromedial surfaces, respectively. The parotid gland receives its blood supply through branches of the ECA, mainly through the posterior auricular artery. The superficial temporal artery provides the transverse facial artery, which travels anteriorly between the zygoma and parotid duct to supply the parotid gland and parotid duct as well as the masseter muscle.

3.1.8 Venous Drainage

The retromandibular vein is formed in the body of the parotid gland by the union of the maxillary and the superficial temporal veins, and provides venous return for the gland, descending superficial to the ECA and deep to the facial nerve before eventually joining the external jugular vein. The retromandibular vein is intimately associated with the facial nerve and is used as a surrogate anatomic landmark to determine whether tumors are in the deep or superficial lobe of the parotid gland. However, there are many variations as regards the surgical anatomy of the retromandibular vein.

3.1.9 Lymphatic Drainage

As a result of late encapsulation during embryological development, the parotid gland, unlike the submandibular and sublingual glands, contains intraparenchymal LNs, with salivary gland structures, usually ducts and less frequency acini, in the intra- and periparotid LNs. Parotid gland LNs lie in the superficial and partly in the deep fascia over the parotid gland. In addition to the parotid gland, they also drain the temple, side of the scalp, external auditory meatus (EAM), middle ear, upper part of the cheek, and parts of the eyelids and orbit.

Lymphatic drainage of the parotid gland follows the venous system, draining to a superficial (fascial) and deep (intraparenchymal) group of LNs before flowing into the upper deep cervical LNs.

3.1.10 Parapharyngeal Space

Tumors of the deep parotid lobe often extend medially into the parapharyngeal space, which is shaped like an inverted pyramid, where the greater cornu of the hyoid bone serves as the apex and the petrous bone of the skull base as the base of the pyramid.

The parapharyngeal space is bound medially by the lateral pharyngeal wall, which consists of the superior constrictor muscles, buccopharyngeal fascia and tensor veli palatine. It is bounded laterally by the ramus of the mandible and the medial pterygoid muscle, anteriorly by the pterygoid fascia and the pterygomandibular raphe and posteriorly by the carotid sheath and pre-vertebral fascia.

A line from the styloid process to the medial portion of the medial pterygoid plate divides the parapharyngeal space into pre- and post-styloid compartments. The pre-styloid one contains the deep parotid lobe, internal maxillary and ascending pharyngeal arteries, and inferior alveolar, lingual, and ATNs. The post-styloid compartment contains the internal jugular vein (IJV), carotid artery, vagus nerve (CN-X), all within the carotid sheath as well as the cranial nerves, glosso-pharyngeal (CN-IX), accessory (CN-XI), and hypoglossal (CN-XII), in addition to the cervical sympathetic chain. Thus, neurogenic tumors or paragangliomas arising from these nerves lie in this post-styloid compartment [6].

3.2 Surgical Anatomy of the Submandibular Gland

The submandibular gland is the second largest major salivary gland and weighs 7–15 g. It is classified as a mixed gland that is predominantly serous with tubular acini. Approximately 90% of acinar cells are serous and only 10% are mucinous. It is located in the submandibular triangle, which is bounded superiorly by the inferior edge of the mandible, inferiorly by the anterior and posterior bellies of the digastrics muscle, and superficially by the platysma. It contains several important neurovascular structures, in addition to the submandibular gland; namely, the marginal mandibular branch of facial nerve, the lingual nerve, the hypoglossal nerve (CN-XII), and the facial artery, as well as LNs that can harbor regional metastases from oral and oropharyngeal primary tumors [2].

The submandibular gland lies on the hyoglossus muscle, superficial to the hypoglossal and lingual nerves, and can be arbitrarily divided into superficial and deep parts or lobes according to its relationship with the mylohyoid muscle.

The superficial lobe lies superficial to the muscle, reaching upward under cover of the mandible and is separated posteriorly from the parotid gland by the stylomandibular ligament. The smaller deep lobe wraps around the posterior aspect of the mylohyoid muscle and its anterior end reaches as far as the sublingual gland. During submandibular sialadenectomy or neck dissection, the mylohyoid muscle must be gently retracted anteriorly to expose the lingual nerve and the submandibular ganglion. The vertical posterior edge of the submandibular gland and the digastric muscle can be used as a boundary between levels I and II of the neck.

3.2.1 Fascia

The submandibular gland is covered by a capsule derived from the middle layer of the deep cervical fascia. The marginal mandibular nerve (MMN) lies superficial to this fascia. Thus, division of the submandibular gland fascia, when oncologically appropriate, is a reliable method for preserving the nerve during neck dissection and/or gland resection.

3.2.2 Submandibular Duct (Wharton's Duct)

The submandibular gland has both mucous and serous cells that empty into ductules, which in turn empty into the submandibular duct (Wharton's duct), which is about 4–5 cm long. It emerges from the anterior end of the deep part of the gland, runs anteriorly between the hyoglossus and mylohyoid muscles on the genioglossus muscle, and opens in the oral cavity on the summit of a small papilla, near the frenulum of the tongue behind the lower incisor tooth. On the hyoglossus muscle, it lies between the hypoglossal and lingual nerves, but at the anterior border of the muscle, it is crossed laterally by the lingual nerve, which then ascends medial to the duct. The sublingual veins lie lateral and the sublingual artery medial to the duct, more anteriorly.

3.2.3 Innervation: Lingual Nerve

The chorda tympani nerve (from CN-VII) unites with the lingual nerve of CN-V3 in the infratemporal fossa before entering the oral cavity to synapse with postganglionic fibers in the submandibular ganglion. The submandibular ganglion is suspended from the lingual nerve and located inferior to the submandibular duct, supplying postganglionic parasympathetic fibers that pass directly to the submandibular and sublingual glands.

The lingual nerve passes forward and downward between the duct and the deep part of the gland before passing medially under the duct opposite the first lower molar. While still lateral to the duct it gives off its sublingual branch, which runs close to the mandible, lateral to the sublingual glands. The lingual nerve crosses Wharton's duct twice lateral to medial and the hypoglossal nerve (CN-XII) travels inferior to the duct [7]. During submandibular sialadenectomy, care should be taken to preserve the lingual nerve as it supplies the general sensation and taste to the anterior two-thirds of the tongue. Branches from the lingual nerve to the submandibular gland are ligated during gland excision.

3.2.4 Arterial Supply: Facial Artery

The submandibular gland is supplied by branches of the facial (main supply) and lingual arteries, branches of the ECA. The facial artery emerges from under the stylohyoid muscle, runs medial to the posterior belly of the digastric muscle, and then hooks over to pass upward deep to the gland. The artery exits the superior border of the gland at the lower border of the mandible (facial notch), around which it curls to enter the face. During resection of the submandibular gland, the facial artery must be sacrificed twice, first at the inferior border of the mandible and again just superior to the posterior belly of the digastric muscle. The lingual artery runs deep to the digastric muscle along the lateral surface of the middle constrictor muscle and then courses anterior and medial to the hyoglossus muscle and gives off branches to the submandibular gland.

3.2.5 Venous Drainage

The submandibular gland is mainly drained by the anterior facial vein (AFV) and to a lesser extent by the venae comitantes of the lingual artery into the internal jugular vein (IJV). The anterior facial vein is in close approximation to the facial artery as it runs posteriorly and inferiorly from the face to the lower aspect of the mandible. Since it lies deep to the MMN, ligation and superior retraction of the AFV can help preserve this important nerve during surgery of the submandibular gland. Venous anatomy can be variable.

3.2.6 Lymphatic Drainage

Lymph nodes draining the submandibular gland are not embedded in the glandular tissue. They are located between the gland and its fascia, in close relation to the facial artery and vein at the superior aspect of the gland, and drain into the deep cervical and jugular chains. These LNs are frequently associated with cancers in the oral cavity. Care should be taken during ligation of the facial vessels and dissection of the lympho-adipose tissue, to preserve the MMN, which runs in close proximity to these structures.

3.3 Surgical Anatomy of the Sublingual Gland

The paired sublingual salivary glands are the smallest of the three major salivary glands, weighing 2–4 g each. Sublingual salivary glands are almond-shaped and lie immediately below the mucous membrane of the floor of the mouth above the mylohyoid muscle lateral to the submandibular duct and lingual nerve. It fills the medial groove or sublingual fossa of the mandible. Superiorly, the gland creates a mucosal elevation (sublingual fold) on the floor of the oral cavity.

According to Batsakis, these are poorly encapsulated glands that do not represent unit organs but, rather, a "mosaic" composed of a large segment (major sublingual gland), which is drained by the sublingual or Bartholin's duct (may connect with the submandibular duct at the sublingual carbuncle), and a group of 8–30 smaller glands (minor sublingual glands), which are drained by several openings (ducts of Rivinus) directly into the oral cavity or into the submandibular duct [8].

The sublingual glands are separated by the paired midline genioglossus and genio-hyoid muscles. A crest of mucous membrane along the frenulum (plica sublingualis) represents the projection of the glands and openings of the sublingual ducts. The blood supply to the sublingual gland comes from the sublingual and submental arteries, and the nerve supply from the chorda tympani and lingual nerves. Lymphatic drainage goes into the submental and submandibular LNs.

3.4 Surgical Anatomy of the Minor Salivary Glands

Minor salivary glands are scattered throughout the oral submucosa, with the exception of the gingiva and anterior hard palate. They are not encapsulated, and each gland possesses one duct draining directly into the oral cavity. Minor salivary glands are predominantly mucinous apart from the purely serous von Ebner glands of the dorsal tongue that surround the circumvallate papillae.

3.5 Clinical and Surgical Implications

- Salivary gland inflammation (sialadenitis) manifests as lymphoid infiltration and destruction of serous and mucinous acini, leading to pain, swelling, and dry mouth; this can be secondary to bacterial or viral infection, autoimmune disorder (e.g., Sjögren's syndrome and IgG4-related disease), impaction of calculi (sialolithiasis), trauma, and irradiation of the facial nerve, preventing ipsilateral hemifacial paralysis.
- Each cellular component of the salivary glands can give rise to benign and malignant lesions that may present as swellings, with or without associated discomfort or pain.
- Accessory parotid tissue is clinically important as salivary gland tumors can arise in this location.
- Dilatation of salivary gland ducts (sialectasis) may be associated with recurrent sialadenitis and typically presents as painful, diffuse parotid gland swelling.
- Xerostomia follows irradiation of the major or minor salivary gland tissues.
- Most (80%) of the salivary gland neoplasms arise in the parotid gland, 80% of these are benign; on the other hand, most neoplasms of the sublingual gland are malignant.
- Salivary gland neoplasms are primary epithelial. Other neoplasms include lymphomas and metastatic malignancies from the skin and soft tissues of the scalp (squamous cell carcinoma, melanoma, angiosarcoma, pleomorphic dermal sarcoma); these are more likely to occur in the parotid gland due to the presence of native LNs.
- Parotidectomy requires precise dissection of the parotid gland to identify and preserve the integrity of the facial nerve. Submandibular sialadenectomy also requires preservation of the MMN.

- Malignant tumors of the parotid gland can involve the facial nerve as the nerve passes through the gland.
- Minor salivary gland neoplasms generally manifest as submucosal nodules and, unlike parotid tumors, are most commonly malignant.

References

1. Kontis TC, Johns ME. Anatomy and physiology of the salivary glands. In: Bailey BJ, editor. Head and neck surgery—otolaryngology. Philadelphia, PA: Lippincott Williams & Wilkins; 2001.
2. Johns ME. The salivary glands: anatomy and embryology. Otolaryngol Clin N Am. 1977;10(2):261–71.
3. Kochhar A, Larian B, Azizzadeh B. Facial nerve and parotid gland anatomy. Otolaryngol Clin N Am. 2016;49:273.
4. Frommer J. The human accessory parotid gland: its incidence, nature, and significance. Oral Surg Oral Med Oral Pathol. 1977;43(5):671–6.
5. Bhattacharyya N, Varvares MA. Anomalous relationship of the facial nerve and the retromandibular vein: a case report. J Oral Maxillofac Surg. 1999;7(1):75–6.
6. Carrau RL, Johnson JT, Myers EN. Management of tumors of the parapharyngeal space. Oncology (Williston Park). 1997;11(5):633–40.
7. Iwai T, Sugiyama S, Oguri S, Mitsudo K. Anatomical relationship between the lingual nerve and submandibular duct. J Craniofac Surg. 2022;33(3):949–50.
8. Batsakis JG. Sublingual gland. Ann Otol Rhinol Laryngo. 1991;100(6):521–2.

Applied Physiology of the Salivary Glands

4

4.1 Introduction

Salivary glands can be classified as serous, mucous, or mixed (sero-mucous). In humans, saliva-synthesizing acinar cells are capable of producing a volume of up to 1.5 L daily, secreted in response to parasympathetic and sympathetic stimulation [1]. Parasympathetic activity favors the production of serous or watery solution while sympathetic activity triggers protein secretion [1, 2]. In serous secretions, the main type of protein secreted is the enzyme alpha-amylase (ptylin) that breaks down starch into maltose and glucose [3], whereas in mucous secretions the main protein secreted is mucin, which acts as a lubricant [4]. Parotid glands are responsible for up to 50% of saliva production upon stimulation [5].

Saliva is a complex secretion; 93% by volume is secreted by the major salivary glands and the remaining 7% by the minor salivary glands. Thus, the major function of the salivary glands is to secrete saliva, which primarily contains the enzymes amylase and lysozyme, IgA and IgG antibodies, inorganic ions, and a variable quantity of mucous. Saliva has a crucial protective and digestive function within the upper aerodigestive cavity, providing mucosal lubrication and dental protection, facilitating taste and speech, initiating enzymatic digestion of carbohydrates, and contributing to oral immunity [6]. Initially isotonic, saliva becomes a hypotonic, bicarbonate-rich solution as it passes through the mitochondria-packed striated ducts that facilitate ion transport.

4.2 Constituents (Composition) of Saliva

Saliva contains both inorganic and organic compounds (Fig. 4.1) and is characterized by its high volume compared to salivary gland weight, high potassium concentration, and low osmolarity. The large relative volume of saliva production is due to its high secretion rate, which can go up to 1 mL/g of salivary gland/minute.

© The Author(s), under exclusive license to Springer Nature Switzerland AG 2024
M. Sakr, *Surgery of the Salivary Glands*,
https://doi.org/10.1007/978-3-031-82069-4_4

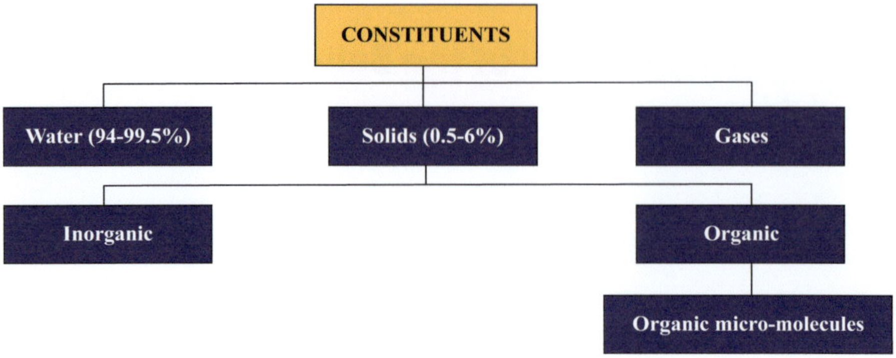

Fig. 4.1 Constituents of saliva secreted by the parotid gland

Saliva contains both inorganic and organic compounds and is characterized by its high volume compared to salivary gland weight, high potassium concentration, and low osmolarity. The large relative volume of saliva production is due to its high secretion rate, which can go up to 1 mL/g of salivary gland/minute.

Saliva is mostly hypotonic to plasma due to the fact that reabsorption of sodium (Na^+) and chloride (Cl^-) is greater than the secretion of potassium (K^+) and bicarbonate ($HCO3^-$) within the salivary ducts.

Several organic compounds present in saliva include α-amylase, lingual lipase, mucus, lysozymes, glycoproteins, lactoferrin, and the IgA secretory piece. Saliva is also comprised of the organic blood group antigens A, B, AB, and O. "Kallikrein" is secreted by the salivary glands during increased metabolic activity. Kallikrein enzymatically converts plasma protein into bradykinin, a vasodilator, in order to increase blood flow to the glands. Saliva contains approximately one-tenth of the total amount of protein found in plasma.

4.3 Functions of Saliva

Salivary functions serve to maintain oral health and create an appropriate ecological balance. Salivary components work in concert in overlapping, multifunctioning roles, which can be simultaneously beneficial and detrimental. The functions of saliva can be summarized as follows.

4.3.1 Digestion of Carbohydrates and Fats

Saliva begins the digestive process. It plays a crucial role in the digestion of carbohydrates and fats through two main enzymes. The first is ptyalin, which is an α-amylase in saliva that cleaves the internal α-1,4-glycosidic bonds of starches to produce maltose, maltotriose, and α-limit dextrins. This enzyme functions at an optimal pH of 7, but rapidly denatures when exposed to a pH less than 4, such as when in contact with the acidic secretions of the stomach. Up to 75% of the carbohydrate content in a meal, however, is broken down by the gastric enzyme because a significant portion of an ingested meal remains unmixed within the oral region, and thus there is a delay in the mixture of gastric juices with the food bolus.

Starch digestion is not slowed in the absence of ptyalin because pancreatic amylase is identical to salivary amylase and is thus able to break down all carbohydrates when in the small intestine.

The second enzyme is produced by the salivary glands of the tongue (lingual lipase), which breaks down triglycerides. Unlike ptyalin, this enzyme is functional within the acidic stomach and proximal duodenum because it is optimally active at a low pH [7].

4.3.2 Lubrication (Mastication, Swallowing, Speech)

The best lubricating components of saliva are mucins: they have the properties of low solubility, high viscosity, high elasticity, and strong adhesiveness. Any intraoral contact between soft tissues, between soft tissues and teeth, or between soft tissues and prostheses benefits from the lubricating capability of saliva supplied largely by these mucins. Mastication, speech, and swallowing and traveling of the bolus down the esophagus all are aided by the lubricating effects of mucins.

4.3.3 Antimicrobial Action (Antibacterial/Antifungal)

Mucins also perform an antibacterial function by selectively modulating the adhesion of microorganisms to oral tissue surfaces, which contributes to the control of bacterial and fungal colonization.

Saliva can prevent microbial growth based on the elements it contains. For example, lactoferrin in saliva binds naturally with iron. Since iron is a major component of bacterial cell walls, removal of iron breaks down the cell wall, which in turn breaks down the bacteria. Antimicrobial peptides such as histatins inhibit the growth of *Candida albicans* and *Streptococcus mutans*. Salivary Immunoglobulin A serves to aggregate oral bacteria such as *S. mutans* and prevents the formation of dental plaque [8].

4.3.4 Protection/Immunity

The antibacterial properties of saliva are due to its many protective organic constituents. The binding glycoprotein for immunoglobulin A (IgA), known as the secretory piece, forms a complex with IgA that is immunologically active against viruses and bacteria.

Lysozyme causes bacterial agglutination and autolysin activation to degrade bacterial cell walls. Lactoferrin inhibits the growth of bacteria that need iron by chelating with the element. Xerostomia, (dry mouth), due to lack of salivation, can lead to chronic buccal mucosal infections or dental caries.

As a seromucous coating, saliva lubricates and protects oral tissues, acting as a barrier against irritants. These irritants include, but are not limited to, proteolytic and hydrolytic enzymes produced in plaque, potential carcinogens from smoking and exogenous chemicals, and desiccation from mouth breathing.

Many agents and viruses are actively excreted in saliva. Mercury poisoning can manifest as stomatitis and lead poisoning by the gingival deposition of lead. The viruses causing rabies and poliomyelitis are excreted into saliva and can be transmitted in this manner.

4.3.5 Buffering Action and Clearance

Saliva also serves as a protective buffer for the mouth by diluting harmful substances and lowering the temperature of solutions that are too hot. It washes out foul-tasting substances from the mouth and neutralizes gastric juice to protect the oral cavity and esophagus [9].

The buffer capacity of both unstimulated and stimulated saliva involves three major buffer systems: the bicarbonate, the phosphate, and the protein buffer systems. These systems have different pH ranges of maximal buffer capacity, the bicarbonate and phosphate systems having pH values of 6.1–6.3 and 6.8–7.0, respectively.

Dilution and removal of substances (oral debris, noxious agents) from the oral cavity is referred to as salivary or oral clearance. Both the act of swallowing and the salivary flow rate are important to this process, and these are the principal ways by which oral bacteria and injurious, noxious agents are eliminated from the mouth. Accordingly, a high salivary flow rate results in a high clearance and vice versa.

The oral sugar clearance becomes extensively prolonged when the whole unstimulated saliva flow rate is below 0.2 mL/min. In addition to clearing sugars, saliva also clears dietary acids and thereby protects the teeth against erosion.

In general, the higher the flow rate, the faster the clearance and the higher the buffer capacity. Dental caries is probably the most common consequence of hyposalivation. A low flow rate combined with a low or moderate buffer effect clearly indicates poor salivary resistance against microbial attack.

4.3.6 Maintenance of Tooth Integrity

Saliva forms a pellicle on the surface of the tooth to prevent wearing. The film contains mucins and proline-rich glycoprotein from the saliva. The proteins (statherin and proline-rich proteins) within the salivary pellicle inhibit de-mineralization and promote re-mineralization by attracting calcium ions [10].

Demineralization occurs when acids diffuse through plaque and the pellicle into the liquid phase of enamel between enamel crystals. A pH of 5–5.5 is the critical pH range for the development of caries. When this occurs, the buffering capacity effect of saliva (increases saliva flow rate) inhibits demineralization.

Saliva can then begin to promote the remineralization of the tooth by strengthening the enamel with calcium and phosphate minerals (remineralization is the process of replacing lost minerals through the organic matrix of the enamel to the crystals) [11].

4.3.7 Taste Sensation

The sense of taste is activated during the initial stage of ingestion of food particles allowing for identification of essential nutrients and of harmful and potentially toxic compounds. Taste is a main stimulant for the formation of saliva. On the other hand, the presence of saliva in the oral cavity is also essential for taste perception, first of all because food particles need to be in solution in order to stimulate taste receptor cells in the taste buds within the lingual papillae (fungiform, foliate, and vallate papillae) [12, 13].

Furthermore, taste sensitivity is related to saliva composition as each receptor cell's upper surface is bathed by the oral fluids. The hypotonicity of saliva enhances the tasting capacity of salty foods and nutrient sources. This enhanced tasting capability depends on the presence of gustin, which binds zinc.

4.3.8 Tissue Repair

Saliva can encourage soft tissue repair by decreasing clotting time, increasing wound contraction, production of growth factors, and other regulatory peptides [14].

Constituents (components) of saliva and their role in relation to functions of saliva are summarized in Table 4.1 [15].

Table 4.1 Saliva constituents and function

Functions	Constituents
Lubrication	Mucins, proline-rich glycoproteins, water
Antimicrobial action	Lysozyme, lactoferrin, lacto-peroxides, mucins, cystins, histatins, immunoglobulins
Mucosal integrity	Mucins, electrolytes, water
Cleansing action	Water
Buffer capacity	Bicarbonates, phosphates, calcium, statherin, fluoride
Mastication and swallowing	Water, mucins
Digestion	Amylase, lipase, ribonucleases, proteases, water, mucins
Taste	Water, gustin (carbonic anhydrase)
Speech	Water, mucin

4.4 Control of Saliva Secretion

The secretion, blood flow, and growth of salivary glands are mostly controlled by both branches of the autonomic nervous system. Even though the parasympathetic nervous system has more influence on the secretion rate of the salivary glands than the sympathetic system, secretion is stimulated by both branches.

4.4.1 Parasympathetic System

Parasympathetic innervation of the major salivary glands follows branches of the facial and glossopharyngeal nerves. Parasympathetic stimulation activates both acinar activity and ductal transport mechanisms, leading to glandular vasodilation and myoepithelial cell contraction. Acetylcholine (ACh) serves as the parasympathetic neurotransmitter that acts on the muscarinic receptors of the salivary glands. The subsequent formation of inositol trisphosphate leads to increased calcium (Ca) concentrations within the cell, released from either intracellular Ca stores or from the plasma. This second messenger significantly affects salivary volume secretion. Glandular secretion is sustained by acetylcholinesterases, which inhibit the breakdown of ACh. The muscarinic antagonist atropine, however, decreases salivation by competing with ACh for the salivary receptor site.

4.4.2 Sympathetic System

Sympathetic supply to the salivary gland is mainly from the thoracic spinal nerves of the superior cervical ganglion. Like parasympathetic innervation, myoepithelial cell contraction also results. Changes in blood flow, however, are biphasic: vasoconstriction due to α-adrenergic receptor activation is followed by vasodilation due to buildup of vasodilator metabolites. Binding of the neurotransmitter nor-epinephrine to α-adrenergic receptor results in the formation of 3′,5′-cyclic adenosine monophosphate (cAMP), which then leads to phosphorylation of various proteins and activation of different enzymes. Increases in cAMP result in increased salivary enzyme and mucus content.

4.4.3 Hormones

Within saliva, K^+ concentrations increase while Na^+ concentrations decrease in the presence of antidiuretic hormone (ADH) or aldosterone. Unlike other digestive glands, however, these two hormones do not affect salivary gland secretion rate. Hormones such as androgens, estrogens, glucocorticoids, and peptides also influence salivary composition.

4.5 Flow Rates of Saliva Secretion

The amount of saliva is affected by the total body fluid volume and so dehydration decreases its amount and one feels thirsty. In normal circumstances, the minimal total unstimulated salivary flow rate is 0.1 mL/min, and the minimal stimulated flow rate is 0.2 mL/min. The maximal stimulated flow rate is 7 mL/min. The 24-h volume of salivary secretion has been estimated to be 500–1500 mL. The greatest volume of saliva is produced before, during, and after meals, reaching its maximum peak at around 12 a.m., and falls considerably at night, while sleeping [16]. Salivary flow in the unstimulated glands is produced primarily by the submandibular glands (65%), with the parotid, sublingual, and minor glands providing 20% and 7–8% of the flow, respectively. Once stimulated, the relative contributions of the parotid and submandibular glands are reversed, with the parotid gland supplying greater than 50% of the flow. The minor salivary glands, independent of stimulation, produce less than 10% of the total flow.

The two main triggers for salivary production are mastication and gustatory stimuli. Acidic foods are the best stimulus and sweet tastes the least. Olfaction is surprisingly a poor secretory stimulus. The presence of food in the mouth, the act of chewing, and nausea all stimulate salivation, while sleep, fatigue, dehydration, and fear inhibit it. Salivary flow rates are independent of age, and flow rates remain constant despite the degeneration of acinar cells during the aging process. Xerostomia in the elderly is probably the result of systemic disease or medication side effects. Salivary gland hypofunction is defined as an unstimulated flow rate less than 0.1 mL/min or a 50% reduction below basal rates if they have been determined [17, 18].

4.6 Applied Physiology

4.6.1 Hyposalivation

A number of physiological circumstances reduce salivary secretion. They include age, the number of teeth in the mouth, male/female, body weight, and the time of day [19, 20]. Reduction in salivation (hyposalivation) may be temporary or permanent. Temporary hyposalivation may result from dehydration, malnutrition, fever, or emotional conditions such as fear and depression. Permanent hyposalivation may result from congenital absence (aplasia) or hypoplasia of salivary glands, sialolithiasis, or Bell's palsy.

Over 400 medicines, many of them in common use, induce salivary gland hypofunction [15]. Head and neck radiotherapy causes irreversible hyposalivation by destroying the glandular parenchyma. The adverse effects start from 4000 rads onward, and the reduction in salivary flow depends on the dose [21]. Some systemic disorders cause progressive destruction of the salivary glands, as in some autoimmune diseases such as Sjögren's syndrome [22].

4.6.2 Xerostomia (Dry Mouth, Pasties, Cotton Mouth)

It results from hyposalivation or aptyalism and may be 1ry or 2ry. The main causes include dehydration due to renal failure, shock, Sjögren's syndrome, trauma to the gland or ducts, post-radiotherapy, and side effects of some drugs, after smoking marijuana.

Xerostomia is usually not a problem until the flow rate is <0.2 mL/min/gland. Patients suffering from xerostomia can experience difficulty with eating, swallowing, speech, the wearing of dentures, trauma to and ulceration of the oral mucosa, taste alteration, poor oral hygiene, a burning sensation of the mucosa, oral infections, including *Candida,* and rapidly progressing dental caries.

4.6.3 Hypersalivation (Pytalism, Sialorrhea, Sialism, Sialosis)

It means excess of saliva secretion and may be physiological or pathological. Physiologically, the greatest salivary secretion takes place during tooth eruption and is linked to hyperstimulation of the peripheral receptors in the oral mucus. Hyperstimulation of salivary secretion also takes place during the first half of pregnancy and during menstruation, as well as resulting from smell and mechanical stimuli such as mastication and taste stimuli such as sourness and sweetness.

The pathological causes of hypersalivation include those of oral origin such as the first stages of wearing dentures, dental pain, tooth decay, or neoplasm if the mouth or tongue, or any inflammatory process in the oral-pharyngeal or digestive regions, particularly in the upper tract. Certain neurological disorders such as parkinsonism, epilepsy, encephalitis, or some tumors can cause hypersalivation, as can exogenous poisoning by lead, bismuth, mercury, silver, gold, or arsenic, and endointoxications such as uremia, certain medicines such as pilocarpin, cholinesterase inhibitors, cholinergic agonists, lithium, iodides, mercury compounds, or L-dopa, hyperparathyroidism, and some stages of serious infectious processes [23].

4.6.4 Drooling

Drooling means "uncontrolled flow of saliva with inability to retain saliva in the mouth." It occurs in the following conditions: during teeth eruption in children, upper respiratory tract infection or nasal allergies in children, dysphagia, tonsillitis, and peri-tonsillar abscess.

4.6.5 Paralytic Secretion of Saliva

Paralytic saliva secretion results from iatrogenic/traumatic severance of the parasympathetic nerve supply. It leads to increased salivary secretion for 3 weeks (known as paralytic secretion) due to the release of large amounts of adrenalin from the adrenal medulla after denervation. This is followed by a reduction in secretion and finally cessation in about the sixth week. Cutting the sympathetic nerve fully (sympathectomy) does not influence paralytic secretion.

4.6.6 Augmented Secretion of Saliva

If the nerves supplying the salivary glands are stimulated twice, the amount of saliva secreted by the second stimulus is larger than that due to the first stimulus. This is explained by the fact that the first stimulus increases the excitability of acinar cells. Hence, when the second stimulus is applied, salivary secretion is augmented.

4.7 Diagnostic Applications of Saliva

Both intra- and extracellular enable the saliva to be reached by some substances that are not among its normal components [24]. The use of saliva in diagnosing several pathological diseases is summarized as follows.

4.7.1 Oral Cavity Infections

The use of saliva in diagnosing dental caries risk is well known owing to the possibility of detecting the presence of *S. mutans* and *Lactobacillus* spp., as well as lactic acid, which causes the subsurface demineralization that causes the onset of the caries lesion [25]. Other infectious diseases of the oral cavity can be diagnosed in this way, such as candidiasis through the presence of *Candida* spp. in the saliva. The presence of peri-odontal pathogenic bacteria can also be diagnosed by this method. Some of these bacteria play a role in increasing the risk of cardiovascular and cerebrovascular diseases [26], pre-term birth, and low birth weight.

4.7.2 Cystic Fibrosis

Cystic fibrosis, a hereditary disease characterized by an alteration in electrolyte transport in the epithelial cells and the secretion of viscous mucus by the glands and epithelia, is linked to raised sodium level, chloride, calcium, phosphate, lipid, and protein contents in the submaxillary saliva. An epidermal growth factor with low biological activity compared to that of healthy persons and raised prostaglandin E2 levels are also found in the saliva of these patients [27].

4.7.3 Celiac Disease

For diagnosing celiac disease, IgA and anti-gliadin antibody detection in saliva shows high specificity and low sensitivity, whereas their determination in serum is highly sensitive and less specific [28].

4.7.4 Sjögren's Syndrome

In Sjögren's syndrome, minor salivary gland biopsy is an accepted diagnostic procedure. A predominant inflammatory infiltrate composed of CD4 lymphocytes is found, together with lowered at-rest and stimulated salivary flow rates. Quantitatively, there are raised concentrations of sodium, chloride, IgA, IgG, lactoferrin, albumin, â2 microglobulin, cystatin C and S, lipids, and inflammation mediators such as prostaglandin E2, thromboxane B2, and interleukin-6. Autoantibodies (IgA, IgG, and IgM) can also be detected in the saliva [29].

4.7.5 Malignancy

In some malignant diseases, tumor markers can be detected in the saliva, such as protein p53 antibodies in patients with oral squamous cell carcinoma, or high levels of defensin-1 positively correlated with the serum levels. The presence of the c-erbB-2 tumor marker in the saliva and blood serum of breast cancer patients and its absence in healthy women is a promising tool for the early detection of this disease. Moreover, in ovarian cancer, the CA 125 marker can be detected in the saliva with greater specificity and less sensitivity than in serum [30].

4.7.6 *Helicobacter Pylori* Detection

Detection of *Helicobacter pylori* in the saliva by polymerase chain reaction (PCR) shows high sensitivity; studies have shown that the oral–oral transmission route for this bacterium may be of considerable importance in developed countries [31]. The presence of antibodies to other infectious organisms such as *Borrelia burgdorferi*, *Shigella,* or *Tenia solium* can also be detected through the saliva.

4.7.7 Viral Diseases

Detection of hepatitis A antigen and hepatitis B surface antigen in the saliva has been used in epidemiological studies, as have that of IgM and IgG type antibodies to both types of hepatitis with 100% sensitivity and specificity [32].

Saliva has also been used to detect antibodies to the rubella, parotitis, and rubeola viruses. In neonates, the presence of IgA is an excellent marker of rotavirus infection. Some studies have suggested that reactivation of herpes virus type 1 infections is related to the pathogenesis of Bell's palsy and that PCR detection of the virus in the saliva would be a suitable method for early detection of reactivations of this illness [33].

Detection of human immunodeficiency virus (HIV) antibody is as precise in saliva as in serum and is applicable in both clinical and epidemiological studies. The presence of HIV virus antibodies and viral components in the saliva can assist in the diagnosis of acute infection, congenital infection, and reactivations of the infection [34].

4.7.8 Monitoring Drug and Alcohol Levels

The determination of certain drugs in saliva depends on their concentration in the blood and their diffusion capacity, lipo-solubility, and molecular size. Saliva has been used to monitor the levels of lithium, carbamazepine, barbiturates, benzodiazepines, phenytoin, theophylline, and cyclosporine. Equally, there is a high correlation between ethanol concentrations in saliva and serum. The presence of thiocyanate in the saliva is an excellent indicator of active or passive smoking. Other drugs such as cocaine or opiates can also be detected in saliva [35].

4.7.9 Detection of Certain Hormones

Detection in the saliva of certain hormones such as cortisol, aldosterone, testosterone, estradiol, or insulin is highly correlated with concentrations in serum. In general, it is the "lipo-soluble" hormones with lower molecular weights that can be detected most reliably in the saliva, which they enter by ultrafiltration or passive diffusion, whereas protein-bound hormones will not be found as there is no active transport into the saliva [36].

References

1. Carolyn A, Cathy E, Julia J, Sivakumar S, Nicky P. Treatment of sialorrhea (excessive saliva) in people with motor neuron disease/amyotrophic lateral sclerosis. Cochrane Database Syst Rev. 2011;5:CD006981.
2. Andrew N, Jo T. Parasympathetic drugs for the treatment of salivary gland dysfunction due to radiotherapy. Cochrane Database Syst Rev. 2015;(10):D003782.
3. Frederic MH, Judi NL, Edwin B. Fundamentals of anatomy & physiology. 9th ed. San Francisco, CA: Pearson Benjamin Cummings; 2012.
4. Michael E, Colin D, Denis O. Saliva and oral health. 4th ed. Little Steine, Hill Farm Lane, Duns Tew, OX: Stephen Hancocks Limited; 2012. p. 1.
5. Iorgulescu G. Saliva between normal and pathological. Important factors in determining systemic and oral health. J Med Life. 2009;2(3):303–7.
6. Nanci A. Ten Cate's oral histology: development, structure, and function. 9th ed. Sparks, NV. Elsevier Inc, Philadelphia, PA: USA; 2018. ISBN 978-0-323-48524-1
7. Anthea M. Human biology and health. 1st ed. Englecliffss, NJ: Prentice Hall; 1993.
8. John T. Immunity in the oral cavity. Newcastle University, UK: British Society for Immunology; 2018.
9. Bechir F, Pacurar M, Tohati A, Bataga SM. Comparative study of salivary pH, buffer capacity, and flow in patients with and without gastroesophageal reflux disease. Int J Environ Res Public Health. 2021;19(1):201.

10. Buzalaf MA, Hannas AR, Kato MT. Saliva and dental erosion. J Appl Oral Sci. 2012;20(5):493–502.
11. Dowd FI. Saliva and dental caries. Dental Clin North Am. 1999;43(4):579–97.
12. Nanci A. Ten Cate's oral histology: development, structure, and function. 6th ed. St. Louis, MO: Mosby; 2003. p. 300–1.
13. Matsuo R. Role of Saliva in the maintenance of taste sensitivity. Crit Rev Oral Biol Med. 2000;11(2):216–29.
14. Mandel ID. The functions of saliva. J Dental Res. 1987;66:623–6.
15. Sreebny L, Baum B, Edgar W, Epstein J, Fox P, Larmas M. Saliva: its role in health and diseases. Int Dent J. 1992;42:291–304.
16. Nauntofte B, Tenevuo JO, Lagerlöf F. Secretion and composition of saliva. In: Fejerskov O, Kidd E, editors. Dental caries. The disease and its clinical management. Oxford: Blackwell Munksgard; 2003. p. 7–29.
17. Johnson LR, editor. Secretion. Amsterdam: Elsevier; 2003.
18. Kontis TC, Johns ME. Anatomy and physiology of the Salivary Glands. In: Bailey BJ, editor. Head and neck surgery—otolaryngology. Philadelphia, PA: Lippincott Williams and Wilkins; 2001.
19. Dodds MW, Jonson DA, Yeh CK. Health benefits of saliva: a review. J Dent. 2005;33:223–33.
20. Cohen-Brown G, Ship JA. Diagnosis and treatment of salivary gland disorders. Quintessence Int. 2004;35:108–23.
21. Andrews N, Griffiths C. Dental complications of head and neck radiotherapy: part 2. Aus Dent J. 2001;46:174–82.
22. Mariette X. Treatment of oral dryness in Sjogren's syndrome. Rev Med Interne. 2004;25:287–93.
23. Meningaud JP, Pitak-Arnnop P, Chikhani L, Bertrand JC. Drooling of saliva: a review of the etiology and management options. Oral Surg Oral Med Oral Pathol Oral Radiol Endod. 2006;101:48–57.
24. Haeckel R, Hanecke P. Application of saliva, sweat and tear fluid for diagnostic purposes. Ann Biol Clin. 1993;51:903–10.
25. Llena MC, Almerich JM, Forner L. Determinación de ácido láctico en el dorso de la lengua. Su relación con la presencia de caries activa. RECOE. 2004;9:303–7.
26. Morrison HI, Ellison LF, Taylor GW. Periodontal disease and risk of fatal coronary heart and cerebrovascular diseases. J Cardiovascular Risk. 1999;6:7–11.
27. Slomiany BL, Aono M, Murty VL, Slomiany A, Levine MJ, Tabaka LA. Lipid compositition of submandibular saliva from normal and cystic fibrosis individuals. J Dent Res. 1982;61:1163–6.
28. Rujner J, Socha J, Barra E, Gregorek H, Madalinski K, Wozniewicz B, et al. Serum and salivary antigliadin antibodies and serum Ig A anti-endomysium antibodies as a screening test for coeliac disease. Acta Pediatr. 1996;85:814–7.
29. Tishler M, Yaron I, Shiraiz I, Levartovsky D, Yaron M. Salivary and serum soluble interleukina-2 receptor in primary Sjögren syndrome. Arch Oarl Biol. 1999;44:305–8.
30. Streckfus C, Bigler L, Tucci M, Thigpen JT. A preliminary study og CA15-3, c-erbβ-2, epidermal growth factor receptor, cathepsin-D, and p53 in saliva among women with breast carcinoma. Cancer Invest. 2000;18:101–9.
31. Loeb MB, Riddell RH, James C, Hunt R, Smaill FM. Evaluation of salivary antibodies to detect infection with Helicobacter pylori. Can J Gastroenterol. 1997;11:437–40.
32. El-Medany OM, El-Din Abdel Wahab KS, Abu Shady EA, Gad El-Hak N. Chronic liver disease and hepatitis C virus in Egyptian patients. Hepatogastroenterology. 1999;46:1895–903.
33. Furuta Y, Fukuda S, Chida E, Takasu T, Ohtania F, Inuyama Y, et al. Reactivation of herpes simples virus type I in patients with Bell's palsy. J Med Virol. 1998;54:162–6.
34. Emmons WW. Accuracy of oral specimen testing for human immunodeficiency virus. Am J Med. 1997;102:15–20.
35. Navazesh M, Denny P, Sobel S. Saliva: a fountain of opportunity. J Calif Dent Assoc. 2002;30:783–8.
36. Kaufman E, Lamster IB. The diagnostic applications of saliva. A review. Crit Rev Oral Biol Med. 2002;13:197–212.

Evaluation of the Parotid Gland

5

5.1 Clinical Evaluation

Despite the availability of modern technology for the diagnosis of parotid gland disorders, great care should be taken during history-taking and physical examination as they still play important roles in the clinical diagnosis of the patient.

5.1.1 History-Taking

Patients with parotid gland disorders usually complain of swelling, pain, xerostomia (dry mouth), foul taste, and occasionally sialorrhea (excessive salivation). Swelling and pain during meals followed by a reduction in symptoms after meals may indicate partial stenosis of the duct. The most common presenting symptom of neoplasms (both benign and malignant) is an asymptomatic swelling. Pain is more common in patients with parotid cancer (10–29%) than those with benign tumors (2.5–4%) [1], but pain itself is not diagnostic of malignancy.

Demographic data (age and gender) are very important. Sjögren's syndrome, for example, is common in menopausal women while mumps usually occurs in children.

Medical profile of the patient may provide helpful clues to diagnosis. Gland dysfunction is often associated with certain systemic disorders such as diabetes mellitus (DM), atherosclerosis, hormonal imbalances, and neurological disorders [2, 3]. A careful dietary history should not be neglected for patients who suffer from chronic dehydration due to bulimia or anorexia or during chemotherapy are at risk for parotitis.

Drug history of the patient should also be considered as salivary function is often affected by certain drugs such as diuretics and other antihypertensive drugs, which may cause xerostomia [2, 3]. History of prior irradiation should be sought since "xerostomia" is a debilitating consequence of radiation therapy to the head and neck.

© The Author(s), under exclusive license to Springer Nature Switzerland AG 2024
M. Sakr, *Surgery of the Salivary Glands*,
https://doi.org/10.1007/978-3-031-82069-4_5

For the evaluation of a parotid mass, it is important to take history of the parotid mass duration, rate of growth and presence of pain, facial paralysis, cervical lymphadenopathy, and eye and joint symptoms. Facial nerve paralysis in a previously untreated patient usually indicates that a tumor is malignant [1].

5.1.2 Physical Examination

Both extraoral and intraoral examinations should be carried out in a systematic way to avoid missing any crucial signs. Bimanual palpation (extraoral with one hand and intraoral with the palmar aspects of the fingertips of the other) must also be performed to properly examine the submandibular glands.

5.1.2.1 Inspection

Extraoral Inspection is performed, with the patient facing in front of the examiner, 3–4 feet away. The examiner should inspect symmetry, color, pulsations, and discharging sinuses on both sides of the patient. Enlargement of the parotid gland may be unilateral or bilateral. Parotitis typically presents as a pre-auricular swelling, but may not be visible if deep in the parotid tail or within the substance of the gland. Overlying skin changes may suggest a granulomatous process or malignancy. Neurological deficits should also be examined. Facial nerve paralysis in conjunction with a parotid mass, for example, should raise the suspicion of a malignant parotid neoplasm.

Intraoral Inspection is done using a torch or headlight. The orifices of the parotid (Stensen's) ducts are inspected opposite the second upper molar tooth and the two sides compared. Saliva may be seen pouring from the nonaffected side only. Intraoral examination should include observations for asymmetry, discoloration, pulsation, and obstructions in the duct orifices. Swelling of the deep lobe of the parotid gland may be seen intraorally and may also displace the tonsil. The minor salivary glands should be examined. The labial, buccal, and posterior palatal mucosa should be dried with an air blower or tissue and pressed to assess the flow of saliva [1].

5.1.2.2 Palpation

With the examiner standing in front of or behind the patient, the patient's head is inclined forward to maximally expose the parotid gland region. Size, tenderness, consistency, mobility, and other features of the parotid gland and associated masses can be easily evaluated with extraoral and intraoral palpation owing to the superficial anatomical location of the gland.

5.1.2.3 Auscultation

Rare clinical entities, such as hemangiomas and other vascular anomalies, may be identified by auscultation during examination.

5.2 Laboratory Studies

5.2.1 Laboratory Tests

Laboratory studies are rarely necessary in the evaluation of salivary gland pathology. Serological evaluation for the human immunodeficiency virus (HIV) can be performed in patients with bilateral parotid cysts (viral sialadenitis). In the setting of suspected infection, material obtained by expressing ductal secretions may also be sent for culture and Gram stain. Mumps titers may be performed if viral parotitis is suspected in the nonimmunized patient. Sjögren's syndrome A and B antibodies (SS-A and SS-B, respectively) may be useful to evaluate for an autoimmune origin. Any patient with pulmonary symptoms or patients who are suspected of having extrathoracic tuberculosis (TB) may have a Mantoux TB test (also referred to as a purified protein derivative test) [4].

5.2.2 Salivary Flow

Most causes of xerostomia (dry mouth) are systemic in nature, but a significant percentage is idiopathic. Dehydration, hospital admission, mental stress, psychopathic emotional states (e.g., depression), fatigue, infection, raised ambient temperature, tranquilizers, ganglionic blockers, and light deprivation decrease salivary flow. In addition, pernicious and iron-deficiency anemia and loss of salivary tissue (due to irradiation, infection, or Sjögren's syndrome) cause decreased flow. After a full course of radiation therapy, flow rates are indefinitely reduced by 95% or more [5].

On the other hand, cigarette smoking, acute stomatitis, heavy metal poisoning, acrodynia, rabies, ingestion of highly seasoned foods, and schizophrenia increase the flow. Chewing on one side of the mouth increases the flow on that side.

5.2.3 Salivary Composition (Sialochemistry)

The composition of saliva changes in disease states, and analysis of saliva for enzymes, electrolytes, hormones, drugs, and immunization status can be performed.

Primary aldosteronism causes a decreased sodium (Na) level with normal potassium (K) content. A "Na-K ratio" of 0.3 or less is diagnostic, below 0.5 is suggestive, and above 1.0 rules out aldosteronism (normal, 1.3) [6]. Low Na-K ratios are also found in Cushing's disease with a mean ratio of 0.5.24. High ratios occur in Addison's disease with a mean ratio of 5.0 [7]. In pregnancy, the submandibular calcium (Ca) concentration is reduced, whereas the Na concentration is reduced and the K concentration is increased in both parotid and submandibular saliva [8].

The salivary glands, like the other exocrine glands, are affected by cystic fibrosis [9]. Total protein, amylase, lysozyme, and glycoprotein concentrations are increased in submandibular, but not in parotid saliva [10]. There is no change in the flow rate in the major glands [11], but there is a significant reduction in the minor glands [12].

Thyroid diseases and their treatment may affect the saliva. The salivary glands concentrate iodine to 40 times the plasma level, regardless of the thyroid-stimulating hormone (TSH) level or the state of thyroid function [13]. Hyperparathyroidism (HPT) causes an increased amount of Ca and phosphorus (P) in saliva, with the levels paralleling the parathormone levels [14]. In cases of essential hypertension, Na concentration and flow rate are decreased [15]. In sarcoidosis, amylase and kallikrein levels are decreased, whereas albumin and lysozyme concentrations are increased [16, 17]. Acute pancreatitis may cause an increase in the amount of amylase. Alcoholic cirrhosis may cause an increased flow rate with increased concentrations of K and amylase [18].

Inflammatory lesions may cause changes in saliva. In acute infections, the Na and K levels approach those of serum [19]. There is also a pronounced decrease in phosphate concentration. Other elements that are increased in amount include glucose, IgA, IgG, IgM, albumin, and transferrin, which leak from plasma, and myeloperoxidase, lactoferrin, and lysozyme, which are produced by the inflammatory infiltrate. IgG dominates the immunoglobulins, reflecting the normal serum pattern rather than the normal salivary pattern, in which IgA dominates.

Irradiation causes also alteration in the composition of saliva with increased amounts of Ca, Na, chloride, and protein and a decrease in bicarbonate. These changes lead to a significant rise in the number of dental caries.

Numerous systemically administered drugs can be detected in saliva, including iodide, heavy metals, thiocyanate, morphine, clindamycin, and rifampin [20]. Digitalis toxicity causes greatly elevated levels of K and Ca, and this study can be used to distinguish between toxic and therapeutic doses [21].

5.3 Imaging Studies

For patients with no specific symptoms (swelling and pain) and unclear physical signs, imaging studies can play an important role in clarifying the etiology of the gland disorder and assist in treatment selection and planning. These include conventional radiology (plain X-ray), sialography, ultrasound (US), computed tomography (CT) scan and CT sialography, magnetic resonance imaging (MRI), and MR sialography.

5.3.1 Conventional Radiography (Plain X-Ray)

Conventional radiography and sialography were widely used in the past, but are rarely used nowadays because of their limited value. For the parotid gland, anteroposterior (AP), tangential, lateral, and lateral oblique plain radiographs may be useful in showing calculi, calcifications, soft-tissue swellings, and bony erosions.

5.3.2 Sialography

The beginnings of the sialographic studies are dated 1902 [22]. Sialography visualizes the ducts and the parenchyma of the salivary gland, after contrast administration into the main salivary duct. For decades, it has been the main diagnostic method in the salivary glands [23].

There are three types of sialography:

- Conventional/fluoroscopic sialography (with or without digital subtraction)
- CT sialography (ultrafast technique)
- MR sialography

5.3.2.1 Conventional Sialography

Technique

Initial series of plain films are taken to identify radio-opaque calculi. A sialogogue (lemon juice or citric acid) is given to dilate the duct orifice. The duct is intubated by means of a blunt-tipped slightly angulated, metal cannula, or fine thin-walled polyethylene catheter with a tapered end. Approximately 0.5–1.5 mL of contrast medium (radio-opaque such as Lipiodol Ultrafluid) or a water-soluble medium, for example, hypaue (sodium diatrizoate), is slowly injected by hand until the duct system is filled. To complete examination, few drops of lemon juice are given to stimulate salivation. After an interval of 10 min, a further plain film is taken, which normally shows most of the contrast medium cleared from the ducts. Any filling defect (e.g., stone), retained sections (e.g., chronic sialadenitis), stricture (e.g., inflammation), extravasation (e.g., Sjögren's syndrome), or irregular borders (e.g., tumor) are noted. Fistulae and abscesses cavities can also be displayed with this technique.

Indications

The main indications of sialography include repeated pain and swelling where ultrasound does not yield any useful findings. It is also indicated in suspected sialolithiasis (or other causes of duct obstruction), chronic sialadenitis (suspected sialectasis), autoimmune diseases (e.g., Sicca syndrome), tumors, and duct lesions [24–29]. It is advised to wait approximately 6 weeks from the moment of inflammatory symptom relief until sialography [27]. Sialography is also excellent in revealing and localizing calcifications close to salivary ducts [30]. It also allows for a high-certainty discrimination of stone location; in the salivary duct or in parenchyma, which is crucial for the choice of the appropriate therapeutic method [24]. However, it is not a method of choice in the diagnosis of salivary gland tumors [31–33].

The diagnostic reliability of sialography has improved after the introduction of "digital subtraction sialography" (DSS) [34]. The use of postprocessing enables for a subtraction of a bony background and contrast enhancement of the salivary ducts [35].

Contraindications

Sialography is contraindicated in case of pregnancy, allergy to iodinated contrast medium, or acute sialadenitis as it can exacerbate and worsen the condition.

Disadvantages

Sialography is an invasive procedure, and its disadvantages include (1) patient's exposure to ionizing radiation and iodine contrast media (with the risk of allergic reactions), (2) pain during contrast medium injection into the salivary ducts, (3) possibility of calculi dislocation toward the inside of the gland, (4) quality of examination results is operator-dependent, (5) movement artifacts, and (6) a substantial failure rate of the procedure (due to cannulation problems, lack of skill, lack of patient compliance, and pain) [29, 36, 37]. In addition, when interpreting sialography, it should be remembered that air bubbles, injected together with the contrast medium, may simulate the presence of the calculi [36].

Complications

Sialography complications include (1) local pain, (2) salivary duct perforation, (3) activation of a dormant inflammation, (4) infection (should be suspected if pain persists for >24 h and antibiotics should be considered in such cases), (5) adverse reactions to iodine contrast medium, and (6) bleeding.

Advantages

Sialography requires a lower X-ray radiation dose compared to CT scan and is more accessible than MRI [38]. Moreover, sialography provides higher spatial resolution for superior diagnostic elucidation (when the procedure is successfully achieved) with accurate delineation of second- and third-order branches.

Owing to its possibilities of a detailed visualization of anatomical and pathological structures of the salivary ducts, sialography enables therapeutic approach in sialoendoscopy for the removal of sialoliths, retrograde displacement of sialoliths to relieve acute obstruction, and dilate strictures [39]. Despite these advantages, sialography being an invasive investigation has largely been replaced by MR sialography.

5.3.2.2 CT Sialography

Technique

The procedure is essentially the same as a conventional sialogram, after which the patient is positioned in a CT in a neutral supine position. Multiplanar data acquisition allows for 3D reconstruction. Intravenous contrast material can be administered for better soft-tissue evaluation, especially for parotid masses.

Advantages

Advantages of CT sialography allow better diagnosis of parenchymal pathology, excellent visualization of the deep lobe, and better subtraction options. Assessment of glands other than the parotids is also possible, and no special positioning of the patient is required.

Disadvantages

CT sialography is an invasive procedure and subjects the patient to radiation. In addition, intravenous atropine is required to minimize run-off of contrast and impair ductal clearance in some cases.

5.3.2.3 MR Sialography

Technique

MRI sialography is a fairly sensitive and reliable method of evaluating the salivary glands. Fast acquisition heavily T2-weighted sequences (e.g., RARE, CISS, FISP, as used in MR cholangio-pancreatography [MRCP] and MR urography) brighten intraluminal fluid and display ductal morphology adequately with no need to inject contrast into the ducts. MR contrast administered intravenously is a useful adjunct.

Advantages

MRI sialography is a noninvasive technique. Its advantages include (1) rapid acquisition, (2) assessment of other glands, (3) excellent delineation of parenchymal pathology, (4) no special positioning required, and (5) no cannulation is required; thus, the risk of air bubbles simulating intraductal calculi is minimized.

Disadvantages

The disadvantages of MR sialography include (1) the known general MRI contraindications such as pacemakers, implants, and claustrophobia, (2) image impairment by dental fillings, implants, and bridges, and (3) first- and second-order branches only can be delineated.

5.3.3 Ultrasonography (US)

Parotid (and submandibular) glands are examined with US using a 7.5 MHz or higher frequency linear array transducer, with patients chin turned away from the side being examined. Both glands have homogeneous echo pattern with scattered echogenic steaks produced by branch ducts converging into the main duct. The external carotid artery (ECA) and retromandibular vein can both be seen. Few lymph nodes (LNs) can be demonstrated within the gland. The entire salivary glands and all lesions have to be evaluated in at least two perpendicular planes during a US examination. The whole neck should also be scanned to assess lymph nodes and search for concomitant or related disease.

Ultrasound (US) remains the initial, noninvasive investigation of choice due to its high resolution, easy availability, and ability to guide needle biopsy. Examination with US and US-guided fine-needle aspiration cytology (FNAC) of the lesions alone may suggest the final diagnosis in most of the clinical settings. Ultrasound can detect around 95% of space-occupying lesions of major salivary glands [40]. Color Doppler can add to the value of US by depicting the blood flow within the lesion. In cases of sialolithiasis, US of the parotid glands is a useful, readily available, noninvasive, and inexpensive option. However, it is sometimes not possible to visualize and analyze the examined lesions completely with US because of their location, for example, deep lobe of the parotid gland or area behind the mandible. In these situations, further imaging examination (CT scan or MRI) is highly recommended and should also be applied in cases of suspected malignant lesions in order to assess possible infiltration of bones or deep structures invisible at US and to evaluate deep-lying LNs [40–43]. On the other hand, dynamic scintigraphy is still the method of choice in the functional evaluation of the salivary glands [44, 45].

5.3.4 Computed Tomography (CT) Scan

The parotid gland has low attenuation due to its high fat content and is therefore easily discernible by CT scanning. Computed tomography scan involves radiation exposure and IV injection of iodinated contrast enhancement, which increases the conspicuity of parotid masses and affords some prediction of their nature. The CT scan should extend from the skull base to the level of the hyoid bone, to demonstrate the facial nerve and ensure that the parotid tail and the high deep cervical and jugulo-digasric LNs have been included. The parotid duct will be demonstrated on thin sections taken parallel to the hard palate.

The main advantage of CT imaging is the two-dimensional view of the salivary gland, which can elucidate relationships to adjacent vital structures, differentiate intrinsic from extrinsic disease, and assess the draining cervical LNs. Differences between intrinsic and extrinsic parotid gland masses, however, are often difficult to assess especially when present in the para-pharyngeal space [46]. CT scan is also extremely valuable in defining abscess formation vs. phlegmon. In addition, several aspects such as detection of calculus, involvement of mandible, and widening of foramina of skull base in case of perineural spread are better seen on CT scan [47]. However, it is limited in evaluating the ductal system unless combined with simultaneous sialography (CT sialography), which is an alternative method of increasing conspicuity of parotid masses, but the technique is invasive and is not widely practiced as MRI is more beneficial [48].

In 2013, Abdel-Wahed et al. reported that in cases that have obstructive salivary gland diseases, it would be advisable to perform "cone beam" CT sialography (CBCT) as the modality of choice in demonstrating the ductal system of the gland and as an alternative to conventional sialography [49]. Drage and Brown [50] were pioneers in reporting cases of CBCT sialography. They concluded that CBCT sialography was superior to conventional sialography and explained that 3D reconstruction could be performed and then viewed from any direction and in any slice thickness, and from which cross-sectional slices might be obtained in any direction [50].

5.3.5 Magnetic Resonance Imaging (MRI)

Magnetic resonance imaging (MRI) allows multiplanar analysis of soft tissues with high-contrast resolution, being an excellent method for both salivary gland observation and for the diagnosis of various glandular disorders, allowing the three-dimensional analysis of the extension of a lesion and its relationship with adjacent anatomical structures [51–53]. It gives excellent soft-tissue contrast of parotid lesions against a fatty background. T1-weighted images with fat suppression and contrast enhancement show the tumor margins and spread accurately, while T2-weighted images give an insight into the internal architecture of the tumor.

Compared with CT, MRI can also contribute to the determination of the lesion stage, having the advantage of not exposing the patient to ionizing radiation since it uses electromagnetic fields to generate images. In addition, MRI provides better contrast resolution, reduces artifacts from dental amulgum, and yields detailed images on several different planes without patient repositioning (multiplaner imaging). However, gadolinium contrast enhancement decreases the conspicuity of some parotid masses.

MRI is more often used for the assessment of para-pharyngeal space abnormalities, especially in discriminating between deep lobe parotid tumors and other lesions, such as schwannoma and/or glomus vagale. Parotid gland masses have low T1 signal, particularly contrasted against the fatty stroma of the parotid. Fat-suppressed T1 sequences are superior in determining the extent of invasion. However, MRI is inferior to CT scanning for the detection of early bone erosion and calcification, the presence of which is important in the diagnosis of pleomorphic adenoma and sialolithiasis. Chronic inflammation of the salivary glands and calculi are not indications for MRI. MR sialography has been described using heavy T2W1, which contrasts ductal fluid against stroma. It is used to evaluate the ductal system of the gland without requiring the use of intravenous/ductal contrast agents via highly fluid-sensitive sequences, so it can also be performed in patients with acute sialadenitis [54].

5.3.6 Algorithm of Imaging

Considering the wide range of diseases that can affect the parotid gland, choosing the best imaging diagnosis method is critical, considering the cost, use of ionizing radiation, accuracy, reliability, and patient satisfaction [54]. In children and pregnant women, US is the examination of choice, especially in lesions involving the superficial part of the parotid gland. Computed tomography (CT) scan is the method used for patients with suspected inflammatory diseases, such as abscesses, calculi, dilation of the major salivary duct, and acute inflammation. On the other hand, MRI is the chosen method for patients with palpable masses and neoplastic suspensions [55].

An algorithm for the imaging of parotid gland swellings, whether cystic or solid, and whether suspected to be inflammatory or neoplastic in origin, is depicted in Fig. 5.1.

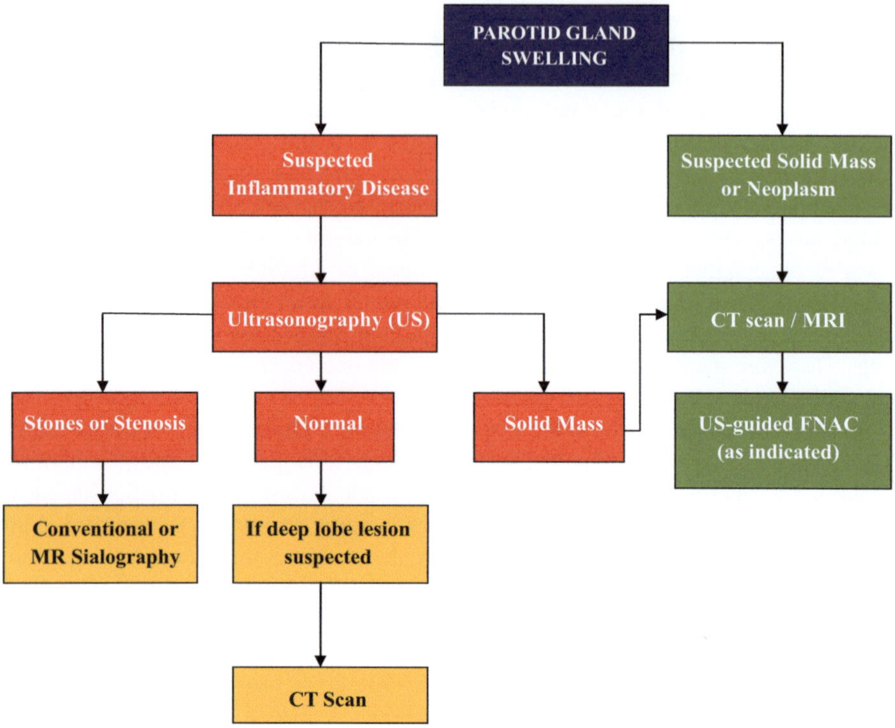

Fig. 5.1 Algorithm of imaging of a parotid gland swelling (FNAC, fine-needle aspiration cytology)

5.4 Endoscopy (Sialoendoscopy)

5.4.1 Introduction

Sialoendoscopy is a nuanced technique of trans-luminal management of obstructive and non-neoplastic pathology of the major salivary glands. It is a minimally invasive technique that inspects the salivary glands using narrow-diameter, rigid, fiberoptic endoscopes, introduced under direct vision through the ductal orifice after its dilatation with a lacrimal probe [56]. It is well tolerated, with minimal complications, and has thus opened up a new frontier for the evaluation and treatment of salivary gland disorders [57].

Direct inspection of the glandular duct and hilum is performed during lavage of the duct. Thus, in one setting, at the time of diagnosis, treatment of benign lesions can be performed [58]. Through a CO_2-laser papillotomy, sialolithectomy can be performed easily. Pharmacotherapy and laser ablation can also be performed. This relatively new technique is an efficient yet simple mode of treatment in the diagnosis and treatment of major salivary gland chronic obstructive sialadenitis (COS) caused by stones (sialoliths), strictures, and mucus plugs.

5.4.2 Indications

Salivary gland stones (sialoliths) are one of the major causes of salivary gland infections (sialadenitis). These types of stones can be found in 1.2% of the general population [59]. The second leading cause of salivary obstruction is from strictures and adhesions, which may result from prior salivary gland infections, including those during childhood such as mumps. Most strictures could be seen in the parotid duct and mostly in the disease process of chronic recurrent sialadenitis. Indications of sialoendoscopy are summarized in Table 5.1.

5.4.3 Preprocedural Preparation

Depending on the obstruction, sialoendoscopy can be conducted under local anesthesia in an outpatient office or in the operating room under general anesthesia. Thus, discussion regarding anesthesia is mandatory. Brief interventions can be under local anesthesia, and topical medications can be used for ductal dilatation; however, sedation and general anesthesia are also utilized. Advantages of general anesthesia are adequate patient compliance and utility for longer procedures or combined approaches of the intra- and extraoral techniques including gland resection. In addition, the patient has to be prepared with instruction for increased self-hydration, gentle salivary gland massage, warm compresses, sialagogues, oral steroids, and analgesics. Perioperatively, aggressive hydration, intravenous antibiotics, and cholinergic agonistic medications are administered [60].

5.4.4 Technique

Generally, the salivary duct opening needs to be either dilated or incised prior to intraoral introduction of the endoscope into the gland through its natural orifice in the oral cavity or by making a small incision in the duct opening. Once the sialoendoscope is in place, saline is utilized to dilate the salivary duct and its branching. Once the endoscopes are introduced into the gland, the internal anatomy is explored either for diagnosis or the treatment of a specific disease entity.

Table 5.1 Indications of sialoendoscopy

Obstructive salivary gland diseases	Secondary salivary stasis
– Sialolithiasis (4–5 mm in diameter) – Sialadenosis – Stenosis – Mucous plugs – Scarring and adhesions – Foreign bodies and polyps	– Autoimmune disorders of saliva glands – Immunoglobulin G4 related to sclerosis – Sjögren's syndrome – Juvenile recurrent parotitis – Masseter muscle hypertrophy-related obstructive parotitis – Radioiodine sialoadenitis

5.4.5 Instrumentation (Equipment)

The ability to perform this technique is the result of the development of miniaturized endoscopic imaging tools. The majority of sialoendoscopes that are currently in use are of the semi-rigid type, which allows for visualization of the diseased process, but the stiffness allows manipulation and navigation of the internal salivary anatomy.

Multiple types of micro-instrumentation are available through many companies, including grasping forceps, biopsy forceps, drills, needles, laser fibers, and lithotripters. Different practitioners utilize different systems according to the experience and clinical training of the surgeon. Sialoendoscopy equipment is listed in Table 5.2.

5.4.6 Contraindications

The only definitive contraindication of sialoendoscopy is active inflammatory or suppurative salivary gland disease. Skill level and access to specialized instrumentation is a relative consideration [61]. Patients with severe trismus and poor access to endoscopic technique are certainly limitations for these procedures.

5.4.7 Complications

Complications can be broadly categorized into patient-related and procedure-related. Patient-related complications are mainly due to acute inflammation, symptomatic intraparenchymal stones, severe distal duct stenosis, coagulopathy, poor patient follow-up, and additional patient-related contraindications. Instrumentation-related complications are ductal trauma, lacerations, ruptures, scarring strictures, and infections. Postprocedural swelling is fairly common, usually within 2 h after the procedure due to the pressure of instrumentation and irrigation. Instrumentation can lead to false lumen, perforation of the ducts, hematoma, extravasation of the irrigant, and pain in the acute setting. Strictures of the duct, pseudo-cystic salivary extravasation phenomena of ranula, neuro-injuries of the lingual and the facial nerve are all documented [62].

Table 5.2 Checklist of sialoendoscopy equipment

– Diagnostic scopes (0.8 mm, 1.0 mm, 1.3 mm diameter)
– Operative scopes (diameters)
– All-in-one type of scope of multiluminal scopes
– Cold lighting source
– Video camera
– Monitor—Wheel-mounted or wall-mounted system
– Irrigation system—a 20-mL syringe filled with saline attached by intravenous catheter
– Wire basket (for extirpation of stones and foreign bodies)
– Grasping forceps
– Balloons—Intraluminal dilators
– Laser fibers (for fragmentation and incisions)
– Microdrills (for fragmentation of sialoliths)

Gland swelling due to papillary infection is the most frequent complication reported at about 23%. All other complications, including nerve injuries, strictures, and salivary fistulas, occur in <5% of cases [60].

5.4.8 Considerations for Success in Sialoendoscopy

Factors to be considered for a successful sialoendoscopy include the following:

- Stone size
- Site—parotid vs. submandibular and ductal pathology location
- Situation—obstructive, stenosis, generalized autoimmune
- Shape—stone(s) and lumen shape
- Shaking—mobility of stones
- Serial instrumentation

5.4.9 Milestones in Sialoendoscopy

- 1990: Konigsberger and Gundlach separately performed sialoendoscopy when they introduced an endoscope into the major salivary glands [63, 64].
- 1991: Katz introduced a 0.8-mm flexible endoscope to diagnose and treat salivary gland stones [65].
- 1994: Nahlieli used a rigid mini-endoscope to diagnose and treat major salivary gland obstructions [66].

5.5 Cytology/Biopsy

5.5.1 Fine-Needle Aspiration Cytology (FNAC)

Fine-needle aspiration cytology (FNAC) with a small-bore needle is a widely used diagnostic tool to evaluate both inflammatory and neoplastic lesions of the salivary glands [26–28]. It is a minimally invasive procedure that does not require anesthesia (can be performed on an outpatient basis) [67–70], well-tolerated, simple, safe, and cost-effective [71, 72]. Moreover, it can be easily repeated in case of nondiagnostic results, thus improving diagnostic precision [67]. FNAC allows for the preoperative diagnosis of histological type in neoplastic lesions, such as benign tumors (e.g., pleomorphic adenoma and Warthin's tumor) [73–82], or to determine the malignancy grade in the case of malignant tumors. Furthermore, FNAC allows for improved patient selection for surgery since it can identify disorders such as reactive lymph nodes (LNs) that might mimic parotid tumors clinically.

Detailed preoperative information is important because histological types such as pleomorphic adenoma and Warthin's tumor, which account for the majority of benign tumors, require different treatments [83–86]. On the other hand, in malignant neoplasms, it is important to diagnose the grade of malignancy to determine subsequent treatment strategies. The prognosis differs significantly between low- or medium-grade and high-grade malignant cancers, and operative strategies, such as facial nerve treatment and indications for cervical LN dissection, vary accordingly [87–95].

The sensitivity of FNAC ranges from 57% to 98%, specificity from 56% to 100%, and accuracy from 78% to 98% [96–106]. The sensitivity and specificity of parotid gland FNA cytology depend on the operator's technique, the quality of the specimen, the pathologist's experience, and the presence and absence of cystic components [73–82, 107, 108]. However, the most relevant aspect for differential diagnosis is the wide variety of histological types of parotid tumors: There are 23 types of malignant tumors and 11 types of benign tumors [109]. Guidance with US improves the yield of FNAC; it increases the diagnostic accuracy by enabling avoidance of necrotic or cystic regions and by targeting of higher yield areas of the lesion for tissue extraction. It also allows the operator to confirm that the needle tip is inserted within the lesion.

In view of the above, in 2018, the Milan System for Reporting Salivary Gland Cytopathology was proposed as a standardized reporting system for the stratification of malignancy grades [110]. However, it does not consider aspects related to the histological type or malignancy grade, so a new classification was developed, referred to as the Osaka Medical College (OMC) classification [111].

5.5.2 Specimen Collection and Processing Procedures

Because FNAC has some disadvantages, core-needle biopsy (CNB) and liquid-based cytology (LBC) were recently introduced as new sample collection and processing procedures, respectively. All three procedures and the advantages and disadvantages of each procedure are summarized in Table 5.3.

5.5.2.1 Fine-Needle Aspiration Cytology (FNAC)

In parotid gland, fine-needle aspiration cytology (FNAC), appropriate specimen collection, and processing are important. In order to obtain samples, a 22- to 23-gauge needle is attached to a 10-cc syringe, and a puncture is made into the mass under ultrasound guidance. Then, the needle is moved back and forth to make sure that it reaches the deepest part of the lesion, and aspiration is performed. For aspiration, pressure is applied by pulling the syringe plunger. Once the aspiration is complete, the negative pressure is released (by returning the syringe plunger to the original position), the needle is removed, and compression is applied to the puncture site. It is advisable to prepare the sample immediately after aspiration; usually, immediately after smearing the cells onto a sliding glass, the sample is fixed with 95% ethanol and then stained with Papanicolaou stain. In addition, the smeared cells are dried, and after methanol fixation, Giemsa staining is performed. In order to improve the rate of correct diagnosis; repuncture is performed if the specimen is

Table 5.3 Advantages and disadvantages of fine-needle aspiration, core-needle biopsy, and liquid-based cytology

Procedure	Advantages	Disadvantages
Fine-needle aspiration	– Rapid, simple, and minimally invasive – Cost-effective	– The rate of inadequate specimen collection is higher
Core-needle biopsy	– High sensitivity and specificity – Immunostaining and molecular biological tests can be performed	– Invasive, possible risk of tumor seeding – Requires skill
Liquid-based cytology	– Cell specimens can be preserved – Better observation of nuclear details and background – Immunostaining and molecular biological tests can be performed	– Costly – Changes may occur in cytomorphological findings and sample background

bloody to ensure that the sample includes tumor cells. If possible, rapid onsite cytodiagnosis should be performed to evaluate the adequacy of the specimen [112].

5.5.2.2 Core-Needle Biopsy (CNB)

Core-needle biopsy (CNB) is a biopsy method in which tissue is removed with a thicker needle (8–20 G) than that used in FNA. Compared with FNA, CNB allows for the collection of larger tissue samples with preserved tissue structure [113], enabling general tissue and immunohistochemical staining and, thus, a more reliable histological diagnosis than is possible with standard cytology. Although CNB is generally considered safe, the use of a thicker needle can increase the risk of complications, such as tumor seeding, facial nerve damage, and hematoma [114–118]. However, according to a review by Shah et al., seeding after CNB in the head and neck region is rare, and the risk of local recurrence is roughly 0.0011% with CNB vs. 0.00012% with FNA, indicating that the risk of seeding is not significantly different between FNA and CNB [119]. In a review by Schmidt et al., the sensitivity, specificity, and rate of inadequate specimen collection of CNB were reported to be 92%, 100%, and 1.2%, respectively, demonstrating that the sensitivity is higher and the rate of inadequate specimen collection is lower than with FNA [120]. Similarly, Cengiz et al. also noted that CNB has a higher diagnosis rate than FNA cytology [121]; the group pointed out the usefulness of CNB but admitted that there is room for argument regarding its risks, such as tumor seeding.

5.5.2.3 Liquid-Based Cytology (LBC)

In LBC, sampled cells are stored as a cell suspension solution, and cytology specimens are prepared later with a special instrument. The specific advantages of this method are that the background contamination with blood can be cleaned, artifacts from air-drying are reduced, quick and proper fixation can be performed, samples can be preserved for a longer time, and specimens can be created with uniform density because the cells are smeared onto a limited circular area of the slide. However, the procedure also has some disadvantages in that cytomorphological, and sample background findings differ from those of conventional specimens because of the decreased cell cluster size and reduced extracellular particles [122–124]. Nevertheless, in addition to being used for the preparation of cytology specimens, the remaining samples can be used for tests such as immunocytochemistry and molecular chemical analysis [125, 126]. Given these advantages, LBC is considered to enable a more accurate diagnosis than is possible with conventional FNA cytology. Kumar et al. examined the use of LBC in parotid tumors and found that, although LBC had comparable specificity and sensitivity to FNAC, it was better for observing nuclear details and background [127]. Another advantage of LBC is that cell blocks can be prepared and used for immunostaining [128].

5.5.3 Ultrasound Core Biopsy (USCB)

The perceived and real diagnostic limitations associated with FNAC have led operators to explore alternative biopsy techniques. USCB is a safe and successful technique for the diagnosis of parotid lesions where FNAC is nondiagnostic [129] and is developing into an established technique. The technique [129, 130] requires an operator, usually a radiologist trained in head and neck US and biopsy techniques. The procedure requires local anesthetic infiltration, a small skin incision, and the use of an automated spring-loaded biopsy device. The throw is deployed under US guidance.

Figure 5.2 shows the biopsy needle within the lesion. The core of tissue is then processed by paraffin section histology. Sections from the core can be used for grading, staging, and immunohistochemical analysis, allowing planning of appropriate operative or nonoperative management. Figures 5.3 and 5.4 show the results of a core biopsy macroscopically and microscopically, respectively. Immunofluorescence analysis is particularly useful for hematological malignancies [129, 130].

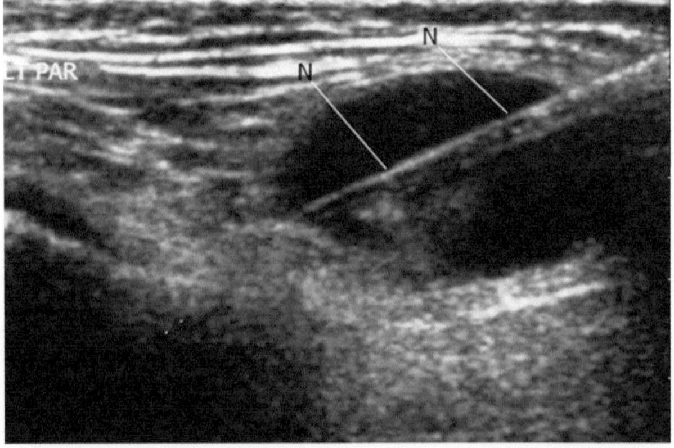

Fig. 5.2 USCB undertaken with spring-loaded biopsy automated device, 22 mm throw, 18G needle (N). Note needle deployed to traverse but not exit the lesion

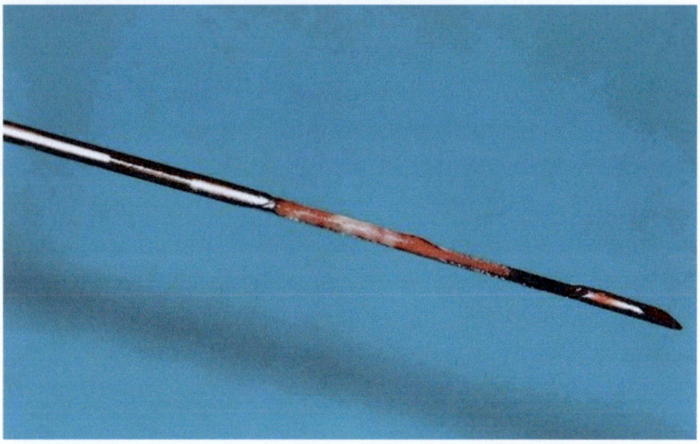

Fig. 5.3 Image of biopsy specimen taken in Fig. 5.2. 18G needle in biopsy tray with overlying needle overlying sheath retracted

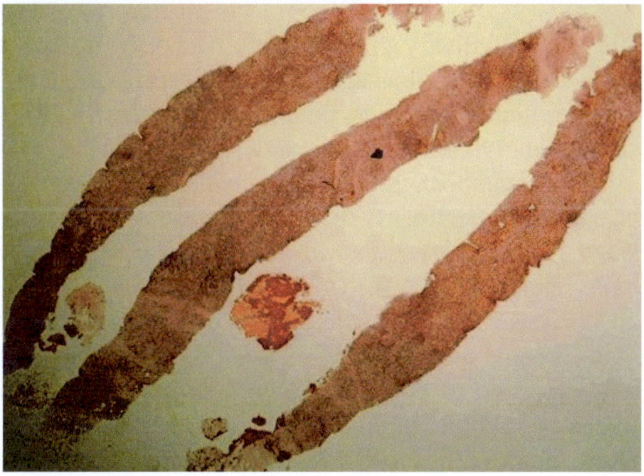

Fig. 5.4 Low-power image of biopsy samples obtained in this case to give an idea of what material is available to the pathologist for reporting and immunohistochemistry—final diagnosis in this case was B cell non-Hodgkin's lymphoma. H&E stain

This technique is already well established in other areas of image-guided biopsy including the breast and abdomen [131] and is now widely accepted by histopathologists and oncologists as a sufficient technique to allow tumor grading and typing [132].

A recent meta-analysis incorporates 12 studies and provides substantial evidence supporting the potentially superior diagnostic yield of USCB over FNAC as it showed a higher sensitivity (96%) and specificity (100%) compared to FNAC, a low complication rate (1.6% hematoma rate) and no variation in accuracy between locations [133]. The low complication rate is attributed to the ability of US to visualize the vessels and allow the operator to infer the position of facial nerve branches. A systematic observational clinico-pathological study demonstrated USCB of salivary gland lesions to have sensitivity 94%, specificity 100%, accuracy 96%, positive predictive value 100%, and negative predictive value 90% [134]. A study by Eom et al. [135] also showed that trainees had a significantly lower accuracy with FNAC than USCB when diagnosing malignant tumors when compared to USCB with lymphomas being diagnosed much more accurately using USCB as reported by Huang et al. [136].

Despite generally favorable outcomes and diagnostic advantages, USCB is not yet considered the reference standard in parotid lesion biopsy and the optimum technique remains controversial. The potential problems with USCB include possible false negative results, complications of a slightly more invasive technique and tumor seeding. Haldar et al. [137] described two cases that were malignant clinically, on imaging and in the resected specimen, but benign on USCB (false negative). Also, some cases of well-differentiated malignancy require direct histological assessment of the whole excised lesion capsule to demonstrate invasiveness; USCB will miss this. This emphasizes that USCB should not be used alone in parotid lesion assessment.

5.5.4 Ancillary Diagnosis in Salivary Gland Cytology

Diagnosing salivary gland tumors by conventional cytology alone is difficult in some cases, so various ancillary diagnostic procedures are used. These procedures include staining methods, fluorescent in situ hybridization (FISH), and reverse transcription polymerase chain reaction (RT-PCR) [138–147].

Most immunostaining and molecular biological tests can be applied to a variety of cytology specimens, such as alcohol-fixed, dry-fixed, and LBC specimens, but using formalin-fixed, paraffin-embedded cell block sections is considered to be more reliable [139, 140, 142]. Immunostaining is used to support differential diagnosis in cases with an unclear diagnosis. Because each tumor can have a wide range of differential diagnoses (e.g., basaloid tumor, eosinophilic tumor, clear cell tumor), it is desirable to perform immunostaining with multiple antibody panels [141]. Recently, specific, highly reproducible gene translocations were found in salivary gland tumors [138–140, 148–152]. Fusion oncogenes and onco-proteins resulting from gene translocations are useful diagnostic markers and can be detected by FISH and RT-PCR. Previously reported gene translocations and fusion oncogenes include the CRTC1/3-MAML2 fusion gene in mucoepidermoid carcinoma and the MYB-NFIB fusion gene in adenoid cystic carcinoma [153–155]. Although these genetic abnormalities are highly specific and can be considered as powerful diagnostic markers, detection of genetic abnormalities, in general, is not always reliable, so certain types of salivary gland tumors should not be excluded only on the basis of genetic testing. In the future, the detection of genetic abnormalities may become useful not only as an indicator for tissue diagnosis and prognosis but also as a target for gene therapy [148, 151].

5.5.5 Frozen Section Biopsy (FSB)

Another salivary gland biopsy technique is intraoperative frozen section biopsy (FSB), which is used in a small number of specialist centers as an alternative to FNAC or where FNAC is not performing well. Results can be telephoned to the surgeon within 20–30 min. This is useful where no preoperative diagnosis is available, for example, in deep parotid lesions not amenable to percutaneous biopsy or for lesions that are suspicious on clinical/imaging assessment but benign or considered nonrepresentative on FNAC/USCB. Intraoperative frozen section can be employed to guide further surgical management while the patient is still on the operating table. A meta-analysis published in 2011 looking at data from 13 studies over a 25-year period described 90% sensitivity, 99% specificity, and good consistency of results across study centers [156].

Intraoperative frozen section (IOFS) cannot be recommended as a first-line diagnostic technique, which cannot be widely supported outside dedicated histopathology units. Most pathologists are reluctant to diagnose complex parotid lesions on the table in the absence of further techniques including immunofluorescence. The pitfalls and failures outlined above for USCB also apply to IOFS. In general, IOFS can be used as an adjunct to the less invasive options described where diagnostic suspicion and uncertainty remain [157].

In parotid surgery, FSB has the following three general roles: clarify the diagnosis, check the resection stump, and determine the presence or absence of nerve and cervical lymph node infiltration [158]. As FNAC became more commonly used for preoperative diagnosis in parotid surgery, opportunities to perform FSB became scarce, and its role shifted from being primarily a tool to differentiate between benign and malignant tumors and diagnose histological type to a method for assessing margins [156]. Although performing FSB may improve preoperative diagnosis in parotid surgery, it remains unclear whether it should always be used or be limited to specific situations. Some authors suggest that FSB is more reliable than FNA cytology and that it should be used on a routine basis to ensure the best patient management [159]; on the other hand, others advocate using FSB only under certain circumstances, such as in cases with uncertain preoperative FNA cytology [160–163].

In their study on the usefulness of FSB for preoperative diagnosis based on FNAC, Choy et al. reported that the risk of malignancy (ROM) increased to as high as 100% when the result of FSB was "malignant" in cases with a diagnosis of atypia of undetermined significance (AUS), salivary gland neoplasm of uncertain malignant potential (SUMP), or suspicious for malignancy (SFM) based on FNAC [160]. Pastorello et al. also found that the use of FSB in specimens diagnosed as nondiagnostic or SUMP by FNAC can increase specificity and positive predictive value [161].

If FNA cytology does reveal a benign diagnosis, such as polymorphic adenoma or Warthin's tumor, the effectiveness of FSB is limited because the risk of malignancy is very low; hence, in such cases, there is likely to be little need for FSB [162]. Disease stage and histological grade are important prognostic factors for parotid cancer, and the histological type and grade of tumors need to be accurately determined before surgery to allow surgeons to decide on the necessary extent of local resection, whether the facial nerve can be preserved or not, and whether neck dissection is necessary. Nishikawa et al. reported that compared with FNA cytology alone, additional FSB increases the accuracy of the histological grade [164]. If malignancy is suspected on FNA cytology, performing FSB concomitantly might allow the appropriate range of resection in parotid cancer surgery to be determined [163].

5.5.6 Classification Systems

5.5.6.1 Milan System

The Milan System was introduced in 2018 as a system for reporting the classification of salivary gland cytology [110]. It divides tumors into six groups with the aim at allowing for the stratification of malignancy grades. Hence, risk of malignancy (ROM) and clinical response are indicated for each category [74–76, 78, 79, 165]. The classes of the Milan System (Table 5.4) are described as follows.

5.5.6.2 Osaka Medical College (OMC) Classification

The OMC Classification was proposed as a cytology classification that better matches clinical needs by incorporating the histological type and malignancy grade. The OMC Classification has 11 categories, and the main difference from the Milan System is that tumors classified as "IVA Neoplasm—Benign" are further classified into histology confirmed (class 4–1) or histology unconfirmed (class 4–2). Moreover, those classified as "VI—Malignant" is divided into three categories: malignant (grade/histology unconfirmed) (class 6–2), malignant (grade confirmed) (class 6–3), and malignant (grade/histology confirmed) (class 6–4) [166].

Table 5.4 Classes of the Milan System

Class	ROM (%)	Description	Clinical measures
I. Nondiagnostic	25	Insufficient specimen in terms of quantity and quality and do not provide useful information for making a diagnosis	Repeat FNAC
II. Non-neoplastic	10	Mucocele—Sialadenitis (acute–chronic including COS–granulomatous, e.g., sarcoidosis)	Re-examine physical and imaging findings are re-examined, and follow-up. If imaging shows changes or symptoms worsen, repeat FNAC
III. AUS	20	Insufficient cytological findings (neoplastic or neoplastic) in terms of quantity and quality for making a diagnosis	Consider other types of clinical information (imaging and physical findings), and decide whether to perform repeat FNA, biopsy, or surgical resection
IV. Neoplasm			
IVA: Benign	≤ 5	Clearly benign (PA and Warthin's tumor in the majority)	Diagnostic imaging then surgical excision are performed
IVB: SUMP	35	Difficult to determine whether it is benign or malignant; vascular and nerve infiltration needs to be diagnosed histologically[a]	Diagnostic imaging then surgical excision, but rapid intraoperative diagnosis should be performed because likelihood of low-grade cancer is high. Accordingly, additional excision (e.g., neck dissection) may be indicated
V. SFM	60	Sample does not have all findings of malignancy, but suggests malignancy as a whole, e.g., specimens contain highly atypical cells	Repeat FNAC, needle biopsy, incision biopsy, surgical resection
VI. Malignant	90	Malignant based on cytological findings alone or in conjunction with an ancillary diagnosis	Extent of local progression should be determined by close examination of CT, MRI, and PET-CT images before surgical excision

ROM risk of malignancy, *FNAC* fine-needle aspiration cytology, *COS* chronic obstructive sialadenitis, *AUS* atypia of undetermined significance, *SUMP* salivary gland neoplasm of uncertain malignant potential, *SFM* suspicious for malignancy, *CT* computed tomography, *MRI* magnetic resonance imaging, *PET* positron emission tomography

[a] Such tumors include basal cell adenoma/basal cell adenocarcinoma, myoepithelial tumors, myoepithelial carcinoma, clear cell tumors, and low-grade malignant tumors with limited atypical features

References

1. Anniko M, Bernal-Sprekelsen M, Bonkowsky V, Bradley P, Iurato S, editors. Otorhinolaryngology, head and neck surgery. Berlin, Heidelberg: Springer; 2010.
2. Graamans K, von der Akker HP. History and physical examination. In: Graamans AK, editor. Diagnosis of salivary gland disorders. Dordrecht: Kluwer Academic Publishers; 1991. p. 1–3.
3. Mason D, Chisholm D. Salivary glands in health and disease, vol. 31. London: WB Saunders; 1975. p. 156.
4. Sidell DR, Shapiro NL. Disorders of salivary glands. In: Puri P, editor. Pediatric surgery. Berlin, Heidelberg: Springer; 2021.
5. Dreizen S, Daley TE, Drane JB, Brown LR. Oral complications of cancer radiotherapy. Postgrad Med. 1977;61:85–92.
6. Lawler DP, Hickler RB, Thorn GW. The salivary sodium-potassium ratio. N Engl J Med. 1962;267:1136–7.
7. Frawley TF, Thurn FW. The relation of the sodium-potassium ratio to adrenal cortical activity. In: Mote JR, editor. Proceedings of second annual ACTH conference. London: Churchill Livingstone; 1951.
8. Marder MX, Wotman S, Mandel ID. Salivary electrolyte changes during pregnancy-I. Normal pregnancy. Am J Obstet Gynecol. 1972;112:233–6.
9. Di Sant' Agnese PA, Davis PB. Research in cystic fibrosis. N Engl J Med. 1976;295(1):481–5.
10. Mandel ID, Kutscher AH, Denning CR, Carolyn R, Denning MD, Robert H, et al. Salivary studies in cystic fibrosis. Am J Dis Child. 1967;113:431–8.
11. Bloomfield J, Rush AR, Allars H, Brown JM. Parotid gland function in children with cystic fibrosis and child control subjects. Pediatr Res. 1976;10:574–8.
12. Kurscher AH, Denning CR, Zegarelli EV, Kessler W, Eriv A, Mandel ID, et al. Capillary tube test for minor salivary gland secretion in cystic fibrosis of pancreas. NY State J Med. 1968;68:2812–3.
13. Mason DK, Harden RM, Alexander WB. The salivary and thyroid glands. Br Dent J. 1967;122:485–9.
14. Weinberger A, Sperling O, DeVries A. Calcium and inorganic phosphate in saliva of patients with primary hyperparathyroidism. Clin Chim Acta. 1974;50:5–7.
15. Niedermeier W, Dreizen S, Stone RE, Spies TD. Sodium and potassium concentrations in the saliva of normotensive and hypertensive subjects. Oral Surg. 1956;9:426–31.
16. Bhoola KD, McNichol NW, Oliver S, Foran J. Changes in salivary enzymes in patients with sarcoidosis. N Engl J Med. 1969;281:877–9.
17. Beeley JA, Chisholm DM. Sarcoidosis with salivary gland involvement: biochemical studies on parotid saliva. J Lab Clin Med. 1976;88:276–81.
18. Abelson DC, Mandel ID, Karmiol M. Salivary studies in alcoholic cirrhosis. Oral Surg. 1976;41:188–92.
19. Masson PL, Heremans JF, Prignot JJ, Wauters G. Immunohistochemical localization and bacteriostatic properties of an iron-binding protein from bronchial mucus. Thorax. 1966;21:538–44.
20. Mandel ID. Sialochemistry in diseases and clinical situations affecting salivary glands. CRC Crit Rev Clin Lab Sci. 1980;12:321–66.
21. Wotman S, Bigger TJ, Mandel ID, Bartelstone HJ. Salivary electrolytes in the detection of digitalis toxicity. N Engl J Med. 1971;285:871–6.
22. White SC, Pharoah MJ. Wydawnictwo Czelej, Wyd I. Mały atlas błędów technicznych i artefaktów w radiografii wewnątrzustnej. Radiologia Stomatologiczna. 2002. pp. 621–628.
23. Forman WH. Subtraction sialography. Radiology. 1977;122(2):533.
24. Białek EJ, Jakubowski W, Zajkowski P, Zopinski KT, Osmolski A. US of the major salivary glands: anatomy and spatial relationships, pathologic conditions, and pitfalls. Radiographics. 2006;26(3):745–63.

25. Yu C, Zheng L, Yang C, Shen N. Causes of chronic obstructive parotitis and management by sialoendoscopy. Oral Surg Oral Med Oral Pathol Oral Radiol Endod. 2008;105(3):365–70.
26. Forman WH. Subtraction sialography. Radiology. 1977;122(2):536–339.
27. Kalk WW, Vissink A, Fred KL, Möller JM, Roodenburg JL. Morbidity from parotid sialography. Oral Surg Oral Med Oral Pathol Oral Radiol Endod. 2001;92(5):572–5.
28. Szolar DH, Groell R, Braun H, Preidler K, Stiskal M, Kern R, et al. Ultrafast computed tomography and three-dimensional image processin of CT sialography in patients with parotid masses poorly defined by magnetic resonance imaging. Acta Otolaryngol. 1996;116(1):112–8.
29. Kalinowski M, Heverhagen JT, Rehberg E, Klose KJ, Wagner HJ. Comparative study of MR sialography and digital subtraction Sialography for benign salivary gland disorders. AJNR Am J Neuroradiol. 2002;23(9):1485–92.
30. Obaid H, Sinha R, Robinson L. Submandibular sialogram performed through a Wharton's duct fistula: technical adaptation of conventional technique. Eur J Radiol. 2006;60(1):56–7.
31. Eyjólfsson O, Nordshus T, Dahl T. Sialography and CT-sialography in the diagnosis of parotid masses. Acta Radiol Diagn (Stockh). 1984;25(5):361–4.
32. Bryan RN, Miller RH, Ferreyro RI, Sessions RB. Computed tomography of the major salivary glands. AJR Am J Roentgenol. 1982;139(3):547–54.
33. Nixon PP, Lancer J, Bradley MJ. Case report: percutaneous Sialography. Clin Radiol. 1998;53(5):381–3.
34. Kalk WW, Vissink A, Spijkervet FK, Bootsma H, Kallenberg CG, Roodenburg JL. Parotid sialography for diagnosing Sjögren syndrome. Oral Surg Oral Med Oral Pathol Oral Radiol Endod. 2002;94(1):131–7.
35. Buckenham TM, George CD, McVicar D, Moody AR, Coles GS. Digital sialography: imaging and intervention. Br J Radiol. 1994;67(798):524–9.
36. Jäger L, Menauer F, Holzknecht N, Scholz V, Grevers G, Reiser M. Sialolithiasis: MR sialography of the submandibular duct—an alternative to conventional sialography and US? Radiology. 2000;216(3):665–71.
37. Becker M, Marchal F, Becker CD, Dulguerov P, Georgakopoulos G, Lehmann W, et al. Sialolithiasis and salivary ductal stenosis: diagnostic accuracy of MR sialography with a three-dimensional extended-phase conjugate-symmetry rapid spin-echo sequence. Radiology. 2000;217(2):347–58.
38. Drage NA, Brown JE, Wilson RF. Pain and swelling after sialography: is it a significant problem? Oral Surg Oral Med Oral Pathol Oral Radiol Endod. 2000;90(3):385–8.
39. Hasson O. Sialoendoscopy and sialography: strategies for assessment and treatment of salivary gland obstructions. J Oral Maxillofac Surg. 2007;65(2):300–4.
40. Gritzmann N, Rettenbacher T, Hollerweger A, Macheiner P, Hubner E. Sonography of the salivary glands. Eur Radiol. 2003;13(5):964–75.
41. Rabinov JD. Imaging of salivary gland pathology. Radiol Clin North Am. 2000;38(5):1047–57.
42. Silvers AR, Som PM. Salivary glands. Radiol Clin North Am. 1998;36(5):941–66.
43. Howlett DC, Kesse KW, Hughes DV, Sallomi DF. The role of imaging in the evaluation of parotid disease. Clin Radiol. 2002;57(8):692–701.
44. Bussels B, Maes A, Flamen P, Lambin P, Erven K, Hermans R, et al. Dose-response relationships within the parotid gland after radiotherapy for head and neck cancer. Radiother Oncol. 2004;73(3):297–306.
45. Roesink JM, Moerland MA, Hoekstra A, Van Rijk PP, Terhaard CH. Scintigraphic assessment of early and late parotid gland function after radiotherapy for head-and-neck cancer: a prospective study of dose-volume response relationships. Int J Radiat Oncol Biol Phys. 2004;58(5):1451–60.
46. Som PM, Biller HF. The combined computerized tomography-sialogram. A technique to differentiate deep lobe parotid tumors from extraparotid pharyngomaxillary space tumors. Ann Otol Rhinol Laryngol. 1979;88(5 Pt 1):590–5.
47. Yousem DM, Kraut MA, Chalian AA. Major salivary gland imaging. Radiology. 2000;216:19–29.

48. Quinn HJ Jr. Symposium: management of tumors of the parotid gland. II. Diagnosis of parotid gland swelling. Laryngoscope. 1976;86(1):22–4.
49. Abdel-Wahed N, Amer ME, Abo-Taleb NS. Assessment of the role of cone beam computed sialography in diagnosing salivary gland lesions. Imaging Sci Dent. 2013;43(1):17–23.
50. Drage NA, Brown JE. Cone beam computed sialography of sialoliths. Dentomaxillofac Radiol. 2009;38:301–5.
51. Hisatomi M, Asaumi J, Yanagi Y, Unetsubo T, Maki Y, Murakami J, et al. Diagnostic value of dynamic contrast-enhanced MRI in the salivary gland tumors. Oral Oncol. 2007;43(9):940–7.
52. Joe VQ, Westesson PL. Tumors of the parotid gland: MR imaging characteristics of various histologic types. AJR Ame J Roentgenol. 1994;163(2):433–8.
53. Burke CJ, Thomas RH, Howlett D. Imaging the major salivary glands. Br J Oral Maxillofac Surg. 2011;49(4):261–9.
54. Afzelius P, Nielsen MY, Ewertsen C, Bloch KP. Imaging of the major salivary glands. Clin Physiol Funct Imaging. 2016;36(1):1–10.
55. Thoeny HC. Imaging of salivary gland tumours. Cancer Imaging. 2007;7(1):52–62.
56. Nahlieli O, Baruchin AM. Sialoendoscopy: three years' experience as a diagnostic and treatment modality. J Oral Maxillofac Surg. 1997;55(9):912–8.
57. Ziegler CM, Hedemark A, Brevik B, Idris M, Isaksen R. Endoscopy as minimal invasive routine treatment for sialolithiasis. Acta Odontol Scand. 2003;61(3):137–40.
58. Nahlieli O, Baruchin AM. Long-term experience with endoscopic diagnosis and treatment of salivary gland inflammatory diseases. Laryngoscope. 2000;110(6):988–93.
59. Rauch SGR. Diseases of the salivary glands. 6th ed. St. Louis, MO: Mosby; 1970. p. 997.
60. Chandra SR. Sialoendoscopy: review and nuances of technique. J Maxillofac Oral Surg. 2019;18(1):1–10.
61. Luers JC, Damm M, Klussmann JP, Beutner D. The learning curve of sialoendoscopy with modular sialoendoscopes—a single surgeon's experience. Arch Otolaryngol Head Neck Surg. 2010;136(8):762–5.
62. Gallo A, Benazzo M, Capaccio P, De Campora L, De Vincentiis M, Fusconi M, et al. Sialoendoscopy: state-of-the-art, challenges and further perspectives. Round table, 101st SIO National Congress, Catania 2014. Acta Otorhinolaryngol Ital. 2015;35:217–33.
63. Konigsberger R, Feyh J, Goetz A, Schilling V, Kastenbauer E. Endoscopic controlled laser lithotripsy in the treatment of sialolithiasis. Laryngorhinootologie. 1990;69:322–3.
64. Gundlach P, Scherer H, Hopf J, Leege N, Müller G, Hirst L, et al. Endoscopic-controlled laser lithotripsy of salivary calculi. In vitro studies and initial clinical use. HNO. 1990;38:247.
65. Katz P. Endoscopy of the salivary glands. Ann Radiol (Paris). 1991;34:110–3.
66. Nahlieli O, Neder A, Baruchin AM. Salivary gland endoscopy: A new technique for diagnosis and treatment of sialolithiasis. J Oral Maxillofac Surg. 1994;52:1240–2.
67. Stewart CJ, MacKenzie K, McGarry GW, Mowat A. Fine-needle aspiration cytology of salivary gland: a review of 341 cases. Diagn Cytopathol. 2000;22:139–46.
68. Zbären P, Schär C, Hotz MA, Loosli H. Value of fine-needle aspiration cytology of parotid gland masses. Laryngoscope. 2001;111:1989–92.
69. Klijanienko J, Vielh P. Fine-needle sampling of salivary gland lesions. II. Cytology and histology correlation of 71 cases of Warthin's tumor (adenolymphoma). Diagn Cytopathol. 1997;16:221–5.
70. David OD, Blaney S, Hearp M. Parotid gland fine-needle aspiration cytology: an approach to differential diagnosis. Diagn Cytopathol. 2007;35:47–56.
71. Alphs HH, Eisele DW, Westra WH. The role of fine needle aspiration in the evaluation of parotid masses. Curr Opin Otolaryngol Head Neck Surg. 2006;14:62–6.
72. O'Donnell ME, Salem A, Badger SA, Sharif MA, Kamalapurkar D, Lieo T, et al. Fine needle aspiration at a regional head and neck clinic: a clinically beneficial and cost-effective service. Cytopathology. 2009;20:81–6.
73. Ahn S, Kim Y, Oh YL. Fine needle aspiration cytology of benign salivary gland tumors with myoepithelial cell participation: an institutional experience of 575 cases. Acta Cytol. 2013;57:567–74.

74. Colella G, Cannavale R, Flamminio F, Foschini MP. Fine-needle aspiration cytology of salivary gland lesions: a systematic review. J Oral Maxillofac Surg. 2010;68:2146–53.
75. Rossi ED, Wong LQ, Bizzarro T, Petrone G, Mule A, Fadda G, et al. The impact of FNAC in the management of salivary gland lesions: institutional experiences leading to a risk-based classification scheme. Cancer Cytopathol. 2016;124:388–96.
76. Liu CC, Jethwa AR, Khariwala SS, Johnson J, Shin JJ. Sensitivity, specificity, and post-test probability of parotid fine-needle aspiration: A systematic review and meta-analysis. Otolaryngol Head Neck Surg. 2016;154:9–23.
77. Hughes JH, Volk EE, Wilbur DC. Pitfalls in salivary gland fine-needle aspiration cytology: lessons from the College of American Pathologists Interlaboratory Comparison Program in Nongynecologic Cytology. Arch Pathol Lab Med. 2005;129:26–31.
78. Griffith CC, Pai RK, Schneider F, Duvvuri U, Ferris RL, Johnson JT, et al. Salivary gland tumor fine-needle aspiration cytology: A proposal for a risk stratification classification. Am J Clin Pathol. 2015;143:839–53.
79. Wei S, Layfield LJ, LiVolsi VA, Montone KT, Baloch ZW. Reporting of fine needle aspiration (FNA) specimens of salivary gland lesions: a comprehensive review. Diagn Cytopathol. 2017;45:820–7.
80. Song IH, Song JS, Sung CO, Roh JL, Choi SH, Nam SY, et al. Accuracy of core needle biopsy versus fine needle aspiration cytology for diagnosing salivary gland tumors. J Pathol Transl Med. 2015;49:136–43.
81. Tyagi R, Dey P. Diagnostic problems of salivary gland tumors. Diagn Cytopathol. 2015;43:495–509.
82. Wang H, Fundakowski C, Khurana JS, Jhala N. Fine-needle aspiration biopsy of salivary gland lesions. Arch Pathol Lab Med. 2015;139:1491–7.
83. Patel DK, Morton RP. Demographics of benign parotid tumours: Warthin's tumour versus other benign salivary tumours. Acta Otolaryngol. 2016;136:83–6.
84. Kawata R, Kinoshita I, Omura S, Higashino M, Nishikawa S, Terada T, et al. Risk factors of postoperative facial palsy for benign parotid tumors: outcome of 1,018 patients. Laryngoscope. 2021;131:E2857–64.
85. Veder LL, Kerrebijn JD, Smedts FM, den Bakker MA. Diagnostic accuracy of fine-needle aspiration cytology in Warthin tumors. Head Neck. 2010;32:1635–40.
86. Witt RL, Eisele DW, Morton RP, Nicolai P, Poorten VV, Zbären P. Etiology and management of recurrent parotid pleomorphic adenoma. Laryngoscope. 2015;125:888–93.
87. Seethala RR. Histologic grading and prognostic biomarkers in salivary gland carcinomas. Adv Anat Pathol. 2011;18:29–45.
88. Westergaard-Nielsen M, Möller S, Godballe C, Grau Eriksen J, Larsen SR, Kiss K, et al. Prognostic scoring models in parotid gland carcinoma. Head Neck. 2021;43:2081–90.
89. Meyer MF, Kreppel M, Meinrath J, Grünewald I, Stenner M, Drebber U, et al. Prediction of outcome by lymph node ratio in patients with parotid gland cancer. Clin Otolaryngol. 2017;42:98–103.
90. Klussmann JP, Ponert T, Mueller RP, Dienes HP, Guntinas-Lichius O. Patterns of lymph node spread and its influence on outcome in resectable parotid cancer. Eur J Surg Oncol. 2008;34:932–7.
91. Eneroth CM, Hamberger CA. Principles of treatment of different types of parotid tumors. Laryngoscope. 1974;84:1732–40.
92. Sinha BK, Buntine DW. Parotid gland tumors. Clinicopathologic study. Am J Surg. 1975;129:675–81.
93. Armstrong JG, Harrison LB, Thaler HT, Friedlander-Klar H, Fass DE, Zelefsky MJ, et al. The indications for elective treatment of the neck in cancer of the major salivary glands. Cancer. 1992;69:615–9.
94. Medina JE. Neck dissection in the treatment of cancer of major salivary glands. Otolaryngol Clin N Am. 1998;31:815–22.
95. Jinnin T, Kawata R, Higashino M, Nishikawa S, Terada T, Haginomori SI. Patterns of lymph node metastasis and the management of neck dissection for parotid carcinomas: a single-institute experience. Int J Clin Oncol. 2019;24:624–31.

96. Frable MA, Frable WJ. Fine needle aspiration biopsy of salivary glands. Laryngoscope. 1991;101:245–9.
97. Cohen EG, Patel SG, Lin O, Oyle JO, Kraus DH, Singh B, et al. Fine-needle aspiration biopsy of salivary gland lesions in a selected patient population. Arch Otolaryngol Head Neck Surg. 2004;130:773–8.
98. Zurrida S, Alasio L, Tradati N, Bartoli C, Chiesa F, Pilotti S. Fine needle aspiration of parotid masses. Cancer. 1993;72:2306–11.
99. Jayaram G, Verma AK, Sood N, Khurana N. Fine needle aspiration cytology of salivary gland lesions. J Oral Pathol Med. 1994;23:256–61.
100. Atula T, Greénman R, Laippala P, Klemi PJ. Fine-needle aspiration biopsy in the diagnosis of parotid gland lesions: evaluation of 438 biopsies. Diagn Cytopathol. 1996;153:185–90.
101. Cristallini EG, Ascani S, Farabi R, Liberati F, Macciò T, Peciarolo A, et al. Fine needle aspiration biopsy of salivary gland, 1985-1995. Acta Cytol. 1997;41:1421–5.
102. Cajulis RS, Gokaslan ST, Yu GH, Frias-Hidvegi D. Fine needle aspiration biopsy of the salivary glands. A five-year experience with emphasis on diagnostic pitfalls. Acta Cytol. 1997;41:1412–20.
103. Al-Khafaji BM, Nestok BR, Katz RL. Fine needle aspiration of 154 parotid masses with histologic correlation: ten-year experience at the University of Texas, MD Anderson Cancer Center. Cancer. 1998;84:153–9.
104. Que-Hee CG, Perry CF. Fine-needle aspiration cytology of parotid tumours: is it useful? ANZ J Surg. 2001;71:345–8.
105. Bajaj Y, Singh S, Cozens N, Sharp J. Critical clinical appraisal of the role of ultrasound guided fine needle aspiration cytology in the management of parotid tumours. J Laryngol Otol. 2005;119:289–92.
106. Carrillo JF, Ramirez R, Flores L, Ramirez-Ortega MC, Arrecillas MD, Ibarra M, et al. Diagnostic accuracy of fine needle aspiration biopsy in preoperative diagnosis of patients with parotid gland mass. J Surg Oncol. 2009;100:133–8.
107. Layfield LJ, Tan P, Glasgow BJ. Fine-needle aspiration of salivary gland lesions. Comparison with frozen sections and histologic findings. Arch Pathol Lab Med. 1987;111:346–53.
108. Mairembam P, Jay A, Beale T, Morley S, Vaz F, Kalavrezos N, et al. Salivary gland FNA cytology: role as a triage tool and an approach to pitfalls in cytomorphology. Cytopathology. 2016;27:91–6.
109. El-Naggar A. WHO classification of tumors of salivary glands. In: El-Naggar AK, Chan JKC, Grandis JR, Takata T, Slootweg PJ, editors. WHO classification of head and neck tumours. Lyon: International Agency for Research on Cancer; 2017. p. 160.
110. Rossi ED, Faquin WC, Baloch Z, Barkan GA, Foschini MP, Pusztaszeri M. The Milan system for reporting salivary gland cytopathology: analysis and suggestions of initial survey. Cancer Cytopathol. 2017;125:757–66.
111. Taniuchi M, Kawata R, Omura S, Haginomori SI, Terada T, Higashino M, et al. A novel clinically-oriented classification of fine-needle aspiration cytology for salivary gland tumors: A 20-year retrospective analysis of 1175 patients. Int J Clin Oncol. 2021;26:326–34.
112. Kakkar A, Kumar M, Subramanian P, Zubair A, Kumar R, Thakar A, et al. Utility of the Milan system for reporting salivary gland cytopathology during rapid on-site evaluation (ROSE) of salivary gland aspirates. Cytopathology. 2021;32:779–88.
113. Yuen HY, Lee Y, Bhatia K, Wong KT, Ahuja AT. Use of end-cutting needles in ultrasound-guided biopsy of neck lesions. Eur Radiol. 2012;22:832–6.
114. Supriya M, Denholm S, Palmer T. Seeding of tumor cells after fine needle aspiration cytology in benign parotid tumor: a case report and literature review. Laryngoscope. 2008;118:263–5.
115. Yamaguchi KT, Strong MS, Shapshay SM, Soto E. Seeding of parotid carcinoma along Vim-Silverman needle tract. J Otolaryngol. 1979;8:49–52.
116. Roussel F, Dalion J, Benozio M. The risk of tumoral seeding in needle biopsies. Acta Cytol. 1989;33:936–9.
117. Douville NJ, Bradford CR. Comparison of ultrasound-guided core biopsy versus fine-needle aspiration biopsy in the evaluation of salivary gland lesions. Head Neck. 2013;35:1657–61.

118. Howlett DC, Menezes LJ, Lewis K, Moody AB, Violaris N, Williams MD. Sonographically guided core biopsy of a parotid mass. AJR Am J Roentgenol. 2007;188:223–7.
119. Shah KS, Ethunandan M. Tumour seeding after fine-needle aspiration and core biopsy of the head and neck—A systematic review. Br J Oral Maxillofac Surg. 2016;54:260–5.
120. Schmidt RL, Hall BJ, Layfield LJ. A systematic review and meta-analysis of the diagnostic accuracy of ultrasound-guided core needle biopsy for salivary gland lesions. Am J Clin Pathol. 2011;136:516–26.
121. Cengiz AB, Tansuker HD, Gul R, Emre F, Demirbas T, Oktay MF. Comparison of preoperative diagnostic accuracy of fine needle aspiration and core needle biopsy in parotid gland neoplasms. Eur Arch Otorrinolaringol. 2021;278:4067–74.
122. Mygdakos N, Nikolaidou S, Tzilivaki A, Tamiolakis D. Liquid based preparation (LBP) cytology versus conventional cytology (CS) in FNA samples from breast, thyroid, salivary glands and soft tissues. Our experience in Crete (Greece) Rom. J Morphol Embryol. 2009;50:245–50.
123. Tripathy K, Misra A, Ghosh JK. Efficacy of liquid-based cytology versus conventional smears in FNA samples. J Cytol. 2015;32:17–20.
124. Suzuki A, Hirokawa M, Higuchi M, Yamao N, Kuma S, Nakamura H, et al. Cytological characteristics of papillary thyroid carcinoma on LBC specimens, compared with conventional specimens. Diagn Cytopathol. 2015;43:108–13.
125. Rossi ED, Raffaelli M, Minimo C, Mule A, Lombardi CP, Vecchio FM, et al. Immunocytochemical evaluation of thyroid neoplasms on thin-layer smears from fine-needle aspiration biopsies. Cancer. 2005;105:87–95.
126. Hashimoto K, Morimoto A, Kato M, Tominaga Y, Maeda N, Tsuzuki T, et al. Immunocytochemical analysis for differential diagnosis of thyroid lesions using liquid-based cytology. Nagoya J Med Sci. 2011;73:15–24.
127. Kumar M, Katiyar S, Sagar M, Kumari M, Goel MM. Liquid-based cytology versus conventional cytology in fine-needle aspirates of salivary gland neoplasms. Indian J Pathol Microbiol. 2018;61:45–9.
128. Rarick JM, Wasman J, Michael CW. The utility of liquid-based cytology in salivary gland fine-needle aspirates: experience of an academic institution. Acta Cytol. 2014;58:552–62.
129. Buckland JR, Manjaly G, Violaris N, Howlett DC. Ultrasound-guided cutting-needle biopsy of the parotid gland. J Laryngol Otol. 1999;113:988–92.
130. Kesse KW, Manjaly G, Violaris N, Howlett DC. Ultrasound-guided biopsy in the evaluation of focal lesions and diffuse swelling of the parotid gland. Br J Oral Maxillofac Surg. 2002;40:384–8.
131. Zinzani PL, Colecchia A, Festi D, Magagnoli M, Larocca A, Ascani S, et al. Ultrasound-guided core-needle biopsy is effective in the initial diagnosis of lymphoma patients. Haematologica. 1998;83:989–92.
132. Burke C, Thomas R, Inglis C, Baldwin A, Ramesar K, Grace R, Howlett DC. Ultrasound-guided core biopsy in the diagnosis of lymphoma of the head and neck. A 9 year experience. Br J Radiol. 2011;84:727–32.
133. Witt BL, Schmidt RL. Ultrasound-guided core needle biopsy of salivary gland lesions: a systematic review and meta-analysis. Laryngoscope. 2014;124:695–700.
134. Pfeiffer J, Ridder GJ. Diagnostic value of ultrasound-guided core needle biopsy in patients with salivary gland masses. Int J Oral Maxillofac Surg. 2012;41:437–43.
135. Eom HJ, Lee JH, Ko MS, Choi YJ, Yoon RG, Cho KJ, et al. Comparison of fine-needle aspiration and core needle biopsy under ultrasonographic guidance for detecting malignancy and for the tissue-specific diagnosis of salivary gland tumors. AJNR Am J Neuroradiol. 2015;36:1188–93.
136. Huang YC, Wu CT, Lin G, Chuang WY, Yeow KM, Wan YL. Comparison of ultrasonographically guided fine-needle aspiration and core needle biopsy in the diagnosis of parotid masses. J Clin Ultrasound. 2012;40:189–94.

137. Haldar S, Mandalia U, Skelton E, Chow V, Turner SS, Ramesar K, et al. Diagnostic investigation of parotid neoplasms: a 16-year experience of freehand fine needle aspiration cytology and ultrasound-guided core needle biopsy. Int J Oral Maxillofac Surg. 2015;44:151–7.
138. Griffith CC, Schmitt AC, Little JL, Magliocca KR. New developments in salivary gland pathology: clinically useful ancillary testing and new potentially targetable molecular alterations. Arch Pathol Lab Med. 2017;141:381–95.
139. Pusztaszeri MP, Faquin WC. Update in salivary gland cytopathology: recent molecular advances and diagnostic applications. Semin Diagn Pathol. 2015;32:264–74.
140. Pusztaszeri MP, García JJ, Faquin WC. Salivary gland FNA: new markers and new opportunities for improved diagnosis. Cancer Cytopathol. 2016;124:307–16.
141. Griffith CC, Siddiqui MT, Schmitt AC. Ancillary testing strategies in salivary gland aspiration cytology: A practical pattern-based approach. Diagn Cytopathol. 2017;45:808–19.
142. Foo WC, Jo VY, Krane JF. Usefulness of translocation-associated immunohistochemical stains in the fine-needle aspiration diagnosis of salivary gland neoplasms. Cancer Cytopathol. 2016;124:397–405.
143. Evrard SM, Meilleroux J, Daniel G, Basset C, Lacoste-Collin L, Vergez S, Uro-Coste E, Courtade-Saidi M. Use of fluorescent in-situ hybridisation in salivary gland cytology: a powerful diagnostic tool. Cytopathology. 2017;28:312–20.
144. Hudson JB, Collins BT. MYB gene abnormalities t(6;9) in adenoid cystic carcinoma fine-needle aspiration biopsy using fluorescence in situ hybridization. Arch Pathol Lab Med. 2014;138:403–9.
145. Moon A, Cohen C, Siddiqui MT. MYB expression: potential role in separating adenoid cystic carcinoma (ACC) from pleomorphic adenoma (PA) diagn. Cytopathology. 2016;44:799–804.
146. Sun T, Akalin A, Dresser K, Fischer AH, Zuo T. The utility of MYB immunohistochemistry (IHC) in fine needle aspiration (FNA) diagnosis of adenoid cystic carcinoma (AdCC). Head Neck Pathol. 2021;15:389–94.
147. Pusztaszeri MP, Sadow PM, Ushiku A, Bordignon P, McKee TA, Faquin WC. MYB immunostaining is a useful ancillary test for distinguishing adenoid cystic carcinoma from pleomorphic adenoma in fine-needle aspiration biopsy specimens. Cancer Cytopathol. 2014;122:257–65.
148. Weinreb I. Translocation-associated salivary gland tumors: A review and update. Adv Anat Pathol. 2013;20:367–77.
149. Skálová A, Stenman G, Simpson RHW, Hellquist H, Slouka D, Svoboda T, et al. The role of molecular testing in the differential diagnosis of salivary gland carcinomas. Am J Surg Pathol. 2018;42:e11–27.
150. Skálová A, Hyrcza MD, Vaneček T, Baněčková M, Leivo I. Fusion-positive salivary gland carcinomas. Genes Chromosomes Cancer. 2022;61:228–43.
151. Andersson MK, Stenman G. The landscape of gene fusions and somatic mutations in salivary gland neoplasms-implications for diagnosis and therapy. Oral Oncol. 2016;57:63–9.
152. Stenman G. Fusion oncogenes in salivary gland tumors: molecular and clinical consequences. Head Neck Pathol. 2013;7(Suppl. 1):S12–9.
153. Tonon G, Modi S, Wu L, Kubo A, Coxon AB, Komiya T, et al. t(11;19)(q21;p13) translocation in mucoepidermoid carcinoma creates a novel fusion product that disrupts a notch signaling pathway. Nat Genet. 2003;33:208–13.
154. Okumura Y, Nakano S, Murase T, Ueda K, Kawakita D, Nagao T, et al. Prognostic impact of CRTC1/3-MAML2 fusions in salivary gland mucoepidermoid carcinoma: A multiinstitutional retrospective study. Cancer Sci. 2020;111:4195–204.
155. West RB, Kong C, Clarke N, Gilks T, Lipsick JS, Cao H, et al. MYB expression and translocation in adenoid cystic carcinomas and other salivary gland tumors with clinicopathologic correlation. Am J Surg Pathol. 2011;35:92–9.
156. Schmidt RL, Hunt JP, Hall BJ, Wilson AR, Layfield LJ. A systematic review and meta-analysis of the diagnostic accuracy of frozen section for parotid gland lesions. Am J Clin Pathol. 2011;136:729–38.

157. Haldar S, Sinnott JD, Tekeli KM, Turner SS, Howlett DC. Biopsy of parotid masses: review of current techniques. World J Radiol. 2016;8(5):501–5.
158. Wong DSY. Frozen section during parotid surgery revisited: efficacy of its applications and changing trend of indications. Head Neck. 2002;24:191–7.
159. Arabi Mianroodi AA, Sigston EA, Vallance NA. Frozen section for parotid surgery: should it become routine? ANZ J Surg. 2006;76:736–9.
160. Choy KCC, Bundele MM, Fu EW, Li H, Gan JYJ, Rao NCL, et al. Risk stratification of parotid neoplasms based on intraoperative frozen section and preoperative fine needle aspiration cytology. Eur Arch Otorrinolaringol. 2022;279:2117–31.
161. Pastorello RG, Rodriguez EF, McCormick BA, Calsavara VF, Chen LC, Zarka MA, et al. Is there a role for frozen section evaluation of parotid masses after preoperative cytology or biopsy diagnosis? Head Neck Pathol. 2021;15:859–65.
162. Suzuki M, Nakaegawa Y, Kobayashi T, Kawase T, Matsuzuka T, Murono S. The role of frozen section biopsy for parotid gland tumour with benign fine-needle aspiration cytology. J Laryngol Otol. 2019;133:227–9.
163. Zbären P, Guélat D, Loosli H, Stauffer E. Parotid tumors: fine-needle aspiration and/or frozen section. Otolaryngol Head Neck Surg. 2008;139:811–5.
164. Nishikawa S, Kawata R, Higashino M, Lee K, Terada T, Kurisu Y, et al. Assessing the histological type and grade of primary parotid carcinoma by fine-needle aspiration and frozen section. Auris Nasus Larynx. 2015;42:463–8.
165. Schmidt RL, Hall BJ, Wilson AR, Layfield LJ. A systematic review and meta-analysis of the diagnostic accuracy of fine-needle aspiration cytology for parotid gland lesions. Am J Clin Pathol. 2011;136:45–59.
166. Taniuchi M, Terada T, Kawata R. Fine-needle aspiration cytology for parotid tumors. Life (Basel). 2022;12(11):1897.

Parotid Injuries and Fistulae

6

6.1 Introduction

A parotid "fistula" is a communication, through which saliva is discharged, between the parotid gland (glandular fistula), or duct (ductal fistula) and the skin externally (external fistula) or to the oral cavity internally (internal fistula). In glandular fistulae, discharge is less than in ductal fistulae and tends to heal spontaneously with conservative treatment, whereas ductal fistulas continuously discharge the saliva, and spontaneous healing is very rare [1].

A "sialocele" is a collection of saliva beneath the skin that occurs if the duct leaks but no fistula forms, or when the glandular substance, but not the duct, is disrupted. An internal parotid fistula commonly presents as a sialocele or an effusion, whereas communication with the skin leads to an external parotid fistula [2].

6.2 Etiology

Causes of the parotid fistula include (1) trauma (penetrating or blunt injury in the region of the parotid gland or as a complication of facial fractures) [3]; (2) improper incision and drainage or spontaneous rupture of a parotid abscess (or sialocele); (3) intraoperative iatrogenic injury of the gland or duct (following surgery in the maxillofacial region or in the temporomandibular joint (TMJ) region, parotidectomy or secondary to drainage of facial/parotid abscess, mandibular osteotomy [4–6], or the use of external pin fixation [7]); (4) complication of parotid duct cannulation during sialography; and (5) malignant tumors invading to the surface [8]. A parotid fistula can also occur as a congenital malformation during fetal development, leading to ectopic accessory parotid gland [9].

© The Author(s), under exclusive license to Springer Nature Switzerland AG 2024
M. Sakr, *Surgery of the Salivary Glands*,
https://doi.org/10.1007/978-3-031-82069-4_6

6.3 Diagnosis

6.3.1 History-Taking

Males are twice as likely to experience parotid duct injury as females, and the mean age of individuals with parotid duct injury is approximately 30 years. Flow through the fistula increases during meals, particularly during mastication, which confirms the diagnosis [9]. Important aspects of history of the wound include the circumstances surrounding the injury, precipitating cause, exact mechanism and site of injury, time of occurrence, and treatment initiated prior to presentation. Other important aspects of the history include tobacco, alcohol, or drug use, tetanus immune status, and comorbid conditions that may place the patient at a higher risk for infection such as diabetes mellitus (DM) and immunosuppression.

6.3.2 Physical Examination

An internal fistula constitutes no consequences and requires no treatment. However, an external fistula connected with large ducts causes extreme discomfort every time the patient has a meal, smells, or even thinks of food, due to excessive outpouring of saliva on the cheek causing skin excoriation (Fig. 6.1). A sialogram will determine whether the fistula is ductal or glandular.

A thorough clinical examination is necessary for proper evaluation of the overall state of health, comorbidities, nutritional status, and mental status of the patient. Important signs/symptoms related to the wound include pain, fever, edema, discharge, and/or odor. Important aspects of wound assessment include location, shape, size, type (blunt or penetrating), depth, drainage (quality, character, odor), presence

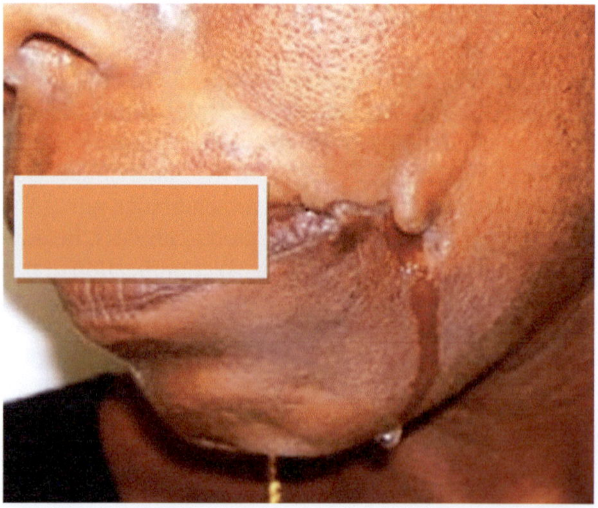

Fig. 6.1 Left external parotid fistula with an outpouring of saliva

of a foreign body (e.g., glass, tooth fragments), loss of tissue, tenderness, asymmetry, surrounding skin (erythema, edema, crepites), and status of the facial nerve.

The parotid duct is 7 cm long and arises from the anterior border of the gland, crosses over the masseter, and turns medially at its anterior border to pierce the buccinator. It travels for a while beneath the buccal mucosa and opens in the papilla opposite the second maxillary molar. The course of the duct can be marked on the surface as the middle third of a straight line drawn from the anterior aspect of the tragus to the midpoint of the upper lip. The duct is accompanied by the buccal branch of the facial nerve and the transverse facial artery during its course, and these structures are at risk of injury during surgery for the duct fistula. Wounds across this line should be assessed meticulously for injury to these structures [9].

An injury classification system that divides the parotid duct into three regions has been devised for parotid duct injuries as follows [10]:

- Site A: posterior to the masseter muscle or intraglandular (glandular)
- Site B: overlying the masseter muscle (masseteric)
- Site C: anterior to masseter muscle (pre-masseteric)

6.3.3 Investigations

Fistulas can usually be diagnosed by history and clinical examination of watery discharge from the fistula during meals or use of the lemon test. In the case of any doubt, serum amylase analysis of the fluid and sialo-fistulography can be done [11].

Computed tomography (CT) scan or fistulography is helpful to look for the extent of the fistula. Fistulography is a radiographic procedure that demonstrates the origin and extent of fistulae. In this method, the tract is filled with a radiopaque contrast medium (70% urografin), usually under fluoroscopic control. Right-angle and oblique projections are occasionally required to demonstrate the full extent of a sinus tract while digital sialography with fistulography demonstrates the precise anatomical location of a fistula [11]. Ultrasonography may also be performed to reveal the fistula and know the condition of the gland and duct.

6.4 Management

Although there is consensus in the literature that "acute" parotid injury must be explored primarily and all injured structures be repaired accurately, the treatment of the "chronic" injury is controversial. Several methods of treatment have been described with varying success and morbidity. Management options include pressure dressings and use of anti-sialagogues [12], total parotidectomy, tympanic neurectomy [13], intraoral transposition of the parotid duct [14], radiation therapy [15], the use of botulinum toxin A [16–18], and the use of fibrin glue [19].

Various treatment modalities to treat the parotid fistula have been advocated if conservative measures fail. Radiation has been used in the past to suppress the gland, but the use of radiation for benign disease is now avoided because of its long-term ill-effects. Some authors advocate the use of anticholinergics to suppress glandular function during healing, but this is not a frequently used modality.

Tympanic neurectomy involves drilling into the temporal bone and disruption of the tympanic nerve, which carries parasympathetic secretory nerve fibers to the parotid gland [20, 21]. This technique aims at reducing salivary flow and causing spontaneous fistula resolution. Although popular in the past, this method tends to be abandoned due to short-term and poor results due to reinnervation of the gland with time [22].

Three operative techniques have been popularized over time. These include repair of the duct over a stent, ligation of the duct, and fistulization of the duct into the oral cavity, which could be done by either T-tube or catheter drainage into the mouth or the drainage of proximal duct by a catheter [11]. Parotidectomy has been discouraged as a treatment modality as postoperative facial palsy is seen in 75% of cases [23].

6.4.1 Nonsurgical Treatment

6.4.1.1 Wound Care/Antibiotic Therapy

Wound care is the cornerstone of therapy. Prophylactic antibiotics should be administered and continued for 5–7 days, but it should be noted that antibiotics cannot avert or cure infections in the setting of poor wound care. Selection of the appropriate antibiotic involves multiple factors including culture results if obtained and available, drug sensitivities, patient age, drug interactions, expected compliance, and renal and hepatic function. The drug of choice is amoxicillin/clavulanate potassium. It is the most effective and economical choice for outpatient therapy, unless contraindicated because of penicillin allergy. Doxycycline is an alternative choice for oral therapy in patients allergic to penicillin.

In rare cases, human saliva contains and occasionally transmits *Clostridium tetani*. Accordingly, all patients should be assessed for their tetanus immune status and immunization should be updated as appropriate.

6.4.1.2 Anticholinergic Agents

Some authors choose to use anticholinergic agents to suppress glandular function during healing or in an attempt to close a fistula or resolve a sialocele spontaneously. A commonly used agent is propantheline bromide (Pro-Banthine), which inhibits the action of acetylcholine at the post-ganglionic nerve endings of the parasympathetic nervous system (adult dose 15 mg PO qid half an hour prior to meals). Absence of reflex stimulation from mastication and chemical stimuli minimizes parotid secretions and allows healing of the injured duct, but this method requires maximum patient compliance for a prolonged time. Anticholinergic drugs are unlikely to be useful if used alone and are associated with numerous side effects such as urinary retention, xerostomia, nausea, vomiting, and vision disturbances.

6.4.1.3 Pressure Dressings

Sialocele and salivary fistula can frequently be managed nonoperatively with antibiotics, pressure dressings, and serial aspiration. Pressure dressings lead to atrophy of the gland as the lobules of the gland are contained in relatively inelastic capsule. The sustained rise in ductal pressure leads to compression of capillaries and veins, resulting in decrease in secretion and gland atrophy [12]. However, there is no adequate proof of their efficacy.

6.4.1.4 Intermittent Serial Aspiration

Intermittent aspiration of sialoceles has led to a resolution in many cases. Anticholinergics may be used to temporarily decrease salivary flow in order to effect healing.

6.4.1.5 Botulinum Toxin A

Botulinum toxin (Botox) type A is one of eight distinct neurotoxins that are known, each with its own immunological specificity [24]. It leads to partial or complete muscle paralysis by inhibiting acetylcholine release at the neuromuscular synaptic end plate. Due to this paralytic function, it has become the mainstay of therapeutic nonsurgical treatment for neuromuscular disorders such as hemifacial spasm, blepharospasm, spasmodic dysphonia, and dystonia [25]. Because this toxin also blocks the release of acetylcholine at the cholinergic synapses of the autonomic nervous system, it also has effects on the cholinergic parasympathetic secreto-motor fibers of the salivary gland. Hence, botulinum toxin has been tested in some autonomic diseases, such as achalasia, hyperhidrosis, and gustatory sweating (Frey's syndrome) [26, 27].

The proposed technique for the use of Botox in the parotid gland, according to the Cologne protocol, requires the reconstitution of the toxin with 4 mL of preservative-free normal saline to obtain a 25 mU/0.1 mL concentration. Between 0.1 and 0.2 mL are injected at each point on the parotid gland. Depending on the size of the gland, 4–10 points are injected into the parotid. The injections are preferably performed under sonographic control with a 7.5 Hz linear transducer. In general, a significant decrease in the salivary production is seen within the first 2 weeks after the injections and the duration of the effect averages between 2 and 3 months. Minimal side effects are seen with this protocol [28].

Botulinum toxin A has been used nowadays, but it has a latency period and requires repeated injections for desired effects and the effects may not last long enough to bring about complete remission of disease. Moreover, it is a costly procedure [29].

6.4.1.6 Fibrin Glue

Fibrin glue has also been used recently; Zwaveling et al. [19] reported treating two cases of post-parotidectomy fistulae treated by injection with fibrin tissue glue (Tissucol Duo 500, Baxter AG, Vienna, Austria). In both patients, the fistulae completely healed within months without complications. They concluded that post-parotidectomy fistulae can be effectively treated with fibrin glue, a simple and safe procedure with no side effects [19]. However, fibrin glue is rendered inactive by saliva, leading to recurrence of the fistula.

6.4.1.7 Hypertonic Saline Sclerotherapy

Hypertonic saline has been used in sclerotherapy in various concentrations. It has also been used for the treatment of varicose veins as an alternative to surgery [30]; and in the head and neck region for treatment of venous malformations with good results [31]. Thermodynamic and physicochemical calculations suggest that these solutions work by causing conformational denaturation of the cell membrane proteins in situ and saline can be diluted to a point where there will be no cellular toxicity. The temperature of the saline can be raised above body temperature (60o) to enhance the fibrosing property of physiological saline [32].

Hot hypertonic saline can be used for the purpose of fistula closure because it is easily available, cost-effective, causes no foreign body reaction or hypersensitivity reaction, nontoxic, and nonirritant to the surrounding structures. In addition, there are no chances of inadvertent injury to facial nerve and its branches and serves the purpose of causing fibrosis of gland parenchyma and spontaneous closure of the fistula with no complications [33].

6.4.2 Surgical Treatment

Copious irrigation of the wound with normal saline solution has been shown to decrease the incidence of wound infection. Careful debridement of devitalized tissue, particulate matter, and clot is necessary to reduce the infection risk and to improve the cosmetic result. Clean, surgically created wound margins allow for faster wound healing and better scarring.

Head and neck wounds, <12 h old and not obviously infected, being in a cosmetically sensitive area, may be closed directly with a low incidence of infection. The low infection rate is probably related to the excellent regional blood supply and infrequency of edema in these areas. For a good cosmetic result, closure is performed in a simple interrupted fashion using fine stitches and avoiding layered closure with buried sutures.

The most important initial step for proper surgical repair is the identification of key structures; namely, the buccal branches of the facial nerve (with the aid of a nerve stimulator intra-operatively if available) and the parotid duct itself. If the buccal branch was transected, repair it with fine sutures (8–0 to 10–0 monofilament is appropriate) under microscopic aid. The distal end of the parotid duct is identified by a silastic tube, placed via cannulation of the intraoral papilla. The proximal parotid duct can usually be identified by the flow of saliva into the wound, with gentle pressure over the gland if necessary. Once all key structures are identified, a decision is made regarding which repair technique to employ.

6.4.2.1 Site C (Distal or Glandular)

Distal lacerations, occurring at site C, may be treated in several ways. If the papilla is uninjured, the proximal portion may be dissected free and reimplanted into the papilla. If the papilla is injured or if the proximal duct does not reach the papilla, the duct may be reimplanted (under magnification) into the oral mucosa posterior to the papilla using fine interrupted absorbable sutures with meticulous approximation of duct epithelium to oral mucosa. If the distal injury is too short to be reimplanted into the oral mucosa without undue tension, then the best decision is to ligate the proximal duct.

6.4.2.2 Site B (Masseteric)

Injuries occurring over the masseter muscle, at site B, are the most common injuries to the parotid duct and may be treated by repair or ligation. If enough length remains, primary anastomosis over a silastic stent, using a single layer of interrupted fine sutures (8–0 to 10–0 monofilament), is performed under magnification. If a portion of the duct is damaged beyond repair or is missing, the proximal and distal ducts should be ligated. Reports of attempts to use a vein graft (saphenous) in such cases have generally found such attempts unsuccessful. Sialendoscopy-assisted repair of a transected Stensen duct in zone B has been reported [34].

6.4.2.3 Site A (Proximal or Pre-Masseteric)

Injuries of the proximal duct near the parotid substance, at site A, are usually best treated by duct ligation as the amount of proximal duct remaining is usually insufficient to result in a useful repair. Laceration of the gland itself without disruption of the parotid duct may be repaired with fine absorbable sutures (5–0 or 6–0 Vicryl).

A drain in the wound bed is recommended to drain any residual salivary leak and prevent early sialocele formation. Drains are removed once drainage is minimal and the skin has become adherent to the operative site. Postoperatively, a compression dressing is placed over the operative field postoperatively for several days. If ductal injury required ligation of the proximal duct, marked temporary swelling of the gland followed by rapid glandular atrophy is expected. If leaking of saliva occurs as in the development of a fistula or sialocele, the pressure dressing should be continued or reinstituted.

In the case of a chronic parotid duct fistula, an intraoral diversion technique to re-establish salivary flow in case of a nonfunctional parotid duct punctum has been described. The fistula tract and the surrounding ellipse of skin are passed in the oral cavity and sutured to the buccal mucosa with 4–0 chromic sutures without the need for stenting. Alternatively, chronic fistula and sialocele have been medically managed with botulinum toxin [18].

6.5 Complications

6.5.1 Persistent Salivary Fistula

If the fistula occurs in the oral cavity, it is of no consequence and requires no further therapy. If the fistula occurs on the overlying skin, the patient experiences saliva dripping down the cheek. Initial expectant management, with or without anticholinergic medications, has led to a resolution in many cases. Other cases have required surgical excision of the fistula tract with repair of the duct or superficial parotidectomy.

6.5.2 Sialocele

Sialocele usually resolves with intermittent aspiration and compression and rarely requires drain placement. Anticholinergics may be beneficial in the treatment of sialoceles. Duct ligation may lead to early edema of the gland with accompanying pain from stretching of the capsule. This usually subsides spontaneously within 1–2 weeks as atrophy of the gland occurs. Infection of the remaining glandular substance may occur as a late complication of duct ligation.

6.5.3 Sialadenitis

Sialadenitis may result from manipulation of the intraoral papilla or from sialography and may require drainage and antibiotics.

6.5.4 Nerve Injury

Facial nerve injury and sensory nerve injury may occur when surgery is conducted in the region of the parotid duct, particularly in cases where trauma and blood extravasation have discolored the tissues and disrupted tissue planes.

References

1. Ajike SO, Omisakin OO. The use of a feeding tube in the treatment of a parotid duct fistula: a case report. J Med Med Sci. 2011;2(8):1014–6.
2. Parekh D, Glezerson G, Stewart M, Esser J, Lawson HH. Post-traumatic parotid fistulae and sialoceles. A prospective study of conservative management in 51 cases. Ann Surg. 1989a;209(1):105–11.
3. Bergstrom L, Hemenway WG. Parotid-antral fistula. Complication of facial fracture. Arch Otolaryngol. 1971;93:519–20.
4. Shapiro DN, Gallo J, Moss M. Subcutaneous parotid effusion after mandibular osteotomy. J Oral Surg. 1978;36:397–8.
5. Goldberg MH, Marco W, Googel F. Parotid fistula: a complication of mandibular osteotomy. J Oral Surg. 1973;31:207–8.
6. Dierks EJ, Granite EL. Parotid sialocele and fistula after mandibular osteotomy. J Oral Surg. 1977;35:299–300.
7. Laskin JL. Parotid fistula after the use of external pin fixation: report of case. J Oral Surg. 1978;36:621–2.
8. Ananthakrishnan N, Parkash S. Parotid fistulas: a review. Br J Surg. 1982;69(11):641–3.
9. Naragund AI, Halli VB, Mudhol RS, Sonoli SS. Parotid fistula secondary to suppurative parotitis in a 13-year-old girl: a case report. J Med Case Rep. 2010;4:249.
10. Dalili Z. Sialography and fistulography of post traumatic fistulae; A case presentation. J Dent. 2005;2(2):70–3.
11. Chow TL, Kwok SP. Use of botulinum toxin type a in a case of persistent parotid sialocele. Hong Kong Med J. 2003;9(4):293–4.

12. Parekh D, Glezerson G, Stewart M, Esser J, Lawson HH. Post-traumatic parotid fistulae and sialoceles. A prospective study of conservative management in 51 cases. Ann Surg. 1989b;209:105–11.
13. Davis WE, Holt GR, Templer JW. Parotid fistula and tympanic neurectomy. Am J Surg. 1977;133:587–9.
14. Doctor VS, Rafii A, Enepekides DJ, Tollefson TT. Intraoral transposition of traumatic parotid duct fistula. Arch Facial Plast Surg. 2007;9:44–7.
15. Robinson AC, Khoury GG, Robinson PM. Role of irradiation in the suppression of parotid secretions. J Laryngol Otol. 1989;103:594–5.
16. Lim YC, Choi EC. Treatment of an acute salivary fistula after parotid surgery: botulinum toxin type A injection as primary treatment. Eur Arch Otorrinolaringol. 2008;265:243–5.
17. Dessy LA, Mazzocchi M, Monarca C, Onesti MG, Scuderi N. Combined transdermal scopolamine and botulinum toxin A to treat a parotid fistula after a face-lift in a patient with siliconomas. Int J Oral Maxillofac Surg. 2007;36:949–52.
18. Arnaud S, Batifol D, Goudot P, Yachouh J. Non-surgical management of parotid gland and duct injuries: interest of botulinum toxin. Ann Chir Plast Esthet. 2008a;53:36–40.
19. Zwaveling S, Steenvoorde P, da Costa SA. Treatment of postparotidectomy fistulae with fibrin glue. Acta Med (Hradec Kralove). 2006;49:67–9.
20. Chitre VV, Premchandra DJ. Recurrent parotitis. Arch Dis Child. 1997;77(4):359–63.
21. Vasama JP. Tympanic neurectomy and chronic parotitis. Acta Otolaryngol. 2000;120(8):995–8.
22. Mandour MA, El-Sheikh MM, El-Garem F. Tympanic neurectomy for parotid fistula. Arch Otolaryngol. 1976;102(6):327–9.
23. Ananthakrishan N, Prakash S. Parotid fistulas: a review. Br J Surg. 1982;69:641–3.
24. von Lindern JJ, Niederhagen B, Appel T, Berge S, Reich RH. New prospects in the treatment of traumatic and postoperative parotid fistulas with type a botulinum toxin. Plast Reconstr Surg. 2002;109:2443–5.
25. Christie A. Infectious disease. London: Churchill Livingstone; 1987.
26. Laskawi R, Drobik C, Schonebeck C. Up-to-date report of botulinum toxin type A treatment in patients with gustatory sweating (Frey's syndrome). Laryngoscope. 1998;108:381–4.
27. Tugnoli V, Eleopra R, Montecucco C, DeGrandis D. The therapeutic use of botulinum toxin. Expert Opin Investig Drugs. 1997;6:1383–94.
28. Van Sickels JE. Parotid duct injuries. Oral Surg Oral Med Oral Pathol. 1981;52(4):364–7.
29. Gordin EA, Daniero JJ, Krein H, Boon MS. Parotid gland trauma. Facial Plast Surg. 2010;26(6):504–10.
30. Parsons ME. Sclerotherapy basics. Dermatol Clin. 2004;22:501–8.
31. Cabrera J, Cabrera J Jr, Olmedo AG, Redondo P. Treatment of venous malformations with sclerosant in microfoam form. Arch Dermatol. 2003;139:1494–6.
32. Chhabra N, Chhabra S, Kapila SA. Use of hypertonic saline in the management of parotid fistulae and sialocele: a report of 2 cases. J Maxillofac Oral Surg. 2009;8:64–7.
33. Rao JKD, Gehlot N, Laxmy V, Vijay Siwach V. Management of parotid fistula using hypertonic saline. Natl J Maxillofac Surg. 2011;2(2):177–80.
34. Koch M, Iro H, Bozzato A, Zenk J. Sialendoscopy-assisted microsurgical repair of traumatic transection of Stensen's duct. Laryngoscope. 2013;123(12):3074–477.

7 Calculi of the Parotid Gland

7.1 Incidence

The incidence of sialolithiasis is estimated at 1 in 10,000 to 1 in 30,000 individuals [1, 2]. Escudier and McGurk [3] stated that, on the basis of hospital admissions due to salivary obstructive symptoms, the incidence is between 1 per 15,000 and 1 per 30,000. The primary age of diagnosis is between 30 and 60 years old, with a higher incidence in males [4]. Sialolithiasis is the most common disorder of major salivary glands [1]. The majority of salivary calculi (80–95%) occur in the submandibular gland, whereas 5–20% are found in the parotid gland [4–10]. The difference in incidence is attributed to a number of factors such as the difference in the composition of the saliva produced by each gland and the dependence of the submandibular (Wharton's) duct, which hinders easy drainage of its viscid secretions. The submandibular gland also produces more alkaline saliva, which predisposes to precipitation of inorganic salts (calcium and phosphate), further leading to salivary stone formation. Sialothiasis rarely affects the sublingual gland and the minor salivary glands (1–2%) [11–13]. The majority of stones are single. In 25% of cases, the stones are multiple [1, 5, 6, 9]. The mean number of stones per patient is 1.67 (range 1–5) [4].

7.2 Composition

Parotid stones are composed of varying ratios of organic and inorganic materials within an inner core. The exact ratios of inorganic material found within a sialolith depend on the chemical environment in which it forms. The inner core is considered the initial sialolith, which subsequently enlarges from the deposition of additional organic and inorganic material, forming the outer lamellae (layers). Inorganic materials include hydroxyapatite, whitlockite, and octacalcium phosphate, with hydroxyapatite (calcium phosphate) being the most prevalent. Organic materials found

© The Author(s), under exclusive license to Springer Nature Switzerland AG 2024
M. Sakr, *Surgery of the Salivary Glands*,
https://doi.org/10.1007/978-3-031-82069-4_7

within sialoliths include glycoproteins, cellular debris, bacteria, and mucopolysaccharides [14, 15].

Studies utilizing scanning electron microscopy and polymerase chain reaction (PCR) showed bacteria within sialoliths, predominantly the *Streptococcus* genus [16, 17]. Bacteria are not present in all sialoliths, suggesting that they are not necessary for their formation.

7.3 Etiology

The etiology of salivary stones formation remains elusive. Factors that are believed to cause salivary stones formation are divided into two major groups: "anatomical," affecting saliva formation or flow (i.e., duct stenosis or inflammation), and "compositional" (i.e., increased calcium content or altered enzyme function). Research examining the geographical distribution of hard water and salivary calculi formation demonstrated no correlation with an increased incidence of salivary stones in areas of increased water hardness [18]. Studies examining the effects of hypercalcemia using animal models demonstrated no evidence of increased salivary stones with hypercalcemia [14]. Additional factors such as decreased fluid intake and pharmacological side effects resulting in decreased salivary production (diuretic use) remain under study. In recent years, tobacco smoking has been discussed as a potential risk factor for the formation of salivary stones. Tobacco may induce inflammation within the salivary ducts and decrease the production of salivary amylase [2, 14].

7.4 Pathogenesis

The exact pathogenesis of sialolithiasis is not well understood, but two dominant etio-pathogenetic theories were suggested. The first theory proposes that there are multiple internal micro-calculi within salivary gland secretory granules. When these micro-calculi get secreted into the salivary ducts, they may act as a nidus for the formation of larger calculi, ultimately forming a sialolith [15]. The second theory suggests that the formation of the salivary gland calculi results from a deposition of calcium salts around a core made of desquamated epithelial cells, foreign bodies, bacteria, or mucus [19].

7.5 Clinical Presentation

Parotid calculi can occur in the gland or Stensen's duct. Sialolithiasis can occur at any age; however, most cases occur in patients in their third to sixth decade. Sialothiasis rarely occurs in children. Clinical presentations of a parotid stone vary from being asymptomatic, to intermittent obstructive parotitis (sialolithiasis is the cause of 42–77% of cases of salivary duct obstruction) [20, 21], to an acute abscess. The patient usually presents with swelling and pain, aggravated by eating, but subsiding within the next hour or so after the meal [22]. A decreased production of the saliva may be observed as well [1, 6, 8, 10, 23].

Physical examination will demonstrate asymmetric swelling of the affected parotid gland. Approximately 60% of parotid stones (and 30% of submandibular stones) will be located distally in their respective ducts. If large enough, these stones may be visually apparent on examination of the oral cavity. Salivary stones typically demonstrate an oval or round shape and a white or yellow color on visual inspection. If not visually apparent, the stones are usually palpable along the anatomical course of the affected salivary duct or gland [24–26].

The annual growth rate of an established stone is about 1 mm per year and the average size is about 3.4 mm (range 1.5–10 mm) and only 7.6% exceeds 15 mm in diameter [4, 27]. The stone size is determined by the long axis, and the majority of stones take the shape of the length of the duct. Calculi within a major duct tend to be smooth and rounded, whereas those within the gland tend to be irregular in shape. Sialoliths weigh 300 mg on average, ranging between 1 mg and 5 g [27].

7.6 Complications

The primary complications of sialolithiasis are the development of sialadenitis, acute or chronic, and atrophy of the affected salivary gland. Obstruction of the salivary glands by a sialolith blocks the flow of saliva, resulting in swelling and pain. Additionally, this blockage of flow prevents the removal of bacteria and debris from the salivary duct, resulting in bacterial infection. If the obstruction is chronic, the blocked flow of saliva will damage the salivary glands' acinar cells, resulting in local inflammation. Without proper treatment, it can result in permanent fibrosis of the gland and atrophy [15]. Other complications of sialolithiasis include ductal ulceration and stricture formation [1, 28].

7.7 Investigations

Calculi must be differentiated from stenosis of the duct caused by repeated trauma and fibrosis. The basic imaging methods of sialolithiasis are plain X-ray images, X-ray sialography, ultrasonography (US), computed tomography (CT) scan, and magnetic resonance imaging (MRI). Sialoendoscopy, which is also a therapeutic method, is becoming increasingly common.

Plain X-rays may reveal larger stones but the soft-tissue image of the cheek makes this method less suited for the detection of smaller ones. Sialograms (contrast radiology of the duct system) are more likely to be able to reveal the stones but still may be difficult to interpret. Other investigative options include US, CT scanning, and MRI, all of which are particularly useful in evaluating masses in the salivary glands. In the USA, a major role in sialolithiasis diagnostics is played by unenhanced CT, while in Europe it is US and digital subtraction sialography [1]. MR sialography is also gaining popularity.

7.7.1 Plain X-Rays

Occlusal and lateral-oblique views demonstrate radio-opaque calculi. Radiolucent calculi are undetectable by plain radiography. It was reported that stones of the submandibular gland produce opacity in 80–90% of cases, while stones of the parotid gland only in 60% (Fig. 7.1) [1, 5, 7]. A single X-ray is normally performed before contrast administration for sialography.

7.7.2 Sialography

Sialography allows examination of the architecture of the salivary gland and duct. Parotid stones are usually imaged through sialography being mostly radiolucent. The sensitivity of conventional sialography in calculi detection ranges from 64% to 100%, while its specificity is from 88% to 100%. Digitalization of that examination, with the use of subtraction (digital subtraction sialography), increased its sensitivity of stone detection up to 96–100%, and its specificity to 88–91.1% [7].

7.7.3 Ultrasonography (US)

Ultrasonography can be used to differentiate between solid and cystic lesions of the gland. It can be used to differentiate intrinsic from extrinsic disease and is helpful in the identification of abscess formation.

Ultrasonography is regarded by some authors as a method of choice in salivary stone diagnostics. In calculi detection, it has a sensitivity of 94%, specificity of 100%, and accuracy of 96% [1, 6, 29]; US has been reported to allow for nonopaque

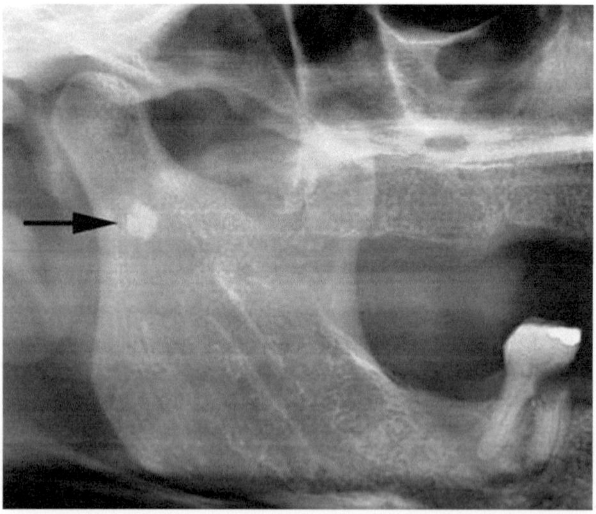

Fig. 7.1 Plain X-ray showing a round radio-opaque shadow (stone) in the parotid (black arrow)

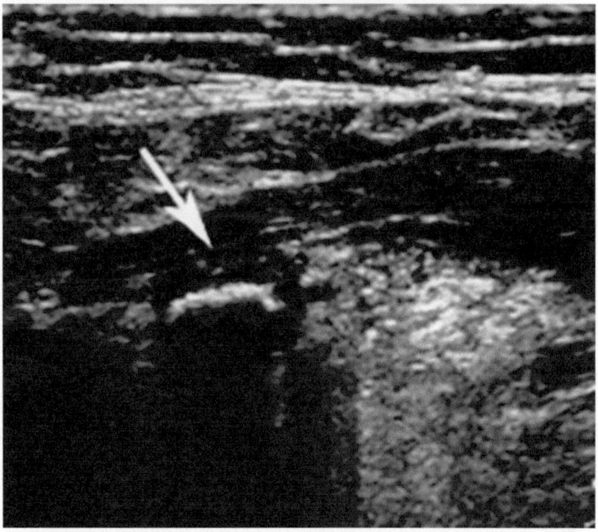

Fig. 7.2 Ultrasound showing a stone (white arrow) with an acoustic shadow behind the calculus

calculi detection with a sensitivity of 80–96% [8, 9]. A typical US image of a stone involves an echogenic, round, or oval structure, producing an acoustic shadow (Fig. 7.2) [1, 8, 10]. Stones in salivary ducts may lead to the distension of the duct above the obstacle, which may be shown on US [9]. Stones smaller than 2 mm may not produce any acoustic shadow [1, 7–9]. Diagnostic mistakes may concern very small stones in intraparenchymal ducts, with no duct distension [1, 6]. Moreover, hyperechogenic air bubbles, mixed with the saliva and simulating stones, may also be misleading [10].

The detection of fine stones may be helped by sialogogue injection, which causes salivary duct dilatation and thus facilitates calculi visualization [1, 8]. In about 50% of the sialolithiasis cases, US images show features of inflammation. Despite many advantages of US, it turns out to be less precise in differentiating a cluster of stones from a single, large stone [6].

7.7.4 Computed Tomography (CT) Scan/CT Sialography

Computed tomography (CT) scan is commonly used for glandular architecture, obstructive location, and visualization of the stones (Fig. 7.3) [30]. It is useful in differentiating intrinsic from extrinsic glandular disease and can be used in defining abscess formation versus phlegmon, but has limited usefulness in the evaluation of ductal system unless combined with simultaneous sialography in addition to patient exposure to ionizing radiation and a relatively high cost of the examination [4].

Similar to the conventional sialography, CT sialography requires cannulation of the duct opening. Moreover, it exposes patients to a higher dose of radiation compared with the conventional sialography. This method allows for simultaneous visualization of the glandular tissue and the salivary ducts. The salivary glands may be

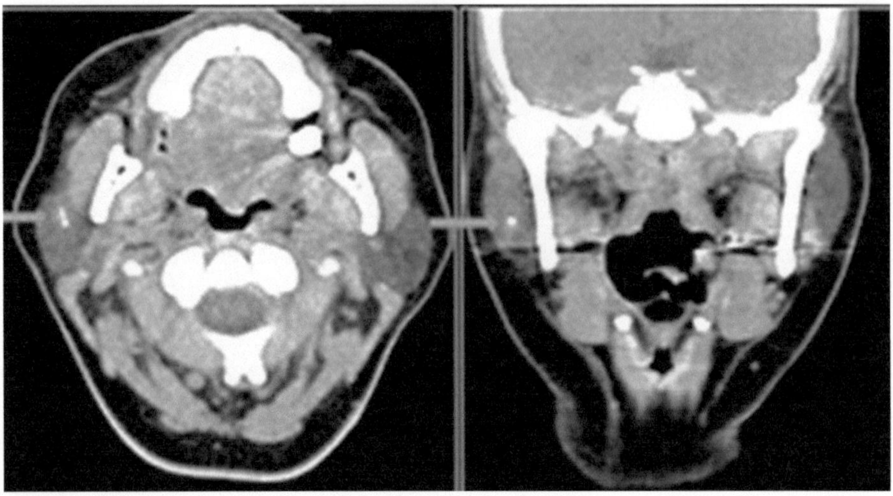

Fig. 7.3 Computed tomography (CT) scan showing a parotid gland calculus (arrow)

shown in 3D reconstruction. However, CT sialography cannot visualize the secondary and the tertiary branches [7].

According to some authors, unenhanced CT scan is the best method in the detection of sialolithiasis, especially in case of painful salivary glands and suspicion of a few, very tiny calculi [1, 6]. A cluster of fine stones is hard to differentiate from one, large stone. That is when CT is recommended [1]. The phenomenon of the postcontrast enhancement in CT should be used in suspicion of an abscess that cannot be detected with US.

Recently, some authors reported encouraging results on the use of the volumetric tomography (alternatively called cone beam computed tomography) in sialolithiasis diagnostics [31]. This method produces high-resolution, 3D images of bony structures of the head and neck, with the use of up to 15 times lower ionizing radiation dose, and being much cheaper [32, 33].

7.7.5 Magnetic Resonance Imaging (MRI)/Magnetic Resonance Sialography (MRS)

Magnetic resonance imaging (MRI) does not allow evaluation of the ductal system, and it is not helpful in defining calcifications. It is an excellent tool for soft-tissue definition (invaluable in instances of suspected neoplasia).

Being a noninvasive method, it does not require cannulation of the salivary duct opening and does not expose patients to ionizing radiation or iodine contrast administration. MR sialography allows for a precise morphological evaluation of the salivary ducts, enabling the visualization of their tertiary branches [34]. Moreover, the examination may be carried out in acute inflammation of the salivary gland. It is considered an alternative to digital subtraction sialography, especially in cases of acute sialoadenitis or failure of salivary opening cannulation [35–38].

Capaccio et al. [34] compared the results of MRS versus US. Examinations were performed before and after stimulation with lemon juice. MRS showed secondary branches of the salivary ducts within submandibular salivary glands and tertiary branches within the parotid glands. MRS allowed visualization of very tiny stones that could not be found with US [34].

According to Becker et al. [38], MRS is a better method for salivary gland evaluation than conventional X-ray sialography or US as it allows visualization of distal salivary ducts [38]. Moreover, by adding extra MRI sequences for parenchymal imaging, it is possible to detect some lesions located outside the system of the salivary ducts (e.g., Warthin's tumor) [5].

Becker et al. [38] compared MRS precision in the detection of calculi compared to conventional sialography, US, and sialoendoscopy. MRS showed a sensitivity of 91%, a specificity of 94–97%, a positive predictive value of 93–97%, and a negative predictive value of 91%. False-negative results were obtained in calculi measuring 2–3 mm, located in undilated salivary ducts. MRS did not distinguish a stone from a dense mucosal plug.

Moreover, amalgam fillings veiled tiny calculi and stenoses of the salivary ducts. Results also revealed that the peripheral salivary ducts could be better visualized with the conventional X-ray sialography than with MRS. The limitation of MRS is also connected with its lower spatial resolution, enabling the differentiation of partial and of complete occlusions of the salivary ducts [36]. In conclusion, MRS is considered a highly effective, noninvasive diagnostic method of visualization of salivary ducts of large salivary glands, especially in cases of acute sialoadenitis.

7.7.6 Sialoendoscopy

The causes of salivary duct stenosis remain unknown by imaging modalities in 5–10% of cases. The diagnostic gap is filled by sialoendoscopy that allows direct visualization of the salivary duct lumen, that is, visualization of calculi, mucosal plugs, foreign bodies, and polyps.

Sialoendoscopy enabled the surgeons to examine the salivary ducts from the inside. Combination of sialoendoscopy with therapeutic procedures increases the frequency of sialography [28]. Some authors recommend dilatation of the ductal openings before performing sialoendoscopy. Others recommend papillotomy [28]. During sialoendoscopy, the operators use very small tools and a camcorder to reach the proximal parts of the salivary ducts. Sialoendoscopy includes performance of the following procedures: calculi removal with the use of the Dormia basket, dilatation of the stenosed salivary ducts with the use of balloons, as well as stenosis correction [20]. At the end of the sialendoscopic procedure, a stent, 2–3 cm long, is left in the salivary duct for 7–10 days to facilitate healing and drainage.

7.8 Differential Diagnosis

In general, the differential diagnosis of a parotid gland swelling includes sialolithiasis, sialadenitis (inflammatory or infectious), and neoplasm. However, the clinical presentation can vary, and the differential diagnosis can be extensive and relies heavily on physical examination findings and clinical history. Conditions that can have a similar presentation include cellulitis, poor dentition and dental abscess formation, infection of the buccal or masticator space, herpes zoster, and neoplasm.

7.9 Treatment

7.9.1 Surgical Treatment

Glandular or ductal stones can be treated with parotidectomy, while those close to the duct orifice are removed by ductal dilation and massage or by longitudinal slitting of the duct and releasing the stone.

7.9.2 External Lithotripsy

New therapeutic modalities use extracorporeal or intracorporeal crushing of the salivary gland calculi. The crushed stones can be flushed out with saliva through natural salivary duct openings [4]. The advent of external lithotripsy in the early 1990s paved the way for conservative treatment of all calculi, with a success rate of 40% in the submandibular gland and 75% in the parotid. Unfortunately, results were discouraging, specifically in patients with large calculi [39–42].

7.9.3 Interventional Sialendoscopy

Interventional sialendoscopy, first described in the 1990s, offered much less invasive therapeutic options and became popular with technological improvements after 2000 [43–47]. It can be used to retrieve stones from the ducts and dilate ductal strictures. The common techniques used to remove the salivary gland stones are the grasping technique using a small wire basket retrieval system, mechanical fragmentation, extracorporeal shockwave lithotripsy (ESWL), and intracorporeal laser fragmentation [48]. According to the size of the stone, the following techniques can be used as shown in Table 7.1.

7.9.3.1 Small Stones (<5 mm)

When the diameter of the stone is 5 mm or less, it can be removed purely by an endoscopic technique (Fig. 7.4), particularly when the stone is located above the muscles that comprise the floor of the mouth. In the presence of strictures or adhesions, the diagnosis and exact location of obstruction are established using a

Table 7.1 Techniques of stone extraction according to stone size

Stone size	Treatment technique
Small (<5 mm)	Extirpation during endoscopy (alone)
Intermediate (5–7 mm)	Needs fragmentation-holmium laser Ho-YAG) or lithotripsy prior to endoscopic extraction
Large (>7 mm)	Needs combined extirpation (endoscopic assisted)

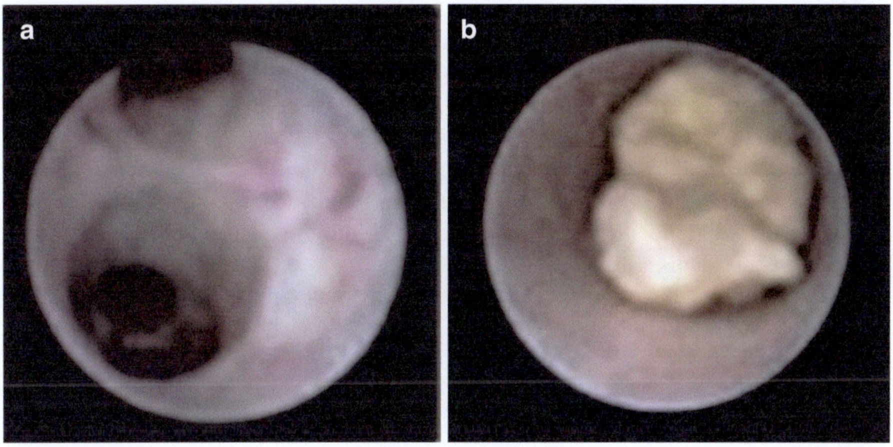

Fig. 7.4 Sialendoscopy showing the interior of the parotid (Stensen's) duct (**a**) and intraductal stones (**b**)

sialogram. The surgeon can use the endoscopic method. The first step is anesthetizing and lavaging the duct with 2% lidocaine and saline solution. If there is no improvement, the surgeon can then insert a dilation balloon, which can be inflated up to 3 mm. The pressure created by the inflation can be sufficient to dilate most strictures. Another technique for dilating strictures is to expand the stricture region with grasping forceps used as a dilator.

7.9.3.2 Intermediate Stones (5–7 mm)

Stones of intermediate size (5–7 mm) and spiculated calcified stones are difficult to remove with sialoendoscopy alone. Other than mechanical microdrills, extracorporeal shockwave lithotripsy (ESWL) and intracorporeal lasers are utilized to fragment the mineralized sialoliths [49]. Following this fragmentation, physiological expulsion of the stones by salivary flow and endoscopic techniques with irrigation are therapeutic. This procedure is more effective with parotid stones compared with submandibular stones. Pregnancy, cardiac pacemaker, and total distal duct stenosis are contraindications to ESWL. Relative contraindications are inflammatory painful glandular swellings. Postprocedural tenderness, petechiae, and swelling are noted on occasion.

There is no overall consensus on the type of laser for endoscopic-assisted laser lithotripsy [50]. Laser causes cavitation fragmentation assisting stone extirpation trans-luminal after application of laser lithotripsy. Ho/YAG laser at pulsed setting with a 2080 nm wavelength carried in a fiber diameter as small as 200 μm is well documented [50]. There are no major contraindications other than poor visibility and iatrogenic injury to adjacent soft tissues in large stones in intraluminal deployment. Nevertheless, success rates of interventional sialendoscopy with intraductal laser fragmentation and basket extraction of calculi remained possible in only 80% of patients [14]. Unsuccessful treatment was attributed to large-sized calculi (6 mm and larger) and associated ductal stenosis [51]. In such cases, the only solution was to remove the gland, with its associated significant morbidity [39–41].

7.9.3.3 Large Stones (>7 mm)

When the diameter is larger than 7 mm, a twofold (endoscopic assisted) approach can also be utilized. The endoscope is introduced and the stone localized, and then dissected and removed through an intraoral approach. After a sialolith is removed from an affected gland, a silastic stent is inserted into the duct for 2–4 weeks for the duration of the healing process of the oral region and until normal function of the gland is restored. This prevents scar formation, which can develop over the ductal opening into the mouth.

7.10 Prognosis

Sialolithiasis has an excellent prognosis, and the majority of patients can be managed conservatively. The minimally invasive procedures have excellent success rates with minimal morbidity compared to traditional surgical techniques. Sialadenectomy for the treatment of sialolithiasis is rarely necessary with modern treatment techniques [52]. However, in cases in which only the calculus is removed, the recurrence rate may be as high as 18% because the underlying cause, which is unknown, has not been corrected.

References

1. Madani G, Beale T. Inflammatory conditions of the salivary glands. Semin Ultrasound CT MRI. 2006;27(6):440–51.
2. Huoh KC, Eisele DW. Etiologic factors in sialolithiasis. Otolaryngol Head Neck Surg. 2011;145(6):935–9.
3. Escudier MP, McGurk M. Symptomatic siloadenitis of sialolithiasis in the English population, and estimate of the cost of hospital treatment. Br Dent J. 1999;186(9):463–6.
4. Drage NA, Brown JE, Escudler MP, McGurk M. Interventional radiology in the removal of salivary calcluli. Radiology. 2000;214(1):139–42.
5. Rabinov JD. Imaging of salivary gland pathology. Radiol Clin North Am. 2000;38(5):1047–57.
6. Yousem DM, Kraut MA, Chalian AA. Major salivary gland imaging. Radiology. 2000;216(1):19–29.
7. Jäger L, Menauer F, Holzknecht N, Scholz V, Grevers G, Reiser M. Sialolithiasis: MR sialography of the submandibular duct—an alternative to conventional sialography and US? Radiology. 2000;216(3):665–71.
8. Koischwitz D, Gritzmann N. Ultrasound of the neck. Radiol Clin North Am. 2000;38(5):1029–45.

9. Alyas F, Lewis K, Williams M, Moody AB, Wong KT, Ahuja AT, et al. Diseases of the submandibular gland as demonstrating using high resolution ultrasound. Br J Radiol. 2005;78(928):362–9.
10. Białek EJ, Jakubowski W, Zajkowski P, Szopinski KT, Osmolski A. US of the major salivary glands: anatomy and spatial relationships, pathologic conditions, and pitfalls. Radiographics. 2006;26(3):745–63.
11. Rabinov K, Weber AL. Radiology of the salivary glands. Boston, MA: GK. Hall Medical Publishers; 1985.
12. Rzymska-Grala I, Stopa Z, Grala B, Gołębiowski M, Wanyura H, Zuchowska A, et al. Salivary gland calculi—contemporary methods of imaging. Pol J Radiol. 2010;75(3):25–37.
13. Andretta M, Tregnaghi A, Prosenikliev V, Staffieri A. Current opinions in sialolithiasis diagnosis and treatment. Acta Otorhinolaryngol Ital. 2005;25(3):145–9.
14. Marchal F, Dulguerov P. Sialolithiasis management: the state of the art. Arch Otolaryngol Head Neck Surg. 2003;129(9):951–6.
15. Harrison JD. Causes, natural history, and incidence of salivary stones and obstructions. Otolaryngol Clin N Am. 2009;42(6):927–47.
16. Teymoortash A, Wollstein AC, Lippert BM, Peldszus R, Werner JA. Bacteria and pathogenesis of human salivary calculus. Acta Otolaryngol. 2002;122(2):210–4.
17. Brady JM, McKinney L, Stanback JS. Scanning electron microscopy of submandibular sialoliths: a preliminary report. Dentomaxillofac Radiol. 1989;18(1):42–4.
18. Sherman JA, McGurk M. Lack of correlation between water hardness and salivary calculi in England. Br J Oral Maxillofac Surg. 2000;38(1):50–3.
19. Marchal F, Kurt AM, Dulguerov P, Lehmann W. Retrograde theory in sialolithiasis formation. Arch Otolaryngol Head Neck Surg. 2001b;127(1):66–8.
20. Nahlieli O, Shacham R, Yoffe B, Eliav E. Diagnosis and treatment of strictures and kinks in salivary gland ducts. J Oral Maxillofac Surg. 2001;59:484–90.
21. Yuasa K, Nakhayama E, Ban S, Kawazu T, Chikui T, Shimizu M, et al. Submandibular gland duct endoscopy. Diagnostic value for salivary duct disorders in comparison to conventional radiography, sialography, and ultrasonography. Oral Surg Oral Med Oral Pathol Oral Radiol Endod. 1997;84(5):578–81.
22. Diebold S, Overbeck M. Soft tissue disorders of the mouth. Emerg Med Clin North Am. 2019;37(1):55–68.
23. Hasson O. Sialoendoscopy and sialography: strategies for assessment and treatment of salivary gland obstructions. J Oral Maxillofac Surg. 2007;65(2):300–4.
24. Koch M, Zenk J, Iro H. Algorithms for treatment of salivary gland obstructions. Otolaryngol Clin N Am. 2009;42(6):1173–92.
25. Arifa SP, Christopher PJ, Kumar S, Kengasubbiah S, Shenoy V. Sialolithiasis of the submandibular gland: report of cases. Cureus. 2019;11(3):e4180.
26. Pachisia S, Mandal G, Sahu S, Ghosh S. Submandibular sialolithiasis: a series of three case reports with review of literature. Clin Pract. 2019;9(1):1119.
27. Avishai G, Ben-Zvi Y, Ghanaiem O, Chaushu G, Gilat H. Sialolithiasis-do early diagnosis and removal minimize post-operative morbidity? Medicina (Kaunas). 2020;56(7):332.
28. Yu C, Zheng L, Yang C, Shen N. Causes of chronic obstructive parotitis and management by sialoendoscopy. Oral Surg Oral Med Oral Pathol Oral Radiol Endod. 2008;105(3):365–70.
29. Wong KT, Ahuja AT, Yuen HY, et al. Ultrasound of salivary glands. ASUM Ultrasound Bull. 2003;6(3):18–22.
30. Chandra SR. Sialoendoscopy: review and nuances of technique. J Maxillofac Oral Surg. 2019;18(1):1–10.
31. Drage NA, Brown JE. Cone beam computed sialography of sialoliths. Dentomaxillofac Radiol. 2009;38(5):301–5.
32. Ludlow JB, Ivanovic M. Comparative dosimetry of dental CBCT devices and 64-slice CT for oral and maxillofacial radiology. Oral Surg Oral Med Oral Pathol Oral Radiol Endod. 2008;106(1):106–14.
33. Scarfe WC, Farman AG, Sukovic P. Clinical applications of cone-beam computed tomography in dental practice. J Can Dent Assoc. 2006;72(1):75–80.

34. Capaccio P, Cuccarini V, Ottaviani F, Minorati D, Sambataro G, Cornalba P, et al. Comparative ultrasonographic, magnetic resonance sialographic, and videoendoscopic assessment of salivary duct disorders. Ann Otol Rhinol Laryngol. 2008;117(4):245–52.
35. Obaid H, Sinha R, Robinson L. Submandibular sialogram performed through a Wharton's duct fistula: technical adaptation of conventional technique. Eur J Radiol. 2006;60(1):56–7.
36. Kalinowski M, Heverhagen JT, Rehberg E, Klose KJ, Wagner HJ. Comparative study of MR sialography and digital subtraction sialography for benign salivary gland disorders. AJNR Am J Neuroradiol. 2002;23(9):1485–92.
37. McGahan JP, Walter JP, Bernstein L. Evaluation of the parotid gland. Comparison of sialography, non-contrast computed tomography and CT sialography. Radiology. 1984;152(2):453–8.
38. Becker M, Marchal F, Becker CD, Dulguerov P, Georgakopoulos G, Lehmann W, et al. Sialolithiasis and salivary ductal stenosis: diagnostic accuracy of MR sialography with a three-dimensional extended-phase conjugate-symmetry rapid spin-echo sequence. Radiology. 2000;217(2):347–58.
39. Aidan P, De Kerviler E, LeDuc A, Monteil JP. Treatment of salivary stones by extracorporeal lithotripsy. Am J Otolaryngol. 1996;17(4):246–50.
40. Capaccio P, Ottaviani F, Manzo R, Schindler A, Cesana B. Extracorporeal lithotripsy for salivary calculi: a long-term clinical experience. Laryngoscope. 2004;114(6):1069–73.
41. Iro H, Zenk J, Waldfahrer F, Benzel W, Schneider T, Ell C. Extracorporeal shock wave lithotripsy of parotid stones. Results of a prospective clinical trial. Ann Otol Rhinol Laryngol. 1998;107(10 Pt 1):860–4.
42. Gutmann R, Ziegler G, Leunig A, Jacob K, Feyh J. Endoscopic and extracorporeal shock wave lithotripsy of salivary calculi. Laryngorhinootologie. 1995;74(4):249–53.
43. Marchal F, Becker M, Dulguerov P, Lehmann W. Interventional sialendoscopy. Laryngoscope. 2000;110(2 Pt 1):318–20.
44. Marchal F, Dulguerov P, Lehmann W. Interventional sialendoscopy. N Engl J Med. 1999;341(16):1242–3.
45. Marchal F, Dulguerov P, Becker M, Barki G, Disant F, Lehmann W. Specificity of parotid sialendoscopy. Laryngoscope. 2001a;111(2):264–71.
46. Marchal F, Dulguerov P, Becker M, Barki G, Disant F, Lehmann W. Submandibular diagnostic and interventional sialendoscopy: new procedure for ductal disorders. Ann Otol Rhinol Laryngol. 2002;111(1):27–35.
47. Nahlieli O, Baruchin AM. Endoscopic technique for the diagnosis and treatment of obstructive salivary gland diseases. J Oral Maxillofac Surg. 1999;57(12):1394–401.
48. Nahlieli O, Nakar LH, Nazarian Y, Turner MD. Sialoendoscopy: a new approach to salivary gland obstructive pathology. J Am Dent Assoc. 2006;137:1394–400.
49. Phillips J, Withrow K. Outcomes of holmium laser-assisted lithotripsy with sialendoscopy in treatment of sialolithiasis. Otolaryngol Head Neck Surg. 2014;150(6):962–7.
50. Gallo A, Benazzo M, Capaccio P, De Campora L, De Vincentiis M, Fusconi M, et al. Sialoendoscopy: state-of-the-art, challenges and further perspectives. Round table, 101st SIO National Congress, Catania 2014. Acta Otorhinolaryngol Ital. 2015;35:217–33.
51. Marchal F. A combined endoscopic and external approach for extraction of large stones with preservation of parotid and submandibular glands. Laryngoscope. 2007;117(2):373–7.
52. Capaccio P, Torretta S, Pignataro L. The role of adenectomy for salivary gland obstructions in the era of sialendoscopy and lithotripsy. Otolaryngol Clin N Am. 2009;42(6):1161–71.

Inflammatory Disorders of the Parotid Gland (Parotitis)

8

8.1 Introduction

Parotitis is inflammation of the parotid gland and is the most common inflammation of the major salivary glands. It can present as a local process or as a manifestation of systemic illness. Parotitis is caused by duct obstruction (such as sialolithiasis), infectious organisms (viruses or bacteria), or inflammatory/autoimmune conditions [such as Sjögren's syndrome, rheumatoid arthritis, systemic lupus erythematosus [SLE], and sarcoidosis]. Parotitis can result in pain and discomfort, glandular enlargement and swelling, dry mouth, and sometimes fever. Predisposing factors include dehydration, malnutrition, immunosuppression, sialolithiasis, oral neoplasms, and medications, causing decreased salivation. Rare complications of parotitis or parotid procedures include osteomyelitis, Lemierre syndrome (extension of infection into the lateral pharyngeal spaces of the neck with subsequent septic thrombophlebitis of the internal jugular vein(s) (IJV)], sepsis, organ failure, and facial paralysis [1, 2].

8.2 Clinical Presentation

8.2.1 History-Taking

Patients with parotitis usually complain of progressive enlargement and pain in one or both glands. Bilateral parotid involvement is typical for mumps and inflammatory conditions, whereas unilateral parotid swelling, pain, and the presence of fever are more suggestive of bacterial cause. In addition, patients will complain of pain with mastication localizing to the parotid and radiating to the ear, often subsiding within 30–60 min after eating.

© The Author(s), under exclusive license to Springer Nature Switzerland AG 2024
M. Sakr, *Surgery of the Salivary Glands*,
https://doi.org/10.1007/978-3-031-82069-4_8

8.2.2 Physical Examination

On examination, the parotid gland typically appears enlarged, edematous, tender, indurated, and warm. When the parotid is gently massaged in a posterior to anterior direction, bacterial parotitis will exhibit purulent drainage from Stensen's duct. In contrast, small yellow crystal chunks favor an autoimmune cause [3]. Acute parotitis is typically tender and warm, whereas chronic autoimmune parotitis is frequently nontender. Sialolithiasis presents with swelling around Stensen's duct, often with a visible or palpable stone.

8.3 Evaluation

8.3.1 Laboratory Studies

In general, parotitis is a clinical diagnosis. If bacterial parotitis is suspected, drainage from Stensen's duct (pus) is sent for Gram stain, culture, and sensitivity. Other laboratory studies are supportive of diagnosis but are nonspecific; these include elevated serum amylase, white blood cell (WBC) count, C-reactive protein (CRP), and erythrocyte sedimentation rate (ESR) levels.

8.3.2 Imaging Studies

Imaging is rarely necessary for the evaluation of parotitis. Ultrasonography (US) might confirm sialolithiasis and can identify abscesses, differentiate between solid and cystic masses within the gland, and identify hypoechoic areas frequently seen in punctate sialectasis [4].

Plain radiography or CT scan, with or without contrast, can confirm sialolithiasis, and rarely multiple parotid calcifications in chronic parotitis, whereas MRI can be used to differentiate between chronic parotitis and neoplastic changes within the gland. In cases of HIV parotitis, MRI can be diagnostic by demonstrating multiple cyst formation.

Sialography is the historical "gold standard" and could provide detailed visualization of the parotid ductal system and acini; however, it is not a common procedure [5]. Instead, sialendoscopy has proven useful in chronic parotitis and juvenile recurrent parotitis cases [6–9].

8.3.3 Biopsy

Incisional or fine-needle biopsy of the parotid tail, performed by an experienced surgeon carefully avoiding the facial nerve, can be sent for culture for suspected infectious source or histopathology useful to determine parotitis etiology. However, a biopsy is not generally needed to make the diagnosis. Lymphoepithelial cysts occur in HIV parotitis, non-caseating granulomata are present in sarcoid parotitis, and lymphocytic invasion with acinar destruction can be characteristic of neoplastic lymphoma.

8.4 Management

8.4.1 Conservative Treatment

Treatment of parotitis is primarily symptomatic control with a focus on the local warm fomentation, gentle glandular massage from posterior to anterior, sialagogues, and adequate hydration. Simple anti-inflammatory analgesics, such as acetaminophen or ibuprofen, are sufficient for discomfort. If purulent drainage is expressed during the glandular massage, culture and sensitivities should be obtained by swab or needle aspiration to guide proper antibiotic therapy [10–12].

8.4.2 Surgical Treatment

Superficial parotidectomy is usually the last resort for chronic parotitis and may involve ligation of the duct or the instillation of methylene violet [13]. Surgery may be necessary for a disfiguring swelling, chronic autoimmune parotitis at risk for neoplastic lymphoma, or adjacent inflammation resulting in facial nerve paralysis.

8.5 Complications

Mumps parotitis can be complicated with inflammatory disorders (orchitis, oophoritis, mastitis, pancreatitis, meningitis, encephalitis, meningoencephalitis, etc.), sensory neural hearing loss, and miscarriage. In rare instances, parotitis can result in septic thrombophlebitis of the IJV (Lemierre syndrome), usually resulting from oro-pharyngeal *Fusobacterium necrophorum* infection) due to proximity and shared venous drainage [14].

Chronic bacterial parotitis can result from chronic autoimmune diseases or untreated acute bacterial infections with resultant glandular ductal inflammation, ductal stenosis, and decreased salivary flow. Rarely, fistula formation can occur. Neoplasms, such as lymphoma, can result from chronic autoimmune parotitis.

Facial paralysis is a rare complication, but can occur from chronic inflammation from Sjögren's syndrome, SLE, or the rare sarcoidosis Heerfordt–Waldenstrom (or uveo-parotid fever) syndrome [15]. Parotid biopsy or surgery can also result in facial nerve injury.

Xerostomia is uncomfortable, interferes with feeding due to alterations in taste (dysgeusia) and chewing process from lack of lubricant necessary for food bolus formation, and may result in malnutrition.

A rare parotitis complication involving hyperhidrosis and numbness on the cheek in front of the ear during salivation (eating or thinking of food) is known as Frey syndrome (auriculotemporal syndrome, also Baillarger or Dupuy or Frey–Baillarger syndrome). It is caused by damage to the auriculotemporal nerve, a branch of the mandibular trigeminal nerve [16]. Eagle syndrome, a pharyngeal foreign body sensation and cervicofacial pain with an elongated styloid process, which is much more commonly caused by trauma or tonsillectomy, can rarely follow acute parotitis [13, 17].

8.6 Prognosis

Parotitis carries a relatively favorable prognosis for all forms, and underlying diseases determine the prognosis. Most cases of parotitis resolve spontaneously or with antibacterial treatment without recurrence or complication. Children may present with juvenile recurrent parotitis that can be symptomatic for days to weeks and may require a partial parotidectomy. Neonatal parotitis can be life-threatening. Rarely, acute bacterial parotitis can lead to osteomyelitis, sepsis, organ failure, and death [18].

8.7 Viral Infections

8.7.1 Mumps (Acute Viral Parotitis)

8.7.1.1 Epidemiology

Universal immunization has made mumps an uncommon disease in developed countries. All children must receive their first measles, mumps, and rubella (MMR) vaccine at 1 year and a second shot at the age of 4–6 years. However, mumps is still found worldwide [19] and is the most common cause of inflammation of the salivary glands [20]. In the absence of vaccination against mumps, 0.1–1.0% of the population is infected each year. The number of cases peaks every 2–5 years [21], with incidence highest in children 5–9 years old [22]. Furthermore, 50% of 4–6 year olds, 90% of 14–15 year olds, and 95% of adults had tested positive to prior exposure to mumps, indicating that nearly all people are eventually infected in unvaccinated populations [23, 24]. Symptoms are more severe in adolescents and adults than in children [25].

Cases of mumps peak in different seasons of the year in different regions. In temperate climates, cases peak in winter and spring, whereas in tropical regions no seasonality is observed [26]. The seasonality of mumps is thought to be caused by several factors; fluctuation in the human immune response due to seasonal factors, such as changes in melatonin levels; behavior and lifestyle changes, such as school attendance and indoor crowding; and meteorological factors, such as changes in temperature, brightness, wind, and humidity [24].

8.7.1.2 Etiology/Transmission

Mumps is a specific acute viral infection caused by mumps virus (MuV), an RNA virus that belongs to the family "Paramyxoviridae" [27]. It is mainly transmitted by inhalation or oral contact with respiratory droplets or secretion [23]. The mumps virus is excreted in saliva from approximately 7 days before to 8 days after the onset of symptoms [24], peaking at the onset of parotitis [23], though it has also been identified in the saliva of asymptomatic individuals [23]. During infection, the virus first infects the upper respiratory tract. From there, it spreads to the salivary glands and lymph nodes (LNs). Infection of the LNs leads to the presence of the virus in blood, which spreads the virus throughout the body.

Mother-to-child has been observed in various forms. MuV has been isolated from newborns of infected mothers. While MuV has been detected in breast milk, it is unclear if the virus can be transmitted through it [23]. Other means of transmission include direct contact with infected droplets or saliva, fomites contaminated by saliva, and possibly urine [28–30]. Most transmissions likely occur before the development of symptoms and up to 5 days after such time [28].

8.7.1.3 Pathogenesis

Many aspects of the pathogenesis of mumps are poorly understood. Following exposure, the virus infects epithelial cells in the upper respiratory tract that express sialic acid receptors on their surface. After infection, the virus spreads to the parotid glands, causing the signature parotitis [31]. It is thought that shortly after infection the virus spreads to LNs, which leads to viremia [23, 24] that lasts for 7–10 days, during which MuV spreads throughout the body [29].

8.7.1.4 Clinical Picture

The incubation period (IP is about 7–25 days, averaging 16–18 days) [19, 24]. Approximately 20–40% [28] of infections are "asymptomatic" or are restricted to mild respiratory symptoms, sometimes with a fever [21]. Over the course of the disease, three distinct phases are recognized; prodromal, early acute, and established acute. The "prodromal phase" typically has nonspecific, mild symptoms such as a low-grade fever, headache, malaise, muscle pain, loss of appetite, and sore throat [32–34]. In the "early acute phase," as the mumps virus spreads throughout the body, systemic symptoms emerge. Most commonly, parotitis occurs during this time period. During the "established acute phase," orchitis, meningitis, and encephalitis may occur, and these conditions are responsible for the bulk of mumps' morbidity [23].

Parotitis is the most common symptom of mumps and occurs in about 90% [21] of symptomatic cases and 60–70% of total infections [29]. In 85% of cases, it affects the school-age children under the age of 15 years. During mumps parotitis, usually both the parotid glands experience painful swelling [29], with unilateral swelling in a small percentage of cases [20]. Parotitis occurs 2–3 weeks after exposure to the virus, within 2 days of developing symptoms, and usually lasts 2–3 days, but it may last as long as a week or longer [23, 33]. In the absence of

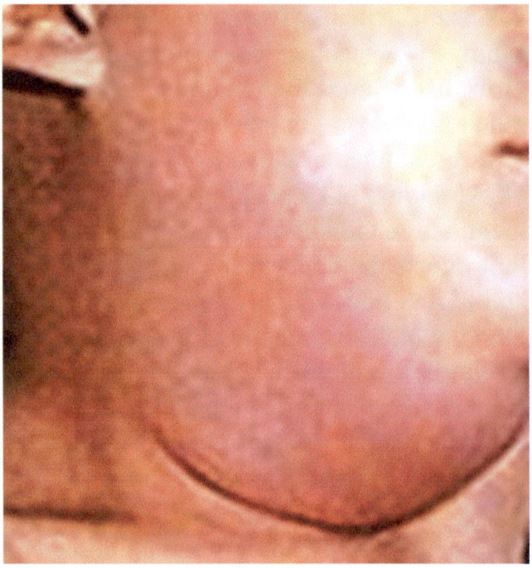

Fig. 8.1 Mumps in a child with a smooth enlargement of the right parotid gland

vaccination, infection normally occurs in childhood, most frequently at the ages of 5–9. Symptoms and complications are more common in males and more severe in adolescents and adults.

The mumps virus causes fever and is considered the most common cause of acute painful profuse swelling of the parotid gland (Fig. 8.1). The gland is soft and tender, but never suppurates. Impingement on the auriculo-temporal and great auricular nerves causes much pain as the gland is pressured during mastication. Symptoms usually resolve within 5–10 days. The parotid duct may become red, swollen, and filled with fluid. Parotitis is usually preceded by local tenderness and occasionally earache [24, 35]. Other salivary glands may also swell. Inflammation of these glands is rarely the only symptom [23].

8.7.1.5 Complications

Inflammatory Conditions

Orchitis

Orchitis is the most common complication of mumps. Pain, swelling, and warmness of a testis appear usually 1–2 weeks [30] after the onset of parotitis, but can occur up to 6 weeks later. During mumps orchitis, the scrotum is tender and inflamed. It occurs in 10–40% of pubertal and postpubertal males who contract mumps. Usually, mumps orchitis affects only one testis but in 10–30% of cases both are affected [30]. Mumps orchitis is accompanied by inflammation of the epididymis (epididymitis), about 85% of the time, typically occurring before orchitis. The onset of mumps orchitis is associated with a high-grade fever, vomiting, headache, and malaise [23, 29]. In prepubertal males, orchitis is rare as symptoms are usually restricted to parotitis [29].

Other Frequent Inflammatory Conditions

A variety of other inflammatory conditions may also occur as a result of mumps virus infection, including [30]:

- Mastitis, in up to about 30% of postpubertal women [22].
- Oophoritis, in 5–10% of postpubertal women, which usually presents as pelvic pain.
- Pancreatitis, in about 4% of cases, which causes severe pain and tenderness in the upper abdomen below the ribs.
- Aseptic meningitis, in 5–10% of cases [36] and 4–6% of those with parotitis, typically occurring 4–10 days after the onset of symptoms. Mumps meningitis can also occur up to 1 week before parotitis as well as in the absence of parotitis. It is commonly accompanied by fever, headache, vomiting, and neck stiffness [31].
- Encephalitis, in <0.5% of cases [36], usually accompanied with fever, altered consciousness, seizures, and weakness. It also can occur in the absence of parotitis [31].
- Meningoencephalitis, commonly accompanied by fever 97% of the time, vomiting 94%, and headache 88.8% of the time [37].
- Nephritis, which is rare because kidney involvement in mumps is usually benign, leads to the presence of the virus in urine.
- Recurrent sialadenitis, which is frequent [19].

Other Rare Inflammatory Conditions

- Other rare inflammatory conditions that may complicate mumps include polyarthritis (affecting at least five joints) [25], polyneuritis, pneumonia [19], acalculous cholecystitis, keratouveitis, thyroiditis, hepatitis, retinitis, corneal endothelitis, transverse myelitis, encephalomyelitis [25], and ascending polyradiculitis [22, 23].
- Rarely, myocarditis and pericarditis can also occur.

Neurosensory Deafness

A relatively common complication of mumps is deafness, which occurs in about 4% of cases [21]. Mumps deafness is often accompanied by vestibular symptoms such as vertigo and repetitive, uncontrolled eye movement.

Hydrocephalus

Fluid buildup in the brain (hydrocephalus) has also been observed and reported as a complication of mumps infection [23, 31].

Miscarriage

In the first trimester of pregnancy, mumps may increase the risk of miscarriage because of fetal endocardial fibroelastosis. Otherwise, mumps is not associated with birth defects [22, 35].

Other Rare Complications

Other rare complications of mumps infection include paralysis, a polio-like disease, seizures, cranial nerve palsies, cerebellar ataxia, arthropathy, autoimmune hemolytic anemia [23], idiopathic thrombocytopenic purpura (ITP), Guillain–Barre syndrome, and hemophagocytic syndrome [29]. Mumps has also been connected to the onset of type 1 diabetes, and, relatedly, the MuV is able to infect and replicate in insulin-producing beta cells [38].

8.7.1.6 Diagnosis

In places where mumps is widespread, diagnosis can be made clinically based on the development of parotitis and history of exposure to someone with mumps. In places where mumps is less common, because parotitis has other causes, laboratory diagnosis may be needed to verify mumps infection [21]. Laboratory findings include leukocytopenia with relative lymphocytosis. Serum amylase peaks in the first week and normalizes by the second or third week. MuV can be isolated from saliva, blood, the nasopharynx, salivary ducts [33], and seminal fluid within 1 week of the onset of symptoms [29], as well as from cell cultures [21].

Soluble antibodies directed against the nucleoprotein core of the virus appear within the final week of infection and disappear within 8 months. Antibodies directed against the outer surface appear several weeks after soluble antibodies and persist for 5 years. Mumps-specific IgM antibodies in serum or oral fluid specimens can be used to identify mumps. IgM quantities peak up to 8 days after the onset of symptoms [21], and IgM can be measured by enzyme-linked immunosorbent assay (ELISA) 7–10 days after the onset of symptoms with a sensitivity ranging from as low as 24–51% [29] to 75% in the first week and 100% thereafter [35]. Antibody titers can also be measured with complement fixation tests (CFTs), hemagglutination assays, and neutralization tests [31]. Real-time reverse transcription polymerase chain reaction (rRT-PCR) can be used to detect MuV RNA from the first day symptoms appear, declining over the next 8–10 days [21].

8.7.1.7 Differential Diagnosis

A differential diagnosis may be used to compare symptoms of mumps infection to other diseases, including allergic reaction, mastoiditis, measles, and pediatric human immunodeficiency virus (HIV) infection and rubella [19].

8.7.1.8 Prevention

Infection with MuV can be prevented with vaccination using live-attenuated viruses [19], either via an individual mumps vaccine [39] or through combination vaccines such as the MMR vaccine (the most common vaccine used in most countries) [21], which also protects against measles and rubella. The spread of the disease can also be prevented by isolating infected individuals and those who are suspected to be infected [40].

8.7.1.9 Treatment

Mumps is usually self-limiting, and no specific antiviral treatments exist, so treatment is aimed at alleviating symptoms and preventing complications. Supportive treatment includes rest, analgesics for pain relief [22], sialagogues, rehydration, eating soft food, and gargling with warm salt water [29, 32]. Antipyretics may be used during the febrile period [22], excluding aspirin when given to children, as it may cause Reye syndrome [33]. Antibiotics may be used as a precaution in cases in which bacterial infection cannot be ruled out and prevent secondary bacterial infection [29, 30]. For seizures, anticonvulsants may be used. In severe neurological cases, ventilators may be used to support breathing [35].

Intramuscular (IM) mumps immunoglobulin (Ig) may be of benefit when administered early in some cases, but it has not shown benefit in outbreaks. Although not recommended, intravenous (IV) Ig therapy may reduce the rates of some complications [29]. Autoimmune-based disorders related to mumps are treatable with IV Ig [22].

8.7.1.10 Prognosis

Prognosis for most people who experience mumps is excellent, even in high-risk groups such as immunocompromised persons, since long-term complications and death are rare. Hospitalization is typically not required [28]. Mumps is usually self-limiting and symptoms resolve spontaneously within 2 weeks as the immune system clears the virus from the body [23, 29]. For most people, infection leads to lifelong immunity against future infection. Reinfections appear to be more mild and atypical than the first infection [29]. The overall case mortality rate of mumps is 1.6–3.8 people per 10,000, and these deaths typically occur in those who develop encephalitis [23].

Mumps orchitis typically resolves within 2 weeks. However, the testicles may be tender for a few more weeks in 20% of cases, and atrophy, or reduction of size, of the involved testicle occurs in 30–50% of orchitis cases, which may lead to hypofertility in 13% of cases, and rarely sterility [23, 29, 30].

Mumps meningitis typically resolves within 3–10 days without long-term complications [33]. The mortality rate of patients with CNS involvement is approximately 1% [24, 35]. Most cases of mumps deafness affect just one ear and are temporary, but permanent hearing loss occurs in 0.005% of infections [22, 23]. Myocarditis and pericarditis that occur as a result of mumps may lead to endocardial fibroelastosis (thickening of endocardium) [22, 35]. With extreme rarity, infertility and premature menopause have occurred as a result of mumps oophoritis [23].

8.7.2 Non-Mumps Viral Parotitis

Parotitis with the same clinical picture as that described for mumps can be caused by other viral agents; namely, coxsackie A and B virus, influenza and parainfluenza (types 1 and 3) viruses, echovirus, cytomegalovirus (CMV), enterovirus, and lymphocytic choriomeningitis virus.

From 2014 to 2015, 256 cases of influenza-related parotitis were observed in 27 states in the USA. Parotitis mainly occurs in patients under the age of 20 years and tends to be painful and unilateral [41].

8.7.3 Human Immunodeficiency Virus (HIV)-Associated Sialadenitis

Human immunodeficiency virus (HIV) may cause parotitis with generalized lymphadenopathy and localized enlargement of parotid glands [42].

8.7.3.1 Pathophysiology

Human immunodeficiency virus (HIV) can result in asymptomatic, firm parotid swelling, more pronounced in children than adults, due to CD8+ lymphocytes responding to HIV or other viruses, such as Epstein–Barr virus (EBV), hepatitis C virus (HCV), cytomegalovirus (CMV), or adenovirus, infiltrating and ultimately depositing in the gland.

8.7.3.2 Clinical Picture

The presentation is in the form of chronic, bilateral enlargement of parotid glands where the glands are painless, hard, and nodular, and the patient is generally asymptomatic. However, the condition may be associated with xerostomia and xerophthalmia, being so similar to the classical Sjögren's syndrome in adulthood. Although both conditions share similar histological characteristics, yet HIV-associated sialadenitis is usually associated with a negative autoantibody screen. Multiple glandular cyst causing gross parotid swelling and facial disfigurement is another pattern of presentation. Approximately 30% of HIV-infected children have been reported to have enlargement of their parotid glands. In addition, patients with HIV are more susceptible to infection with CMV and adenoviruses as causative agents for non-mumps parotitis [43, 44].

8.7.3.3 Investigations

Useful imaging tools include ultrasound (US), computed tomography (CT) scan, and magnetic resonance imaging (MRI). The latter two demonstrate the characteristic "Swiss cheese" appearance of multiple large cystic lesions (Fig. 8.2). They can also guide fine-needle aspiration (FNA), which reveals serous fluid with the presence of lymphocytes and macrophages. As the parotid gland contains many LNs at different levels, they might be enlarged as the HIV virus mainly affects the lymphoid tissue.

8.7.3.4 Treatment

Treatment of HIV parotitis may include antiviral therapy, low-dose radiation, or partial parotidectomy to reduce glandular size and improve the cosmetic appearance; it is the sole indication of surgery [43–46].

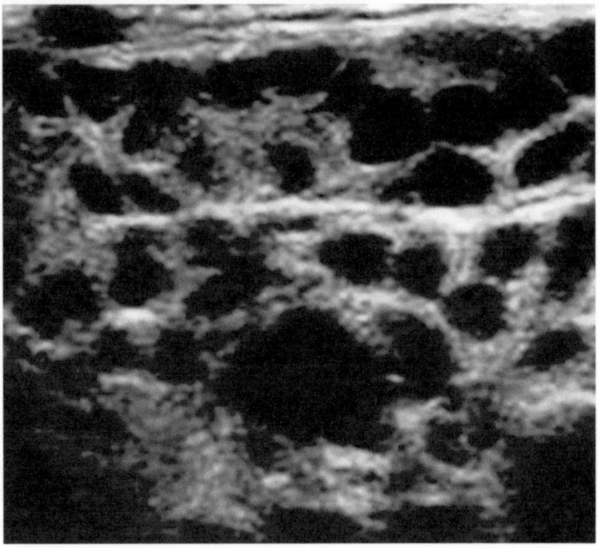

Fig. 8.2 Magnetic resonance imaging (MRI) showing the characteristic "Swiss cheese" appearance of multiple large cystic lesions of human immunodeficiency virus (HIV) parotitis

8.8 Bacterial Infections

8.8.1 Acute Bacterial Parotitis/Acute Suppurative Parotitis (Abscess) [12]

8.8.1.1 Epidemiology

Acute bacterial parotitis is uncommon and has a similar male–female ratio, but it especially concerns the extremes of age. In the elderly population, it is a significant risk, particularly after abdominal surgery, and can be fatal if it occurs in neonates if left without treatment [47]. It is more common in older patients because they often take medications with an atropine effect, causing reduced salivary flow and predisposing them to ascending infection. Acute bacterial parotitis accounts for an estimated 0.01–0.02% of hospital admissions, and occurs in 0.002–0.04% of postoperative patients [10]. Acute neonatal parotitis is rare, with a prevalence of <4 per 10,000 admissions [48].

8.8.1.2 Etiology/Causative Organisms

The infective organism can be any of the following bacteriae: *Staphylococcus aureus*, *Streptococcus viridans*, penicillin-resistant coagulase-positive *Staphylococcus*, *Streptococcus pneumonia*, beta-hemolytic *Streptococcus*, methicillin-resistant *Staphylococcus aureus* (MRSA), or Gram-negative germs, such as *coli*. Studies have shown the presence of 30–40% of anaerobic bacteria; bacteroides, pepto-streptococcus, fusobacteria. In Southeast Asia, *Pseudomonas pseudomallei* from contaminated water have been reported [49]. *Mycobacterium tuberculosis* (TB) is a rare cause of parotitis seen in immunocompromised patients with delayed diagnosis. Hospitalized or immunosuppressed patients may develop candida parotitis. In many cases, the infection is a mixed one.

8.8.1.3 Pathophysiology

A ductal valve creates a unidirectional flow of saliva out of the gland, preventing bacteria from entering. However, this valve may sometimes become incompetent and result in ascending retrograde bacterial infection. Dehydration caused by septicemia, after major surgery, bad oral hygiene, or "drying" medications, such as atropine, antihistamines, and psychotropic agents, which decrease salivary production and flow, can increase the risk of parotitis from either infectious or inflammatory causes. Sialolithiasis is a common condition where calculi formed from inorganic crystals can obstruct the gland duct, although less common in the parotid than submandibular glands due to serous rather than mucoid saliva. Bacteria trapped behind a high-grade obstruction can proliferate and result in acute suppurative parotitis [50]. In the hospital setting, both methicillin-resistant *Staphylococcus aureus* (MRSA) and atypical infections, such as candida, should be considered. However, sometimes the condition is totally idiopathic.

Parotid glands are affected more frequently than submandibular glands. One of the possible reasons is that the bacteriostatic activity of the saliva secreted by the parotid gland is inferior to that secreted by the submandibular gland as the former is predominantly serous and thus lacks the protective constituents (IgA, sialic acid, and lysozomes) seen in mucinous secretions of the other salivary glands.

8.8.1.4 Clinical Presentation

Acute suppurative parotitis is more commonly seen in diabetics. The patient generally complains of anorexia, fever, tachycardia, and malaise. Over several hours, the local condition starts with a swelling, which is very tender, hot, and with throbbing pain that is exacerbated by mastication. The gland size may reach 3–4 times larger than that of the normal gland, which is usually diffuse but may localize to the lower pole. The skin overlying the gland is red, edematous, and tethered (Fig. 8.3). Movements of the ipsilateral temporomandibular joint (TMJ) are restricted and painful. Upper deep cervical LNs are enlarged and tender.

The parotid gland, being enclosed in a dense capsule, is liable to fulminating inflammation and necrosis due to increased tension within this tightly closed fascial compartment. Fluctuation is difficult to elicit and is never waited for. Pus may exude from the duct orifice on massage of the gland, which is in spite of being painful at the moment; it relieves the pressure inside the ductal system and thence the pain. Diseases of the parotid gland cause pain to be referred to the ear, the TMJ, and the external auditory meatus (EAM). This is due to the overlapping of sensory branches of various nerves serving the regions of the parotid bed, ear, and TMJ. Infections of the parotid gland may be confused with toothache as a result of trigeminal nerve (CN-V) involvement. An inflamed parotid papilla (parotid duct orifice in the oral cavity) provides clue to diagnosis.

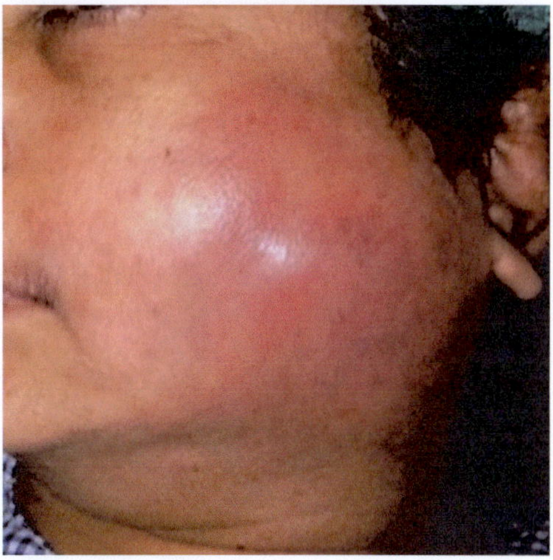

Fig. 8.3 Large left parotid abscess with erythematous, edematous, and tethered overlying skin in a 41-year-old woman

A parotid abscess may be complicated by local spread in the form of cellulitis, chronicity due to inadequate management, development of a fistula, septicemia, and rupture into the EAM or along the carotid sheath.

8.8.1.5 Evaluation

Acute bacterial parotitis is a clinical diagnosis. If drainage from Stensen's duct is present, a specimen is sent for Gram stain, culture, and sensitivity of bacterial parotitis. Serum amylase level will be elevated in many cases, but is nonspecific. Amylase level is less likely to rise in Sjögren's syndrome or parotid tumors. Elevated inflammatory markers, such as white blood cell (WBC) count, C-reactive protein (CRP), and erythrocyte sedimentation rate (ESR), are supportive, but also nonspecific.

Sialography is contraindicated during acute infection and US or CT scan (Fig. 8.4) may be needed; however, the diagnosis is mostly done on clinical grounds.

8.8.1.6 Prophylaxis/Treatment

Prophylaxis against the development of acute suppurative parotitis is considered much safer through adopting good oral hygiene, preventing dehydration, and early adequate correction of electrolyte imbalance.

As an early treatment of any inflammatory condition affecting the parotid gland, one should use warm local fomentations, IV antibiotics (for 7–10 days) [12], anti-inflammatory agents, and analgesics. In community-acquired bacterial parotitis, the first-line treatment is with anti-staphylococcal penicillin (nafcillin, oxacillin), first-generation cephalosporin (cefazolin), vancomycin, or clindamycin for suspected MRSA [51]. For healthcare-associated parotitis, cefoxitin, ertapenem, or ampicillin/sulbactam, with levofloxacin, clindamycin, or piperacillin-tazobactam can be used as alternatives. For patients at high risk of MRSA, vancomycin should be started or linezolid or daptomycin use as alternatives. In case of dental infection,

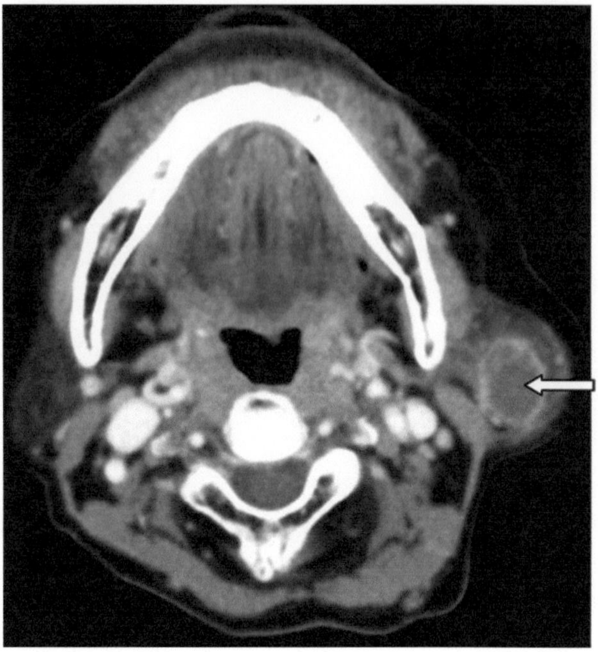

Fig. 8.4 Contrasted computed tomography (CT) scan showing parotid abscess with hypodense content and contrast enhancement (white arrow)

parotitis should prompt the use of clindamycin or metronidazole (anaerobic coverage) and ceftriaxone or piperacillin-tazobactam as an alternative. In neonates, where acute parotitis can be life-threatening, antibiotics are usually IV gentamicin or levofloxacin and anti-MRSA anti-staphylococcal antibiotics. If clinical improvement does not take place within 48 h, parotidectomy may be necessary. The rare parotitis from extrapulmonary tuberculosis responds well to anti-tuberculous medications.

When suppuration ensues (known by throbbing pain, hectic fever, aspirated pus, or US-identified abscess formation), formal drainage under general anesthesia becomes necessary. For decompression of the parotid (Hilton's method), do not wait for fluctuation. Under general anesthesia, a vertical incision is done in the skin down to the parotid capsule. The capsule in then incised transversely along the course of the branches of the facial nerve to avoid their injury. Pus is evacuated, a drain is put in the lower part of the incision for 24–72 h, then closure is achieved. Complications of this procedure include parotid fistula and facial nerve injury. Alternatively, the skin incision may be made low to avoid injury of the lower branch of the facial nerve.

8.8.2 Chronic Bacterial Parotitis

Chronic bacterial sialadenitis is rare in the parotid gland. It may result from improper treatment of acute parotitis, presence of stones in the duct, or stenosis of Stenson's duct due to injury [52]. The more common factor is decreased salivary flow, which could be secondary to inflammation [53]. In most cases, the chronic disease is either autoimmune or idiopathic, with superimposed bacterial infection, and should not be regarded as a chronic bacterial infection. In chronic, nonspecific parotitis, patients may experience painful parotid inflammation lasting for hours to weeks with relatively asymptomatic periods.

8.8.3 Actinomycosis

Actinomycosis affects LNs adjacent to salivary glands, mimicking a salivary gland infection. The pathogen is *Actinomyces israelii*, *A. proprionica*, *A. viscosus*, or *A. odontolyticus*. Infection may be acute, subacute, or chronic. The "acute" form is associated with suppuration, the "subacute" with a slightly tender and tumor-like mass attached to the mandible, and the "chronic" with marked induration that may be misdiagnosed as a neoplasm. The finding of pollen grain-like "sulfur granules" on clinical examination or "sulfur grounds" on pathological evaluation is pathognomonic of this condition. Treatment of the acute phase is surgical, with eventual drainage of the exudates and administration of broad-spectrum antibiotics [54].

8.8.4 Cat Scratch Disease (CSD)

Cat scratch disease is caused by a Gram-negative bacillus called *Bartonella henslae*. The disease originally involves LNs adjacent to salivary glands, which may be secondarily involved by continuous spread. It results from contact with cats, and children or young adults are the most often involved. Laboratory tests include specific PCR or serology. Antibiotics do not seem to shorten the course of the disease, but may be given as prophylaxis against secondary bacterial infection. The affected LNs disappear spontaneously within a few months [55, 56].

8.9 Recurrent Parotitis of Childhood

Recurrent parotitis of childhood, also known as chronic punctate parotitis, is a distinct clinical entity of unknown etiology and unsure prognosis. It is the most frequent nonviral disorder of salivary glands in children [42]. Suggested etiologies include congenital malformation of the parotid ducts, primary or secondary infections, and local manifestations of systemic immunological disease.

The clinical picture comprises fever, malaise, and rapid swelling of one or both parotid glands and pain, which is made worse by mastication. This usually lasts from 3 to 7 days followed by a quiescent period of weeks to several months. The condition may rarely start as early as 4 months of age, but usually children present between the ages of 3 and 6 years and usually resolve around puberty. Diagnosis is made by obtaining typical history and physical examination. Sialography may be confirmatory. It shows a characteristic punctate sialectasis likened to a "snow storm" (Fig. 8.5) that persists until adult life. Sialendoscopy may show diffuse reduction of

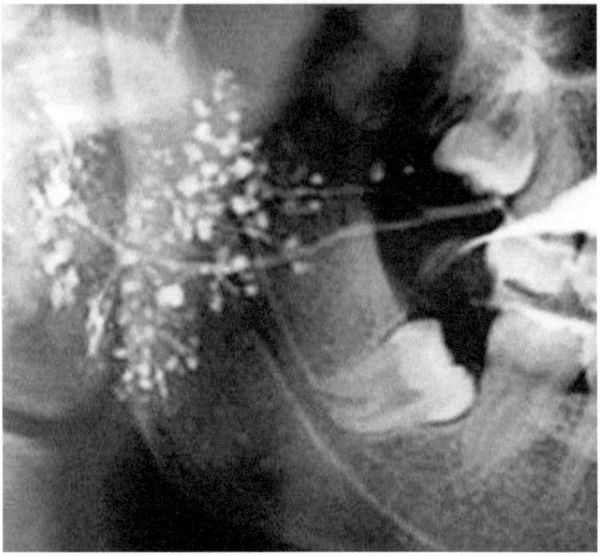

Fig. 8.5 Sialography showing the duct that is normal in course and caliber with dots and blobs appearance at the terminal ductules, the characteristic punctate sialectasis (snow storm appearance)

the caliber of Stensen's duct, associated sometimes with multiple localized stenoses and may be salivary calculi. Endoscopy may also show sialectasia (dilated ductules and acini). Sialendoscopy has proven recently to be effective therapeutically through injection of antiseptic solutions in some cases [42].

No specific treatment is available; however, therapeutic options include good oral hygiene, prophylactic low-dose antibiotics for several months or even years, especially if recurrence is frequent, anti-inflammatory agents, sialendoscopy, and total conservative parotidectomy [57].

8.10 Papillary Obstructive Parotitis

8.10.1 Etiology/Pathophysiology

Although there are many recognized causes of obstructive parotitis, papillary obstruction due to trauma to the parotid papilla through either an overextended upper denture flange or a fractured upper molar tooth is merely the most common of all. Subsequent edema, then fibrosis of the papilla, obstructs salivary flow, especially at meal times, in intermittent, then chronic forms, respectively.

8.10.2 Clinical Presentation

The patient suffers from an intermittent painful swelling of the parotid gland, accumulating over minutes after the start of meal. If stenosis ensues, the symptoms will not resolve except by a papillotomy. Obstructive parotitis is less common than obstructive submandibular sialadenitis.

8.10.3 Evaluation

A study by Wu et al. (2015) indicated that scintigraphy might play an important role in diagnosing chronic obstructive parotitis [58].

8.10.4 Treatment

Sialolithiasis can resolve with warm compresses, massage, and sialagogues (sour food or lemon candy), but occasionally requires extraction. After local anesthesia with topical or infiltrated lidocaine, the duct can be dilated or filleted with scissors and massaged to squeeze out the stone. Extracorporeal shockwave lithotripsy (ESWL) to fragment the stone before extraction or interventional sialoendoscopy by otolaryngology specialists are options for refractory cases [59].

8.11 Granulomatous Sialadenitis

Granulomatous sialadenitis can result from tuberculosis (TB), mycosis, sarcoidosis, or duct obstruction from calculi or malignant tumors. In the latter instance, granulomas result from rupture of ducts and may contain small pools of mucin.

8.11.1 Tuberculosis (TB)

Tuberculosis (TB) infrequently leads to parotitis, but is not considered an important cause, except that around 25% of patients are found to have pulmonary tuberculosis that could infect their associates. *Mycobacterium tuberculosis* and atypical mycobacterium both affect LNs adjacent to salivary glands or intraglandular LNs. The patient may suffer from one or more of the systemic manifestations of TB such as low-grade fever, night sweating, and anemia. The gland is firm and nodular, but may become cystic with sinuses and little pain [60]. Polymerase chain reaction (PCR) is the best preoperative laboratory diagnostic tool, but diagnosis is only confirmed with histopathology after parotidectomy, if needed. Specific treatment includes multidrug anti-TB therapy for an average of 1 year, together with exposure to direct sunlight, good aeration, and well-balanced nutrition, to enhance general health and immunity [60, 61].

8.11.2 Sarcoidosis

Sarcoidosis is a systemic disease that can cause parotid gland inflammation, but is less commonly seen than the involvement of the lungs, LNs, and skin [62]. Its etiology remains unclear, but several hypotheses have been made, including autoantigens and infectious organisms. It resembles TB but with non-caseating granulomas. Salivary glands are usually affected, and specifically the parotid glands.

Symptoms include xerostomia, and chronic, nontender swelling of both parotid glands with minimal symptoms or inflammation. Sometimes, the disease may present as a "tumor" and the diagnosis is only made after surgical excision of the presumed tumor; the sarcoid pseudo-tumor.

Heerfordt–Waldenström syndrome is a rare form of sarcoidosis that involves parotid enlargement, anterior uveitis, facial palsy, and fever (uveo-parotid fever). It affects young patients in their third decade [63].

Laboratory diagnosis of sarcoidosis is made through amylase, kallikrein, and the ACE test. Radiological and histological evidence of non-caseous epithelial granulomas is confirmatory. Corticosteroids are the best therapeutic option.

8.12 Autoimmune Sialadenitis

In autoimmune parotitis such as Sjögren's syndrome (or rheumatoid arthritis), an antigen–antibody complex is endocytosed into epithelial cells, processed into a human leukocyte antigen (HLA) expressed on the cell surface, and recognized by specific CD4 T-lymphocytes, which release cytokines and chemotactic factors augmenting more CD4 activation. B-lymphocytes enter the acini and produce antibodies presenting antigens to CD4 T-cells, with resultant oligoclonal expansion and acinar destruction that can increase the risk of neoplastic transformation. These autoimmune causes result in chronic parotitis, often termed also "chronic punctate parotitis." Chronic parotitis eventually results in scar tissue, stricture, and sialectasis [64].

8.12.1 Mikulicz Disease (MD)

Mikulicz disease (MD) is an autoimmune disease that is characterized by chronic, symmetrical, bilateral enlargement of all salivary and lacrimal glands. It is named after Johann von Mikulicz Radecki and is also called "benign lymphoepithelial lesion" or "myoepithelial sialadenitis." The disease almost always occurs in association with another underlying disease such as TB, leukemia, syphilis, or SLE. Patients may experience recurring fever. There is lymphocytic infiltration, parenchymal atrophy, and myoepithelial islands.

Mikulicz disease affects the parotid glands in 85% and the submandibular glands in 15% of cases, occurring more among women (60–80%) with a mean age of 50 years and causing firm, diffuse enlargement of the affected gland. Patients are usually asymptomatic, but may complain of mild pain and are at a higher risk of developing lymphomas. Some authors believe that it should be considered a form of Sjögren's syndrome (SS). Actually the main clinical difference between MD and SS is the preservation of the lacrimation and salivation in MD due to much less gland cell apoptosis than that found in SS [65].

8.12.2 Sjögren's Syndrome (SS)

Sjögren's syndrome (SS), named after the Swedish ophthalmologist Henrik Samuel Conrad Sjögren, is an autoimmune disorder involving the parotid glands more frequently than the submandibular glands.

Females are affected more than males (10:1). It leads to xerostomia and keratoconjunctivitis sicca due to the progressive destruction of both salivary and lacrimal glands. The diseased gland is occasionally enlarged and is occasionally painful. In most cases, discomfort is modest and related to dry mouth and eyes. Secondary bacterial ascending infection may occur due to xerostomia.

Computed tomography (CT) scan and MRI show bilateral parotid enlargement with heterogeneously enhancing parenchyma. The CT scan may show a honey-comb appearance with low-density foci in a generally enhancing gland (Fig. 8.6).

Histologically, "primary" SS is characterized by massive progressive lymphocytic infiltration, acinar cell destruction, and ductal epithelial cell proliferation affecting all salivary and lacrimal glands. "Secondary" SS differs in that it is associated with a connective tissue disorder, symptoms are less severe, and the incidence of lymphomatous transformation (most commonly monocytoid B-cell lymphoma) is also less [65].

There is no known specific treatment available to stop Sjögren Sjogren's syndrome, and thus, management is totally "symptomatic" (Table 8.1). Artificial tears and periodic ophthalmological examination are mandatory to avoid corneal ulcerations. Artificial salivary substitutes are available, and their importance increases in the dentate patient where fluoride should be added as well. Usually the patient consumes a large amount of water daily, carrying a bottle of water with him all the time [66].

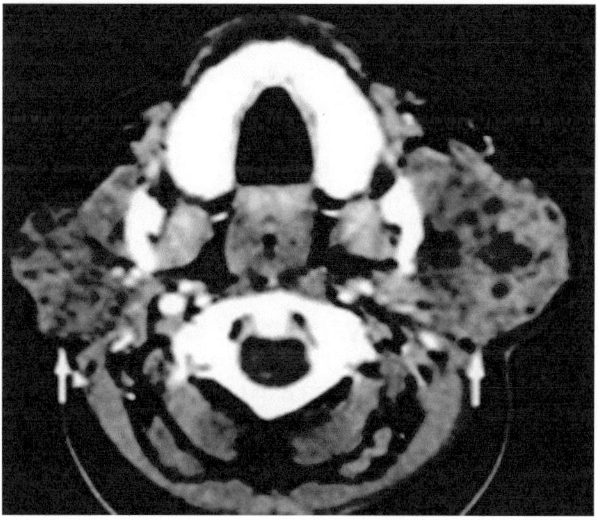

Fig. 8.6 Computed tomography (CT) scan showing honey-comb appearance in a bilaterally enlarged parotid gland (Sjögren's syndrome)

Table 8.1 Symptomatic treatment of Sjögren's syndrome

Dry eyes	Dry mouth	Dry nasal mucosa
– Lubricants: Artificial tears, ointments – Punctal plugs – Lateral tarsorrhaphy	– Saliva substitutes: Sprays, rinses – Salivary stimulation: Hard candy, pilocarpine – Cholinergic agents: Cevimeline hydrochloride – Special toothpaste, oral gel – Active dental care	– Saline nasal sprays – Lavage

8.12.3 Benign Lymphoepithelial Lesion [Myoepithelial Sialadenitis (MESA)]

Myoepithelial sialadenitis (MESA) mostly affects women over 50 years of age. Patients present with a diffusely enlarged, firm, and often painful parotid gland, which is bilateral in 20% of cases. Sialography shows sialectasia, which ranges from punctuate to cavitary. Management is usually surgical (parotidectomy) to establish a final diagnosis.

Histopathological examination of the excised gland carries the very same previously described histopathological features of Sjögren Sjogren's syndrome, and so the differentiation between both is only done on clinical grounds. Prolonged follow-up of such patients is mandatory as 20% of them will develop lymphoma at a certain time [67].

8.12.4 Other Autoimmune Sialadenitis

8.12.4.1 Wegener's Granulomatosis

Wegener's granulomatosis is an autoimmune disease characterized by upper and lower respiratory and renal disease. The most common salivary gland to be involved is the parotid gland [63]; however, this occurs in <1% of the cases [68].

8.12.4.2 Kimura's Disease

Kimura's disease occurs typically in young Asian males and is characterized clinically by painless lymphadenopathy of the head and neck region, including periparotid and intraparotid LNs [63, 67, 69].

8.12.4.3 Chronic Sclerosing Sialadenitis

Chronic sclerosing sialadenitis presents as a firm, localized, swelling of the salivary gland mimicking a neoplasm, most commonly involving the submandibular gland. It may be associated with autoimmune extrasalivary disease such as primary sclerosing cholangitis, and idiopathic retroperitoneal fibrosis [67].

8.13 Uncommon Causes of Parotitis

Uncommon causes of parotitis can include (1) trauma, (2) surgery (such as manipulation during carotid endarterectomy), (3) drug exposure (such as iodides, heavy metals, phenylbutazone, and thiouracil), and (4) radiation therapy, especially whole-brain radiation therapy can lead to parotitis [70].

References

1. Greenberg JS, Breiner MJ. Anatomy, head and neck: auriculotemporal nerve. Treasure Island, FL: StatPearls Publishing; 2023.
2. Alhajj M, Babos M. Physiology, salivation. Treasure Island, FL: StatPearls Publishing; 2023.
3. Majdoub I, Kallel S, Hsairi M, Snoussi M, Charfi M, Ben Halima A, et al. Primary Sjögren syndrome in a child. Arch Pediatr. 2017;24(12):1249–52.
4. Schapher M, Goncalves M, Mantsopoulos K, Iro H, Koch M. Transoral ultrasound in the diagnosis of obstructive salivary gland pathologies. Ultrasound Med Biol. 2019;45(9):2338–48.
5. Tucci FM, Roma R, Bianchi A, De Vincentiis GC, Bianchi PM. Juvenile recurrent parotitis: diagnostic and therapeutic effectiveness of sialography. Retrospective study on 110 children. Int J Pediatr Otorhinolaryngol. 2019;124:179–84.
6. Jáuregui E, Kiringoda R, Ryan WR, Eisele DW, Chang JL. Chronic parotitis with multiple calcifications: clinical and sialendoscopic findings. Laryngoscope. 2017;127(7):1565–70.
7. Erkul E, Gillespie MB. Sialendoscopy for non-stone disorders: the current evidence. Laryngoscope Investig Otolaryngol. 2016;1(5):140–5.
8. Erkul E, Çekin E, Güngör A. Long-term outcomes of sialendoscopy in the management of sialolithiasis and idiopathic chronic sialadenitis with ductal scars. Turk Arch Otorhinolaryngol. 2019;57(2):75–80.
9. Canzi P, Occhini A, Pagella F, Marchal F, Benazzo M. Sialendoscopy in juvenile recurrent parotitis: a review of the literature. Acta Otorhinolaryngol Ital. 2013;33(6):367–73.
10. Fattahi TT, Lyu PE, Van Sickels JE. Management of acute suppurative parotitis. J Oral Maxillofac Surg. 2002;60(4):446–8.
11. Brook I. The bacteriology of salivary gland infections. Oral Maxillofac Surg Clin North Am. 2009;21(3):269–74.
12. Brook I. Acute bacterial suppurative parotitis: microbiology and management. J Craniofac Surg. 2003;14(1):37–40.
13. van der Lans RJL, Lohuis PJFM, van Gorp JMHH, Quak JJ. Surgical treatment of chronic Parotitis. Int Arch Otorhinolaryngol. 2019;23(1):83–7.
14. Alabraba E, Manu N, Fairclough G, Sutton R. Acute parotitis due to MRSA causing Lemierre's syndrome. Oxf Med Case Rep. 2018;2018(5):omx056.
15. Denny MC, Fotino AD. The Heerfordt-Waldenström syndrome as an initial presentation of sarcoidosis. Proc (Bayl Univ Med Cent). 2013;26(4):390–2.
16. Ellies M, Laskawi R. Diseases of the salivary glands in infants and adolescents. Head Face Med. 2010;6:1.
17. Permpalung N, Suksaranjit P, Chongnarungsin D, Hyman CL. Unveiling the hidden eagle: acute parotitis-induced eagle syndrome. N Am J Med Sci. 2014;6(2):102–4.
18. Vorrasi J, Zinberg G. Concomitant suppurative parotitis and condylar osteomyelitis. J Oral Maxillofac Surg. 2017;75(3):543–9.
19. Davison P, Morris J. Mumps. In: StatPearls. Treasure Island, FL: StatPearls Publishing; 2023.
20. Kessler AT, Bhatt AA. Review of the major and minor salivary glands, part 1: anatomy, infectious, and inflammatory processes. J Clin Imaging Sci. 2018;8:47.
21. Lam E, Rosen JB, Zucker JR. Mumps: an update on outbreaks, vaccine efficacy, and genomic diversity. Clin Microbiol Rev. 2020;33(2):e00151–19.

22. Shu M, Zhang YQ, Li Z, Liu GJ, Wan C, Wen Y. Chinese medicinal herbs for mumps. Cochrane Database Syst Rev. 2015;2015(4):CD008578.
23. Rubin S, Eckhaus M, Rennick LJ, Bamford CG, Duprex WP. Molecular biology, pathogenesis and pathology of mumps virus. J Pathol. 2015;235(2):242–52.
24. Su SB, Chang HL, Chen AK. Current status of mumps virus infection: epidemiology, pathogenesis and vaccine. Int J Environ Res Public Health. 2020;17(5):1686.
25. Senanayake SN. Mumps: a resurgent disease with protean manifestaitons. Med J Aust. 2008;189(8):456–9.
26. Beleni AI, Borgmann S. Mumps in the vaccination age: global epidemiology and the situation in Germany. Int J Environ Res Public Health. 2018;15(8):1618.
27. Koenig KL, Shastry S, Mzahim B, Almadhyan A, Burns MJ. Mumps virus: modification of the identify-isolate-inform tool for frontline healthcare providers. West J Emerg Med. 2016;17(5):490–6.
28. Kutty PK, Kyaw MH, Dayan GH, Brady MT, Bocchini JA, Reef SE, et al. Guidance for isolation precautions for mumps in the United States: a review of the scientific basis for policy change. Clin Infect Dis. 2010;50(12):1619–28.
29. Davis NF, McGuire BB, Mahon JA, Smyth AE, O'Malley KJ, Fitzpatrick JM. The increasing incidence of mumps orchitis: a comprehensive review. BJU Int. 2010;105(8):1060–5.
30. Masarani M, Wazait H, Dinneen M. Mumps orchitis. J R Soc Med. 2006;99(11):573–5.
31. Junghanss T. Manson's tropical diseases. 23rd ed. Oxford: Elsevier/Saunders; 2013. p. 261.
32. National Center for Biotechnology Information. Mumps. ADAM Medical Encyclopedia. Archived from the original on 17 October 2014. Retrieved 30 October 2020.
33. Marlow M, Haber P, Hickman C, Patel M. Mumps. Centers for Disease Control and Prevention (CDC). CDC Retrieved 30 October 2020.
34. Rima B, Balkema-Buschmann A, Dundon WG, Duprex P, Easton A, Fouchier R, et al. ICTV virus taxonomy profile: paramyxoviridae. J Gen Virol. 2019;100:1593–4.
35. Gupta RK, Best J, MacMahon E. Mumps and the UK epidemic 2005. BMJ. 2005;330(7500):1132–5.
36. Latner DR, Hickman CJ. Remembering mumps. PLOS Pathog. 2015;11(5):e1004791.
37. Kanra G, Isik P, Kara A, Cengiz AB, Seçmeer G, Ceyhan M. Complementary findings in clinical and apidemiologic features of mumps and mumps meningoencephalitis in children without mumps vaccination. Pediatr Int. 2004;46(6):663–8.
38. Smatti MK, Cyprian FS, Nasrallah GK, Al-Thani AA, Almishal RO, Yassine HM. Viruses and autoimmunity: a review on the potential iinteraction and molecular mechanisms. Viruses. 2019;11(8):762.
39. Noda A, Sakai T, Tsuchiya M, Oyanagi G, Obara T, Mano N. Characteristics of adverse events following immunization reporting in children: the Japanese adverse drug event report database. MDPI. 2020;8:357. https://www.mdpi.com/2076-393X/8/3/357
40. Levine DA. Vaccine-preventable diseases in pediatric patients: a review of measles, mumps, rubella, and varicella. Pediatr Emerg Med Pract. 2016;13(12):1–20.
41. Woolley AL. Salivary gland diseases in children. Curr Opin Otolaryngol Head Neck Surg. 1996;4(6):385–91.
42. Santra G. HIV parotitis. J Assoc Physicians India. 2009;57:517.
43. Huang RD, Pearlman S, Friedman WH, Loree T. Benign cystic vs. solid lesions of the parotid gland in HIV patients. Head Neck. 1991;13(6):522–7.
44. Schiodt M, Greenspan D, Levy JA, Nelson JA, Chernoff D, Hollander H, et al. Does HIV cause salivary gland disease? AIDS. 1989;3(12):819–22.
45. Schwarze-Zander C, Draenert R, Lehmann C, Stecher M, Boesecke C, Sammet S, et al. Measles, mumps, rubella and VZV: importance of serological testing of vaccine-preventable diseases in young adults living with HIV in Germany. Epidemiol Infect. 2017;145(2):236–44.
46. Shivhare P, Shankarnarayan L, Jambunath U, Basavaraju SM. Benign lymphoepithelial cysts of parotid and submandibular glands in a HIV-positive patient. J Oral Maxillofac Pathol. 2015;19(1):107.

47. Decembrino L, Ruffinazzi G, Russo F, Manzoni P, Stronati M. Monolateral suppurative parotitis in a neonate and review of literature. Int J Pediatr Otorhinolaryngol. 2012;76(7):930–3.
48. Spiegel R, Miron D, Sakran W, Horovitz Y. Acute neonatal suppurative parotitis: case reports and review. Pediatr Infect Dis J. 2004;23(1):76–8.
49. Dance DA, Davis TM, Wattanagoon Y, Chaowagul W, Saiphan P, Looareesuwan S, Wuthiekanun V, White NJ. Acute suppurative parotitis caused by Pseudomonas pseudomallei in children. J Infect Dis. 1989;159(4):654–60.
50. Kao WK, Chole RA, Ogden MA. Evidence of a microbial etiology for sialoliths. Laryngoscope. 2020;130(1):69–74.
51. Raad II, Sabbagh MF, Caranasos GJ. Acute bacterial sialadenitis: a study of 29 cases and review. Rev Infect Dis. 1990;12(4):591–601.
52. Arriaga MA, Myers EN. The surgical management of chronic parotitis. Laryngoscope. 1990;100(12):1270–5.
53. Harbison JM, Liess BD, Templer JW, Zitsch RP, Wieberg JA. Chronic parotitis: a challenging disease entity. Ear Nose Throat J. 2011;90(3):E13–6.
54. Belmont MJ, Behar PM, Wax MK. Atypical presentations of actinomycosis. Head Neck. 1999;21(3):264–8.
55. Ben Slama L, Hasni W, Royer B. Cat-scratch disease localisation in the parotid gland. Rev Stomatol Chir Maxillofac. 2008;109(3):183–6.
56. Malatskey S, Fradis M, Ben-David J, Podoshin L. Cat-scratch disease of the parotid gland: an often-misdiagnosed entity. Ann Otol Rhinol Laryngol. 2000;109(7):679–82.
57. Baurmash HD. Chronic recurrent parotitis: a closer look at its origin, diagnosis, and management. J Oral Maxillofac Surg. 2004;62(8):1010–8.
58. Wu CB, Xi H, Zhou Q, Zhang LM. The diagnostic value of technetium 99m pertechnetate salivary gland scintigraphy in patients with certain salivary gland diseases. J Oral Maxillofac Surg. 2015;73(3):443–50.
59. Koch M, Schapher M, Mantsopoulos K, von Scotti F, Goncalves M, Iro H. Multimodal treatment in difficult sialolithiasis: role of extracorporeal shock-wave lithotripsy and intraductal pneumatic lithotripsy. Laryngoscope. 2018;128(10):E332–8.
60. Thakur J, Thakur A, Mohindroo N, Mohindroo S, Sharma D. Bilateral parotid tuberculosis. J Glob Infect Dis. 2011;3(3):296–9.
61. Ozcan C, Apa DD, Aslan G, Gulhan S, Gorur K. Mycobacterium tuberculosis infection within parotid gland Warthin tumor. J Craniofac Surg. 2008;19(6):1561–5.
62. Banks GC, Kirse DJ, Anthony E, Bergman S, Shetty AK. Bilateral parotitis as the initial presentation of childhood sarcoidosis. Am J Otolaryngol. 2013;34(2):142–4.
63. Mandel L, Surattanont F. Bilateral parotid swelling: a review. Oral Surg Oral Med Oral Pathol Oral Radiol Endod. 2002;93(3):221–37.
64. Capaccio P, Canzi P, Gaffuri M, Occhini A, Benazzo M, Ottaviani F, et al. Modern management of paediatric obstructive salivary disorders: long-term clinical experience. Acta Otorhinolaryngol Ital. 2017;37(2):160–7.
65. Fox RI. Sjogren's syndrome. Lancet. 2005;366(9482):321–31.
66. Petrone D, Condemi JJ, Fife R, Gluck O, Cohen S, Dalgin P. A double-blind, randomized, placebo-controlled study of cevimeline in Sjogren's syndrome patients with xerostomia and keratoconjunctivitis sicca. Arthritis Rheum. 2002;46(3):748–54.
67. Peel R. Diseases of the salivary gland. In: Barnes L, editor. Surgical pathology of the head and neck. New York, NY: Marcel-Dekker; 2001. p. 634–757.
68. Fauci AS, Haynes BF, Katz P, Wolff SM. Wegener's granulomatosis: prospective clinical and therapeutic experience with 85 patients for 21 years. Ann Intern Med. 1983;98(1):76–85.
69. Som PM, Biller HF. Kimura disease involving parotid gland and cervical nodes: CT and MR findings. J Comput Assist Tomogr. 1992;16(2):320–2.
70. Cairncross JG, Salmon J, Kim JH, Posner JB. Acute parotitis and hyperamylasemia following whole-brain radiation therapy. Ann Neurol. 1980;7(4):385–7.

9 Sialadenosis (Sialosis) of the Parotid Gland

9.1 Definition

Sialadenosis (sialosis) is a chronic, bilateral, diffuse, noninflammatory, non-neoplastic swelling of the major salivary glands that primarily affects the parotid glands, but occasionally involves the submandibular glands and rarely the minor salivary glands [1]. There are differing uses of the term "sialosis" in the literature. Some consider "sialosis" to be synonymous with "sialadenosis." Others such as Katz et al. (2009) consider sialosis as an umbrella term to "designate all chronic diseases of the salivary glands that are not infections or neoplasms" [2].

9.2 Etiology

The causes of sialadenosis can be categorized into (1) nutritional such as alcoholism, cirrhosis, cystic fibrosis, bulimia, anorexia nervosa, kwashiorkor, and pellagra. Any disorder that affects digestion of food over a prolonged period can result in sialosis, and malnutrition may contribute to sialosis in alcoholics, (2) endocrinal (diabetes mellitus, thyroid disorders such as acromegaly, pregnancy, gonadal dysfunction, following oophorectomy), and (3) neurochemical/drugs [vegetative state, lead and mercury poisoning, iodine, thiouracil (anti-thyroid), isoproterenol (sympatho-mimetic), and phenothiazines] [3–6]. Among the wide range of drugs that may induce sialosis, antihypertensive agents are prominent [1]. However, in many cases sialosis can be "idiopathic" and no underlying disorder can be detected.

© The Author(s), under exclusive license to Springer Nature Switzerland AG 2024
M. Sakr, *Surgery of the Salivary Glands*,
https://doi.org/10.1007/978-3-031-82069-4_9

9.3 Pathogenesis

The proposed pathogeneses of sialosis include prolonged malnutrition with resultant glandular atrophy and fatty replacement. Sialadenosis is also thought to be a neurosecretory disorder. Diabetic neuropathy may be the clue causing acinar cell atrophy, in some cases.

Ultrastructural and animal experimental studies point to a disturbance in the autonomic innervation of salivary glands (autonomic neuropathy). This is considered to be the initiating factor for sialadenosis [4, 5, 7–9].

Multiple emetic episodes (bulimia) cause autonomic neuropathy. With sympathetic nerve impairment, individual acinar cells enlarge because of zymogen granule engorgement. One explanation is that the sympathetic nerve supply to the secreting acinar cell is concerned with the production and secretion of zymogen, the precursor of amylase. Because of sympathetic nerve dysfunction, there may be an increase in zymogen storage in the cell, owing to increased production, decreased secretion of the granules, or both. The ensuing cellular enlargement, which is evidenced by fine-needle aspiration biopsy (FNAB), leads to the clinically visible bilateral parotid gland enlargement [4, 5, 7–9].

9.4 Pathology

Grossly, there is only diffuse enlargement of the affected gland. Histologically, the condition is characterized by acinar hypertrophy and fatty infiltration (Fig. 9.1) [10]. Zymogen granules are increased in size and number by light and electron microscopy [9]. No inflammation or fibrosis can be detected, which differentiates sialadenosis from sialadenitis. While amyloidosis may also present with diffuse enlargement of the salivary glands, histologically, there will be interstitial fibrosis as well as the characteristic pale amyloid deposition that can be demonstrated with a Congo red stain [11].

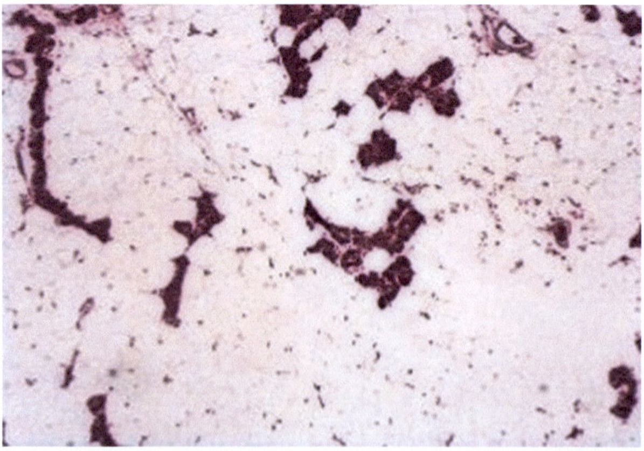

Fig. 9.1 Microscopy showing atrophy of parotid parenchymal tissue and increased intraglandular fat. Inflammatory infiltrates are absent

Characteristic histopathological pictures were identified in diabetic [12, 13] and alcoholic sialosis [12, 14]. Diabetics with sialosis were found to have smaller acini, greater fatty infiltration in the glandular stroma, and normal-appearing epithelium, while alcoholic sialosis identified a reduction in the proportion of fatty tissue of stroma with an enlargement in ductal epithelium felt to contribute to an increased caliber of the striated ducts. Also noted in alcoholic sialosis are the accumulation of secretory granules in the acinar cells' cytoplasm and enlarged excretory ducts.

9.5 Clinical Presentation

Sialadenosis is usually bilateral and has an equal sex distribution. Most of the patients are between 40 and 70 years of age. There is painless, soft, and diffuse enlargement of both parotid glands, giving the patient a striking facial feature, known as the "hamster-like appearance." In some instances, parotid enlargement can be tender.

9.6 Investigations/Diagnosis

9.6.1 Laboratory Tests

Blood tests may reveal hyperglycemia (diabetes mellitus) and abnormal liver function tests (cirrhosis, alcoholism). Sialochemistry may show increased serum potassium and calcium levels.

9.6.2 Imaging Studies

Clinical picture, coupled with imaging studies, is sufficient to establish the diagnosis in the majority of cases. Imaging may include ultrasound, computed tomography (CT) scan, magnetic resonance imaging (MRI), and/or sialography. Ultrasonography (US) will show enlarged, hyperechoic parotid glands (bilateral), without focal lesions or increased blood flow. Computed tomography (CT) scan may show normal or enlarged glands (Fig. 9.2), normal density throughout most of the disease, diffusely dense and large end-stage glands, greater fatty infiltration in diabetic sialadenosis, and reduction in fatty tissue in alcoholic sialadenosis. Sialography, on the other hand, will show sparse peripheral ducts.

9.6.3 Biopsy

Fine-needle aspiration biopsy (FNAB) or open biopsy has been supported by some authors to help establish the diagnosis of sialosis. In general, biopsy is rarely indicated, but the concern about tumor or processes other than sialosis may warrant a

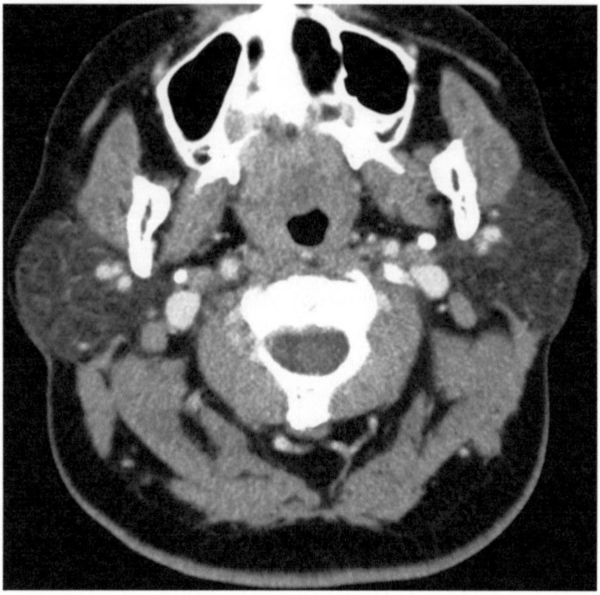

Fig. 9.2 Computed tomography (CT) scan showing bilateral enlargement of both parotid glands

tissue diagnosis. A novel approach for obtaining a biopsy has been proposed by Mignogna et al. (2004) by doing a minor salivary gland biopsy through a palatal approach to confirm the diagnosis. Biopsy will show hypertrophy of acinar cells to almost twice the normal diameter with small, round, and basally situated nuclei, and cytoplasm packed with enzyme granules, along with "areas of fatty infiltration" [6].

9.7 Treatment

Usually no specific treatment is necessary. Treatment in the form of controlling the underlying disorder or withdrawing the incriminated drug helps sialosis to resolve. There is usually little morbidity associated with the condition itself, and surgery (superficial parotidectomy) is resorted to only in case of significant disfigurement and cosmetic complaint.

In some instances, anorexic or bulimic patients may seek advice about removal of the glands. Anorexia or bulimia would need to be treated first before any such surgery could be contemplated. Mehler and Wallace (1993) [15], and more recently, Park et al. (2009) [16] reported that pilocarpine has proved to be beneficial in the treatment of sialadenosis in "bulimic" patients.

References

1. Scully C, Bagan JV, Eveson JW, Barneard N. Turner Fioan: Sialosis: 35 cases of persistent parotid swelling from two countries. Br J Oral Maxillofac Surge. 2008;46:468–72.
2. Katz P, Hartl DM, Guerre A. Clinical ultrasound of the salivary glands. Otolaryngol Clin N Am. 2009;42(6):973–1000.

3. Peel R. Diseases of the salivary gland. In: Barnes L, editor. Surgical pathology of the head and neck. New York, NY: Marcel-Dekker; 2001. p. 634–757.
4. Chilla R. Sialadenosis of the salivary glands of the head. Studies on the physiology and pathophysiology of parotid secretion. Adv Otorhinolaryngol. 1981;26:1–38.
5. Donath K. Sialadenosis of the parotid gland. Ultrastructural, clinical and experimental findings in disturbances of secretion (author's transl). Veroff Pathol. 1976;103:1–122.
6. Mignogna MD, Fedele S, Lo Russo L. Anorexia/bulimia-related sialadenosis of palatal minor salivary glands. J Oral Pathol Med. 2004;33(7):441–2.
7. Chilla R, Witzemann V, Opaitz M, Arglebe C. Possible involvement of parotid beta-adrenergic receptors in the etiology of sialadenosis. Arch Otorhinolaryngol. 1981;230(2):113–20.
8. Donath K, Seifert G. Ultrastructural studies of the parotid glands in sialadenosis. Virchows Arch A Pathol Anat Histol. 1975;365(2):119–35.
9. Donath K, Spillner M, Seifert G. The influence of the autonomic nervous system on the ultrastructure of the parotid acinar cells. Experimental contribution to the neurohormonal sialadenosis. Virchows Arch A Pathol Anat Histol. 1974;364(1):15–33.
10. Gupta S, Sodhani P. Sialadenosis of parotid gland: a cytomorphologic and morphometric study of four cases. Anal Quant Cytol Histol. 1998;20(3):225–8.
11. Eversole L. Salivary gland pathology. In: Fu Y, Wenig BM, Abemayor E, Wenig BL, editors. Head and neck pathology: with clinical correlations. Philadelphia, PA: Churchill-Livingstone; 2001. p. 242–91.
12. Chen S, Benjamin C, Myssiorek D. An algorithm approahc to diagnosin bilateral parotid enlargement. Otolaryngol Head Neck Surg. 2013;148(5):732–9.
13. Carda C, Mosquera-Lloreda N, Salom L, Gomez de Ferraris ME, Peydró A. Structural and functional salivary disorders in type 2 diabetic patietns. Med oarl patol Oral Cir Bucal. 2006;11:E309–14.
14. Merlo C, Bohl L, Carda C, Gómez de Ferraris ME, Carranza M. Parotid sialosis: morphometrical analysis of the glandular parenchyme and stroma among diagbetic and alchoholic patients. J Oral Pathol Med. 2010;39:10–5.
15. Mehler PS, Wallace JA. Sialadenosis in bulimia. A new treatment Arch Otolaryngol Head Neck Surg. 1993;119(7):787–8.
16. Park KK, Tung RC, de Luzuriaga AR. Painful parotid hypertrophy with bulimia: a report of medical management. J Drugs Dermatol. 2009;8(6):577–9.

Benign Cystic Lesions of the Parotid Gland

10

10.1 Etiology/Classification

10.1.1 Unilateral or Bilateral?

Cysts of the parotid gland represent a clinical dilemma. The causes of cystic parotid lesions, which may be bilateral or unilateral, are summarized in Table 10.1. Apart from the cystic forms of benign and malignant neoplasms, cysts of the parotid gland may be the presentation of a variety of diseases. Such non-neoplastic cysts are uncommon and represent 2–5% of all salivary gland lesions [1]. A “first branchial arch” anomaly must be considered when one encounters a case of parotid cyst [2].

“Sialoceles” result from trauma to the parotid gland or duct. Dermoid cysts [3] and hydatid cysts [4] have also been reported in the parotid, though exceptionally rare.

Parotid duct cysts, also known as sialocysts, simple cysts, and retention cysts, result from obstruction of the parotid duct due to various causes [3, 5, 6]. They are true cysts lined by epithelium, unlike “mucocele,” which is lined by granulation tissue [6]. Parotid duct cysts should not be confused with duct ectasia (Fig. 10.1).

10.1.2 Congenital or Acquired?

As reported in the literature, cystic lesions of the parotid may be congenital or acquired as follows.

10.1.2.1 Congenital Cysts

Congenital cysts of the parotid gland are of three types:

© The Author(s), under exclusive license to Springer Nature Switzerland AG 2024
M. Sakr, *Surgery of the Salivary Glands*,
https://doi.org/10.1007/978-3-031-82069-4_10

Table 10.1 Cystic parotid lesions

Bilateral	Unilateral
– Warthin's tumor – Benign lymphoepithelial lesions of HIV – Sjoören's syndrome – Sialocele	– Warthin's tumor – Sialocele – First branchial cleft cyst (parotid lymphoepithelial cyst) – Parotid lymphangioma – Parotid mature cystic teratoma – Necrotic LN(s), especially from SCC – Infected LN(s)

HIV human immunodeficiency virus, *LN* lymph node, *SCC* squamous cell carcinoma

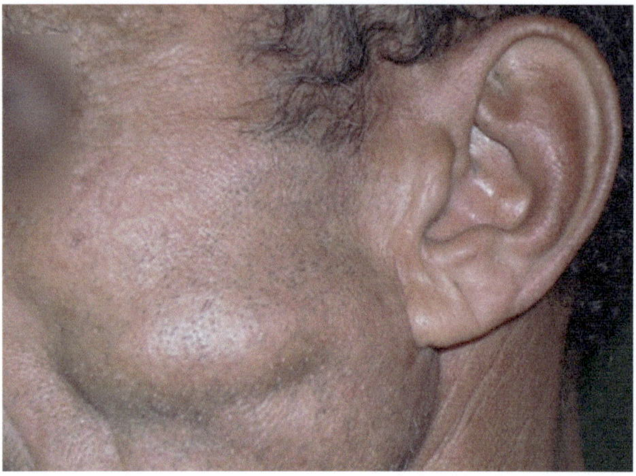

Fig. 10.1 Left parotid duct ectasia, simulating a parotid cyst, in a 41-year-old man

- *Dermoid cyst*: It consists of keratinizing squamous epithelium with associated skin appendages and is treated by complete removal with preservation of the facial nerve.
- *Congenital ductal cyst*: It is generally seen in infancy. No therapy is required unless repeated infections occur [7].
- *Cysts of the first branchial groove* (Fig. 10.2): First branchial cleft cysts develop as a result of incomplete fusion of the cleft between the first and second branchial arches. They account for <1% of all branchial arch anomalies. There are two distinct anomalies: types I and II. Type I anomalies are purely ectodermal while type II anomalies exhibit ectodermal and mesodermal elements. Type II anomaly is more common than type I and incorporates some portion of the first and second arch as well as the cleft. Type I is a duplication anomaly of the membranous external auditory canal. It appears histologically as a cyst lined by squamous epithelium. Clinically, it presents as a cystic mass or fistula posterior to the pinna and concha. The cyst is usually superior to the main trunk of the facial nerve and ends in a cul-de-sac on or near a bony plate at the level of the mesotympanum. Complete excision during a quiescent period, with preservation of the facial nerve, is curative. Type II lesions represent a duplication of both membranous and cartilaginous portions of the external auditory canal. It may occur from the pre-auricular area to the hyoid bone. Regardless of the location, the tract is inti-

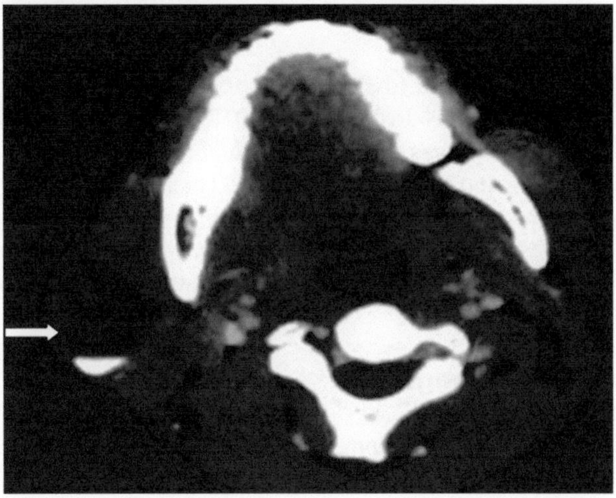

Fig. 10.2 Branchial cleft cyst. Axial CT images showing a large hypodense lesion in the right parotid gland (arrow) with calcific content in the dependent portion

mately associated with the facial nerve. It contains skin as well as adnexal structures and cartilage and may be associated with the parotid gland. Most frequently it is associated with fistulae in the concha or external auditory canal as well as fistulous openings in the neck. As with type I, treatment entails complete excision during a quiescent period, with preservation of the facial nerve [8].

10.1.2.2 Acquired Cysts

Acquired cysts may be due to neoplasms, a benign lymphoepithelial lesion, trauma, parotitis, calculi, duct obstruction, or mucus extravasation [9]. Furthermore, the presence of a cyst does not preclude the possibility of a neoplasm, especially a pleomorphic adenoma, an adenoid cystic carcinoma, a mucoepidermoid carcinoma, or Warthin's tumor. These are the most common parotid tumors and most commonly cystic. For an acquired cyst with an identifiable underlying cause, the latter should be treated first. If that fails, the cyst should then be excised.

Mucoceles and mucus-retention cysts usually involve minor salivary glands and not the parotid gland, occurring mostly in the lips, buccal mucosa, and ventral tongue. Mucus-retention cysts are true cysts with an epithelial lining and result from partial duct obstruction. Complete duct obstruction leads to glandular atrophy [10]. Mucoceles do not possess an epithelial lining (i.e., pseudo-cysts). They represent mucus extravasation into the soft tissue.

10.2 Benign Lymphoepithelial Cyst (BLEC)

10.2.1 Definition

The term "lymphoepithelial cyst" was introduced in 1958 by Bernier and Bhaskar. They stressed that this lesion is not an embryologic remnant and defined it as "solitary or multiple cysts within lymph nodes (LNs) associated with salivary glands" [11].

10.2.2 Incidence

Lymphoepithelial (the so-called branchial) cysts within the parotid gland are rare. As mentioned by Joshi et al. in 2018, the first reported case of branchial cyst in the parotid gland was in 1895 by Hildebrant. Since then, over 100 cases of this type were reported in the literature [12]. The ages of patients ranged from 16 to 69 years, with a mean age of 44 years. Such cysts were found to be three times more frequent in males than in females. The majority of cases were unilateral, with a greater number arising in the right parotid gland rather than the left gland [12–16].

10.2.3 Pathogenesis

The origin and development of benign lymphoepithelial cysts (BLECs) is a controversial subject; thus, many theories have been suggested. Bernier and Bhaskar postulated that BLECs arise from cystic changes in parotid gland epithelium that become entrapped in the cervical and parotid LNs during embryonic life [11]. Accordingly, lymphoepithelial cysts are considered distinct entities from the lymphoepithelial lesions. Other authors favor remnants of the branchial arch as the origin of BLECs, and indeed, many cases have been reported as "branchial cysts." Still, others believe it to be probably a dysontogenetic benign cyst that originated from the epithelial remnants retained in lymphoid tissues during the embryogenesis or from branchial cleft epithelium [11, 17–20]. It has been widely recognized that BLEC is a common cause of parotid gland enlargement in patients infected with human immunodeficiency virus (HIV) infection. There are two peculiarities that distinguish the cyst associated with HIV: frequent bilateral occurrence and multicystic appearance observed in computed tomography (CT) scan or magnetic resonance imaging (MRI) [21–23].

10.2.4 Types

The main types of lymphoepithelial cysts that can be found in the parotid gland are as follows:

- Simple cysts, comparable with both the extravasation and retention type of mucocele.
- Larger BLECs, which are mainly congenital, but also reported in patients with acquired immunodeficiency syndrome (AIDS).
- A polycystic disease of the parotid gland, a developmental disorder, which is seen bilaterally, especially in females.
- Cystic tumors.

A review of 100 cases of non-neoplastic disease of the parotid gland found "parotid cyst" to be the most common (10%). Histologically, seven were simple cysts and three were BLECs in that review [24–26].

10.2.5 Clinical Presentation

The clinical diagnosis of a parotid cyst is often based on a slowly enlarging painless lump in the parotid region; the examination not always confirming the cystic nature of the lesion. Patients with BLECs most commonly present in the fifth decade of life, with equal distribution among males and females. Although duct obstruction appears to be the cause, the source of the obstruction is often not apparent. Most lesions in the parotid gland present as a slowly enlarging, painless, and swelling affecting the gland. It is a smooth-surfaced cyst with normal overlying skin that is freely moveable over the mass, and with normal function of the facial nerve and no associated regional lymphadenopathy [12, 21, 27]. Hence, the diagnosis is seldom made preoperatively and sometimes a superficial parotidectomy is needed [12, 13, 27, 28].

In the last few years, such cysts have been found in increasing numbers in patients with acquired immunodeficiency disease (AIDS), and in the patients belonging to the AIDS risk groups [21–23].

10.2.6 Site and Progression

The most common sites for BLECs are in the lateral cervical area. The parotid gland is the preferential site for these cysts to occur, and this is probably due to the presence of intraparotid LNs in the glands, which are absent in all the other salivary glands. However, in the review of 468 cases of branchial cyst from the file of the Armed Forces Institute of Pathology, only five cases were located in the parotid area. In addition, a review of 149 cases of branchial cysts reported that only 14 cases were found at the upper part of the neck above the angle of the mandible [17, 27, 28].

Benign lymphoepithelial cysts (BLECs) can grow to large sizes and may lead to disfigurement. The BLECs may be single or multiple, and may be unilateral or bilateral [29].

10.2.7 Investigations

10.2.7.1 Laboratory Studies

Investigations are important for the diagnosis and treatment planning of BLECs. The most important laboratory study for a BLEC is to rule out HIV infection, usually by ELISA-based test [29]. The aspirate of a BLEC of the parotid gland shows a high protein content, which is characteristic of the lesion.

10.2.7.2 Imaging Studies

Ultrasound (US) is useful in showing cystic nature of the lesion [25]. Computed tomography (CT) scan and magnetic resonance imaging (MRI) provide a clear image of the lesion and reveal intraparotid cystic masses. Magnetic resonance imaging will show a well-defined, thin, smooth-walled cystic lesion within the

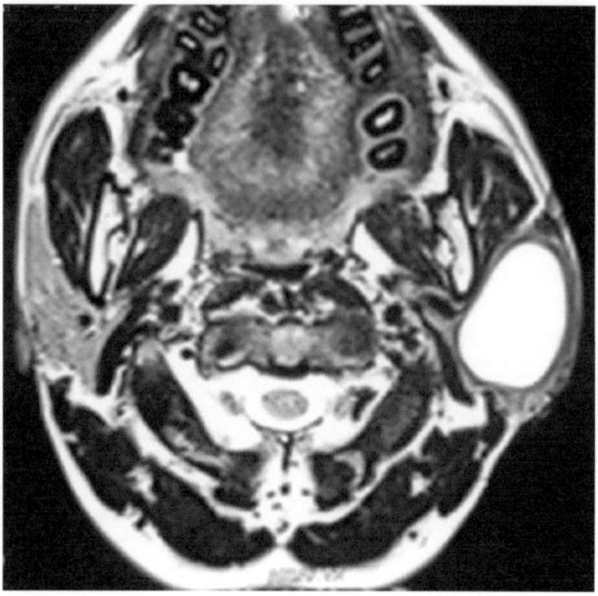

Fig. 10.3 Magnetic resonance imaging (MRI) of the neck showing a well-defined, thin, smooth-walled cystic, hyperintense, lesion within the superficial part of the parotid gland

superficial part of the parotid gland measuring (Fig. 10.3). The fluid content of the lesion is hyperintense on T1 as well as T2-weighted imaging, suggestive of high proteinaceous or hemorrhagic content with no solid component [29].

10.2.7.3 Cytology/Histology

Fine-needle aspiration cytology (FNAC) of the mass is useful in certain cases of BLECs [26]. It will show a proteinaceous fluid, and in the presence of infection, a cellular smear consisting of inflammatory infiltrate predominantly with neutrophils, lymphocytes, and cystic macrophages against a proteinaceous background.

The definitive diagnosis of the cystic lesion of the parotid gland depends solely on histopathological examination. Within the category of BLECs, various types of epithelium have been described. The most frequent has been squamous, but variable combinations of cuboidal, columnar, ciliated columnar, and mucin-producing epithelia also have been reported. In addition, rare examples of squamous epithelium containing sebaceous differentiation have been documented [11, 17]. The characteristic histopathological pattern is that of a glandular or squamous epithelium-lined cleft surrounded by abundant lymphoid tissue with prominent germinal centers, with some specimens even containing salivary gland tissue and ducts (Fig. 10.4) [30].

10.2.8 Differential Diagnosis

The differential diagnosis of parotid BLEC includes Warthin's tumor, intramuscular benign hemangioma (IMH), branchial cleft cyst, and lymphoma. The imaging modality of choice is MRI as it helps in characterizing the lesion. The IMHs are typically multiloculated and resemble a "bunch of grapes." They are iso-intense on

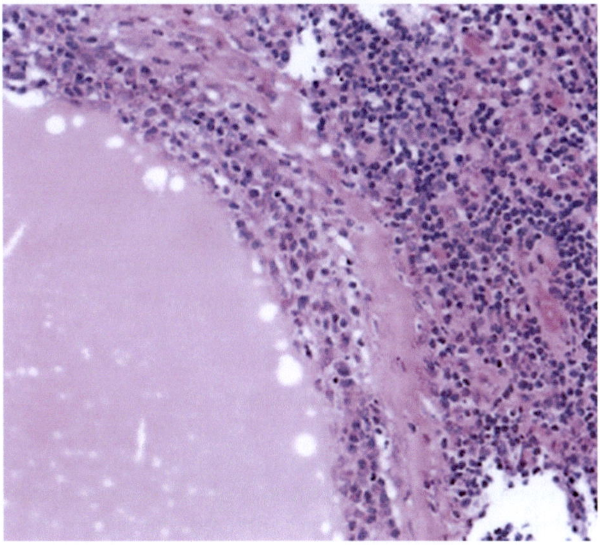

Fig. 10.4 Microscopic picture of a benign lymphoepithelial cyst (BLEC) showing a cystic cavity line by thin epithelium and connective tissue with germinal centers

T1-WI and hyperintense on T2-WI and show a heterogeneous peripheral enhancement after contrast administration. Warthin's tumors show a similarly low signal on T1-WI and moderate-to-high signal on T2-WI with, however, no rim enhancement after contrast injection [30].

Thus far, BLECs have neither been known to recur nor metastasize. For this reason, it is important that they should be differentiated from aggressive lesions, especially cystic low-grade mucoepidermoid carcinoma. The potential for this problem in differential diagnosis is underscored by the recent report of a low-grade mucoepidermoid carcinoma arising within an intraparotid LN [11, 17].

10.2.9 Treatment

While the etiology of benign parotid cysts is controversial, the treatment is not. As the diagnosis is seldom made preoperatively, superficial parotidectomy or complete excision with a sufficient margin of normal tissue surrounding is usually done [14, 21, 27]. Superficial parotidectomy should be performed as a curative treatment when a conservative approach cannot safely remove the lesion.

10.3 Sialocele/Parotid Cyst

10.3.1 Etiology

Disruption of the parotid duct or parenchyma results in extravasation of saliva into the glandular or periglandular and subcutaneous tissues [31]. When the rate of saliva accumulation within these areas surpasses the body's capacity to reabsorb it, a sialocele can form. The cause might be facial trauma (assault, traffic accident, sports injury, etc.) or parotid surgery (parotidectomy), or less commonly, infection [31].

10.3.2 Pathology

Duct cysts are unilocular and may grossly contain mucoid material, or sialoliths in long-standing cases. Histologically, they are lined by a cuboidal, columnar, or squamous epithelium, though oncocytic metaplasia may be seen in older patients. However, these cysts are not associated with lymphoid elements [32].

10.3.3 Clinical Presentation

Sialocele is relatively benign and may present with no symptoms apart from a swelling (lump) in the parotid region (Fig. 10.5). On palpation, the lesion may be soft and mobile and unless secondary infected, the patient has no pain, fever, chills, or erythema of the skin [33]. However, if the sialocele is left untreated it can be associated with the following complications [34]:

- Pain due to the accumulation of saliva and stretching/compression of surrounding tissues.
- Infection due to the stagnation of salivary flow rate.
- Interference with speech or chewing.

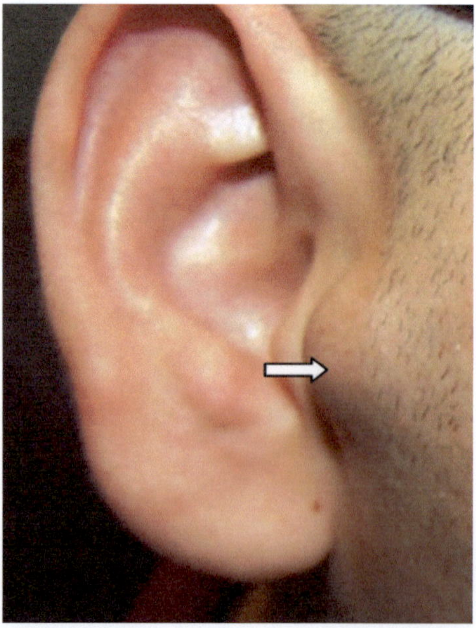

Fig. 10.5 Parotid cyst presenting as a lump (cyst) in front of the tragus of the right ear (arrow) of a 38-year man

- A significantly large facial swelling with an undesirable cosmetic change.
- Extraoral fistula formation.
- Recurrence (rare) due to incomplete excision [32].

10.3.4 Evaluation

The diagnosis is complex and involves a combination of thorough history and clinical assessment of the patient, image analysis, and fine-needle aspiration. Imaging studies include sialography, US, CT scan, and MRI [33]. If aspiration is performed, the aspirated fluid is usually a clear yellow and contains amylase (around 10,000 units/L, in contrast to fluid from a seroma). Imaging with ultrasound (US) will clearly demonstrate the cystic nature of the parotid lesion and accurately measure its exact size (Fig. 10.6).

Computed tomography (CT) scan can also delineate the parotid lesion. CT may show details of the area, such as a single- or multiloculated cystic lesion with regular margins and lower density of the surrounding tissues (Fig. 10.7). It also provides anatomical relations to the surrounding structures. The CT differential diagnosis would include retention cyst, sialodochitis, branchial cleft cyst, and lymphoepithelial cyst [31].

Sialography may increase the sialocele's pressure causing rupture and fistulae, although this is not a commonly observed complication [35]. Fine-needle aspiration is a standard technique that permits sampling and the fluid may be submitted for further investigation.

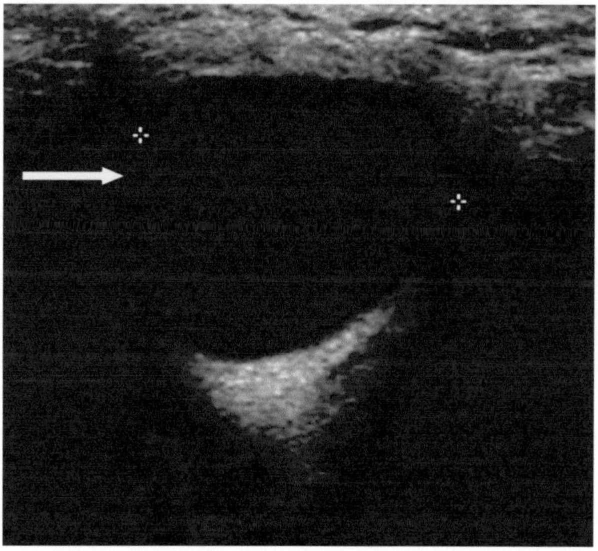

Fig. 10.6 Ultrasound of the parotid gland showing a simple parotid cystic lesion (arrow)

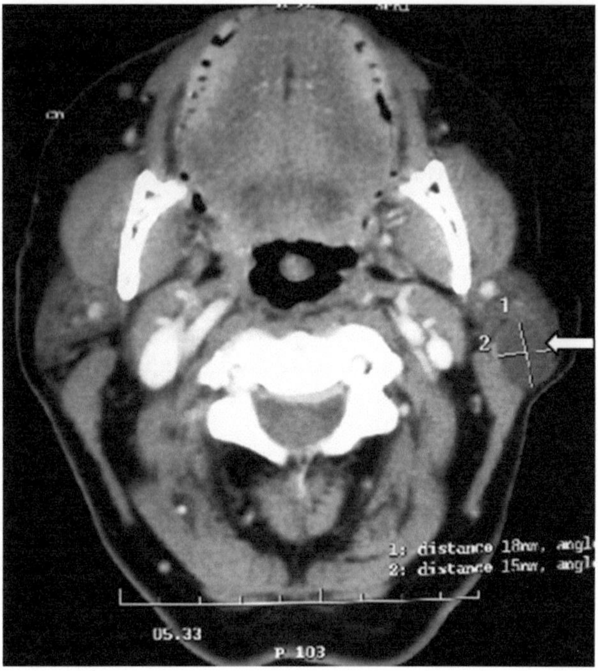

Fig. 10.7 Computed tomography (CT) scan showing a parotid cystic lesion and its dimensions (white arrow)

10.3.5 Treatment

Surgical treatment includes repair or reconstruction of the duct, creation of a controlled internal fistula, superficial or total parotidectomy, parasympathetic denervation, and ductal ligation [34].

Adequate surgical management of a parotid cyst entails (1) precise removal of the affected parotid gland pathology, (2) proper management of the remaining glandular tissue and associated ductal structures, and (3) close postoperative management and care to prevent complications.

The parotid cyst should be meticulously dissected (Figs. 10.8 and 10.9) and resected, thereby preventing potentially serious complications such as facial paralysis, taste distortion, and disfigurement. Once resection of the cyst or affected salivary gland has been completed, proper management of the remaining glandular tissues is crucial to avoid sialocele formation. Proper postoperative care is comprised of close follow-up and dietary modifications. The surgical site is closely followed up for proper drain management, wound healing, quality of scar formation, and infection prevention.

Special compressive dressings and small drains are placed at the surgical site to promote proper fluid drainage as well as to close off any potential areas where saliva can accumulate. In addition to suppressing sialocele formation, this deters bacterial accumulation and infection. Dietary modifications are also prescribed to prevent the production of excess saliva during the healing phase.

It should be remembered that sialoceles that are treated by anticholinergic drugs, radiation, drainage, or aspiration are associated with a high rate of recurrence because

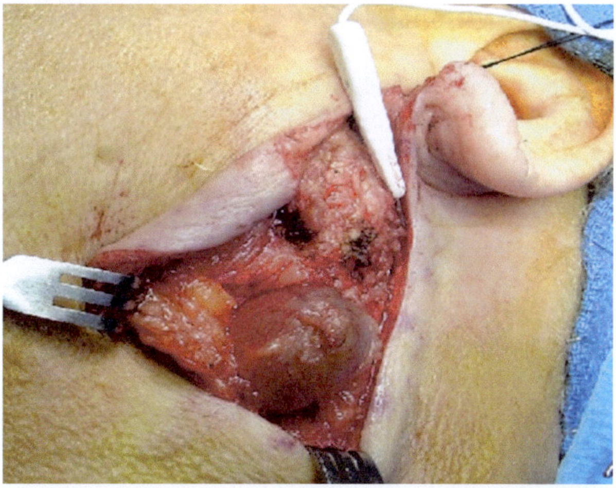

Fig. 10.8 Intraoperative dissection of a left parotid cyst (sialocele)

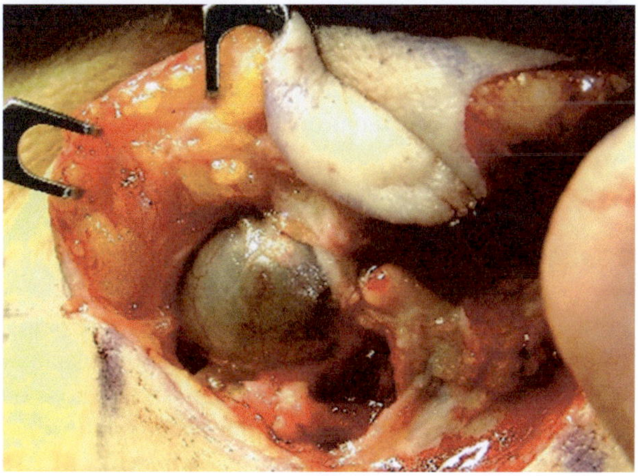

Fig. 10.9 Intraoperative dissection of a right parotid cyst (sialocele)

the mechanism that initially led to the formation of the sialocele has not been treated. Botulinum toxin injections have also been used to manage this condition [36]. It causes temporary chemical denervation of the cholinergic nerve fibers and has been used successfully. It is a highly effective, safe, and noninvasive method [37–39].

10.4 Epidermal/Epidermoid Cyst of the Parotid Gland

10.4.1 Definition/Synonyms

The epidermal cyst is a common, benign skin lesion that develops out of ectodermal tissue, consisting of epithelial-lined cavities, which are filled with viscous or semi-solid epithelial degradation products [40]. The several synonyms are epidermal cyst, epidermoid cyst, epidermal inclusion cyst, infundibular cyst, and keratin cyst [41].

10.4.2 Incidence

Epidermal/epidermoid cysts are common lesions occurring in the skin [42]. However, epidermal cysts of the oral cavity are a very rare entity and only 1.6–6.9% of all epidermal cysts are thought to be located in the oral cavity [43]. Primary epidermal cysts of salivary glands appear to be very rare, and literature search for the past three decades revealed only a very few cases in parotid gland [44] and some cases in submandibular gland [42, 45, 46].

10.4.3 Etiology/Pathogenesis

Epidermal cysts usually occur secondary to obstruction while dermoid cysts arise from developmental epithelial remnants or they are secondary to traumatic implantation of epithelial fragments [47].

The exact pathogenesis of salivary epidermal cyst is uncertain, but it may have arisen from developmental branchial pouch analogue epithelium, which can occur in salivary gland [48] or could be due to obstruction in salivary duct within the substance of the gland leading to epithelial lining cavity filled with viscous semi-solid epithelial degradation product [44]. The cysts clinically are painless swellings.

10.4.4 Clinical Presentation

Epidermal cyst of the parotid gland is a very rare benign cystic lesion and is seen in young to middle-aged adults [41]. The patient usually complains of painless swelling in the parotid region. The swelling is of insidious onset and gradual progression. There is no history of fever, difficulty in swallowing, or any discharge from the swelling. On examination, there is a localized, ovoid, swelling in the parotid region without any attachment to the overlying skin or involvement of facial nerve [41]. There is usually normal skin color and no lifting of the ear lobe, or surface discharge. On palpation, the swelling is soft or cystic in consistency, no-tender, non-pulsatile, and is movable below the skin. If the cyst stays for longer time, it might get infected, forming sinus or fistulas [44].

10.4.5 Investigations/Diagnosis

The diagnosis of an epidermal cyst in the parotid gland is very essential and could be easily mistaken for a salivary gland abscess, neoplasm, and other cysts [49]. Malignant lesions are frequently suspected when there is a rapid enlargement with associated lymphadenopathy or facial nerve paralysis [41, 50]. Diagnosis of an epidermal cyst in the parotid gland can be proven by various investigations like US, CT scan, and FNAC [51, 52].

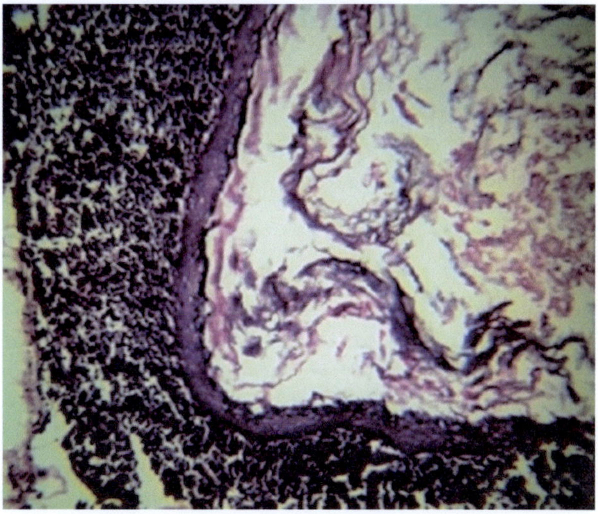

Fig. 10.10 Histopathology of epidermal/epidermoid cyst of the parotid gland showing stratified squamous epithelium with an intraluminal laminated keratinized material. H&E stain

Ultrasound will show a hyperechoic cystic lesion in the right parotid region with no vascularity in the lesion and no evidence of calculi in the duct or glands. Histopathological examination of the cyst is required for the confirmation of diagnosis. Histologically, an epidermal cyst has stratified squamous epithelial lining and is usually filled with cheesy material or keratin (Fig. 10.10), but a dermoid or epidermoid cyst contains skin adnexa or other epidermal structures like sebaceous gland or hair follicle. Implantation dermoid is not derived from epidermal appendages and may contain a foreign body [43], even though it appears very similar to an epidermoid cyst.

10.4.6 Differential Diagnosis

The differentials of an epidermal cyst in the parotid region may include branchial cleft cyst, which is "congenital," or may be "acquired" due to inflammation, obstruction, neoplasm, calculi, and trauma [41].

10.4.7 Treatment

Treatment of an epidermal cyst in the parotid gland is by surgical intervention in the form of superficial parotidectomy so that the cyst is removed in toto [53]. However, the treatment could be surgical excision of the cyst, with great care to be taken not to rupture the cyst, which can lead to postoperative inflammation, and also to preserve the vital structures during surgery [44]. Recurrence is very rare.

10.5 Dermoid Cyst of the Parotid Gland

10.5.1 Classification of Dermoid Cysts

Back in 1937, New and Erich [54], on the basis of hypothesized pathogenesis and histopathological appearance, classified dermoid cysts into the following three categories:

- *Congenital dermoid cysts of teratoma type*: These arise from the embryonic germinal layers. Depending on the dormant layer, they can contain skin, hair, teeth, etc. They are almost always limited to the ovaries and testes.
- *Acquired dermoid cysts*: These are inclusion cysts due to traumatically implanted skin in the deeper tissues. They occur on the hands and the other exposed parts of the body.
- *Congenital inclusion dermoid cysts*: These develop from inclusions of displaced dermal cells along the lines of embryologic fusion. This category is further subdivided into four subgroups: (1) cysts around the eyes and orbits, originating along the naso-optic groove; (2) those around the nose, resulting from intrusion of the fronto-nasal plate; (3) those around the floor of the mouth, and in submental and submaxillary regions, originating from the first and second branchial arches; and (4) those around the suprasternal, suboccipital, thyroidal, lower lip and palate, most of which occur along the mid-ventral or mid-dorsal lines of the body.

10.5.2 Incidence

Dermoid cysts of the head and neck are rare benign lesions that usually present as a midline neck mass and rarely appear in the lateral region. Approximately 7% of all dermoid cysts are seen in the head and neck region [55], and 80% predominantly occur in the orbit, floor of mouth, and nose [54, 56, 57]. These locations are the fusion sites of many embryonic structures and hence prone to dermoid cyst formation [58]. Dermoid cyst in parotid gland is extremely rare, with less than 25 cases reported in the literature worldwide. In general, cystic lesions account for 2–5% of all parotid gland lesions [59].

10.5.3 Etiology

Etiologically, dermoid cystic lesions are either congenital or acquired [60]. Congenital lesions are most often ectodermal in origin and include branchial cleft cysts/lymphoepithelial cysts. Acquired cysts can be due to obstructions, neoplasms, calculi, and traumatic implantation of epithelium in deeper layers [60].

10.5.4 Pathology

Dermoid cysts are benign, closed, epithelium-lined cavities that can form anywhere in the body. The term "dermoid cyst" is a broad term commonly used interchangeably to describe epidermoid, dermoid, and teratoid cysts [3, 61]. These are the three histopathological variants of the dermoid cyst and differ by the content of their lining. Epidermoid cysts originate from ectoderm and are lined by a stratified squamous epithelium. They contain trapped keratin debris. Dermoid cysts, or true dermoid cysts, contain elements from both ectodermal and mesodermal origin (but not endodermal), and are lined by stratified squamous epithelium with cutaneous adnexal structures such as sebaceous glands, sweat glands, and hair follicles (Fig. 10.11). Teratoid cysts contain elements derived from all three germ layers (ectoderm, mesoderm, and endoderm), and their lining varies from stratified squamous to ciliated pseudostratified columnar epithelium [62, 63].

10.5.5 Clinical Presentation

More than 50% of dermoid cysts in the head and neck region are usually detected by the age of six, though approximately one third are present at birth [64]. Dermoid cysts generally are painless swellings (Fig. 10.12) without infiltration into the surrounding important structures such as the facial nerve or skin or fixation to the deeper structures. There are no physical examination findings that can differentiate dermoid cysts from other entities.

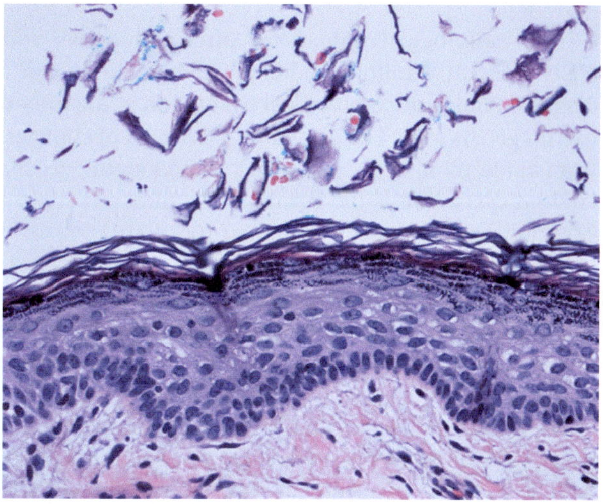

Fig. 10.11 Histopathology of a dermoid cyst: the cyst wall lined by stratified squamous epithelium with granular layer and loose keratin flakes in the lumen. H&E stain

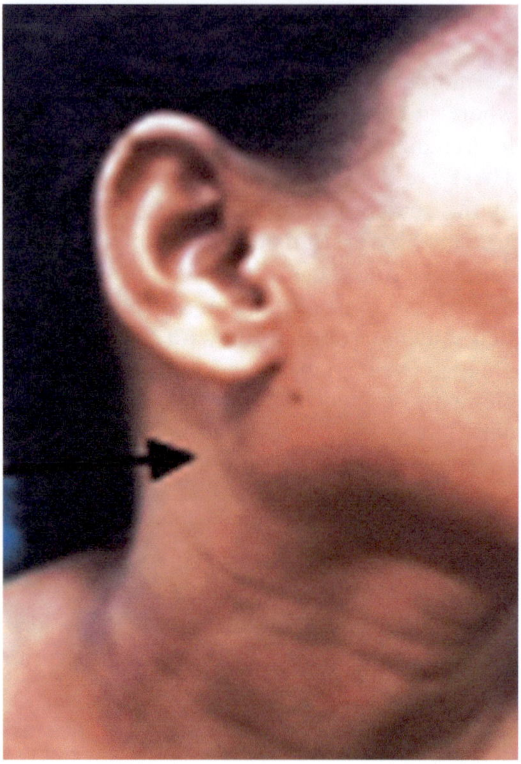

Fig. 10.12 A mass in the right parotid gland in a 37-year-old woman (arrow). It proved to be a dermoid cyst

10.5.6 Diagnosis/Differential Diagnosis

Clinico-radiological evaluation is often ambiguous, which makes preoperative diagnosis difficult. Multiple radiological modalities can help provide a preoperative diagnosis but histopathological evaluation is the only modality to provide a definitive diagnosis [65]. The presence of dermal appendages differentiates dermoid cysts from epidermoid cysts, and a lack of endoderm structures differentiates them from teratoid cysts. Often, the dermoid cyst lumen is filled with sebaceous material and keratin debris, with occasional hair [66, 67].

Ultrasonography (US), CT scan, MRI, and FNAC can be performed. Ultrasound is able to differentiate between solid, vascular, and cystic lesions. Both MRI and CT scan may give an idea about the location and relations of the mass with the surrounding tissue, but cannot give a final preoperative diagnosis.

Magnetic resonance imaging (MRI) of a dermoid cyst typically depicts a cystic mass, hypointense on T1-weighted images and hyperintense on T2-weighted ones with peripheral enhancement on contrast (Fig. 10.13). Some dermoid cysts have variable signal intensity on T1-weighted images, which may be hyperintense because of the presence of sebaceous lipid [68].

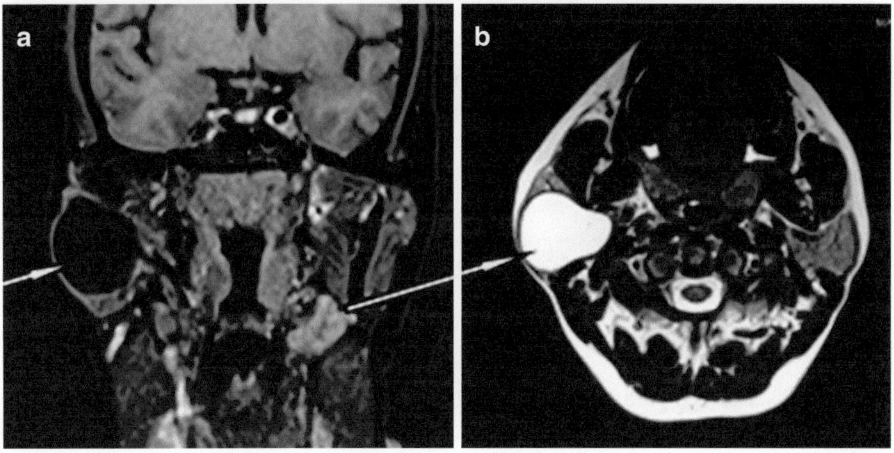

Fig. 10.13 MRI showing (**a**) hypointense mass on T1 image and (**b**) hyperintense on T2. Fat planes are preserved

Fine-needle aspiration cytology (FNAC) may provide reliable information on cystic lesions if there are supporting radiological findings, but can also be misleading because some well-differentiated squamous cell carcinomas and malignant lesions showing squamous metaplasia may share the benign-looking cytological features with dermoid cysts. Hence, the definitive diagnosis should always be made by histopathological examination [60, 69].

As a cystic lesion, a dermoid cyst can mimic other parotid cystic lesions clinically and radiologically. Differential diagnosis includes mucous retention cyst, unilateral obstruction of the parotid duct, benign mesenchymal tumors (e.g., lipoma, fibroma, hemangioma, or neurofibroma), branchial cleft cyst, benign parotid gland tumors (e.g., pleomorphic adenoma or Warthin's tumor), and malignant parotid gland tumors (e.g., mucoepidermoid tumor) [58, 59].

10.5.7 Treatment

Superficial parotidectomy is the standard surgical approach and is generally performed for the treatment of intraparotid dermoid cyst, unless the lesion is embedded deeply within the gland, in which case total parotidectomy should be performed [3]. However, there have been a few cases in which isolated cystectomy (enucleation) was the treatment of choice as it was easily dissected in toto without sacrificing the superficial lobe [70–72] In all kinds of surgical intervention, careful dissection of the facial nerve from the cyst wall is of paramount importance to prevent its injury, which may potentially cause neurological deficits [71]. Moreover, whatever type of surgical approach is taken, it is essential to remove the cyst in total with the capsule intact [73]. This is due to certain risks associated with incomplete resection, notably infection, recurrence, and even malignant transformation [66]. Although malignant transformation has not been documented in dermoid cysts originating within the parotid gland, it has been observed in the submental and sublingual regions of the head and neck at a rate of around 5% [74]. Considering the possibility of malignant transformation of dermoid cysts in the parotid, complete surgical excision is the recommended treatment of choice [74–76].

10.6 Hydatid Cyst of the Parotid Gland

10.6.1 Introduction

Hydatid disease is a parasitic infestation (known as hydatidosis or echinococcosis) caused by larval stage of the cestode tapeworm *Echinococcus granulosus*. It affects both animals and humans. It is transmitted to humans by ingestion of contaminated food and water, which contain eggs of *E. granulosus*. Humans are intermediate hosts that contain larval stage (hydatid cyst), while carnivores such as dogs are definitive hosts that contain the adult worms of *E. granulosus* [77].

10.6.2 Pathogenesis

After the ingestion of *E. granulosus* eggs, the oncospheres pass through the small intestine to portal venous circulation and enter the liver. Then the oncospheres (or developing cysts) can pass to the heart and systemic circulation and settle in any organ such as parotid gland. Parotid hydatid cyst may be primary or secondary. The "primary" hydatid cysts of parotid result from the direct settlement of cysts in the gland only without the involvement of other organs. However, the "secondary cysts" of parotid are more common and may result from surgical rapture of primary cysts of the liver [78, 79].

10.6.3 Sites/Clinical Picture

Hydatidosis (echinococcosis) can affect any organ of body, but affects mainly the liver (70% of cases) because it is the first organ encountered after the passage of hydatid eggs through the small intestine. Less frequently, hydatidosis can affect the lungs (20%) and other organs (10%) such as the brain, spleen, and bone. Primary hydatid cyst of the parotid gland is extremely rare [77, 78, 80–84], even in endemic sheep- and cattle-raising areas of the world, notably, the Mediterranean countries, South America, the Middle East, and Australia [85–88]. Despite its rarity, hydatid cyst must be included in the differential diagnosis of cystic swelling of salivary glands, especially in those with a history of hepatic hydatid cysts.

Hydatid cyst larvae grow slowly, about 1–2 cm/year [89]. Regarding symptomatology, hydatid cysts are asymptomatic and may remain unnoticeable for years till they become large enough to be clinically detectable or cause compression of vital structures [84].

10.6.4 Classification

Regarding the WHO classification of hydatid cysts [90] whether it is in the liver, lung, or parotid, hydatid cysts are classified according to the morphology on US into five cystic echinococcosis (CE) types as follows:

- CE1: unilocular simple cyst with double line
- CE2: multi-septate cyst
- CE3: cyst with detached membranes (CE3a) or contain daughter cysts (CE3b)
- CE4: heterogeneous hypoechoic and hyperechoic content, no daughter cysts
- CE5: cyst with calcified walls

10.6.5 Diagnosis

Preoperative diagnosis of this rare lesion in the parotid gland is very important since hydatid disease and malignant diseases of the parotid gland may present in the same way. The most important factor in the diagnosis of hydatid disease of parotid is the high index of suspicion about its possibility [86, 87].

Some biochemical parameters may be elevated in cases of parotid hydatid cysts, although they were not specific. *E. granulosus* is a parasitic infection that may produce eosinophilia and leukocytosis. The frequency with which eosinophilia is encountered is 25% in the literature [91]. Enzyme-linked immunosorbent assay (ELISA) and immune hemagglutination (IHA) are the most common serological tests; however, negative serology does not exclude the diagnosis [85–88].

Diagnosis can be easily established by considering the geographical region and with the help of the serological tests and imaging studies such as US and preferably CT scan, which has been shown to be a valuable method for establishing the appropriate diagnosis (Fig. 10.14) [92]. It confirms the site, size, and number of cysts. Fine-needle aspiration cytology (FNAC) is controversial in suspected cases of parotid hydatid cysts [82, 83].

Definite diagnosis is certainly confirmed by histopathological examination of the cyst (Fig. 10.15) and the whole surgical specimen in case of parotidectomy [77] (Fig. 10.16).

10.6.6 Differential Diagnosis

Other congenital and acquired cystic lesions of parotid gland should be differentiated from this rare entity. Congenital cysts include dermoid and epidermoid cysts, first branchial cleft cysts, and cystic hygromas. Dermoid and epidermoid cysts may be located

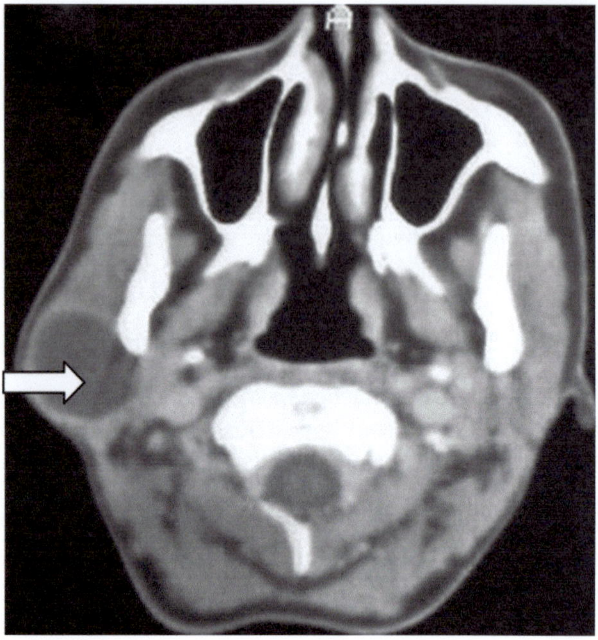

Fig. 10.14 Axial computed tomography (CT) scan of the head and neck region demonstrating a well-defined cystic hypodense lesion in the parotid gland (arrow) that proved postoperatively to be a hydatid cyst

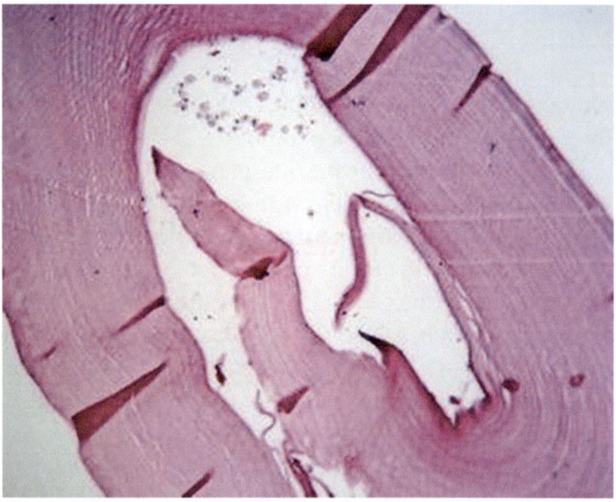

Fig. 10.15 Histopathology of the specimen showing the characteristic features of hydatid cyst. H&E stain

within the parotid and submandibular glands. First branchial cleft cysts are also commonly seen as smooth, nontender, and fluctuant masses in the periauricular area and parotid glands. Uncommonly, cystic hygroma of the parotid gland may present as an asymptomatic, soft, fluctuant mass. It appears hypodense on CT scans, low- to intermediate-signal intensity on T1- and high signal intensity on T2-weighted MRI images.

The acquired cysts include those of lymphoepithelial origin and those resulting from obstruction, infection, or tumors. A high degree of correlation has been demonstrated between HIV seropositivity and the presence of multicentric parotid

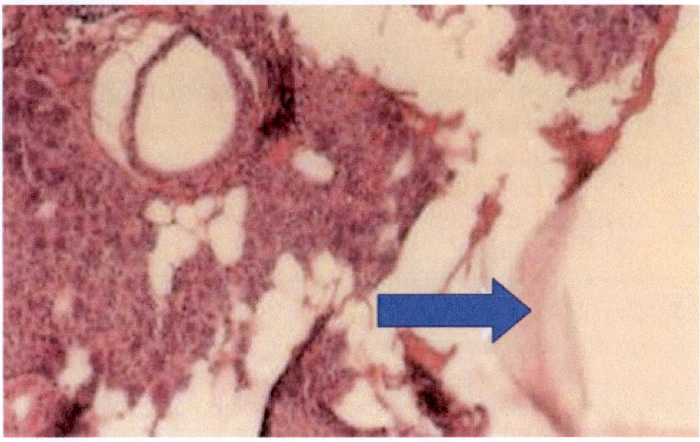

Fig. 10.16 Histopathology of the specimen showing parotid gland tissue and a portion of hydatid cyst (arrow) adjacent to the parotid gland normal tissue. H& stain

benign lymphoepithelial cysts, but the presence of these cysts is not confined to HIV infection and may be associated with chronic infection, autoimmune diseases such as Sjögren's syndrome, systemic lupus erythematosus (SLE), polyarthritis nodosa, polymyositis, and scleroderma and even seen in the idiopathic states [93].

10.6.7 Treatment

Although there are several modalities for the treatment of hydatid cyst, including medical therapy, surgical excision, and minimally invasive techniques [such as puncture-aspiration-injection-respiration (PAIR)], superficial parotidectomy with removal of hydatid cysts is the treatment of choice in parotid hydatid cysts. The major advantage of surgery compared with other methods of treatment is the complete removal of the cysts and their fluid. Operative access is chosen according to the number, size, and location of cysts, nature of complications, and previous surgery. Although it is a typical parotidectomy procedure, avoidance of cyst rapture should be considered as much as possible by using subcapsular dissection and decompression of cyst if too large. The most serious complication of the parotid hydatid cyst is rupture of cysts and seeding of daughter cysts locally or to other organs, as well as anaphylaxis. The complications after superficial parotidectomy are usually mild and temporary, with almost no recurrences [94].

Medical treatment with benzimidazole group drugs, such as albendazole and mebendazole, is necessary in disseminated cases, in patients in whom surgery is high risk, as well as in the pre- and postoperative periods [94]. Presurgery treatment with albendazole may facilitate a complete removal of germinal layer cells. Blood count and transaminases must be checked routinely after the operation, and albendazole started and continued for about 2 months [88, 92, 93].

PAIR has been proposed as an alternative to surgery. In this method, complete aspiration is performed after US-guided percutaneous puncture; the residual cavity is then filled with a protoscolicide, usually ethanol, and reaspirated soon after that. Akhan et al. presented the first case of hydatid cyst of the parotid gland treated percutaneously by using PAIR technique and concluded that it seems to be effective and can be a safe alternative treatment to surgery [95].

References

1. Williams NS, Bulstrode C, O'Connell PR. Bailey & Love's short practice of surgery. 25th ed. London: Hodder Arnold; 2008.
2. Tripti Maithani AP, Acharya S. Congenital agenesis of unilateral parotid gland with ipsilateral type I first branchial cleft anomaly: a rare presentation. Egyptian J Ear Nose Throat Allied Sci. 2014;15:53–6.
3. Yigit N, Karslioglu Y, Yildizoglu U, Karakoc O. Dermoid cyst of the parotid gland: report of a rare entity with literature review. Head Neck Pathol. 2015;9(2):286–92.
4. Kara T, Arpaci RB, Vayisoglu Y, Serinsoz E, Gursoy D, Ozgur A, et al. Hydatid cyst of parotid gland: an unusual case diagnosed by fine needle aspiration biopsy. Turk Patoloji Derg. 2014;4:1–4.
5. Eversole L. Salivary gland pathology. In: Fu Y, Wenig BM, Abemayor E, Wenig BL, editors. Head and neck pathology: with clinical correlations. Philadelphia, PA: Churchill-Livingstone; 2001. p. 242–91.
6. Batsakis JG, Raymond AK. Sialocysts of the parotid glands. Ann Otol Rhinol Laryngol. 1989;98(6):487–9.
7. Work WP. Cysts and congenital lesions of the parotid gland. Otolaryngol Clin N Am. 1977;10:339–43.
8. Finn DG, Buchalter IH, Sarti E, Romo T, Chodosh P. First branchial cleft cysts: clinical update. Laryngoscope. 1987;97(2):136–40.
9. Work WP, Hecht DW. Non-neoplastic lesions of the parotid gland. Ann Otol Rhinol Laryngol. 1968;77:462–7.
10. Sela J, Ulmansky M. Mucous retention cyst of salivary glands. J Oral Surg. 1969;27:619–23.
11. Bernier JL, Bhaskar SN. Lymphoepithelial lesions of salivary glands; histogenesis and classification based on 186 cases. Cancer. 1958;11:1156–79.
12. Fujibayashi T, Itoh H. Lymphoepithelial (so-called branchial) cyst within the parotid gland. Report of a case and review of the literature. Int J Oral Surg. 1981;10:283–92.
13. Kumar KM, Soni R, Sravan C, Indira V. Diagnostic misdiagnosis of lymphoepithelial cyst of the parotid in a HIV patient. Indian J Basic Appl Med Res. 2014;3:362–6.
14. Camilleri AC, Lloyd RE. Lymphoepithelial cyst of the parotid gland. Br J Oral Maxillofac Surg. 1990;28:329–32.
15. Skouteris CA, Patterson GT, Sotereanos GC. Benign cervical lymphoepithelial cyst: report of cases. J Oral Maxillofac Surg. 1989;47:1106–12.
16. Elliott JN, Oertel YC. Lymphoepithelial cysts of the salivary glands. Histologic and cytologic features. Am J Clin Pathol. 1990;93:39–43.
17. Weidner N, Geisinger KR, Sterling RT, Miller TR, Yen TS. Benign lymphoepithelial cysts of the parotid gland. A histologic, cytologic, and ultrastructural study. Am J Clin Pathol. 1986;85:395–401.
18. Gnepp DR, Sporck FT. Benign lymphoepithelial parotid cyst with sebaceous differentiation—cystic sebaceous lymphadenoma. Am J Clin Pathol. 1980;74:683–7.
19. Richardson GS, Clairmont AA, Erickson ER. Cystic lesions of the parotid gland. Plast Reconstr Surg. 1978;61:364–70.
20. Peel R, Gnepp DR. Diseases of the salivary glands. In: Barnes L, editor. Surgical pathology of the head and neck. New York, NY: Marcel Dekker; 1985. p. 550–2.
21. Alves CA, Ribeiro Júnior O, Borba AM, Souza SC, Naclério-Homem MG. Parotid lymphoepithelial cyst in non-HIV patient. J Clin Exp Dent. 2011;3(Suppl 1):e400–3.
22. Marmary Y, Gomori JM, Nitzan DW. Lymphoepithelial parotid cysts as presenting symptom of immunodeficiency virus infection: clinical, sialographic, and magnetic resonance imaging findings. J Oral Maxillofac Surg. 1990;48:981–4.
23. Maynard JD. Solitary cysts of the parotid. Br J Surg. 1988;75:1043.
24. Droese M. Cytological diagnosis of sialadenosis, sialadenitis, and parotid cysts by fine-needle aspiration biopsy. Adv Otorhinolaryngol. 1981;26:49–96.

25. Ward-Booth RP, Williams ED, Faulkner TP, Earl PD. Ultrasound: a simple noninvasive examination of cervical swellings. Plast Reconstr Surg. 1984;73:577–81.
26. Nisha VA, Parthiban J, Manigandan T, Amudhan A, Saravanakumar B. Infected parotid cyst –a case report with review of literature. Biosci Biotech Res Asia. 2014;11:165–7.
27. Rahman S, Shaari R, Hassan R. Parotid lymphoepithelial cyst: a case report. Arch Orofac Sci. 2006;1:71–5.
28. Rickles NH, Little JW. The histogenesis of the branchial cyst. II. A study of the lining epithelium. Am J Pathol. 1967;50:765–77.
29. Joshi J, Shah S, Agarwal D, Khasgiwal A. Benign lymphoepithelial cyst of parotid gland: review and case report. J Oral Maxillofac Pathol. 2018;22(Suppl 1):S91–7.
30. Mhawej R, Richa T, Melkane AE. Benign lymphoepithelial cyst of unusual location: a case report. Acta Otolaryngol Case Rep. 2016;1:110–2.
31. Araujo MR, Centurion BS, Albuquerque DF, Marchesano LH, Damante JH. Management of a parotid sialocele in a young patient: case report and literature review. J Appl Oral Sci. 2010;18(4):432–6.
32. Peel R. Diseases of the salivary gland. In: Barnes L, editor. Surgical pathology of the head and neck. New York, NY: Marcel-Dekker; 2001. p. 634–757.
33. Canosa A, Cohen MA. Post-traumatic parotid sialocele: report of two cases. J Oral Maxillofac Surg. 1999;57(6):742–5.
34. Witt RL. The incidence and management of siaolocele after parotidectomy. Otolaryngol Head Neck Surg. 2009;140(6):871–4.
35. Langdon JD. Complications of parotid gland surgery. J Maxillofac Surg. 1984;12(5):225–9.
36. Capaccio P, Paglia M, Minorati D, Manzo R, Ottaviani F. Diagnosis and therapeutic management of iatrogenic parotid sialocele. Ann Otol Rhinol Laryngol. 2004;113(7):562–4.
37. Parekh D, Glezerson G, Stewart M, Esser J, Lawson HH. Post-traumatic parotid fistulae and sialoceles. A prospective study of conservative management in 51 cases. Ann Surg. 1989;209(1):105–11.
38. Pereira KD, Smith SL, Mitchell RB. Parotid sialocele in a 10-year-old girl. Ear Nose Throat. 2007;86(1):27–8.
39. Vargas H, Galati LT, Parnes SM. A pilot study evaluating the treatment of postparotidectomy sialoceles with botulinum toxin type a. Arch Otolaryngol Head Neck Surg. 2000;126:421–4.
40. Burkitt HG, Quick CRG, Gatt DT. Essential surgery: problems, diagnosis and management. London: Churchill Livingstone, Langmans; 1990.
41. Hegde PN, Prasad HLK, Kumar YS, Sajitha K, Roy PS, Raju M, et al. A rare case of an epidermoid cyst in the parotid gland—which was diagnosed by fine needle aspiration cytology. J Clin Diagn Res. 2013;7(3):550–2.
42. Dutt SN, Hock YL, Saleem Y, Bhat N, East DM. Epidermoid cyst of the submandibular gland. Indian J Otolaryngol Head Neck Surg. 2000;52(4):378–9.
43. Sanglee C, Kaunkin H. Iatrogenic epidermoid cyst in the parotid gland: a case report. J Korean Assoc Oral Maxillofac Surg. 2011;37:237–40.
44. Kar R, Thorawade V, Jagade M, Attakkil A, Kedar S, Rohe D, et al. An unusual case of epidermal cyst in submandibular space. Int J Otolaryngol Head Neck Surg. 2014;3:213–5.
45. Prepageran N, Rahmat O, Kuljit S. Epidermal cyst of submandibular gland. Med J Malaysia. 2005;60(4):483–4.
46. Janarthanam J, Mahadevan S. Epidermoid cyst of submandibular region. J Oral Maxillofac Pathol. 2012;16(3):435–7.
47. Baschinsky D, Hameed A, Kehyani S. Fine needle aspiration cytological features of dermoid cyst of parotid gland. A report of two cases. Diagn Cytopathol. 1999;20(6):387–8.
48. Rosai J. Major and minor salivary glands. In: Mosby RJ, editor. Ackermans surgical pathology. 8th ed. St Louis, MO: Mosby; 1996. p. 815–56.
49. Tuffin JR, Theaker E. True lateral dermoid cyst of the neck. Int J Oral Maxillofac Surg. 1991;20(5):275–6.
50. Streppel M, Thomas JP, Stennert E, Guntinas-Lichius O, Wagner M. Infected epidermoid cyst as cause of peripheral facial palsy. A case report. Laryngorhinootologie. 2001;80(10):617–9.

51. Turetschek K, Hospodka H, Steiner E. Epidermoid cyst of the floor of the mouth: diagnostic imaging by sonography, computed tomography and magnetic resonance imaging. Br J Radiol. 1995;68(806):205–7.
52. Mukunyadzi P. Review of fine-needle aspiration cytology of salivary gland neoplasms, with emphasis on differential diagnosis. Am J Clin Pathol. 2002;118:S100–15.
53. Ganesan A, Nandakumar GK. Epidermal cyst of parotid gland: a rarity and a diagnostic dilemma. Case Rep Dentist. 2015;2015:856170, 1–3
54. New GB, Erich JB. Dermoid cysts of the head and neck. Surg Gynecol Obstet. 1937;65:48–55.
55. Moody AB, Avery CM, Harrison JD. Dermoid cyst of the parotid gland. Int J Oral Maxillofac Surg. 1998;27(6):461–2.
56. Taylor BW, Erich JB. Dermoid cysts of nose. Mayo Clin Proc. 1967;42(8):488.
57. Smirniotopoulos JG, Chiechi MV. Teratomas, dermoids, and epidermoids of the head and neck. Radiographics. 1995;15(6):1437–55.
58. Islam S, Hoffman GR. Parotid dermoid cyst: a rare entity. J Laryngol Otol. 2009;123(2):1–4.
59. Choi EC, Jin JB, Kim JY, Hong WP, Kim MJ, Park YK. Dermoid cyst of the parotid gland. Yonsei Med J. 1988;29(2):199–203.
60. Naujoks C, Handschel J, Braunstein S, Emaetig F, Depprich R, Meyer U, et al. Dermoid cyst of the parotid gland—a case report and brief review of the literature. Int J Oral Maxillofac Surg. 2007;36(9):861–3.
61. Keane A, Warrick J, Andrews GA, Choi KY. Pediatric dermoid cyst of the parotid: case report and review of the literature. Otolaryngol Case Rep. 2021;18:100258.
62. Jham BC, Duraes GV, Jham AC, Santos CR. Epidermoid cyst of the floor of the mouth: a case report. J Can Dent Assoc. 2007;73(6):525–8.
63. Rosen D, Wirtschafter A, Rao VM, Wilcox TO Jr. Dermoid cyst of the lateral neck: a case report and literature review. Ear Nose Throat J. 1998;77(125):129–32.
64. Pryor SG, Lewis JE, Weaver AL, Orvidas LJ. Pediatric dermoid cysts of the head and neck. Otolaryngol Head Neck Surg. 2005;132(6):938–42.
65. Alhusain ZZ, Witczak K, Shabaik A. Dermoid cyst of the parotid gland: case report of a rare entity and review of the literature. Am J Case Rep. 2023;24:e939411.
66. Sahoo NK, Choudhary AK, Srinivas V, Kapil T. Dermoid cysts of maxillofacial region. Med J Armed Forces India. 2015;71(2):389–94.
67. Siddiqui B, Faridi SH, Ahmad SS, Khan R. A rare case of a dermoid cyst of parotid gland. Int Arch BioMed Clin Res. 2016;2:83–6.
68. Mukunyadzi P. Review of fine-needle aspiration cytology of salivary gland neoplasms, with emphasis on differential diagnosis. Pathol Patterns Rev. 2002;118(1):S100–15.
69. Baschinsky D, Hameed A, Keyhani-Rofagha S. Fine-needle aspiration cytological features of dermoid cyst of the parotid gland: a report of two cases. Diagn Cytopathol. 1999;20(6):387–38811.
70. Dwivedi G, Gupta V, Patnaik U, Kumar M, Sood A, Upadhyay M. Dermoid cyst of the parotid gland: a rare entity. Indian J Otolaryngol Head Neck Surg. 2019;71(1):809–12.
71. Damar M, Erdem D, Dinç AE, Biskin S, Bahadir B. Dermoid cyst of the parotid gland. ENT Case. 2015;1(3):191–4.
72. Yang C, Wang X, Zhang S, Wu D. Dermoid cyst of the parotid gland location. J Craniofac Surg. 2020;31(7):e698–e99.
73. Vavro M, Horák S, Dvoranová B, Čierna Z, Babál P, Kobzová D, et al. Rare location of a dermoid cyst in the parotid gland: a case report. Prague Med Rep. 2022;123(3):193–8.
74. Gold BD, Sheinkopf DE, Levy B. Dermoid, epidermoid, and teratomatous cysts of the tongue and the floor of the mouth. J Oral Surg. 1974;32:107–11.
75. Jayasuriya NS, Siriwardena S, Tilakaratne WM, Parthiepan S. Malignant transformation of a long-standing submental dermoid cyst to a carcinosarcoma: a case report. J Med Case Rep. 2017;11(1):11.
76. Devine JC, Jones DC. Carcinomatous transformation of a sublingual dermoid cyst: a case report. Int J Oral Maxillofac Surg. 2000;29:126–7.

77. Darabi M, Varedi P, Mohebi AR, Mahmoodi S, Varedi P, Nabavizadeh SA, et al. Hydatid cyst of the parotid gland. Oral Maxillofac Surg. 2009;13(1):33–5.
78. Karahatay S, Akcam T, Kocaoglu M, Tosun F, Gunhan O. A rare cause of parotid swelling: primary hydatid cyst. Auris Nasus Larynx. 2006e;33(2):227–9.
79. Pakala T, Molina M, Wu GY. Hepatic echinococcal cysts: a review. J Clin Transl Hepatol. 2016;4(1):39–46.
80. Kasliwal N, Pachori G, Indushekar V, Sharma K. Primary hydatid cyst of parotid gland—an aspirate with a clue to diagnosis. Int J Med Sci Pub Health. 2016;5(1):152–4.
81. Hassan QA. Primary hydatid cyst of parotid gland: a rare case diagnosed by computed tomography. Al-Kindy College Med J. 2017;13:2.
82. Kara T, Arpaci RB, Vayisoğlu Y, Serinsöz E, Gürsoy D, Özgür A, et al. Hydatid cyst of parotid gland: an unusual case diagnosed by fine needle aspiration biopsy. Turk Patoloji Derg. 2017;33(2):171–4.
83. Arora VK, Chopra N, Singh P, Venugopal VK, Narang S. Hydatid cyst of parotid: report of unusual cytological findings extending the cytomorphological spectrum. Diagn Cytopathol. 2016;44(9):770–3.
84. Diwan R, Mogra N, Purohit M. Primary hydatid cyst of the parotid gland. BMJ Case Rep. 2015;2015:bcr2014209217.
85. Rajendra Gopal SV, Mahadeva Sastry N, Venkataramana G. Hydatid cyst of parotid. A case report. Indian J Pathol Microbiol. 1985;28:75–6.
86. Emamy H, Asadian A. Unusual presentation of hydatid disease. Am J Surg. 1976;132:403–5.
87. Saxena SK, Chaudhary SK, Saxena GR, Rao S. Hydatid cyst of the parotid gland (a case report). J Postgrad Med. 1983;29:105–6.
88. Tekin M, Osma U, Yaldiz M, Topcu I. Preauricular hydatid cyst: an unusual location for echinoccosis. Eur Arch Otorrinolaringol. 2004;261:87–9.
89. Moradi M, Rampisheh Z, Roozbehani M, Razmjou E. A retrospective study of hydatid cysts in patients undergoing liver and lung surgery in Tehran, Iran. Heliyon. 2019;5(6):e01897.
90. WHO Informal Working Group International classification of ultrasound images in cystic echinococcosis for application in clinical and field epidemiological settings. Acta Trop. 2003;85:253–61.
91. Botezatu C, Mastalier B, Patrascu T. Hepatic hydatid cyst—diagnose and treatment algorithm. J Med Life. 2018;11(3):203–9.
92. Kalovidouris A, Gouliamos A, Andreou I, Ioannovits I, Levett J, Vlahos I, et al. Primary hydatid disease of the infratemporal fossa and the parotid gland. Radiologe. 1985;25:235–6.
93. Mafee MF. Salivary glands. In: Valvassori GE, Mafee MF, Carter BL, editors. Imaging of the head and neck. 2nd ed. New York, NY: Thieme; 2005. p. 625–81.
94. Rasool Hammoodi SA, Aftan KT, Ali MR. Hydatid cysts of parotid glands- diagnosis, treatment and recurrences. Int J Surg Protoc. 2021;25(1):135–40.
95. Akhan O, Ensari S, Ozmen M. Percutaneous treatment of a parotid gland hydatid cyst: a possible alternative to surgery. Eur Radiol. 2002;12:597–9.

Parotid Gland Tumors: Overview and Classification

11

11.1 Introduction

Parotid gland neoplasms may be benign or malignant, and malignant tumors can be primary or metastatic. Due to the epithelial and the nonepithelial histology of the affected organ, many histological types of parotid tumors with variable biological behavior are possible, although some are rare [1]. The distinction between tumor types can be difficult, particularly when based fine needle aspiration (FNA). The commonest benign tumor of the parotid gland [pleomorphic adenoma (PA)] has a malignant transformation potential, and, although considered benign, there is a propensity for recurrence after treatment [2].

Malignant salivary gland tumors usually present after the sixth decade of life, whereas benign lesions present in the fourth to fifth decade of life. Benign lesions tend to be more common in women while malignant lesions tend to occur with equal frequency in both genders. The majority of salivary gland tumors occur in the parotid; about 10% occur in the submandibular gland and <5% occur in the minor salivary glands. Most parotid gland tumors are benign, while those occurring in the submandibular gland and the minor salivary glands are more likely to be malignant. The overall 5-year survival of malignant salivary disease depends on the stage of the disease but has been reported to be around 70%.

11.2 Epidemiology

Approximately 300 cases per year of primary salivary gland malignancy are registered in the United Kingdom, of which fewer than 10 occur in children [3]. The worldwide incidence is estimated to be 0.5–3.0 per 100,000 per year, accounting for about 5% of all head and neck malignancies [4, 5]. Patients with malignant neoplasms typically present in their sixth decade.

© The Author(s), under exclusive license to Springer Nature Switzerland AG 2024
M. Sakr, *Surgery of the Salivary Glands*,
https://doi.org/10.1007/978-3-031-82069-4_11

11.3 Etiology

The "multicellular theory" for the development of salivary gland tumors states that "each tumor type forms from a specific differentiated cell of origin within the salivary gland unit." Excretory stem cells give rise to muco-epidermoid and squamous cell carcinomas, while intercalated stem cells can lead to pleomorphic adenomas, adenoid cystic carcinomas, oncocytomas, adenocarcinomas, and acinic cell carcinomas.

Radiation exposure has been linked to parotid gland carcinomas 15 years after the event. Cigarette smoking and alcohol have also been linked to Warthin's tumor of the parotid gland. In addition, a link between occupational exposure to silica dust and nitrosamines and salivary tumor gland has been reported [6].

Several oncogenes have been implicated in salivary gland tumors. Mutations of P53, MDM2, Bcl-2, and ras have been found in both benign and malignant lesions.

11.4 Clinical Presentation

11.4.1 History-Taking

The usual complaint of patients with a parotid tumor is a slow-growing painless mass. Rapid growth, pain, skin tethering or ulceration, cervical lymphadenopathy, and facial nerve paralysis are all suggestive of malignancy. Tumors low in the tail of the parotid gland can easily be confused with an upper cervical lymph node (LN) or other lateral swellings of the neck. Bilateral parotid tumors are most common in Warthin's tumors and human immunodeficiency virus (HIV)-related lympho-epithelial cysts. Taking a detailed history is important in treating patients with parotid lumps, as infectious, autoimmune, and inflammatory processes may masquerade as neoplasms.

11.4.2 Physical Examination

All patients with a mass in the parotid gland should have an inspection and palpation of the mass itself. Oral examination should include inspection of Stenson's duct orifice, which is situated opposite the upper second molar. Facial nerve assessment is mandatory, as is neck LN palpation. Facial nerve palsy may indicate a malignant lesion with infiltration into the nerve. The head and neck skin should also be checked for cancers since the parotid gland is a common site for metastases from squamous cell carcinomas (SCCs) arising in the skin of the head and neck.

11.5 Work-Up (Investigations)

11.5.1 Imaging

Ultrasonography (US) provides invaluable information about the site, size, and nature of parotid tumors and the presence of any significant cervical lymphadenopathy [7]. The position of a tumor in the superficial or deep aspect of the parotid gland is established by the identification of its relation to the retromandibular vein. Ultrasound-guided fine-needle aspiration biopsy (FNAB) improves the adequacy rate. In experienced hands, this can distinguish malignant from benign disease in 80–90% of cases. Cross-sectional imaging is not essential in straightforward benign tumors, but magnetic resonance imaging (MRI) of a parotid tumor is useful in the assessment and delineation of anatomical structures, extension into the deep lobe, and relation to the facial nerve. If the patient is suspected of having metastatic spread, the use of F-18 fluoro-deoxyglucose positron emission tomography (PET) scan is useful. Recently, the use of a technetium scan aided with lemon juice stimulation has been used to diagnose Warthin's tumor.

11.5.2 Fine-Needle Aspiration Biopsy (FNAB)

The primary diagnostic tool for parotid gland lesions is FNAB, but its role in differentiating benign from malignant disease still carries some controversy. It is a relatively painless procedure, has few complications, and may prevent an ill-advised and often ill-fated incisional or excisional biopsy of a parotid mass. However, it is far from straightforward with issues regarding aspiration technique, adequacy of the specimen, cytological expertise, and limitations of the interpretation. If the result of FNA is at variance with other findings, then clinical judgment should prevail. It is also important to be aware that false-positive results can occur, leading to misdiagnosis of malignant lesions.

11.6 Treatment

11.6.1 Benign Tumors (BTs)

Superficial parotidectomy with identification, exposure, and preservation of the facial nerve was traditionally the preferred procedure. It is now generally accepted that an adequate margin in BTs is a cuff of 1–2 mm. There is thus an increasing recognition that an operation less than the traditional procedures is acceptable such as partial superficial or hemi-superficial parotidectomy. An extracapsular dissection for benign pathology, away from the main branches of the facial nerve, is an option, and even endoscopically assisted parotidectomy can be effective in selected patients. A "lumpectomy" is not considered an appropriate procedure for benign tumors of the parotid gland due to high recurrence rates. Complications from parotid surgery include a scar, facial nerve injury, hematoma, seroma, salivary fistula, and Frey's syndrome (gustatory sweating) [8].

11.6.2 Malignant Tumors (MTs)

In small, low-grade superficial parotid tumors, a superficial parotidectomy with a margin of at least 1.5 cm may suffice, but otherwise, a total conservative parotidectomy is advised with resection of adjacent neck structures if necessary to achieve an en bloc resection. A functioning facial nerve should be preserved unless found to be infiltrated with the tumor itself at the time of resection. If the nerve is sacrificed, then primary nerve grafting should be performed. The greater auricular nerve (GAN) as a donor is an option, but it may be involved, so the sural nerve from the leg may be preferred [8].

Neck dissection should be carried out in patients with clinical or radiological evidence of nodal disease. A prophylactic selective neck dissection (levels I–III) should be performed for patients with high-stage (T3/T4) disease-free clinically high-grade tumors.

Parotid gland MTs respond poorly to chemotherapy, with adjuvant chemotherapy used only for palliation. Adjuvant radiotherapy is recommended for large tumors (>4 cm), patients with incomplete or close margins, recurrent disease, perineural and vascular invasion, nodal disease, in metastatic disease, and is usually indicated for adenoid cystic carcinomas and high-grade tumors [9].

11.7 Histological Classification

A good rule of thumb to remember is the rule of 80 s; that is, 80% of all salivary tumors are in the parotid, 80% of parotid tumors are benign, and 80% of the benign tumors that arise in the parotid are pleomorphic adenomas. Warthin's tumor is the second most common benign lesion. The most common malignant tumor is muco-epidermoid carcinoma (MEC), followed by acinic cell carcinoma, and adenoid cystic carcinoma.

Tumors of the salivary glands are relatively uncommon and represent less than 2% of all head and neck neoplasms. The WHO histological classification of salivary gland tumors now includes over 40 variants as well as tumor-like lesions (e.g., salivary gland cysts). These include the following [10]:

11.7.1 Benign Epithelial Tumors

- Pleomorphic adenoma (PA) (mixed salivary tumor)
- Myoepithelioma

- Basal cell adenoma
- Warthin's tumor (adenolymphoma, papillary cystadenoma lymphomatosum)
- Oncocytoma
- Canalicular adenoma
- Sebaceous adenoma
- Lymphadenoma: sebaceous, non-sebaceous
- Duct papilloma: inverted duct papilloma–intraductal papilloma–sialadenoma papilliferum
- Cystadenoma

11.7.2 Malignant Epithelial Tumors

- Acinic cell carcinoma (ACC)
- Mucoepidermoid carcinoma (MEP)
- Adenoid cystic carcinoma (AdCC)
- Polymorphous low-grade adenocarcinoma (PLGA)
- Epithelial–myoepithelial carcinoma
- Clear cell carcinoma, not otherwise specified
- Basal cell adenocarcinoma
- Sebaceous carcinoma
- Sebaceous lymphadenocarcinoma
- Cystadenocarcinoma
- Low-grade cribriform cystadenocarcinoma
- Mucinous adenocarcinoma
- Oncocytic carcinoma
- Salivary duct carcinoma
- Adenocarcinoma, not otherwise specified
- Myoepithelial carcinoma
- Carcinoma ex-pleomorphic adenoma (CEPA)
- Carcinosarcoma (malignant mixed salivary tumor)
  Metastasizing pleomorphic adenoma
- Squamous cell carcinoma
- Small cell carcinoma (SCC)
- Large cell carcinoma
- Lymphoepithelial carcinoma
- Sialoblastoma

11.7.3 Soft-Tissue Tumors

- Hemangioma
- Lymphangioma
- Lipoma

Table 11.1 Simplified WHO classification of salivary gland tumors

Benign	Malignant	Hematolymphoid	Nonepithelial
– **Pleomorphic** adenoma – Warthin's tumor (adenolymphoma) – Myoepithelioma – Basal cell adenoma – Oncocytoma – Cystadenoma	– Mucoepidermoid carcinoma – Adenoid cystic carcinoma – Acinic cell carcinoma, adenocarcinoma – Squamous cell carcinoma – Undifferentiated carcinoma – Carcinoma ex-pleomorphic adenoma – Polymorphous low-grade carcinoma	– Hodgkin's lymphoma – Diffuse large B-cell lymphoma – Extranodal marginal zone-B-cell lymphoma	– Hemangioma, – Lymphangioma, – Neurofibromas

11.7.4 Hematolymphoid Tumors

- Hodgkin's lymphoma
- Diffuse large B-cell lymphoma
- Extranodal marginal zone B-cell lymphoma

11.7.5 Secondary Tumors

A simplified classification of parotid gland tumors is presented in Table 11.1. They include benign, malignant, hematolymphoid, and nonepithelial tumors. Carcinomas can further be classified as high-grade, low-grade, or mixed, the latter indicating a variable behavior depending on the histological picture.

References

1. Lyu HX, Wang ZR, Gao YQ, Yu M, Li BQ, Zhang ZB. Clinical pathologic analysis on 3 724 cases of salivary gland tumors. Zhonghua Kou Qiang Yi Xue Za Zhi. 2019;54(1):10–6.
2. Hu YH, Li W, Zhang CY, Xia RH, Tian Z, Wang LZ, et al. Prognostic nomogram for disease-specific survival of carcinoma ex pleomorphic adenoma of the salivary gland. Head Neck. 2017;39(12):2416–24.
3. Sood S, McGurk M, Vaz F. Management of salivary gland tumours: United Kingdom national multidisciplinary guidelines. J Laryngol Otol. 2016;130(S2):S142–9.
4. Pinkston JA, Cole P. Incidence rates of salivary gland tumors: results from a population-based study. Otolaryngol Head Neck Surg. 1999;120(6):834–40.
5. Stenner M, Klussmann JP. Current update on established and novel biomarkers in salivary gland carcinoma pathology and the molecular pathways involved. Eur Arch Otorhinolaryngol. 2009;266(3):333–41.

6. Straif K, Weiland SK, Bungers M, Holthenrich D, Keil U. Exposure to nitrosamines and mortality from salivary gland cancer among rubber workers. Epidemiology. 1999;10(6):786–7.
7. Zengel P, Notter F, Clevert DA. VTIQ and VTQ in combination with B-mode and color Doppler ultrasound improve classification of salivary gland tumors, especially for inexperienced physicians. Clin Hemorheol Microcirc. 2018;70(4):457–66.
8. Sethi RKV, Deschler DG. National trends in inpatient parotidectomy: a fourteen-year retrospective analysis. Am J Otolaryngol. 2018;39(5):553–7.
9. Wang K, Pearlstein KA, Moon DH, Mahbooba ZM, Deal AM, Wang Y, et al. Assessment of risk of xerostomia after whole-brain radiation therapy and association with parotid dose. JAMA Oncol. 2019;5(2):221–8.
10. Seifert G, Sobin LH. The world health organization's classification of salivary gland tumors. A commentary on the second edition. Cancer. 1992;70(2):379–85.

Benign Tumors of the Parotid Gland

12

12.1 Background

Benign tumors (BTs) of salivary glands occur mostly in the parotid gland, and most of them are pleomorphic adenomas (PAs), which affect both genders equally. The benign tumor usually presents as a slowly growing painless mass in front of the tragus of the ear, below the ear lobule, or in the upper part of the neck, arising from the superficial lobe of the gland, which represents 80% of the cases. Less commonly, the mass presents as a cheek mass overlying the masseter, arising from the accessory parotid lobe. If the tumor arises from the deep lobe, it presents as a parapharyngeal mass with a completely different clinical presentation. In this instance, the patient will complain of snoring and difficulty in swallowing. Physical examination will reveal a soft palate and tonsillar, firm, diffuse bulge.

Warthin's tumor is the second most common benign lesion. The tumor is more common in men than women and is known to be bilateral in 10–15% of cases. It has been linked to smoking and presents after the fourth decade of life. Oncocytomas are rare tumors that occur in older patients. These lesions are firm and identified using electron microscopy. Monomorphic adenomas may feel like Pas, but lack the pleomorphic features. These slow-growing lesions are likely to occur also in the minor salivary glands.

12.2 Pleomorphic Adenoma (PA)

12.2.1 Epidemiology

Pleomorphic adenoma (PA), the most common salivary gland tumor, is also known as benign mixed tumor (BMT) because of its dual origin from epithelial and myoepithelial elements [1–3]. It represents 75–80% of all benign parotid tumors, predominantly affecting the superficial lobe; however, it may also affect the

© The Author(s), under exclusive license to Springer Nature Switzerland AG 2024
M. Sakr, *Surgery of the Salivary Glands*,
https://doi.org/10.1007/978-3-031-82069-4_12

submandibular and minor salivary glands. The annual incidence of PA is approximately 2–3.5 cases per 100,000 individuals [4]. Its incidence is slightly higher in females than in males (2:1 ratio) and affects individuals of all ages, most commonly patients between 30 and 50 years of age [5–7]. Though uncommon, it has been reported in the first two decades of life. It is uncommon to be bilateral [8]. It is usually a solitary lesion, although synchronous or metachronous involvement of two or more salivary glands can occur. It may also occur in combination with other tumors, mostly Warthin's tumor.

12.2.2 Etiology

The exact etiology of PA is unknown, but the incidence of this tumor has been increasing in the last 15–20 years in relation to the exposure of radiation. One study suggests that oncogenic simian virus (SV40) may play a role in the onset or progression of PA. Prior head and neck irradiation is also a risk factor for the development of these tumors [9].

Approximately 70% of PAs have cytogenetic alterations that likely play a major role in tumorigenesis and can be categorized into four groups: (1) tumors with 8q12 rearrangements, (2) those with 12q13–15 rearrangements, (3) those with miscellaneous clonal changes, and (4) those that are karyotypically normal [10, 11].

12.2.3 Pathology

Pleomorphic adenoma has a highly variable appearance, hence the name "pleomorphic." It has a pleomorphic matrix, with a noncystic cut section that may show some islets of cartilage. Microscopically, it is formed of epithelial cells intermingled with a pleomorphic stroma; fibrous, myxomatous, and pseudo-cartilaginous (Fig. 12.1). It is categorized into four types as follows [12]: (1) principally myxoid, (2) mixed myxoid and cellular components in equal proportions, (3) predominantly cellular, and (4) extremely cellular.

Epithelial elements are usually of polygonal, spindle, or stellate-shaped cells, which may be arranged to form duct-like structures, sheets, clumps, or interlacing strands. The ducts and tubules are seen usually exhibiting an outer lining in addition to an inner cuboidal epithelial cell layer. This outer myoepithelial cell layer (or layers) merges into the surrounding stroma, which also contains dispersed or clumped myoepithelial element cells. Areas of squamous metaplasia and epithelial pearls can be found. Pleomorphic adenoma is a well-defined tumor, but lacks a true capsule and is surrounded by a fibrous pseudo-capsule of variable thickness. The tumor extends through normal glandular parenchyma in the form of finger-like pseudopodia. These microscopic extensions account for the high risk of recurrence in cases treated with simple enucleation or surgical resections performed with inadequate surgical margins.

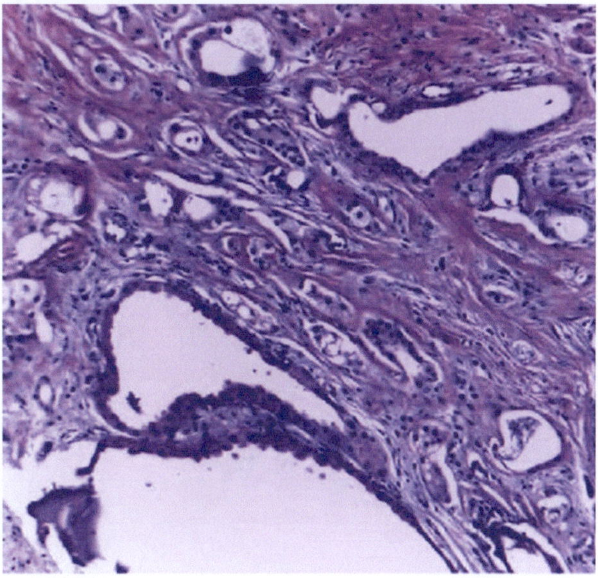

Fig. 12.1 Pleomorphic adenoma (PA): biphasic population of epithelial and mesenchymal cells. Epithelial cells assume tubular profiles, cords, or nests. Stroma is myxoid. (H&E, ×100)

Pleomorphic adenoma carries a malignant potential of 5–10%. The presence of hyalinized stroma is the most predictive histological parameter for malignant transformation. The tumor may rarely metastasize without having the histological features of malignancy, but this almost always occurs after inadequate surgical excision, possibly due to altered anatomy secondary to surgery, which gave access to vascular and lymphatic channels.

12.2.4 Clinical Presentation

The patient usually presents with a solitary, painless, slowly growing, spherical mass, of variable size ranging from pea size to a large mass [13–15] as shown in Figs. 12.2 and 12.3. The mass usually lies over the angle of the mandible and below the lobule of the ear (Fig. 12.4). However, a swelling of the lower pole of the parotid gland may present on the lateral side of the neck, below and behind the angle of the mandible, giving rise to clinical diagnostic difficulty (Fig. 12.5).

Symptoms and signs of the neoplasm depend mainly on tumor size, location, and potential to undergo malignant transformation. The patient's complaint is usually disfigurement. The mass is of heterogonous consistency and mobile, being neither attached to the skin nor to the deep structures. Bosselation of the tumor is demonstrable if it is bigger than 3 cm. A fibrous capsule may not be apparent, but the tumor is clearly demarcated from surrounding tissues.

While most PAs occur in the superficial lobe of the parotid gland (80%), the deep lobe can be involved (20%) [16–18]. It may present as an oral retro-tonsillar or parapharyngeal mass, which is visible or usually palpable, and is clearly demonstrable by imaging. Extensions of deep lobe PAs are the most common tumors of the

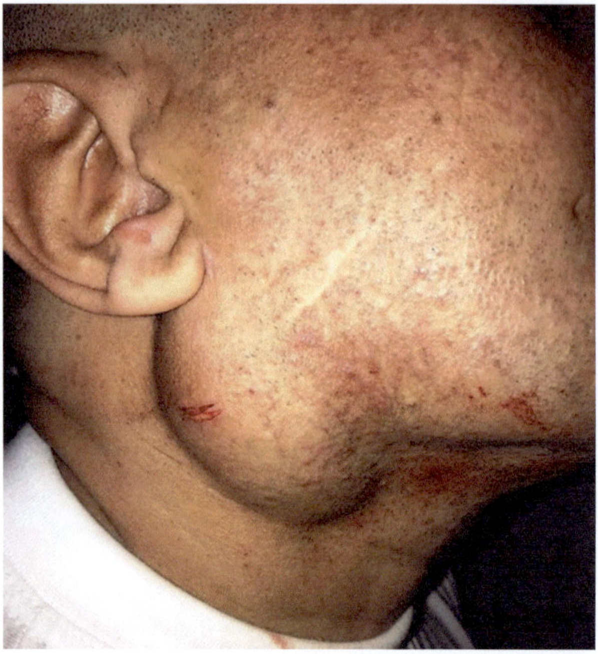

Fig. 12.2 Lateral view showing a large right-sided pleomorphic adenoma (PA) of the parotid gland in a 46-year-old man. Note displacement of the right ear lobule

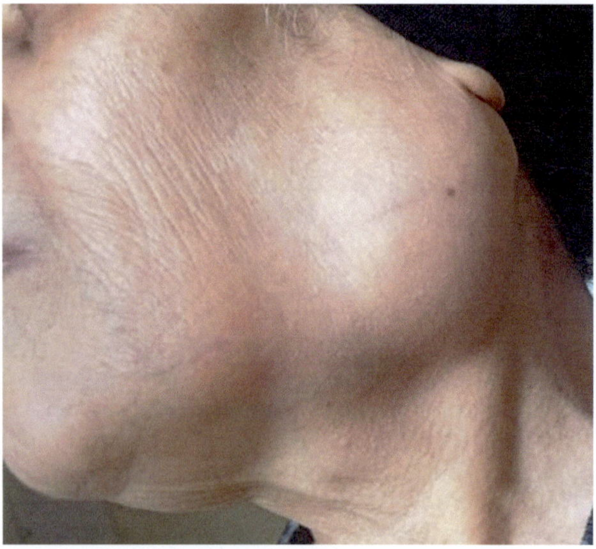

Fig. 12.3 Lateral view showing a large left-sided pleomorphic adenoma (PA) of the parotid gland in a 51-year-old woman. Note displacement of the left ear lobule

para-pharyngeal space constituting 40% of tumors in this region [8, 18]. The draining lymph nodes (LNs) are not enlarged and the facial nerve is always intact. However, signs of facial nerve weakness can occur when the tumor is large or if it undergoes malignant change. Rapid enlargement of a tumor nodule should also raise a concern for malignant change.

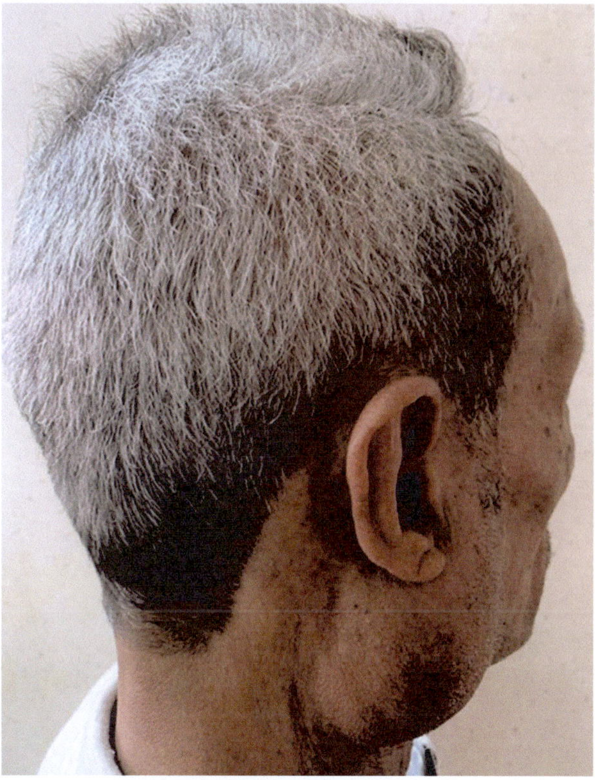

Fig. 12.4 Lateral view showing the pleomorphic adenoma (PA) in its typical position over the angle of the mandible and below the lobule of the ear

12.2.5 Investigations/Diagnosis

The diagnosis of PA is made by both imaging studies and tissue sampling, which includes fine-needle aspiration (FNA) and core-needle biopsy, which can be done in an outpatient setting. These procedures are associated with very low tumor seeding rates [4, 19].

12.2.5.1 Imaging

As for any parotid mass, ultrasonography (US), CT scan, and MRI (preferably with diffusion-weighted and perfusion sequences) are the best imaging tools. Digital subtraction angiography (DSA) can also be considered.

Ultrasonography (US)

On US, pleomorphic adenomas characteristically appear hypoechoic in texture. They usually show a lobulated distinct border with or without posterior acoustic enhancement. Ultrasound-guided biopsy or FNA are minimally invasive and cost-effective procedures.

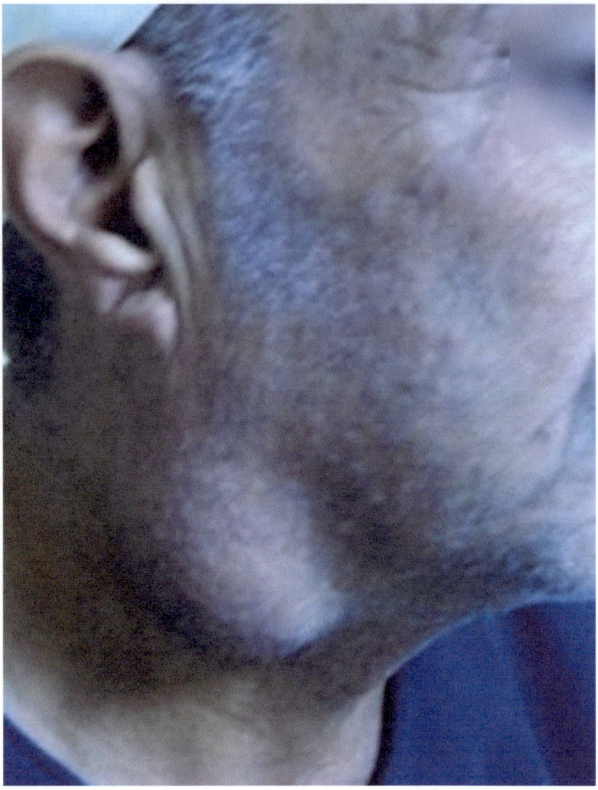

Fig. 12.5 Lateral view showing a pleomorphic adenoma (PA) arising below and behind the angle of the mandible, not related to the ear lobule in a 57-year-old man. It has to be differentiated from other lateral neck swellings

Computed Tomography (CT) Scan

On CT examination, a PA usually appears as a smoothly marginated or lobulated homogeneous soft-tissue density globular mass (Fig. 12.6). Necrosis can be seen in larger masses. Few foci of calcification are common. Smaller tumors show early homogeneous prominent enhancement while in the case of larger tumors enhancement is less marked and delayed.

Magnetic Resonance Imaging (MRI)

The MRI is similar to CT scan; smaller masses appear well-circumscribed and homogeneous, whereas larger tumors appear heterogeneous. Images are seen as follows:

- T1: usually of low intensity.
- T2: usually of very high intensity (Fig. 12.7) (especially myxoid type) and often has a rim of decreased signal intensity on T2-weighted images representing the surrounding fibrous capsule.
- T1 C+ (gadolinium, Gd): usually demonstrates homogeneous enhancement.

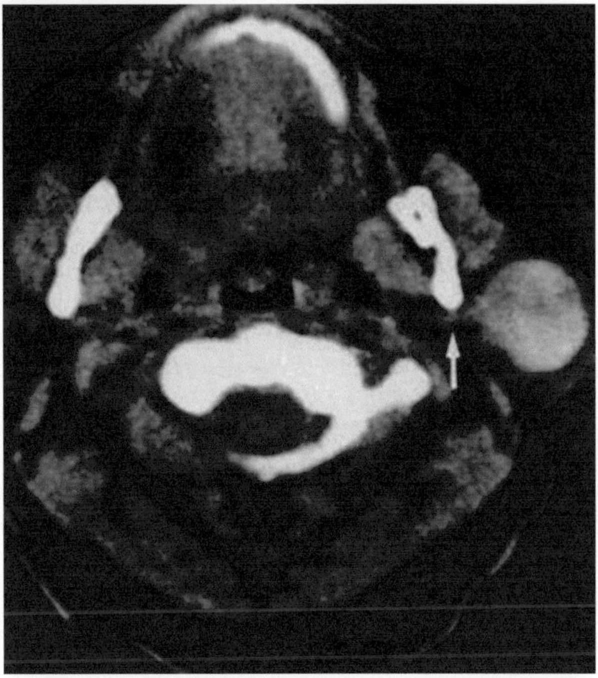

Fig. 12.6 Computed tomography (CT) scan showing a pleomorphic adenoma (PA) of the left parotid gland as a large, high-density, sharply marginated tumor in the superficial lobe of gland. Proximity to retromandibular vessels (arrow) indicates lateral relation to the facial nerve

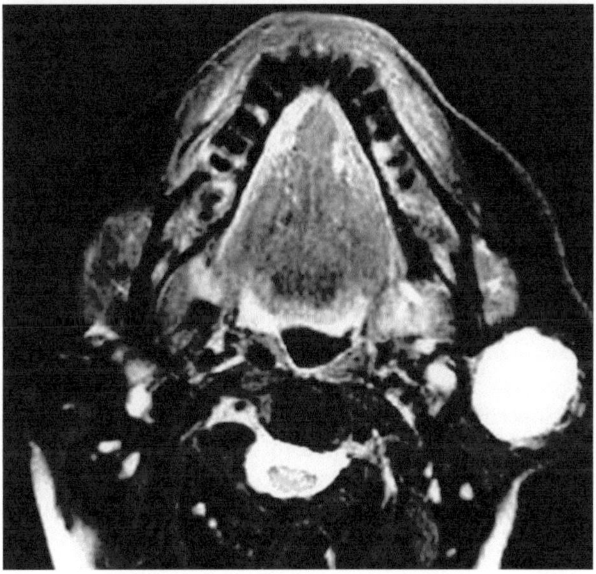

Fig. 12.7 Magnetic resonance imaging (MRI) of the parotid gland—T2 axial MRI showing a case of pleomorphic adenoma (PA), in the left parotid gland as a well-circumscribed, T2-bright mass

The presence of either T2 hypointensity or ill-defined margins after contrast administration can be a simple MRI malignancy test for parotid tumors, with a sensitivity and specificity of 0.70 and 0.73, respectively.

Post-contrast short tau inversion recovery (STIR) images help delineate the perineural spread of tumor in case of malignant change.

12.2.5.2 Cytology/Biopsy

Fine-needle aspiration cytology (FNAC) is a well-recognized method for obtaining preoperative diagnosis and is advised to be done after imaging for the fear of hemorrhage. Many studies showed that the use of flow cytometry as a biological parameter for the prediction of recurrence in PAs should be considered. Tumors of a larger size showed a higher percentage of cells in the S-phase fraction and probably a greater tendency for recurrence [20].

The smears obtained from FNA can determine whether the tumor is malignant in nature with an approximate sensitivity of 90%. Core-needle biopsy is more invasive, but provides more accurate histological typing of the tumor with a diagnostic accuracy of around 97%. Immunohistochemistry (IHC) may prove to be supportive in delineating the different cell components.

12.2.6 Differential Diagnosis

Differentials for PA include Warthin's tumor, parotid nodal metastasis, facial nerve schwannoma, myoepithelioma, mucoepidermoid and adenoid cystic carcinomas, and a large variety of other neoplasms nonspecific to salivary glands. Histopathology remains the gold standard in differentiating them all.

12.2.7 Treatment

Pleomorphic adenomas harbor a small risk of malignant transformation. The malignant potential is proportional to the time the lesion is in situ (1.5% in the first 5 years, 9.5% after 15 years). Therefore, surgical excision is warranted in almost all cases. Other risk factors of malignancy include advanced age, radiation therapy, large size, and recurrent tumors.

Superficial or total conservative parotidectomy with preservation of the facial nerve is usually performed for the treatment of PAs. The skin incision can be the classical lazy-S incision or recently one can resort to the cosmetically better face-lift incision. Flaps are raised and the facial nerve trunk is exposed at the stylomastoid foramen, and all its five terminal branches are followed to the muscles to avoid injury. The incidence of recurrence following surgery varies depending on the surgical technique used, surgeon's experience, and duration of patients' follow-up [21]. In general, a recurrence rate of $<1\%$ is considered acceptable. Recurrent PAs have a higher likelihood of a second recurrence of about 6–15% [22]. Uninodular recurrences have a better outcome than multinodular recurrences [23, 24].

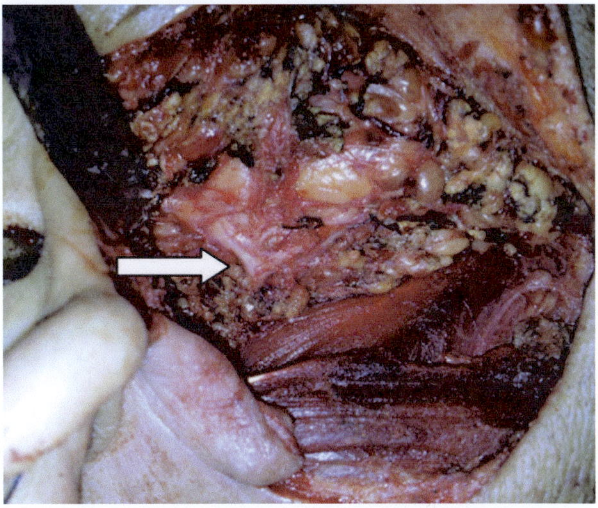

Fig. 12.8 Dissection of the main trunk of the facial nerve and only one division related to the parotid mass (arrow)

Partial superficial parotidectomy and extracapsular dissection (ECD) are other recognized options of resection [25–27]. Partial superficial parotidectomy entails dissection of the main trunk of the facial nerve and only one division with its terminal branches (Fig. 12.8). Enucleation is never done for its high recurrence rate.

12.3 Warthin's Tumor (Adenolymphoma)

12.3.1 Introduction

Warthin's tumor, also known as "papillary cystadenoma lymphomatosum," "adenolymphoma," and "cystadenolymphoma," is a benign cystic tumor of the parotid gland containing abundant lymphocytes and germinal centers (LN-like stroma). It is named after the pathologist Aldred Scott Warthin, who described two cases in 1929. Warthin's tumor represents 2–15% of all primary epithelial tumors of the parotid gland. Extraparotid Warthin's tumor is very rare; it may occur in the periparotid LN, nasopharynx, eyelid, and oral cavity. Warthin's tumor is histologically characterized by a dense lymphoid stroma and a double layer of oncocytic epithelium with a papillary and cystic architectural pattern. Its etiology is still controversial [28].

12.3.2 Epidemiology

Warthin's tumor is the most common "monomorphic" adenoma of the major salivary glands. It accounts for about 2–15% of all parotid tumors [29]. It is the second most frequent benign neoplasm of the salivary glands after pleomorphic adenoma (PA) and is bilateral in 5–10% of cases (Fig. 12.9), but the two masses usually are at different times. Warthin's tumor is the most common "parotid tail" mass

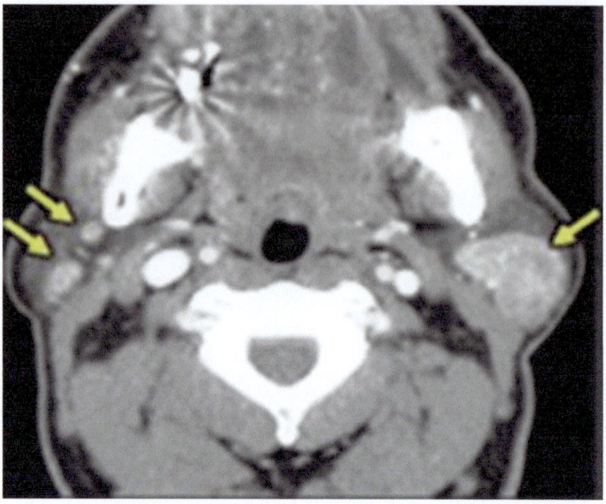

Fig. 12.9 Computed tomography (CT) scan showing bilateral parotid tail masses (yellow arrows)

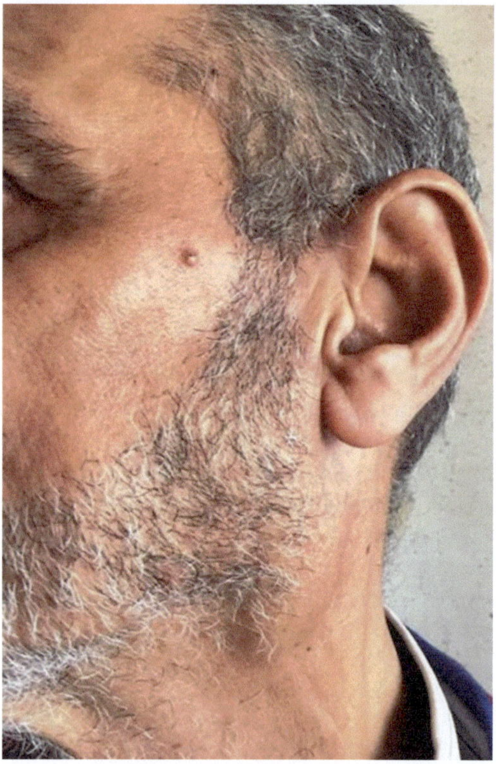

Fig. 12.10 Lateral view showing a tumor in the left parotid tail, not related to the ear lobule in a 60-year-old man

(Fig. 12.10). It occurs almost exclusively in the parotid gland, affecting males more than females (8:1); however, the ratio has decreased drastically during the past 50 years to 2:1 [30, 31]. This gender predilection shift is referred to that it is highly linked to smoking. Smokers have an eight times higher incidence of developing Warthin's tumors than nonsmokers [32]. The mean age is 62 years. Patients are rarely below 40 years [33, 34]. In women, the peak incidence is in the sixth decade, whereas it is in the seventh decade in men [35]. Autoimmune disease or exposure to radiation increases the risk of Warthin's tumor progression.

12.3.3 Etiology

The etiology of Warthin's tumor has not yet been fully established. Some authors suggested that this benign neoplasm arises as a result of some tumorigenic effect on epithelial inclusions located in the LNs adjacent to or in the parotid gland [36]. Etiological factors of Warthin's tumor include Epstein–Barr virus (EBV) infection, tobacco, autoimmune disease, ionizing radiation, and chronic inflammation [37–39]. However, several questions remain regarding the male predominance in Warthin's tumors and why smoking should predominantly affect the parotid gland rather than the intraoral minor salivary glands [37, 40]. Malignant transformation of Warthin's tumor is extremely rare and accounts for only 0.3% of cases [41].

12.3.4 Pathogenesis/Pathophysiology

Warthin's tumor is the only benign neoplasm of salivary glands associated with smoking [42]. The origin of this tumor is still debated despite the numerous theories concerning its histogenesis mentioned in the literature [35, 43]. Initially, Hildebrand (1895) proposed that the lesion may be remnants of the branchial pouches and a variant of the lateral cervical cyst [40]. Later, Albrech and Artz proposed the heterotropic origin of Warthin's tumor from the neoplastic proliferation of salivary gland ducts present within intra- or para-parotid LNs. This theory is widely accepted and was sustained by IHC findings, which demonstrated that basal and luminal epithelial cells of Warthin's tumor bear characteristics similar to those of the basal cells and striated duct cells of the excretory duct of the salivary gland [35]. Only a small subset of Warthin's tumors present the (t11,19)(q21,p13) translocation and expression of the chimeric genes.

These Warthin's tumors are often classified as infarcted or metaplastic tumors [44]. Some authors suggested that the different histological subtypes of Warthin's tumor (epithelial predominance, mixed, lymphoid predominance) may result from staged pathogenetic development in which the lymphoid predominance subtype constitutes the early stage, followed by the mixed and the epithelial predominance subtypes [45, 46]. This spectrum of modifications could be triggered by different and mostly unidentified pathogenetic factors, such as tobacco smoking, autoimmune disorders, or EBV infection [37]. The latter was detected in very close association with multiple/bilateral Warthin's tumors, in comparison with solitary tumors [47]. Different theories of Warthin's tumor according to various authors are summarized in Table 12.1.

Table 12.1 Theories of Warthin's tumor arranged chronologically according to various authors

Authors (reference)	Year	Theory
Hildebrand [48] q	1895	The tumor may be a variant of lateral cervical cyst and remnants of the branchial pouches
Albrech and Artz [48] q	1910	Heterotropic originated from neoplastic proliferation of salivary gland ducts present within intraparotid or para-parotid lymph nodes
Warthin [48] q	1929	The tumor arose from heterotrophic pharyngeal endoderm (further, Hevenor and Clark) specified ectopic Eustachian tube endoderm to be the tissue of origin
Thompson and Bryant [49]	1950	The presence of parotid ductal epithelium in lymph nodes in the immediate vicinity of the parotid gland is responsible for the development of the tumor
Allegra [50]	1971	The lesion results from "hypersensitivity," that is, oxyphilic metaplasia of striated ducts followed by papillary formations with secretion leading to cyst formation
Chung et al. [51]	1986	Smoking—Numerous chemical irritants of tobacco such as benzopyrened, arsenic, N-nitrosoguanidine, etc., affect the aberrant salivary gland tissue in the lymph node, resulting in metaplasia of glandular tissue
Scully [52]	1988	Epstein–Barr virus (EBV) might infect ductal epithelial cells and the release of EBV gene products/cytokine by infected cells might activate lymphoid tissue, which will result in a polyclonal B-cell response

q quoted ref

Finally, there is still a debate whether Warthin's tumor is a true neoplasm or not. The clinical behavior of the lesion as the total lack of recurrence and low malignant transformation rate of this tumor further support the view that it is non-neoplastic. In fact, only one study has shown clonal abnormalities, while most have not. Recent immunohistochemical and molecular studies showed no clonal allelic losses, suggesting that Warthin's tumor is a non-neoplastic lesion [53, 54].

12.3.5 Pathology

12.3.5.1 Macroscopic Picture

Grossly, Warthin's tumor is a well-circumscribed, spherical to oval, reddish brown mass with a "true capsule." On cut section, there are solid areas and multiple cysts with papillary projections. The cystic spaces often contain mucoid creamy brown (or white) fluid resembling "motor oil" [55].

12.3.5.2 Cytology

Smears characteristically show oncocytic epithelial cells without atypia admixed with polymorphous lymphocytes and cellular debris. Mucinous differentiation and squamous cells with mixed inflammation and cytological are rarely encountered [56, 57]. For preoperative assessment of Warthin's tumor, FNAC is a useful method. However, its accuracy is controversial compared with other methods. Confirmation of diagnosis with certainty relies on histopathological examination.

12.3.5.3 Microscopic Picture

Microscopically, Warthin's tumor is composed of varying proportions of papillary-cystic structures. It is comprised of a papillary proliferation lined by a double layer composed of surface columnar oncocytic epithelium and a smaller basal layer of small cuboidal cells with myoepithelial characteristics. The surrounding stroma contains a highly ordered lymphoid architecture with germinal centers similar to an actual LN (Fig. 12.11). Some foci of mucous, ciliated, sebaceous, and squamous cells can be present in Warthin's tumors. A granulomatous reaction can be seen in some cases [58]. Infarcted or metaplastic tumors may have marked mucinous or squamous metaplasia and stromal reaction, which may present diagnostic challenges.

When Warthin's tumor arises in a cervical LN, it may be mistaken for metastatic carcinoma, particularly from a papillary thyroid carcinoma (PTC). Malignant transformation is extremely rare (<1%). The diagnosis of malignant transformation of Warthin's tumor to carcinoma relies on the (1) presence of a Warthin's tumor, (2) presence of transitional zones from a benign oncocytic to a malignant epithelium, (3) presence of an infiltrating growth in the surrounding lymphoid tissue, and (4) exclusion of metastasis to lymphoid stroma from another primary carcinoma. The lymphoid component may lead to lymphoma.

12.3.5.4 Immunohistochemical Study

On immunohistochemistry (IHC), the epithelial component is immunoreactive for cytokeratin cocktail while the lymphoid portion shows kappa- and lambda-chain polyclonality.

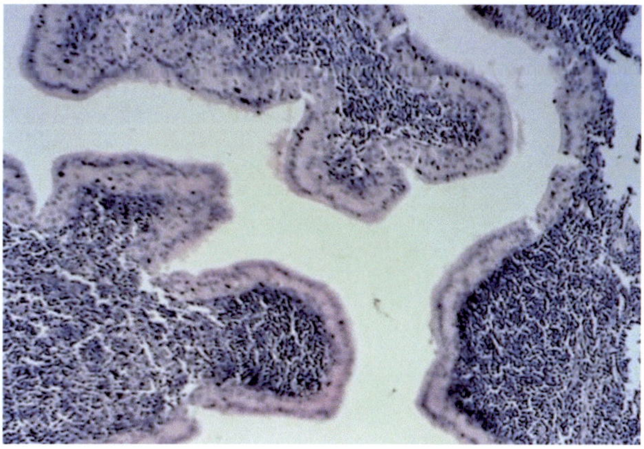

Fig. 12.11 Warthin's tumor composed of papillary structures lined by oncocytic epithelial cells. The core of the papillae is occupied by dense lymphoid aggregates. (H&E ×200)

12.3.6 Clinical Picture

Clinically, Warthin's tumor presents as a rounded or an ovoid, nodular, painless, freely mobile, slow-growing mass, fluctuant to firm at palpation. It is usually 1–3 cm in diameter on average (Fig. 12.12) and rarely attains a larger size (Fig. 12.13) [59]. It has a smooth surface, homogeneous consistency, and is sometimes cystic (30%). It can be unilateral, bilateral, or multicentric or multifocal (20%), and may be fixed to the overlying skin [60]. Warthin's tumor is asymptomatic in 90% of cases, but rarely, infarcted tumors may cause pain and heaviness in the mouth [32]. Ear ringing, ear pain, and hearing loss have been reported in some cases [61].

12.3.7 Imaging Studies

Imaging features of Warthin's tumors show that they are often multicentric (20%) and are usually small (1–4 cm). They have a typically heterogeneous appearance on all modalities, often with cystic components (30%). The tendency to undergo cystic change is greater than any other salivary gland tumor [62, 63].

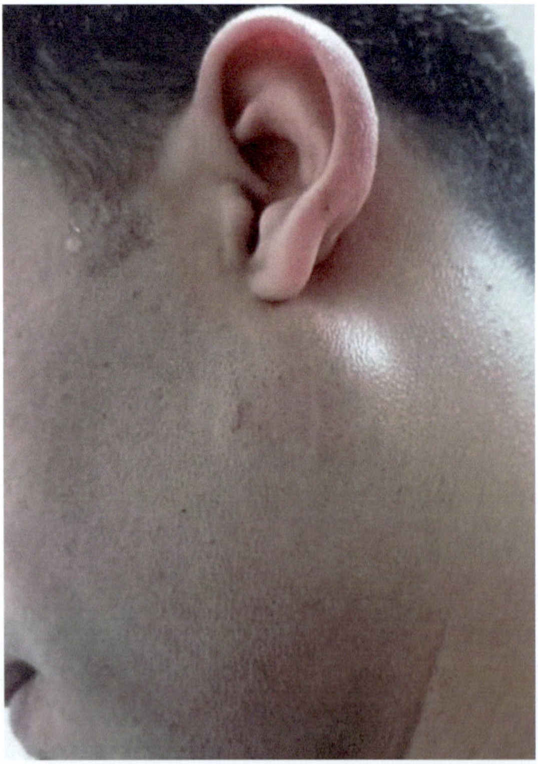

Fig. 12.12 Left adenolymphoma presenting as a small (2 cm), smooth, mass in a 27-year-old man

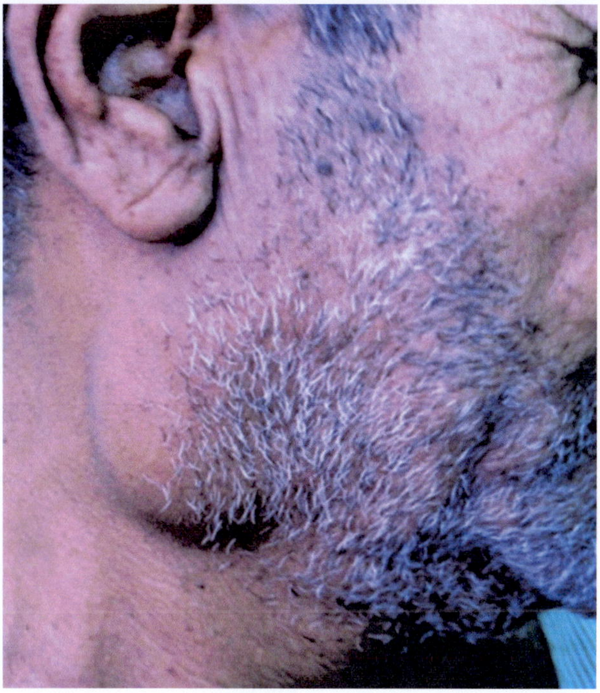

Fig. 12.13 Lateral view showing a right adenolymphoma presenting as a relatively large, smooth mass in a 61-year-old man

12.3.7.1 Ultrasonography (US)

High-resolution US is considered to be the modality of first choice for the detection of salivary gland neoplasms. However, US is unable to evaluate that portion of the parotid gland situated deep in the mandible. Ultrasonographic examination of salivary gland masses in general should include evaluation of the contralateral gland and cervical LNs. If the lesion requires to be identified before surgery, ultrasound-guided FNAC may be performed.

In Warthin's tumors, US reveals a well-defined mass with multiple anechoic areas or an anechoic mass, with posterior acoustic enhancement at the lower pole of the parotid [64] (Fig. 12.14). Nevertheless, the pattern may vary, and fast growth secondary to infection may occur. In some cases, multiple septa and the thickness of intratumoral fluid give a heterogeneous echogenic pattern [65].

Moreover, tumors that are large (e.g., >5 cm) tend to have a higher proportion of cystic content than smaller lesions and in some cases can be composed almost entirely of cystic material. Warthin's tumors are often hypervascular.

12.3.7.2 Computed Tomography (CT) Scan

The classical appearance of Warthin's tumor on CT scanning is a well-defined, heterogeneous, solid/cystic lesion within the superficial lobe of the parotid/parotid tail with moderate enhancement (Fig. 12.15). The mass is usually well-defined with no calcification and can be often seen bilaterally. Cystic changes appear as intralesional lower attenuation. The presence of a mural nodule is strongly suggestive of Warthin's tumor.

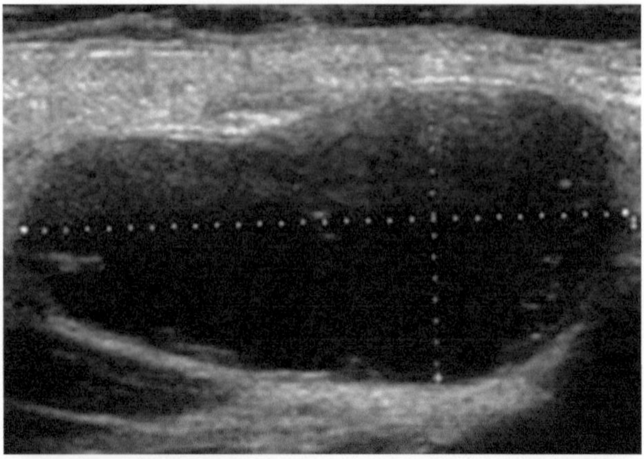

Fig. 12.14 Ultrasonography of the parotid gland showing Warthin's tumor as an ovoid well-defined mass with multiple anechoic areas

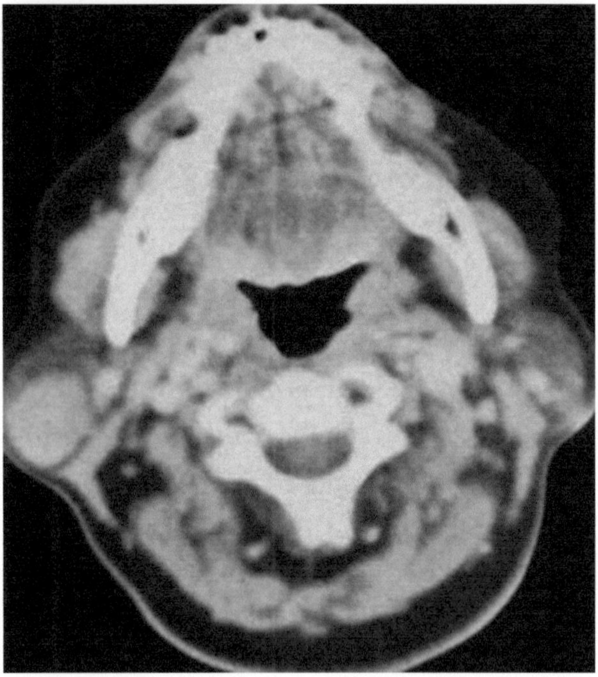

Fig. 12.15 Computed tomography (CT) scan with intravenous contrast injection showing Warthin's tumor as a sharply marginated, high-density lesion in the tail of the right parotid gland

12.3.7.3 Magnetic Resonance Imaging (MRI)

On MRI examination, Warthin's tumors are often seen as encapsulated lesions that show low or intermediate T1-weighted signal features with cyst containing cholesterol components that contain focal high signal [66]. The neoplasm shows heterogeneous and variable intermediate signal intensity on T2-weighted images [67]. The solid portion is predominant in Warthin's tumors, and small cystic parts are seen in approximately 30% of cases with thin uniform walls without enhancement. Well-defined contour is a crucial finding in distinguishing benign parotid tumors from

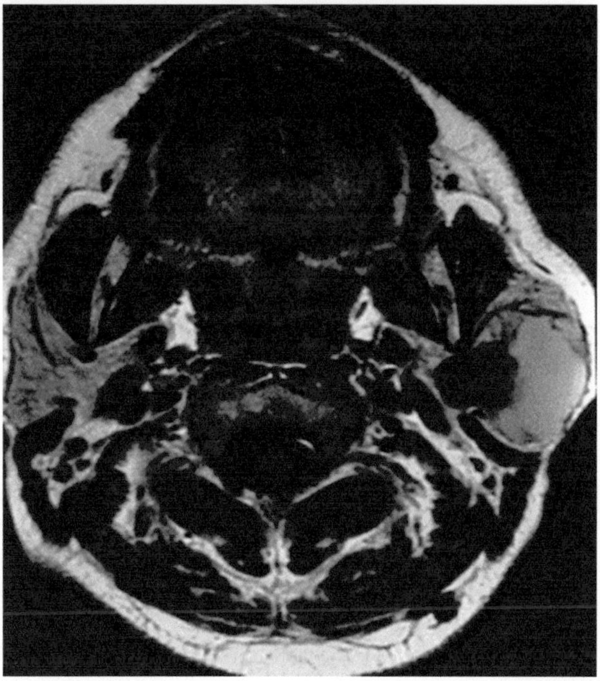

Fig. 12.16 Magnetic resonance imaging (MRI—T1) showing Warthin's tumor as a solid cystic tumor of the left parotid gland with low/intermediate T1-weighted signal features

malignant neoplasms. This can be well identified by MRI as well as content of the mass owing to higher soft-tissue resolution [67]. On MRI with gadolinium contrast (T1C + Gd), cystic components do not take up contrast while solid parts usually enhance [68] (Fig. 12.16).

12.3.7.4 Nuclear Medicine

Warthin's tumors often show uptake with 99Tc-pertechnetate, thallium, and FDG-PET [69]. It is the only parotid tumor that can give a "hot spot" in 99Tc scan.

12.3.8 Differential Diagnosis

The histological differential diagnosis of Warthin's tumor includes the following:

- Lymph node metastases: Usually, there is a marked cellular atypia. LN metastases are devoid of the bilayered, oncocytic epithelial element.
- Sebaceous lymphadenoma: It is devoid of the bilayered, oncocytic epithelial element.
- Cystadenoma of salivary glands: It can be oncocytic; however, it is devoid of lymphoid stroma and usually has small, multilocular cystic spaces.
- Lympho-epithelial cysts.

The possible imaging differential considerations of Warthin's tumor include the following:

- Pleomorphic adenoma (PA).
- Other parotid gland tumors: muco-epidermoid carcinoma (MEC)–adenoid cystic carcinoma (ACC)–acinic cell carcinoma.
- Parotid nodal metastasis.
- Parotid non-Hodgkin lymphoma (NHL).
- Sjögren's syndrome.

12.3.9 Treatment

The optimal treatment of Warthin's tumor is surgical excision, which can be easily performed owing to the superficial location of the tumor. Some surgeons prefer "superficial parotidectomy" to avoid rupture of the tumor capsule, whereas others choose "extracapsular dissection" [36]. Some authors recommended "enucleation" as the best treatment modality for this tumor as it is well-capsulated and does not recur, though a recurrence rate of 2% has been reported [70]. Another study reported that superficial parotidectomy reduces the recurrence rate of Warthin's tumor significantly because of its possible multicentricity [71]. The best treatment option for Warthin's tumor located in the deep lobe is total conservative parotidectomy with preservation of the facial nerve and its branches.

12.3.10 Prognosis/Complications

Warthin's tumor has a favorable prognosis and local recurrence rate is low; when recurrence does occur, it is probably due to multifocal tumors or inadequate excision. Malignant transformation of Warthin's tumor is very rare (0.3%); however, there are a few reported examples in both the epithelial and the lymphoid component. In such cases, a close follow-up of the patients is mandatory to detect metastases. The most frequent histological types of malignant transformation in a Warthin's tumor are MEC, squamous cell carcinoma (SCC), undifferentiated carcinoma, oncocytic adenocarcinoma, and adenocarcinoma.

12.4 Basal Cell Adenoma (BCA)

12.4.1 Epidemiology

Basal cell adenoma (BCA) of the salivary gland is a rare neoplasm that consists of a monomorphic population of basaloid epithelial cells and accounts for approximately 1–2% of all salivary gland tumors [72, 73]. It tends to occur in adults over the age of 50 years [74–76], with a female-to-male ratio of 2:1 [77].

It usually occurs in the parotid gland (75%), much less commonly in the submandibular gland (5%) [78], and rarely in the minor salivary glands with the exclusion of canalicular adenomas, which were previously categorized with BCA [79, 80].

12.4.2 Pathology

The BCA was once considered to be a type of "monomorphic adenoma." However, since 1991, according to the "Salivary Glands Tumours Histological Classification" of the World Health Organization (WHO), the name of this lesion was changed to BCA, excluding the word "monomorphic" [81].

Histologically, BCA is characterized by the presence of uniform and regular basaloid cells. These cells have two different morphologies that are intermingled. One group consists of small cells with little cytoplasm and intensive basaloid rounded nuclei that are usually located in the periphery of the tumoral nests or islands. The other group is formed of large cells with abundant cytoplasm and pale nuclei that are located in the center of the tumoral nests. A basal membrane-like structure rounds these tumoral nests, separating them from the surrounding connective tissue [82]. There were no mitotic figures or perineural invasion.

12.4.3 Clinical Presentation

Basal cell adenoma typically presents as a slowly growing, solitary, firm, freely mobile, painless (asymptomatic) mass. Frequently, this encapsulated tumor does not exceed 3 cm of largest diameter (Fig. 12.17). It is usually superficial within the glandular body, and a brownish appearance is usually observed [83].

A special variant of BCA, the membranous type (dermal analog tumor) has a propensity for multifocality and can be associated with multiple trichoepitheliomas and cylindromas (Brooke–Spiegler syndrome).

12.4.4 Diagnosis

Because BCAs may have solid and cystic components, the imaging findings such as CT scan have been described as relatively nonspecific. The diagnosis of this entity must be established by a histological study, which characteristically demonstrates the presence of uniform and regular basaloid cells with no mitotic figures or perineural invasion.

Generally, biopsy is accepted as the most accurate method to obtain the diagnosis, although some authors advocate for FNA if physical access to the tumor is available. Histopathologically, BCA has four growth patterns; solid, trabecular (Fig. 12.18), tubular, and membranous subtypes.

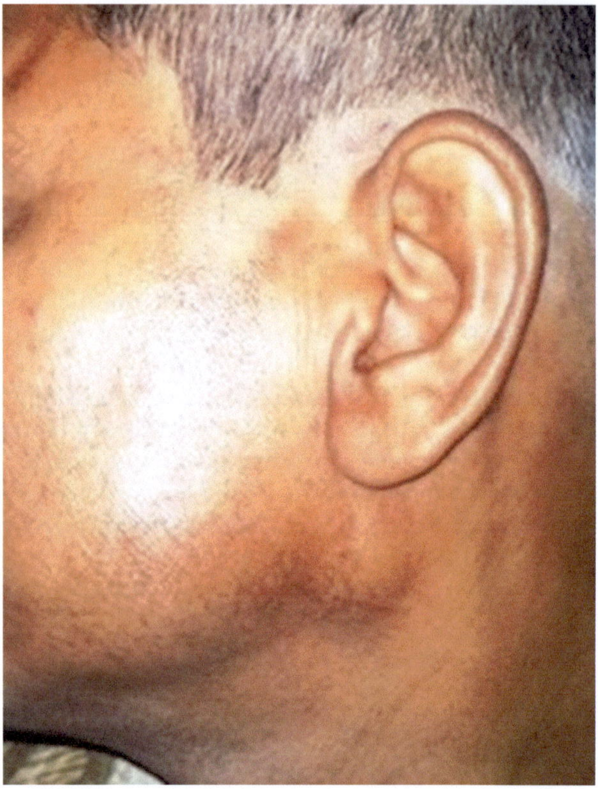

Fig. 12.17 Preoperative photograph showing small, well-demarcated swelling in left parotid gland of a 48-year-old man. Postoperative histology showed a basal cell adenoma (BCA)

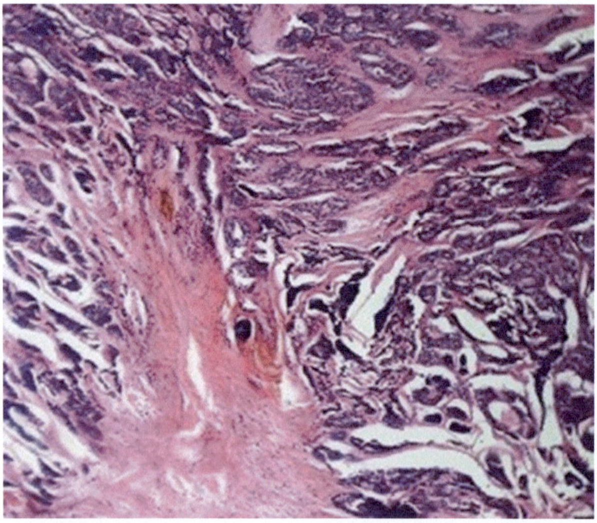

Fig. 12.18 Histopathology of basal cell adenoma showing monotonous cellular growth with cells having round to ovoid hyper-chromatic nuclei with eosinophilic to amphophilic cytoplasm and indistinct cell border (basaloid cell). The tumor shows a trabecular pattern. H&E stain

12.4.5 Differential Diagnosis

Among the malignant tumors of the parotid gland, adenoid cystic carcinoma (ACC) is the lesion that shows the most histological similarities to the BCA, suggesting that the latter is the benign homolog of ACC [84]. However, characteristics such as integrity of the basal layer, absent of very low number of mitoses, and slow growth are typical of a benign lesion.

Basal cell adenocarcinoma is another malignant tumor that shares histological features with the BCA. Both exhibit myoepithelial differentiation, reactivity patterns indicative of ductal epithelium, and closely similar immunohistochemical profiles. Basal cell adenocarcinoma is distinguished from BCA by the histological features of invasion, mitotic activity, and neural or vascular involvement [81, 85, 86]. The differential diagnosis must also include pleomorphic adenoma, the most common benign tumor, and other parotid gland benign tumors such as the canalicular adenoma and sebaceous adenoma.

12.4.6 Treatment

The primary treatment of BCA is surgical excision by means of a superficial or total parotidectomy according to location of the tumor. Extracapsular excision (ECD) is another option. It is performed in cases in which there is involvement of minor salivary glands in the oral mucosa [87].

12.4.7 Prognosis

Prognosis of BCA is generally excellent. Recurrence rate is low, except for the membranous subtype, which may recur in about 25% of cases. Malignant transformation is rare, again favoring the membranous subtype [30, 88, 89].

12.5 Canalicular Adenoma (CA)

12.5.1 Definition

Canalicular adenoma (CA) was recognized as a distinct salivary gland neoplasm based on its unique clinical and histological features. In the latest WHO histological classification of head and neck tumors [90], CA is defined as “a benign salivary gland tumor composed of monomorphous epithelial ductal cells arranged in anastomosing cords within cell-poor vascular stroma.”

12.5.2 Epidemiology

Canalicular adenoma is a rare tumor comprising <1% of all salivary tumors [30, 88, 89]. The mean age is 65 years, with a female-to-male ratio of 1.8:1 [30, 91]. It rarely affects the parotid glands [30]. The minor salivary glands of the upper lip are the ones most commonly involved (80%) followed by the buccal mucosa [89] and palate [92].

12.5.3 Pathology

Histologically, canalicular adenoma is one of the "monomorphic adenomas" in which the architectural pattern tends to be consistent [93]. The neoplasm is usually encapsulated and consists of columnar cells in a loose connective tissue stroma [94]. Several tumor cell nuclei may show detectable nucleoli, and the stroma may contain some capillaries. A "canalicular type pattern" is usually observed (Fig. 12.19) where the cavities are either optically blank or contain a pale eosinophilic material, possibly of stromal extracellular matrix type.

12.5.4 Clinical Presentation

Canalicular adenoma typically presents as painless, slowly growing, submucosal nodule. Rarely, multiple/multifocal canalicular adenomas may occur and present clinically with multiple discrete masses, typically occurring in the upper lip and buccal mucosa.

12.5.5 Management and Prognosis

Surgical excision is the management of choice for CA, and prognosis is excellent. Its specific histological features, however, are difficult to detect on FNA and its

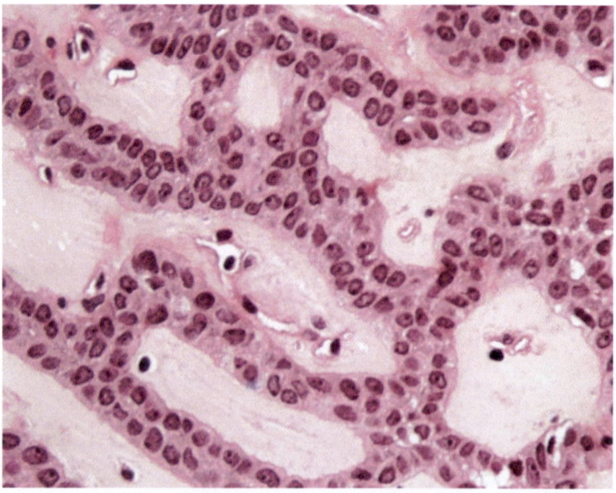

Fig. 12.19 Histopathology of a canalicular adenoma showing the tumor composed of anastomosing, frequently bilayered cords of tumor cells. A canalicular-type pattern is observed. The cavities are optically blank or contain a pale eosinophilic material. H&E stain

multifocal nature can lead to recurrence. This is extremely rare and must be considered in the clinical management. Some of these recurrences may be considered separate tumors [30, 95]. Malignant transformation is also extremely rare. However, CA appears similarly to malignant polymorphous low-grade adenocarcinoma (PLGA) or BCA upon FNA and histological analysis [96, 97]. Therefore, a combination of biopsy, imaging, pathological analysis, and IHC is required to differentiate between similar benign salivary gland tumors and improve diagnostic accuracy [98].

12.6 Myoepithelioma

12.6.1 Definition/Terminology

Myoepithelioma is a rare, benign tumor composed almost exclusively of "myoepithelial" cells. The "epithelial" component should be <5% (some authors consider even focal epithelial differentiation sufficient to label the tumor as pleomorphic adenoma [PA]) [99]. Monomorphic histology and rare or absent ductal structures in myoepithelioma differentiate it from PA.

Formerly, myoepithelioma was considered a variant of PA. It was recognized as a distinct entity by the WHO in 1991 [100]. The terms "myoepithelial cell tumor" and "myoepithelial adenoma" are not recommended.

12.6.2 Epidemiology

Myoepithelioma accounts for about 1% of all salivary gland neoplasms [101]. It represents 2.2% of major and 5.7% of minor salivary gland neoplasms, respectively [101]. The parotid gland is the most common site affected (40–50%), followed by the minor salivary glands (in the palate) (~21%) [101, 102]. There have been rare instances of submandibular gland myoepitheliomas [73, 102]. Neoplastic myoepithelial cell tumors can be found in nearly all exocrine gland tissues.

Myoepithelioma of the parotid gland occurs in older people with a peak incidence in the third to fourth decades (range 8–85 years) [103, 104] and is composed more often of spindle and epithelial cells [105]. Myoepithelioma of minor glands occurs in slightly younger individuals and is composed of plasmacytoid cells [105]. There is no gender predilection [101].

The overwhelming majority of myoepitheliomas are benign in nature, but malignant transformation can take place in recurrent and untreated cases [100, 101, 106].

12.6.3 Etiology

Myoepithelial cells are contractile cells originating from the ectoderm, found in normal tissues with secretory function that aids in excreting glandular secretions [107]. Common stem cell with a bidirectional differentiation into epithelial or myoepithelial cell is hypothesized to be the cell of origin; the varied histological types (spindle, plasmacytoid, epithelioid, clear, and oncocytic) exhibited by myoepitheliomas can be attributed to the various stages in the differentiation from a cell that has the potential to differentiate into epithelial cells [108].

Myoepitheliomas and pleomorphic adenomas (PAs) are hypothesized to exist along a continuum, with a shared chromosome 12q cytogenetic abnormality [109].

12.6.4 Pathophysiology

Myoepitheliomas arise from neoplastic myoepithelial or basket cells located between the basement membrane and the basal plasma membrane of acinar or ductal/luminal cells. Accumulation of p53 and overexpression of KIT receptor have been implicated in malignant progression [107].

12.6.5 Pathology

12.6.5.1 Gross Appearance

Grossly, the mass may reach up to 5 cm in size. It appears encapsulated (in the parotid gland but not in minor salivary glands). It is solid, but may have cystic changes, with a tan or yellow-tan glistening cut surface and absent grossly myxoid or chondroid areas [110].

12.6.5.2 Cytology Description

On FNAC, monotonous spindle cell, plasmacytoid cells, or epithelioid cells are seen with no glandular or ductal cells [111]. Nuclear grooves and intranuclear cytoplasmic inclusions may be seen, with no marked pleomorphism or mitoses.

12.6.5.3 Microscopic (Histological) Picture

Histologically, the tumor is formed of spindled, epithelioid, plasmacytoid, clear, or oncocytic cells; most tumors are composed of a single-cell type, but combinations may occur [101]. In the parotid, it is seen well-circumscribed or encapsulated with a thin capsule. The stroma, when present, may be hyalinized, fibrous (Fig. 12.20), myxoid, or mucoid; lipomatous stroma may rarely be seen. Myoepithelial cells are thought to have contractile units that aid in excreting glandular secretions [100, 106].

The architectural pattern may be solid (non-myxoid), myxoid, reticular (canalicular-like), or mixed patterns of myoepithelial cells with no ductal differentiation. Mucinous myoepithelioma is rarely reported; it contains abundant intracellular mucin material, which may be mistaken for signet-ring cell adenocarcinoma of the parotid gland with positive myoepithelial markers and should be distinguished from secretory myoepithelial carcinoma [112].

12.6.5.4 Histological Subtypes

Subtypes of myoepitheliomas are classified by cell morphology into (1) spindle (interlacing fascicles with a stroma-like appearance), (2) plasmacytoid/hyaline (polygonal cells with eccentric nuclei and dense, nongranular or hyaline, abundant eosinophilic

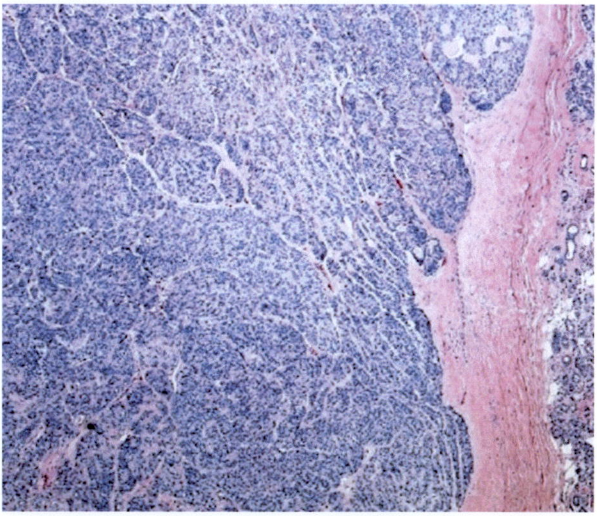

Fig. 12.20 Histopathology of myoepithelioma showing myoepithelial cells arranged in a fascicular nested pattern separated by "fibrous" (collagenic) stroma. H&E stain × 40

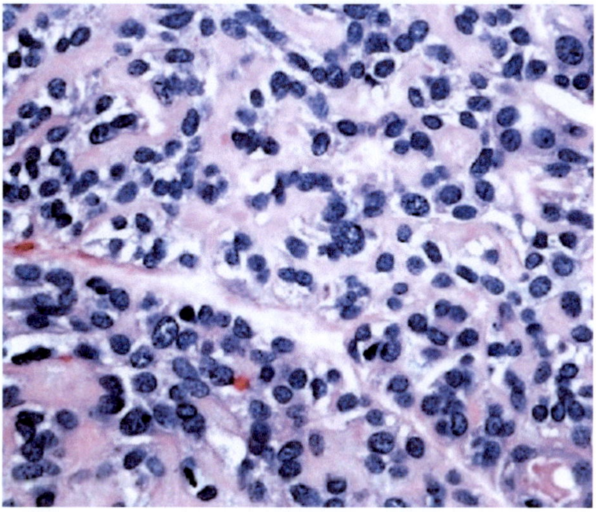

Fig. 12.21 Histopathology of myoepithelioma showing an "epithelioid" pattern of uniform cells with central small nuclei with fine chromatin, inconspicuous nucleoli, and an eosinophilic cytoplasm. There is a mild degree of nuclear atypia without mitosis. H&E stain × 40

cytoplasm), (3) epithelioid (nests or cords of round to polygonal cells, with centrally located nuclei and a variable amount of eosinophilic cytoplasm) (Fig. 12.21), and (4) clear (polygonal cells with abundant optically clear cytoplasm, containing large amounts of glycogen but missing mucin or fat) [113]. Of those subtypes, spindle cell type is the most common (65%) followed by plasmacytoid (20%) [73].

12.6.6 Clinical Features

Myoepithelioma usually presents as a slow-growing, well-circumscribed, painless mass with no distinctive clinical features [113]. The usual age of presentation is

40–50 years, affecting both genders equally [101]. It recurs locally if incompletely removed [114]. The "clear cell" variant may have an unpredictable clinical course despite being histologically benign [115].

12.6.7 Imaging Studies

12.6.7.1 Computed Tomography (CT) Scan

Epithelioma is located chiefly in the superficial lobe and abutted on the capsule of the gland. On CT scan, it is seen as a well-circumscribed, enhancing mass lesion with smooth or lobulated margins [116]. It may contain enhancing nodules and nonenhancing areas of linear bands, slit-like-shaped or of cystic configuration.

12.6.7.2 Magnetic Resonance Imaging (MRI)

The typical MRI studies show a well-defined, homogeneous, lobulated, isointense, and hyperintense mass on T1- and T2-weighted imaging, respectively [117]. There is inhomogeneous enhancement, apparent diffusion coefficient, different from Warthin's tumor and similar to PA [118].

12.6.8 Differential Diagnosis

Differentials of myoepithelioma of the parotid gland include the following:

- Myoepithelial carcinoma: It is characterized by (1) invasive growth pattern (infiltrative and destructive growth), (2) high cell proliferative activity [119], (3) necrosis, (4) spindle morphological characteristics in nodal and distant metastasis [119], (5) cell pleomorphism, and (6) lack of myofilaments [106, 113]. Myoepithelial carcinoma can also occur de novo. Carcinoma only comprises approximately 10% of all myoepithelial neoplasms [102].
- Basal Cell Adenoma (BCA): Ductal (Epithelial) Cells Are Present.
- Pleomorphic adenoma (PA): Fibromyxoid stroma and ductal structure are present. Immunohistochemical analysis can aid in the diagnosis with immunoreactivity to S-100, cytokeratin (specifically 7 and 14), p63, GFAP, calponin, and myogenic markers (actin, myosin) [73, 113, 120].
- Spindle Cell Soft-Tissue Neoplasms: Keratin Negative.
- Plasmacytoma: It shows perinuclear clearing and is positive for plasma cell markers, such as CD138.

12.6.9 Treatment

Complete surgical excision with a free margin recommended for myoepithelioma [101]. Regular follow-up is necessary to evaluate for local recurrence. The role of chemoradiation is not well established due to the rarity of this neoplasm [102, 121].

12.6.10 Prognosis

Prognosis is generally favorable; recurrences are relatively rare and are usually the result of incomplete excision [122]. Malignant transformation to myoepithelial carcinoma has been reported, but seems to be extremely rare [120], and has been attributed to the overexpression of c-kit receptors and p53 mutations.

12.7 Cystadenoma

12.7.1 Definition/Terminology

Cystadenoma is a rare, benign, cystic salivary tumor that resembles Warthin's tumor, though with different clinicopathological features. Unlike Warthin's tumor, there is a slight female predilection, no association with smoking [30, 123], and is not exclusive for the parotid gland, though it is affected in nearly half of the cases. It may be unilocular or multicystic, and the cyst is frequently lined by papillary projections.

Terms that are not recommended include lymphocyte-poor Warthin's tumors, monomorphic adenoma, cystic duct adenoma, and intraductal papillary hyperplasia. The subtypes include oncocytic cystadenoma and mucinous cystadenoma.

12.7.2 Epidemiology/Sites

Cystadenoma comprises 1–4% of all salivary gland neoplasms. It affects women more than men, most commonly in the fifth to seventh decades of life, with a mean age of 57 years [124]. Approximately 45% of adenomas affect the parotid gland; clinically indistinguishable from other primary benign cystic parotid gland lesions. Other sites include the lip and buccal mucosa (mimicking mucocele) [125] and rarely the supra-glottic larynx [126].

12.7.3 Pathology

12.7.3.1 Gross Appearance

Grossly, cystadenoma is seen as a well-circumscribed lesion with uni- or multicystic spaces within the parotid gland tissue.

12.7.3.2 Cytology

On FNAC, cohesive groups of epithelial cells are seen. Oncocytic variants will have ample granular cytoplasm, well-defined cell borders and central nuclei. Squamous differentiation may be seen as well. Squamous or mucinous differentiation should bring a low-grade MEC in the differential diagnosis [127].

12.7.3.3 Microscopic (Histological) Picture

Histologically, cystadenoma is demonstrated as a uniloculated or, more commonly, a multiloculated cystic lesion (Fig. 12.22). It is well-circumscribed, with peripheral entrapment of benign parotid gland tissue. The simple papillary architecture (Fig. 12.23) should not have complex architecture, mitoses, or atypia, and the lining epithelial cells are commonly a mixture of columnar, cuboidal, and oncocytic cells.

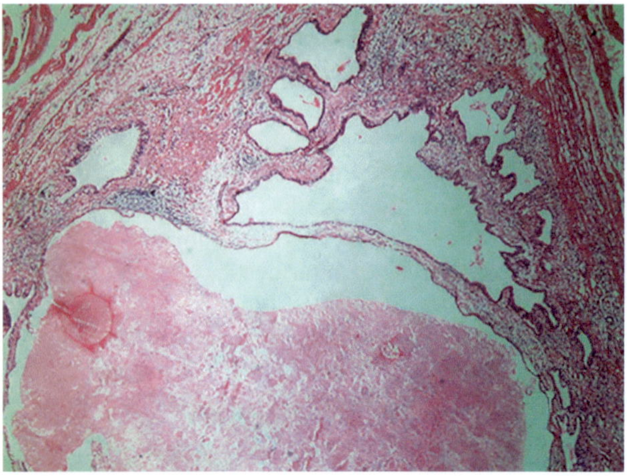

Fig. 12.22 Histopathology showing multiple cystic spaces of papillary cystadenoma with peripheral compression of parotid tissue. H&E × 40

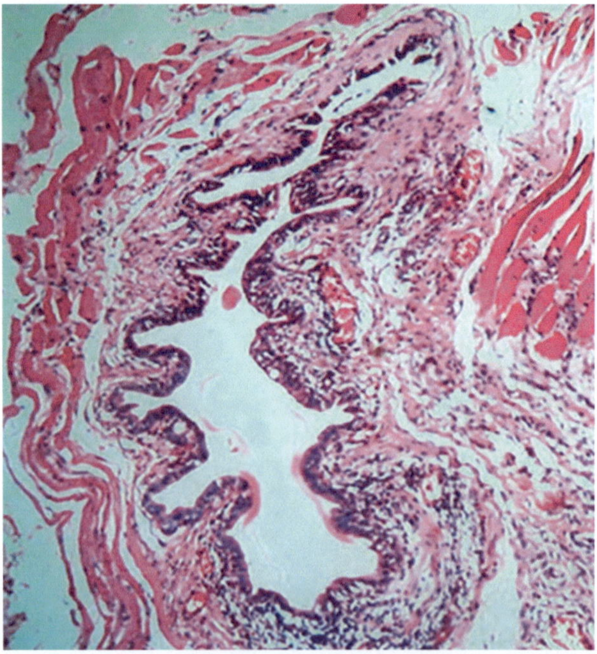

Fig. 12.23 Histopathology showing low-power view of papillary cystadenoma of the parotid gland with intraluminal papillary projections. H&E × 100

Mucinous, squamous, and, rarely, ciliated cells may also be seen. Mucinous cystadenoma is rare; lacks architectural and nuclear atypia. Unicystic MEC should be considered in the differential diagnosis.

Prominent multiloculated/multicystic growth pattern gives a low-power appearance of more lumens than epithelial cells. Simple papillary projections and true papillae are common; however, complex papillary tufting should alert the pathologist to other differential diagnoses such as intraductal carcinoma. Immunohistochemical stains are useful to rule out macrocystic secretory carcinoma and intercalated type intraductal carcinoma [128–130].

12.7.4 Clinical Features

In the parotid gland, cystadenoma usually presents as a painless, slow-growing mass or lump (in minor salivary glands, it mimics mucocele). It usually occurs in adults and has a slightly higher incidence in women [28, 130].

12.7.5 Imaging Studies

Cysadenoma of the parotid gland appears a cystic or solid, well-circumscribed mass on US, CT scan, or MRI with a clear capsule. It may appear cystic or solid due to internal hemorrhage or infection without internal flow. The capsule may show contrast enhancement if infected.

12.7.6 Differential Diagnosis

- Ductal ectasia: Ductal dilation due to obstruction or stones. Squamous metaplasia, duct wall fibrosis, hyalinization, and inflammatory infiltrate may be seen.
- Cystic oncocytic MEC: Nuclear atypia, infiltrative border, and three cell types of MEC (mucous cells, epidermoid cells, and intermediate cells) [131].
- Warthin's tumor: Bilayer of oncocytic cells and prominent inflammatory infiltrate in papillary cores are seen.
- Cystic oncocytic myoepithelioma: Myoepithelial in origin and usually with no papillary architecture.
- Macrocytic secretory carcinoma: Characteristic ETV6-NTRK3 translocation. Eosinophilic or vacuolated cytoplasm is evident. Positive for CK7, GATA3, mammaglobin, SOX10, and S100.
- Low-grade apocrine intraductal carcinoma: Resembles apocrine intraductal carcinoma of the breast with monotonous population of neoplastic cells usually filling the duct space with large nuclei and prominent nucleoli. It may have cribriform, micropapillary, or solid growth pattern.
- Intraductal papilloma: Unicystic lesion that resembles intraductal papilloma of the breast with arborizing fibrovascular cores lined by ductal epithelial cells. The

papillary projections of intraductal papilloma partially or completely fill the lumen, whereas the papillary projections of papillary cystadenoma usually occupy the lumen to a limited degree [132].

- Salivary duct cyst/oncocytic salivary duct cyst: It results from obstruction; most common sites are labial and buccal mucosa. It may represent a true developmental cyst, rather than secondary cyst formation due to obstruction.
- Intercalated duct type of intraductal carcinoma: Prominent complex or arborizing papillae and tufting.
- Mucocele: Reactive extravasation of mucin lined by compressed granulation tissue containing muciphages and inflammatory cells. It is not a true cyst with epithelial lining, although adjacent ductal epithelium may be seen. It is most commonly found in the lower labial mucosa/buccal mucosa.

12.7.7 Treatment

In general, complete surgical excision of cystadenoma of the parotid is indicated and considered curative [133].

12.7.8 Prognosis

Prognosis of cystadenoma is excellent. Recurrence is rare; only a few cases of recurrences have been reported in the literature. No malignant transformation of papillary cystadenoma has been reported; however, there is a reported case of malignant transformation of mucinous cystadenoma in the minor salivary glands [133].

References

1. Mc Loughlin L, Gillanders SL, Smith S, Young O. The role of adjuvant radiotherapy in management of recurrent pleomorphic adenoma of the parotid gland: a systematic review. Eur Arch Otorrinolaringol. 2019;276(2):283–95.
2. Lee JH, Kang HJ, Yoo CW, Park WS, Ryu JS, Jung YS, Choi SW, Park JY, Han N. PLAG1, SOX10, and Myb expression in benign and malignant salivary gland neoplasms. J Pathol Transl Med. 2019;53(1):23–30.
3. Meshram GG, Kaur N, Hura KS. Pediatric pleomorphic adenoma of the parotid: case report, review of literature and novel therapeutic targets. Children (Basel). 2018;5(9):127.
4. Zhan KY, Khaja SF, Flack AB, Day TA. Benign parotid tumors. Otolaryngol Clin N Am. 2016;49(2):327–42.
5. Buenting JE, Smith TL, Holmes DK. Giant pleomorphic adenoma of the parotid gland: case report and review of the literature. Ear Nose Throat J. 1998;77(8):634–40.
6. Honda T, Yamamoto Y, Isago T, Nakazawa H, Nozaki M, Hirayama T. Giant pleomorphic adenoma of the parotid gland with malignant transformation. Ann Plast Surg. 2005;5(5):524–7.
7. Kici S, Peytral C. Giant pleomorphic adenoma of the parotid gland: a case report and review of the literature. Ann Otolaryngol Chir Cervicofac. 2001;118(5):330–2.
8. Eveson JW, Kusafuka K, Stenman G, al. e. Pleomorphic adenoma. In: Barnes EL, Eveson JW, Reichart P, Sidransky D, editors. Pathology and classification of head and neck Tumours. Lyon: IARC; 2005.

9. Gündüz AK, Yeşiltaş YS, Shields CL. Overview of benign and malignant lacrimal gland tumors. Curr Opin Ophthalmol. 2018;29(5):458–68.
10. Kas K, Voz ML, Roijer E, Astrom AK, Meyen E, Stenman G, et al. Promoter swapping between the genes for a novel zinc finger protein and beta-catenin in pleiomorphic adenomas with t(3;8)(p21;q12) translocations. Nat Genet. 1997;15(2):170–4.
11. Voz ML, Astrom AK, Kas K, Mark J, Stenman G, Van de Ven WJ. The recurrent translocation t(5;8)(p13;q12) in pleomorphic adenomas results in upregulation of PLAG1 gene expression under control of the LIFR promoter. Oncogene. 1998;16(11):1409–16.
12. Chaplin AJ, Darke P, Patel S. Tyrosine-rich crystals in pleomorphic adenomas of parotid glands. J Oral Pathol. 1983;12(5):342–6.
13. Lee KC, Chan JK, Chong YW. Ossifying pleomorphic adenoma of the maxillary antrum. J Laryngol Otol. 1992;106(1):50–2.
14. Seifert G, Donath K, Schafer R. Lipomatous pleomorphic adenoma of the parotid gland. Classification of lipomatous tissue in salivary glands. Pathol Res Pract. 1999;195(4):247–52.
15. Skalova A, Starek I, Simpson RH, Kucerova V, Dvorackova J, Curik R, et al. Spindle cell myoepithelial tumours of the parotid gland with extensive lipomatous metaplasia. A report of four cases with immunohistochemical and ultrastructural findings. Virchows Arch. 2001;439(6):762–7.
16. Seifert G, Donath K. Multiple tumours of the salivary glands—terminology and nomenclature. Eur J Cancer B Oral Oncol. 1996;32 B(1):3–7.
17. Yu GY, Ma DQ, Zhang Y, Peng X, Cai ZG, Gao Y, et al. Multiple primary tumours of the parotid gland. Int J Oral Maxillofac Surg. 2004;33(6):531–4.
18. Eveson JW, Cawson RA. Salivary gland tumours. A review of 2410 cases with particular reference to histological types, site, age and sex distribution. J Pathol. 1985;146(1):51–8.
19. Kato H, Kawaguchi M, Ando T, Mizuta K, Aoki M, Matsuo M. Pleomorphic adenoma of salivary glands: common and uncommon CT and MR imaging features. Jpn J Radiol. 2018;36(8):463–71.
20. Junquera L, Alonso D, Sampedro A, Fresno F, Albertos JM, Lopez-Arranz JS. Pleomorphic adenoma of the salivary glands: prospective clinicopathologic and flow cytometric study. Head Neck. 1999;21(7):652–6.
21. Ayoub OM, Bhatia K, Mal RK. Pleomorphic adenoma of the parotid gland: is long-term follow-up needed? Auris Nasus Larynx. 2002;29(3):283–5.
22. Henriksson G, Westrin KM, Carlsoo B, Silfversward C. Recurrent primary pleomorphic adenomas of salivary gland origin: intrasurgical rupture, histopathologic features, and pseudopodia. Cancer. 1998;82(4):617–20.
23. Klintworth N, Zenk J, Koch M, Iro H. Postoperative complications after extracapsular dissection of benign parotid lesions with particular reference to facial nerve function. Laryngoscope. 2010;120(3):484–90.
24. Orita Y, Hamaya K, Miki K, Sugaya A, Hirai M, Nakai K, et al. Satellite tumors surrounding primary pleomorphic adenomas of the parotid gland. Eur Arch Otorrinolaringol. 2010;267(5):801–6.
25. Zbaren P, Vander Poorten V, Witt RL, Woolgar JA, Shaha AR, Triantafyllou A, et al. Pleomorphic adenoma of the parotid: formal parotidectomy or limited surgery? Am J Surg. 2013;205(1):109–18.
26. Bradley PJ. 'Metastasizing pleomorphic salivary adenoma' should now be considered a low-grade malignancy with a lethal potential. Curr Opin Otolaryngol Head Neck Surg. 2005;13(2):123–6.
27. Fukushima M, Miyaguchi M, Kitahara T. Extracapsular dissection: minimally invasive surgery applied to patients with parotid pleomorphic adenoma. Acta Otolaryngol. 2011;131(6):653–9.
28. Mathur A, Mehrotra ML, Dhaliwal U. Warthin's tumour of the eye lid. Indian J Ophthalmol. 1989;37(4):193.
29. Nishikawa H, Kirkham N, Hogbin BM. Synchronous extra-parotid Warthin's tumour. J Laryngol Otol. 1989;103(8):792–3.

30. Tawfik O, Namiq A. Tumors of the salivary glands. Washington DC: Armed Forces Institute of Pathology; 1996.
31. Simpson RHW, Eveson JW. Warthin. In: Barnes EL, Eveson JW, Sidransky D, editors. Pathology and classification of head and neck tumours. Lyon: IARC; 2005. p. 263–5.
32. Snyderman C, Johnson JT, Barnes EL. Extraparotid Warthin's tumor. Otolaryngol Head Neck Surg. 1986;94(2):169–1675.
33. Kotwall CA. Smoking as an etiologic factor in the development of Warthin's tumor of the parotid gland. Am J Surg. 1992;164(6):646–7.
34. Pinkston JA, Cole P. Cigarette smoking and Warthin's tumor. Am J Epidemiol. 1996;144(2):183–7.
35. Rehani S, Bishen KA, Sagari S. Warthin's tumour: a case report and review on pathogenesis and its histological subtypes. J Clin Diagn Res. 2014;8(9):ZD37-40.
36. Maiorano E, Lo Muzio L, Favia G, Piattelli A. Warthin's tumour: a study of 78 cases with emphasis on bilaterality, multifocality and association with other malignancies. Oral Oncol. 2002;38(1):35–40.
37. Gallo O, Bocciolini C. Warthin's tumour associated with autoimmune diseases and tobacco use. Acta Otolaryngol. 1997;117(4):623–7.
38. Cennamo A, Falsetto A, Gallo G, Lanna M, Calleri G, Di Giacomo D. Warthin's tumour in the parotid gland (an inflammatory or a neoplastic disease?). Chir Ital. 2000;52(4):361–7.
39. Kristensen S, Tveterås K, Friedmann I, Thomsen P. Nasopharyngeal Warthin's tumour: a metaplastic lesion. J Laryngol Otol. 1989;103(6):616–9.
40. Kale AD, Prasad UC. Re: Yu et al. Smoking and the development of Warthin's tumour of the parotid gland. Br J Oral Maxillofac Surg. 1999;37(3):245.
41. Therkildsen MH, Christensen N, Andersen LJ, Larsen S, Katholm M. Malignant Warthin's tumour: a case study. Histopathology. 1992;21(2):167–71.
42. Kotwall CA. Smoking as an etiologic factor in the development of Warthin's tumor of the parotid gland. Am J Surg. 1992;164(6):646–7.
43. Thompson AS, Bryant HC. Histogenesis of papillary cystadenoma lymphomatosum (Warthin's tumor) of the parotid salivary gland. Am J Pathol. 1950;26(5):807–49.
44. Bullerdiek J, Haubrich J, Meyer K, Bartnitzke S. Translocation t(11;19)(q21;p13.1) as the sole chromosome abnormality in a cystadenolymphoma (Warthin's tumor) of the parotid gland. Cancer Genet Cytogenet. 1988;35(1):129–32.
45. Aguirre JM, Echebarría MA, Martínez-Conde R, Rodriguez C, Burgos JJ, Rivera JM. Warthin tumor. A new hypothesis concerning its development. Oral Surg Oral Med Oral Pathol Oral Radiol Endod. 1998;85(1):60–3.
46. Seifert G, Bull HG, Donath K. Histologic subclassification of the cystadenolymphoma of the parotid gland. Analysis of 275 cases. Virchows Arch A Pathol Anat Histol. 1980;388(1):13–38.
47. Santucci M, Gallo O, Calzolari A, Bondi R. Detection of Epstein-Barr viral genome in tumor cells of Warthin's tumor of parotid gland. Am J Clin Pathol. 1993;100(6):662–5.
48. Ellis GL, Auclair PL. Surgical pathology of salivary glands. Philadelphia, PA: Saunders WB Co., Ltd.; 1991. p. 187–201.
49. Chaudhry AP, Gorlin RI. Papillary cystadenoma Lymphomatosum (adenolymphoma): a review of literature. Am J Surg. 1958;95(6):923–31.
50. Allegra SR. Warthin's's tumour: a hypersenstivity disease? Ultrastructural, light and immunofluorescent study. Hum Pathol. 1971;2:403–20.
51. Chung YEA, Khoo MLC, Heng MKD, Hong GS, Soo KC. Epidemiology of Warthin's's tumour of the parotid gland in an Asian population. Br J Surg. 1999;86:661–4.
52. Scully C. Viruses and salivary gland disease: are there any associations? Oral Surg Oral Med Oral Pathol. 1988;66:179–83.
53. Honda K, Kashima K, Daa T, Yokoyama S, Nakayama I. Clonal analysis of the epithelial component of Warthin's's tumour. Hum Pathol. 2003;31:1377–80.
54. Teymoortash A, Werner JA. Tissue that has lost its track: Warthin's's tumour. Virchows Arch. 2005;446:585–8.

55. Köybaşioğlu FF, Önal B, Han Ü, Adabağ A, Şahpaz A. Cytomorphological findings in diagnosis of Warthin tumor. Turk J Med Sci. 2020;50(1):148–54.
56. Schindler S, Nayar R, Dutra J, Bedrossian CW. Diagnostic challenges in aspiration cytology of the salivary glands. Semin Diagn Pathol. 2001;18(2):124–46.
57. Kawasaki T, Kanamaru T, Shingaki S, Mizutani H, Nakajima T. Cytologic study of salivary gland tumors. Int J Oral Surg. 1980;9(1):68–73.
58. Chen SL, Hwang CC, Liu YC, Chen WT, Yang SW. Warthin's tumor with necrotizing tuberculous granulomatous inflammation causing severe facial nerve adhesion in parotid gland: a case report and literature review. Medicine (Baltimore). 2020;99(7):e18763.
59. Párraga-Linares L, Aguirre-Urízar JM, Berini-Aytés L, Gay-Escoda C. Papillary cystoadenoma lymphomatosum (Warthin-like) of minor salivary glands. Med Oral Patol Oral Cir Bucal. 2009;14(11):e597–600.
60. van der Wal JE, Davids JJ, van der Waal I. Extraparotid Warthin's tumours—report of 10 cases. Br J Oral Maxillofac Surg. 1993;31(1):43–4.
61. Psychogios G, Vlastos I, Thölken R, Zenk J. Warthin's tumour seems to be the most common benign neoplasm of the parotid gland in Germany. Eur Arch Otorrinolaringol. 2020;277(7):2081–4.
62. Choi DS, Na DG, Byun HS, Ko YH, Kim CK, Cho JM, et-al. Salivary gland tumors: evaluation with two-phase helical CT. Radiology. 2000;214(1):231–6.
63. Harnsberger HR, Glastonbury CM, Michel MA, Bernadette L, Branstetter BF. Diagnostic imaging: head and neck. Philadelphia, PA: Lippincott Williams & Wilkins; 2010.
64. Kim J, Kim EK, Park CS, Choi YS, Kim YH, Choi EC. Characteristic sonographic findings of Warthin's tumor in the parotid gland. J Clin Ultrasound. 2004;32(2):78–81.
65. Shimizu M, Ussmüller J, Hartwein J, Donath K. A comparative study of sonographic and histopathologic findings of tumorous lesions in the parotid gland. Oral Surg Oral Med Oral Pathol Oral Radiol Endod. 1999;88(6):723–37.
66. Minami M, Tanioka H, Oyama K, Itai Y, Eguchi M, Yoshikawa K, et al. Warthin tumor of the parotid gland: MR-pathologic correlation. AJNR Am J Neuroradiol. 1993;14(1):209–14.
67. Alibek S, Zenk J, Bozzato A, Lell M, Grunewald M, Anders K, et al. The value of dynamic MRI studies in parotid tumors. Acad Radiol. 2007;14(6):701–10.
68. Ikeda M, Motoori K, Hanazawa T, Nagai Y, Yamamoto S, Ueda T, et-al. Warthin tumor of the parotid gland: diagnostic value of MR imaging with histopathologic correlation. AJNR Am J Neuroradiol. 2004;25(7):1256–62.
69. Uchida Y, Minoshima S, Kawata T, Motoori K, Nakano K, Kazama T, et al. Diagnostic value of FDG PET and salivary gland scintigraphy for parotid tumors. Clin Nucl Med. 2005;30(3):170–6.
70. Batsakis JG. Carcinoma ex papillary cystadenoma lymphomatosum. Malignant Warthin's tumor. Ann Otol Rhinol Laryngol. 1987;96(2 Pt 1):234–5.
71. Teymoortash A, Krasnewicz Y, Werner JA. Clinical features of cystadenolymphoma (Warthin's tumor) of the parotid gland: a retrospective comparative study of 96 cases. Oral Oncol. 2006;42(6):569–73.
72. Lee DK, Chung KW, Baek CH, Jeong HS, Hyen Y, Son IS. Basal cell adenoma of the parotid gland characteristic of 2-phase helical computed tomography and magnetic resonance imaging. J Comput Assist Tomogr. 2005;29:884–8.
73. Testa D, Galera F, Insabato L, Vassallo A, Mesolella M, Galli V. Submandibular gland myoepithelioma. Acta Otolaryngol. 2005;125(6):664–6.
74. Batsakis JG, Brannon RB, Sciubba JJ. Monomorphic adenomas of major salivary glands: a histologic study of 96 tumours. Clin Otolaryngol. 1981;6:129–43.
75. Gök Ü, Sakallıoğlu Ö, Dağlı AF. Basal cell adenoma of the parotide gland: case report. Fırat Tıp Dergisi. 2006;11:150–2.
76. Main JHP, Orr JA, McGurk FM, McComb RJ, Mock D. Salivary gland tumour: review of 642 cases. J Oral Pathol. 1976;5:88–102.
77. Eveson JW, Cawson RA. Tumours of the minor (oropharyngeal) salivary glands: a demographic study of 336 cases. J Oral Pathol. 1985;14(6):500–9.

78. Zarbo RJ. Salivary gland neoplasia: a review for the practicing pathologist. Mod Pathol. 2002;15(3):298–323.
79. Yu G, Ussmueller J, Donath K. Histogenesis and development of membranous basal cell adenoma of the salivary gland. Zhonghua Kou Qiang Yi Xue Za Zhi. 2000;35(1):31–3.
80. Yu GY, Ubmuller J, Donath K. Membranous basal cell adenoma of the salivary gland: a clinicopathologic study of 12 cases. Acta Otolaryngol. 1998;118(4):588–93.
81. Siefert G, Sobin LH. Histological classification of salivary gland tumours. In: World health organization, international histological classification of tumours. Berlin: Springer; 1991.
82. Nagao K, Matsuzaki O, Saiga H, Sugano I, Shigematsu H, Kaneko T, et al. Histopathologic studies of basal cell adenoma of the parotid gland. Cancer. 1982;50:736–45.
83. Bernacki EG, Batsakis JG, Johns ME. Basal cell adenoma: distinctive tumor of salivary glands. Arch Otolaryngol. 1974;99:84–8.
84. Klijanienko J, Vielh P. Adenomas. In: Klijanienko J, Vielh P, editors. Salivary gland tumors, chapter 6. Basel: Karger; 2000. p. 22–47.
85. Ferreiro JA. Immunohistochemistry of basal cell adenoma of the major salivary glands. Histopathology. 1994;24:539.
86. Mintz GA, Abrams AM, Melrose RJ. Monomorphic adenomas of major and minor salivary glands. Oral Surg Oral Med Oral Pathol. 1982;53:375.
87. Kanaujia SK, Singh A, Nautiyal S, Ashutosh K. Basal cell adenoma of parotid gland: case report and review of literature. Indian J Otolaryngol Head Neck Surg. 2015;67(4):430–3.
88. Daley TD, Gardner DG, Smout MS. Canalicular adenoma: not a basal cell adenoma. Oral Surg Oral Med Oral Pathol. 1984;57(2):181–8.
89. Ferreiro JA. Canalicular adenoma. In: Barnes EL, Eveson JW, Reichart P, Sidransky D, editors. Pathology and classification of head and neck tumours. Lyon: IARC; 2005. p. 267.
90. El-Naggar AK, Chan JKC, Takata T, Grandis JR, Slootweg PJ. The fourth edition of the head and neck World Health Organization blue book: editors' perspectives. Hum Pathol. 2017;66:10–2.
91. Suarez P, Hammond HL, Luna MA, Stimson PG. Palatal canalicular adenoma: report of 12 cases and review of the literature. Ann Diagn Pathol. 1998;2(4):224–8.
92. Rousseau A, Mock D, Dover DG, Jordan RC. Multiple canalicular adenomas: a case report and review of the literature. Oral Surg Oral Med Oral Pathol Oral Radiol Endod. 1999;87(3):346–50.
93. Samar ME, Avila RE, Fonseca IB, Anderson W, Fonseca GM, Cantín M. Multifocal canalicular adenoma of the minor labial salivary glands. Int J Clin Exp Pathol. 2014;7(11):8205–10.
94. Thompson LD, Bauer JL, Chiosea S, McHugh JB, Seethala RR, Miettinen M, Müller S. Canalicular adenoma: a clinicopathologic and immunohistochemical analysis of 67 cases with a review of the literature. Head Neck Pathol. 2015;9(2):181–95.
95. Sciubba JJ, Brannon RB. Myoepithelioma of salivary glands: report of 23 cases. Cancer. 1982;49(3):562–72.
96. de Ru JA, van Leeuwen MS, van Benthem PP, Velthuis BK, Sie-Go DM, Hordijk GJ. Do magnetic resonance imaging and ultrasound add anything to the preoperative workup of parotid gland tumors? J Oral Maxillofac Surg. 2007;65(5):945–52.
97. Seethala RR. Basaloid/blue salivary gland tumors. Mod Pathol. 2017;30(s1):S84–S954.
98. Griffith CC, Pai RK, Schneider F, Duvvuri U, Ferris RL, Johnson JT, et al. Salivary gland tumor fine-needle aspiration cytology: a proposal for a risk stratification classification. Am J Clin Pathol. 2015;143(6):839–53.
99. Gore CR, Panicker N, Chandanwale S, Singh BK. Myoepithelioma of minor salivary glands—a diagnostic challenge: report of three cases with varied histomorphology. J Oral Maxillofac Pathol. 2013;17(2):257–60.
100. Barnes L, Eveson JW, Reichart P, Sidransky D. Tumor of the salivary glands. In: Barnes L, Eveson JW, Reichart P, Sidransky D, editors. World health organization classification of tumors. Pathology and genetics of head and neck tumors. Lyon: IARC Press; 2005. p. 209.
101. Iguchi H, Yamada K, Yamane H, Hashimoto S. Epithelioid myoepithelioma of the accessory parotid gland: pathological and magnetic resonance imaging findings. Case Rep Oncol. 2014;7(2):310–5.

102. Nayak JV, Molina JT, Smith JC, Branstetter BF 4th, Hunt JL, Snyderman CH. Myoepithelial neoplasia of the submandibular gland: case report and therapeutic considerations. Arch Otolaryngol Head Neck Surg. 2003;129(3):359–62.
103. Begin LR, Black MJ. Salivary-type myxoid myoepithelioma of the sinonasal tract: a potential diagnostic pitfall. Histopathology. 1993;23(3):283–5.
104. Begin LR, Rochon L, Frenkiel S. Spindle cell myoepithelioma of the nasal cavity. Am J Surg Pathol. 1991;15(2):184–90.
105. Choi CH, Chu YC, Kim L, Choi SJ, Park IS, Han JY, et al. Myoepithelial carcinoma of soft tissue: a case report and review of the literature. Korean J Pathol. 2014;48(6):413–7.
106. Kermani W, Belcadhi M, Ben Ali M, Sriha B, Bouzouita K. Myoepithelioma of the vallecula: a case report. Ear Nose Throat J. 2011;90(7):E9–E11.
107. Jeng YM, Lin CY, Hsu HC. Expression of the c-kit protein is associated with certain subtypes of salivary gland carcinoma. Cancer Lett. 2000;154(1):107–11.
108. Mochizuki Y, Omura K, Tanaka K, Sakamoto K, Yamaguchi A. Myoepithelioma of the parotid gland presenting as a retroauricular cutaneous nodule: a case report. J Clin Diagn Res. 2013;7(6):1165–8.
109. el-Naggar AK, Lovell M, Callender DL, Ordonez NG, Killary AM. Cytogenetic analysis of a primary salivary gland myoepithelioma. Cancer Genet Cytogenet. 1999;113(1):49–53.
110. Nair BJ, Vivek V, Sivakumar TT, Joseph AP, Varun BR, Mony V. Clear cell myoepithelioma of palate with emphasis on clinical and histological differential diagnosis. Clin Pract. 2014;4(1):628.
111. Gayathri B, Kalyani R, Harendra Kumar M, Azeem Mohiyuddin S. Fine-needle aspiration findings in epithelioid myoepithelioma of the parotid gland: a diagnostic pitfall. J Oral Maxillofac Pathol. 2014;18(1):131–3.
112. Gnepp DR. Mucinous myoepithelioma, a recently described new myoepithelioma variant. Head Neck Pathol. 2013;7(Suppl 1):S85–9.
113. Sheldon WH. So-called mixed tumours of the salivary glands. Arch Pathol Lab Med. 1943;35:1–20.
114. Maiorano E, Altini M, Favia G. Clear cell tumors of the salivary glands, jaws, and oral mucosa. Semin Diagn Pathol. 1997;14(3):203–12.
115. Rossai J. Major and minor salivary glands. In: Rosai J, editor. Ackerman's surgical pathology. St. Louis, MO: Mosby; 1996. p. 834–5.
116. Wang S, Shi H, Wang L, Yu Q. Myoepithelioma of the parotid gland: CT imaging findings. Head Neck. 2008;29(7):1372–5.
117. Seifert G. World Health Organization Classification of Tumours. Histological typing of salivary gland tumors. 2nd ed. Berlin: Springer; 1991.
118. Habermann CR, Arndt C, Graessner J, Diestel L, Petersen KU, Reitmeier F, et al. Diffusion-weighted echo-planar MR imaging of primary parotid gland tumors: is a prediction of different histologic subtypes possible? AJNR Am J Neuroradiol. 2009;30(3):591–6.
119. Nagao T, Sugano I, Ishida Y, Tajima Y, Matsuzaki O, Konno A, et al. Salivary gland malignant myoepithelioma: a clinicopathologic and immunohistochemical study of ten cases. Cancer. 1998;83(7):1292–9.
120. Batsakis JG, Kraemer B, Sciubba JJ. The pathology of head and neck tumors: the myoepithelial cell and its participation in salivary gland neoplasia, part 17. Head Neck Surg. 1983;5(3):222–33.
121. Barnes L, Appel BN, Perez H, El-Attar AM. Myoepitheliomas of the head and neck: case report and review. J Surg Oncol. 1985;28(1):21–8.
122. Savera AT, Sloman A, Huvos AG, Klimstra DS. Myoepithelial carcinoma of the salivary glands: a clinicopathologic study of 25 patients. Am J Surg Pathol. 2000;24(6):761–74.
123. Waldron CA, el-Mofty SK, Gnepp DR. Tumors of the intraoral minor salivary glands: a demographic and histologic study of 426 cases. Oral Surg Oral Med Oral Pathol. 1988;66(3):323–33.
124. Brandwein M, Huvos A. Laryngeal oncocytic cystadenomas. Eight cases and a literature review. Arch Otolaryngol Head Neck Surg. 1995;121(11):1302–5.

125. Skalova A, Michal M. Cystadenoma. In: Barnes EL, Eveson JW, Sidransky D, editors. Pathology and classification of head and neck Tumours. Lyon: IARC; 2005. p. 273–4.
126. Gilcrease MZ, Nelson FS, Guzman-Paz M. Tyrosine-rich crystals associated with oncocytic salivary gland neoplasms. Arch Pathol Lab Med. 1998;122(7):644–9.
127. Lim CS, Ngu I, Collins AP, McKellar GM. Papillary cystadenoma of a minor salivary gland: report of a case involving cytological analysis and review of the literature. Oral Surg Oral Med Oral Pathol Oral Radiol Endod. 2008;105(1):e28–33.
128. Tjioe KC, de Lima HG, Thompson LD, Lara VS, Damante JH, de Oliveira-Santos C. Papillary cystadenoma of minor salivary glands: report of 11 cases and review of the English literature. Head Neck Pathol. 2015;9(3):354–9.
129. Beena VT, Thomas JK, Sabu P, Manju SM, Sreela KK, Ravikumar K. Papillary cystadenoma of salivary glands: report of two rare cases and review of literature. Oral Maxillofac Pathol J. 2017;8(1):28–31.
130. Agaimy A. Papillary neoplasms of the salivary duct system: a review. Surg Pathol Clin. 2021;14(1):53–65.
131. Fonseca FP, de Andrade BA, Lopes MA, Pontes HA, Vargas PA, de Almeida OP. P63 expression in papillary cystadenoma and mucoepidermoid carcinoma of minor salivary glands. Oral Surg Oral Med Oral Pathol Oral Radiol. 2013;115(1):79–86.
132. Skalova A, Michal M. Cystadenoma. In: Barnes EL, Eveson JW, Reichart P, Sidransky D, editors. World Health Organization classification of tumours. Pathology and genetics, head and neck tumours. Lyon: IARC Press; 2007. p. 273–4.
133. Girotra C, Padhye MN, Mahajan P, Nair A. A rare case report of mucinous cystadenoma with immunohistochemical—analysis and review of literature. J Maxillofac Oral Surg. 2015;14(Suppl 1):426–34.

13 Recurrent Pleomorphic Adenoma

13.1 Introduction

The standard surgical treatment of pleomorphic adenoma (PA) is an open parotidectomy [1], which is associated with a recurrence rate (RR) below 2–3% [2]. By contrast, in earlier studies, the RR following enucleation was as high as 40% [3, 4].

In general, the incidence of recurrence of PA following surgery varies depending on the tumor characteristics, surgical technique used, experience of the surgeons, the duration of patient's follow-up, and clinical integrity. The meta-analysis by Colella et al. (2015) showed that the RR varies according to the type of surgery from 1% to 8% [5]. A recent publication (2016) from a Danish registry covering close to 5500 patients followed for 15 years and treated with formal parotidectomy reported a 2.9% incidence of recurrent PA and the rate of malignant transformation 3.3% [6].

Recurrent PA following surgery (or any other treatment) usually presents as a recurrent swelling at the primary site, with or without local symptoms; a mass or multiple masses, pain, ulcer, facial palsy, dyspnea, diplopia, or dysphonia depending upon the primary site of origin.

13.2 Causes of Recurrence

13.2.1 Pathology-Related Variables

13.2.1.1 Multicentricity

Pleomorphic adenomas (PAs) were considered "unifocal" in the major salivary glands; however, surgeons and pathologists no longer support this theory.

13.2.1.2 Histopathological Subtype

In PA, epithelial and glandular elements intermingle with various amounts of mucoid, myxoid, or chondroid extracellular stroma. Seifert et al. [7] proposed a

© The Author(s), under exclusive license to Springer Nature Switzerland AG 2024
M. Sakr, *Surgery of the Salivary Glands*,
https://doi.org/10.1007/978-3-031-82069-4_13

classification of PA based on relative composition of cellular and stroma components: (1) hypocellular or stroma-rich or myxoid (50–80% of stroma), (2) classical with balanced content (30–50% stroma), and (3) hypercellular (<30% stroma). Myxoid PA accounts for more than half of the cases, the classical subtype for one-third, and the remaining 15% were hypercellular. They noticed that recurrences were more frequent in the hypocellular (myxoid) subtype [7], an observation previously reported by others [8, 9]. By examining 31 recurrent PAs, Stennert et al. [10] found a predominance of myxoid histology (80.6%; 25/31). This tendency was confirmed (89.2%; 58/65) in a more recent report by Wittekindt et al. [11], as well as by others [12–14].

13.2.1.3 Capsular Integrity/Bare Area

There is a consensus that, in the major salivary glands, PAs are enclosed by a "capsule" formed by a layer of fibrous tissue (Fig. 13.1a) [15]. The presence of incomplete or "bare" capsule (Fig. 13.1b) as a source of recurrence has been previously discussed in the 1950s and 1960s [16, 17]. The bare area is not always exposed to the facial nerve and may occur at any location along the tumor surface. The surgeon should carry out a wide local excision with the tumor contained within as much normal tissue as is possible. The bare area or deep surface of the tumor can lie against the cartilaginous external auditory meatus (EAM), styloid process, facial nerve, or masseter muscle.

Absence of encapsulation of PA is found in 20–50% of pathology specimen. A somewhat related parameter is the amount of tumor surface with an incomplete capsule, and this was estimated by Stennert et al. (2001) to be approximately 4% [18].

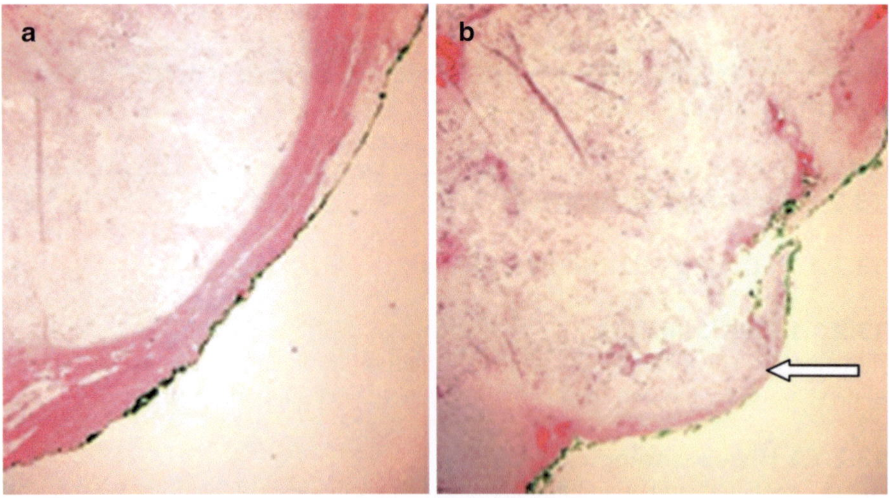

Fig. 13.1 Integrity of the capsule of pleomorphic adenoma of the parotid gland. (**a**) Capsular integrity preserved (intact capsule); (**b**) capsular integrity not preserved (ruptured capsule) (white arrow)

Naeim et al. [8] were probably the first to relate incompleteness of encapsulation to the pathological subtype of PA; they reported that 69% of myxoid PAs had incomplete capsules versus 30% of classic subtypes and 18% of hypercellular subtypes. Most authors [13, 14, 18–21] confirm more frequent incomplete capsules in myxoid PA, although the statistical differences were not always significant. Stennert et al. [18] described more extensive areas of incomplete capsule in the myxoid type, reaching up to 28% of the whole tumor circumference.

13.2.1.4 Capsular Thickness

The capsule of PA may vary in thickness from 5 to 250 μm as described by Stennert et al. [18]; this variation may occur on the surface of the same tumor. Myxoid PA is described as being at the lower end (5 μm) of the spectrum and cellular PA at the higher one (250 μm). Similar results were reported by Naeim et al. [8], Webb and Eveson [19], and Zbären and Stauffer [20]. Because many PAs have a nodular surface, there is always the possibility of a nodule attached by a narrow stalk becoming separated from the main tumor mass, thus giving rise to a recurrence.

13.2.1.5 Pseudopodia

"Pseudopodia" (microscopic finger-like formations of tumor tissue extending beyond the main mass of tumor and separated from it by fibrous tissue, but still localized within the main tumor capsule) (Fig. 13.2) are a significant risk factor for local recurrence of PAs [22, 23]. This is known as "capsule penetration," which occurs earlier and is more common in the bosselation process [24]. In capsular perforation, the tumor cells perforate the capsule and lie adjacent to the normal parotid tissue. Subcapsular splitting may be no more than a dehiscence resulting from perioperative handling, and the presence of blood within the split would support this hypothesis. Another publication [25] confirmed that no tumor has a smooth surface, and all tumors have a "bare area."

Pseudopodia were found in 28% of PA in Stennert's series [18], in 40% of PA by Zbären and Stauffer [20], and in 54% by Park et al. [13]. No clear correlation was found between pseudopodia and PA subtype [13, 14, 18]. Henriksson et al. [23]

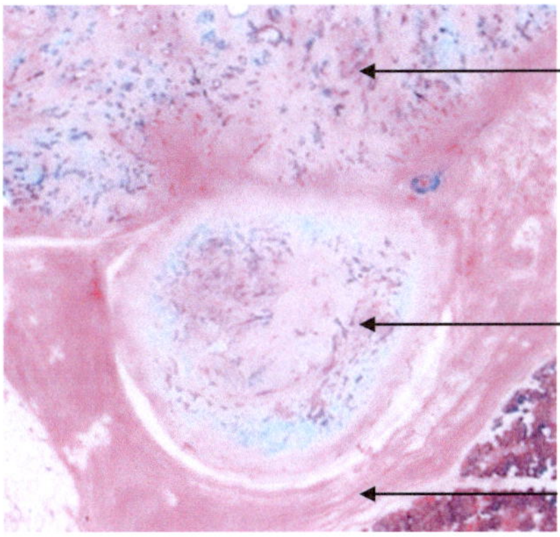

Fig. 13.2 Histopathology of a pleomorphic adenoma (PA) showing pseudopodia formation consisting of acini in lobules embedded in myxoid matrix protruding into the adjacent soft tissue. Capsule thickness ranges from thin to thick. H&E ×200

observed pseudopodia in 5 of 9 (55.6%) PAs with subsequent recurrence and in 16 of 197 (8.1%) without subsequent recurrence. However, this series was not limited to the parotid gland. No such difference was found by Park et al. [13].

13.2.1.6 Satellite Nodules

Satellite nodules are "distinct tumor nodules in the vicinity of the main tumor lump, but separated from it by salivary or fat tissue without any direct connection" (Fig. 13.3). Orita et al. [26] and Li et al. [21] evaluated the distance between the main tumor and satellite nodules and found a maximum of 5.0 and 8.5 mm, respectively.

Satellite nodules were found in 15% [13, 20] to 28% [18] of PA. There is no correlation between histological PA subtype and occurrence of satellite nodules [13, 20, 21]. Park et al. [13] reported an increased prevalence of satellite nodules in patients with recurrent PA; 6 of the 10 patients (60%) versus only 10% in nonrecurrent PAs.

13.2.1.7 Tumor Size

The relation between PA tumor size and capsular integrity was examined by Li et al. [21]. They reported that larger tumors (>4 cm) more often exhibited incomplete capsules, although the difference was not statistically significant. Similar findings were described by Webb and Eveson [19] and Zbären and Stauffer [20]. A significant correlation between the size of tumor and satellite nodules was reported by several authors, with larger PA exhibiting more often satellite nodules [13, 20, 21].

In the Riad et al. [27] series, the mean PA diameter was 32.8 mm and recurrence of PA was related to tumor size, with a mean tumor diameter of 30 mm in nonrecurrent PA and of 43 mm in the recurrent PA. Similarly, in the Ghosh et al. [28] series, all recurrences occurred in tumors larger than 2.5 cm. On the other hand, Henriksson et al. [23] could not correlate tumor size and recurrence.

13.2.1.8 Other Pathological Variables

Bankamp and Bierhoff [15] evaluated the proliferation index of recurrent and nonrecurrent PAs by the MIB-1 antibody immunohistochemistry (IHC) against the cell proliferation-associated nuclear antigen (Ki-67 antigen). They reported that a

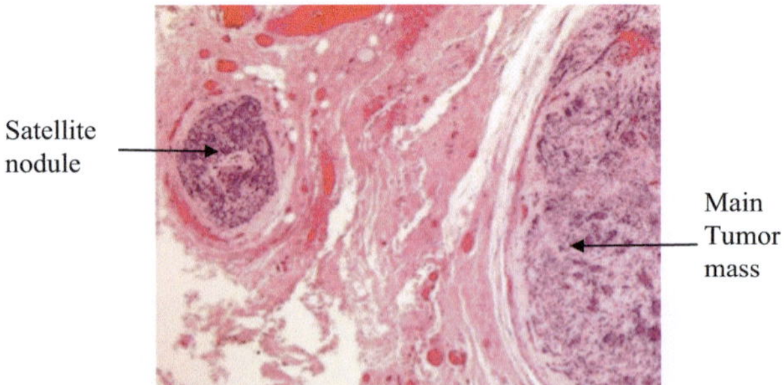

Fig. 13.3 Histopathology of pleomorphic adenoma (PA) showing a satellite nodule separated from the main tumor mass

statistically significant difference was present with a proliferation index of 4.67 ± 3.14 for recurrent PA and 2.34 ± 1.83 for nonrecurrent PA. Higher MIB-1 expression was also found by Glas et al. [29] and Stennert et al. [10], but the differences were not statistically significant.

The presence of multiple nodules in recurrent PA prompted Stennert et al. [10] to suspect a lymphatic spread. This hypothesis was tested by IHC for vascular endothelial factors C and D (VEGF-C and VEGF-D), which are ligands for endothelial tyrosine kinase receptor VEGFR-3, known to primarily mediate lymphangiogenesis. The results were inconclusive and did not support the hypothesis of local lymphangiogenic spread.

A higher expression of mucin 1 (MUC1) glycoprotein and especially of the MUC1/DF3 glycoform by immunostaining was found in recurrent PA and was the only variable significant in multivariate analysis [12]. Only 8% of nonrecurrent PA showed some immunostaining for MUC1/DF3 [12]. Other studies confirmed the progressively increased staining for MUC1/DF3 from normal salivary gland to nonrecurrent PA, recurrent PA, and carcinoma ex PA [30, 31]. In addition, the staining pattern appeared different in recurrent and nonrecurrent PA [30].

13.2.2 Surgery-Related Variables

13.2.2.1 Enucleation

Local excision or "enucleation" was a practice recommended in the 1970s and 1980s as the primary treatment of parotid PA followed by postoperative radiotherapy (RT) [32, 33]. These procedures fell out of favor many years ago, but advocates are resurgent again, suggesting that in "expert hands" using extracapsular dissection, benign tumors can be removed safely by techniques much less invasive than a formal parotidectomy [34, 35]. However, an RR of 2% has been associated with this procedure. Other authors continue to discourage minimal margin surgery in the parotid gland [10, 36–38].

Unfortunately the capsule surrounding PA is at best a "pseudo-capsule" that allows for bits of tumors to be left behind at enucleation surgery or allows spillage during handling or manipulation during surgery, possibilities that have been discussed by many authors [39–41]. If the tumor has been enucleated with obvious rupture or documented spillage, then the proper course of treatment is a formal "parotidectomy."

13.2.2.2 Resection Margin

Riad et al. [27] collected prospective data on 182 parotidectomies. The resected margins ranged between 0 and 26 mm, with a mean of 5.8 mm. Tumor recurrence was inversely related to the safety margin with an average of 1.3 mm in recurrent PA (n = 18) and of 6.0 mm in nonrecurrent PA. Furthermore, the safety margin was inversely correlated with tumor size.

Ghosh et al. [28] reviewed the slides of 83 PAs with prolonged follow-up (mean 12.5 years) and noted an RR of 6.02% (5/83). They classified the specimen margins

(0; <1 mm; >1 mm) and amount of close margins relative to the specimen circumference (focal as <10% and wide as >10%). All recurrences were in the widely exposed capsule group, and most recurrences were found in margins either 0 or <1 mm (18%) versus 1.8% if larger margins were obtained. Positive margins were also seen as the source of recurrence by Buchman et al. back in 1994 [42]. In case of positive resection margin, the term "residual disease" rather than "recurrence" may be more accurate.

13.2.2.3 Extension of Tumor into Other Areas

Extension of tumor into other areas, which may go unrecognized at the time of surgery has been cited [43, 44] and suggested to be the cause of recurrence. For instance, the tumor may become wedged between the mastoid process and the body of the mandible.

13.2.2.4 Tumor Puncture (Rupture) and Spillage

Puncture or rupture of the tumor, because of overzealous traction, instrument compression, rough handling, or poor surgical technique, with spillage into the surgical wound are factors that have been thought to predispose to recurrence. The interior of a PA is usually soft and gelatinous, and it is these myxoid and friable cellular tumors that are at the highest risk for rupture [25]. Tumor puncture is described as a "breach in the tumor capsule during surgery and described in the pathological report." Spillage consists of "spread in the surgical field of tumor content."

The incidence of tumor puncture during parotidectomy is unclear, although Henriksson et al. [23] reported an incidence of 14% with a higher incidence of recurrences though not statistically significant (7% versus 4%). High incidence of recurrences with tumor spillage (11% versus 5%) was reported by Ghosh et al. in 2003 [32] and the difference was not significant. In the more recent study by Riad et al. [27], all the seven tumors (100%) that recurred were punctured, while there was an incidence of 11% of puncture in nonrecurrent PAs. Spillage was reported in seven patients and four developed a recurrence. Park et al. [13] concluded that the risk of recurrence is more than 14-fold higher (4% vs. 30%) if the tumor had ruptured during surgery.

Buchman et al. [42] found that recurrence did not necessarily follow tumor spillage, although different treatment options including radiation were employed preventively to avoid recurrence. Likewise, Natvig and Soberg [45], in their 11–25-year follow-up study, suggested that there is no correlation between tumor capsule rupture and recurrence of PA. However, these studies do not fully explain the most frequent finding of multiple nodules rather than solitary, isolated recurrences. These observations suggest that rupture of the capsule of the tumor and spillage of tumor cells are still the most likely factors contributing to tumor recurrence.

13.2.2.5 Implantation of Tumor Cells

Implantation of tumor cells may take place along the tract of a suction drain or at the point of egress from the skin in cases of tumor rupture. Recurrences tend to be found within the surgical scar or on either side of it, marking the entry and exit points of the suture needle [43]. Soiling and contamination of instruments and gloves from an unrecognized microrupture may also give rise to recurrence.

13.2.2.6 Misdiagnosis

Many clinicians still believe that a small mass in the pre-auricular area is more likely to be a lymph node (LN) or a sebaceous cyst than a PA. This belief results in an incisional biopsy or a local enucleation, followed by the discovery days later that the lesion was actually a PA. The clinician often elects to follow a "watch and wait" policy, and the recurrence becomes evident years later.

13.2.2.7 Preoperative Biopsy

Preoperative biopsy or intraoperative sampling of the tumor may lead to soiling of the surrounding tissues and create a potential risk of recurrence. A survey of 34 internationally recognized head and neck oncologists concluded that the routine use of fine-needle aspiration cytology (FNAC) does not alter the treatment of a discreet mass in the parotid [46].

13.2.2.8 Poorly Designed Incisions

The incision in parotid surgery may be poorly designed, usually too small, limiting complete exposure of the tumor mass, and as a consequence, the surgeon may cut across the posterior border or outer surface of the tumor when the flap is being raised [47].

13.2.3 Patient-Related Variables

13.2.3.1 Age

The younger age at the initial presentation of patients who later present a recurrence is well established [6, 11, 12, 48–50]; patients who will later exhibit a recurrent PA tend to be 20 years younger at initial presentation. There are several possible explanations for this observation; PAs in younger patients may be more aggressive than that in older patients [25], alternatively, as younger patients have a longer lifespan, they are at a greater risk of developing recurrence. On the other hand, this relationship between younger age and recurrence of PAs was not confirmed in some series [27].

13.2.3.2 Gender

Wittekindt et al. (2007), in their analytical study of 108 consecutive patients with recurrent PA, observed that gender has an influence on the potential of PA to recur with a predilection for the female gender [11]. This was also shown by Zbaren et al. in 2007 [20], and more recently, by Valstar et al. from the Netherlands [51], Andersean et al. from Denmark [6], Espinoaa et al. [52], and Aro et al. [53]. However, other authors showed no such influence of gender on PA recurrence [2, 13, 27].

13.3 Clinical Course

In the parotid gland, there is frequently history of a formal parotidectomy with a large scar or a smaller scar in the pre-auricular area suggesting local surgery, most commonly involving the lower pole of parotid.

Recurrence of PA is a complex problem, occurring 1–15 years after the initial operation [11, 43, 50, 54], and in relatively young patients [11, 48–50]. Recurrences are best classified clinically as uninodular (solitary isolated lump), multinodular, or with multiple nodules extending above and below the scar. The recurrence is often multinodular (50-100%) [10, 50]. Maran et al. [43] reported 63.2% recurrences of multinodular tumors in their series of recurrent parotid tumors. A solitary palpable single nodule is almost always discovered at microscopy to be a small cluster of nodules lacking even the most rudimentary capsule.

Recurrent PAs are associated with an increased rate of postoperative complications, especially facial nerve paralysis (2–20%) [10, 11], further recurrences [10, 11], and malignant degeneration (0–16%) [6, 50, 55, 56].

13.4 Assessment

Assessment of recurrent disease must include computed tomography (CT) scan and/or magnetic resonance imaging (MRI), and probably ultrasound (US). Several authors recommended MRI as the preferred imaging method in recurrent PA [34, 57]. It is superior in detecting multinodularity, but the smallest nodules still remain undetectable [58]. In superficial lesions, US and US-guided FNAC are usually utilized. The latter (FNAC) is mandatory to ensure that the tumor presenting is still a PA as errors initially may have occurred or pathological changes may have developed in the interval between original surgery and the current presentation. The sensitivity of FNAC for detecting salivary gland neoplasms is generally around 83% [58], and even higher for PA [59, 60]. However, FNAC does not seem to be adequate in defining the eventual malignant nature of a recurrent tumor since the sensitivity of FNAC for detecting carcinoma-ex PA was only 47% [53, 61]. Heaton et al. (2013) have shown that FNAC combined with MRI can offer a highly confident preoperative diagnosis of PA [59].

The pathological recurrence is usually much bigger and more extensive than clinically suspected [10] and the revision surgery is rather difficult and time consuming. The risk of trauma to the facial nerve is high and may be difficult to identify even with nerve monitoring. If traumatized, the facial nerve may never recover normal function, and even may be permanently paralyzed.

The skin may need to be replaced if recurrences invade or are adherent to the skin. Should the patient have had prior adjuvant radiotherapy or further recurrences, further surgery if offered will be more difficult than anticipated.

13.5 Treatment

13.5.1 Impact of Recurrence on Management Treatment

Treatment of recurrent PA (RPA) remains a challenge, and some tumors may even be incurable. Even expert surgeons consider parotidectomy of recurrent PA as one of the most challenging head and neck procedures. Delays in treatment may also increase the size of the recurrent tumor and thus increase treatment-related complications [62].

Myssiorek et al. [63] reported that only 67% of patients with recurrent PAs ultimately achieved tumor-free status after surgery. Although initial recurrence of PA can occur as long as 20 years following the first surgery, most subsequent recurrences are known to develop within 2–5 years [32, 54]. In the parotid gland, recurrences deep to the facial nerve, which would include recurrences in the para-pharyngeal space, are less likely to be controlled by further surgery than recurrences lateral to the nerve [64].

Patients with more than one recurrence were significantly younger than patients who have had only one recurrence [65]. Once a patient has a second recurrence, the tumor appears to become more aggressive. Subsequent recurrences are more likely and appear more quickly than the initial recurrence [54], and the likelihood of histological malignant degeneration is also greater [32, 66, 67].

Treatment of the recurrent PA is determined by the age and physical health of the patient, the number of previous operations, and the anatomical extent of the recurrence. Preoperative assessment must include imaging and biopsy.

13.5.2 Options of Treatment

Available options for recurrences confirmed as benign by FNAC include the following:

No treatment for the elderly and infirmed; very small tumors, isolated recurrence, or enormous tumors with complex anatomical involvement.

Local excision of a solitary recurrence including the overlying scar (rarely feasible).

Superficial parotidectomy and facial nerve dissection for the recently enucleated tumor of small size and limited to the superficial lobe in which there has been no attempt to locate the facial nerve [33, 65].

Total parotidectomy with facial nerve dissection and preservation; the overlying scar is excised in continuity [65].

Total parotidectomy with resection of the involved nerve and immediate nerve graft with or without replacement of overlying skin.

Any of these surgical procedures followed by radiotherapy (RT) [68, 69].

Radiotherapy alone after FNAC confirmation of PA may be used, after full patient and family consent.

13.6 The Facial Nerve

Radical excision with sacrifice of the facial nerve has been advocated for the treatment of recurrent PA, but morbidity is naturally high. Even if the nerve is grafted, a House–Brackman grade III is as good a result as one gets [70–72]. Several authors expressed reservations about forfeiting neural integrity in the presence of benign disease and recommended parotidectomy with dissection and preservation of the facial nerve [63, 67]. Facial nerve injury is more likely if the tumor is deep, is in multiple sites, or if extensive scar tissue is present. It also depends on the extent of previous surgery and whether the facial nerve was paralyzed previously but recovered. Facial nerve paralysis after the first operation for recurrent PA is approximately 15%. There is a greater risk of permanent nerve damage with each ensuing operation (30% chance of permanent nerve injury after three operations).

Additional surgery for recurrent PA increases the risk of facial nerve paralysis [11, 53, 57]. The likelihood of a "temporary" facial nerve weakness for 6 months was 27% at the first operation, 14% after the second, and rose to 33% at the third attempt. The likelihood of permanent paralysis rose from 27% after the first surgery to 29% at the second surgery [54]. In a series of 126 patients from the Mayo Clinic [67], rates of tumor recurrence after one operation were 32.3%, 7.1% after two operations, and 1.6% after three. After all procedures, partial facial nerve paralysis was recorded in 13.5% of patients and total paralysis in 5.5%. In 24 patients who had had multiple operations, the rate of facial nerve paralysis was 53% (38% temporary and 15% permanent). In another series of 42 patients [66], all patients had multinodular, nontender, recurrent nodules following 1–4 prior surgical procedures, and six patients had been treated with RT. In 30 patients, the facial nerve was preserved. Ten patients had House–Brackmann Facial Nerve Grading grades I–II, 14 patients had grades III–IV, and 6 patients had grades V–VI. In the 12 patients who had the facial nerve sacrificed, the facial nerve function was grades III–IV in only five and grades V–VI in seven.

The use of "loupes" and operating "microscope" as well as "continuous facial nerve monitoring" have greatly helped with minimizing permanent paralysis of the facial nerve after revision surgery for recurrent PA [73, 74]. In such cases, facial nerve monitoring resulted in reduced facial nerve deficit and faster recovery [75, 76].

13.7 Risk of Malignant Transformation

The risk of malignant transformation of recurrent PA is said to increase with time. In the literature, this incidence has varied from <10% to as much as 40% [68]. In a series, 2 out of 36 (6.9%) patients treated for multiple recurrences developed malignant disease. In another series, 2 out of 40 (5%) patients [77] developed carcinoma ex-pleomorphic adenoma (CEPA) and died of disseminated metastases to the lung and bone. Thus, patients with recurrent PA require thorough investigation and biopsy to confirm the true nature of the persistent clinical benign disease to exclude malignant change, prior to recommencing treatment [67].

A retrospective series of 35 patients treated surgically for first recurrence of a PA of the parotid gland were seen over a 15-year period, with a minimum follow-up of 7 years. Loco-regional control was 77% and malignant transformation was 5.7% [78].

Factors associated with a higher change of malignant transformation in PA of the parotid gland [53] (Fig. 13.4a, b) were age >40 years at initial treatment, male gender, nodules >2 cm in diameter, tumors of the deep lobe [77], solitary nodules, more frequent recurrences (>4) [79], and having had >1 previous operation. Malignant tumors were reported in nine (7.1%) patients. In 2009, Suh et al. [80] reported risk factors for malignant transformation of recurrent PA include an age of over 45 years and multiple recurrences. It must be remembered that patients who have been treated with RT for recurrent PA also continue to have a risk of malignancy [81, 82].

An appraisal of CEPA or carcino-sarcoma confirms that there is a malignant change in both the epithelial and mesenchymal elements [83, 84]

The enigma of the metastasizing PA needs to be considered. It seems to be associated with incomplete surgery or enucleation, leading to multiple recurrences that appear to be a prerequisite for the development of distant metastasis [85]. The evidence is overwhelming that this is associated with persistent disease at the following sites: 95% associated with the parotid gland followed by the submandibular gland (4%) and minor salivary glands (1%). This should be considered a low-grade malignancy, but has lethal potential and can be associated with a fatal outcome [86]. In a case series by Nouraei et al. [87], 42 patients had sufficient data to analyze. The mean presentation-to-metastasis latency was 16 years. Bone was the most common

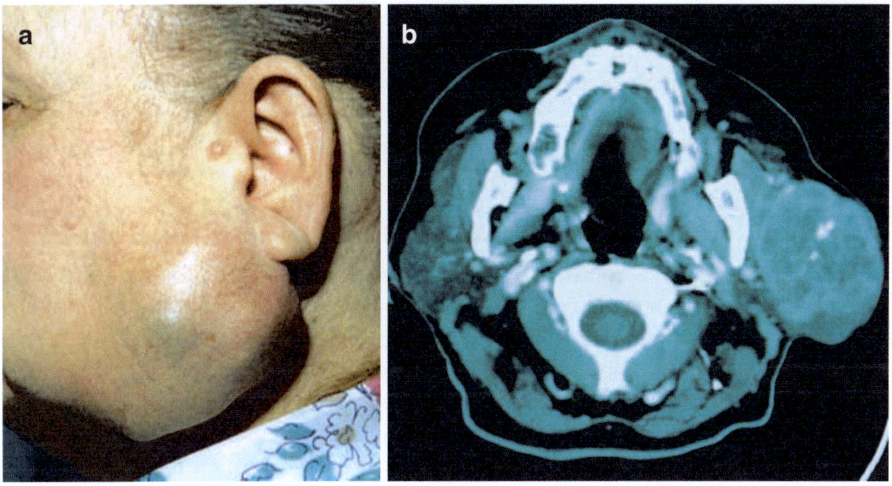

Fig. 13.4 (**a**) A 65-year-old woman with a 20-year history of a 7 × 5 cm mass in the parotid gland with a recent history of rapid increase in size and pain. Parotidectomy revealed carcinoma ex-pleomorphic adenoma. The patient was treated with adjunctive postoperative radiotherapy, had local and regional control, but died of distant metastasis within 2 years. (**b**) CT scan of the same patient with carcinoma ex-pleomorphic adenoma

site for metastases (45%), followed by the head and neck (43%) and lungs (36%). There was significant morbidity and mortality from distant metastases with 5-year disease-specific and disease-free survival of 58% and 50%, respectively [87].

13.8 The Role of Radiotherapy (RT)

The role of radiotherapy (RT) remains controversial in the management of primary or recurrent PA [45, 65, 68]. Radiotherapy should be considered if there has been tumor spillage or residual tumor following reoperation [77, 88]. Some surgeons do not treat with RT for first-time recurrence [68] because of its ineffectiveness in preventing further recurrences as well as concerns about subsequent morbidity [20, 64].

In a series of patients, a decision was made not to sacrifice the facial nerve in 17 of 21 patients and performed instead a subtotal excision of recurrent PA followed by postoperative RT. Sixteen of the 17 patients (94%) remained free of clinical recurrence, with an average follow-up of 5.9 years [89]. The dose of RT ranged from 50 to 67 Gy (average 50.5 Gy). It is thus recommended that certain patients who have undergone surgery and who had ominous clinical and pathological presentations should receive postoperative RT [64].

In a large series of 187 patients from the Christie Hospital, Manchester, UK [81], all had PAs of the parotid gland treated by surgery and postoperative RT by one of two techniques. Until 1976, "needle implant" was used, to a dose of 60 Gy, and after that time, external beam radiotherapy (EBRT) using mega-voltage linear accelerators using an inclined plane to avoid the eyes was used. The tumor dose was 50 Gy in 15–16 fractions. This treatment followed surgery for incomplete excision or tumor spillage. The median age was 46 year, and the median follow-up for all patients was 14 years. A total of 115 patients had RT after their first operation, with an RR of 0.9% (1/115); of the 115 cases, there were two cases of radio-necrosis, facial palsy, Frey's syndrome, and salivary fistula (one patient each). Also, 72 patients had radiotherapy delayed until one or more recurrences had been surgically treated. Nine of these patients (12.5%) developed yet another recurrence after radiotherapy. There were 2 cases of radio-necrosis, 4 cases of facial palsy, 16 cases of Frey's syndrome, and 1 case of malignant change.

Recurrence after RT continued after 20 years of follow-up. It is recommended that patients having unsatisfactory surgery due to spillage at surgery or residual tumor left behind should have RT immediately, rather than delaying treatment until local recurrence occurs, because of the increased morbidity and the higher complication incidence of yet further recurrences. A similar treatment plan has been recommended at Princess Margaret Hospital, Toronto, Canada, with treatment to 45 Gy in 20 fractions over 4 weeks, using an ipsilateral technique encompassing the parotid bed. Using this approach, the authors report the long-term control of tumor to be in excess of 90% [69].

The use of "neutron RT" has been recommended for the management of recurrent PA of the parotid gland [90, 91]. The indications included gross residual disease and multirecurrent multinodular disease. The actuarial 15-year loco-regional control was 76% for patients with gross residual disease versus 100% for those with microscopic disease [53]. The use of neutron therapy may be considered an alternative to further surgery when patients present with >2 recurrences, with a functioning facial nerve, and with a tumor < 5 cm as there is less likely resultant damage to the facial nerve.

The long-term risks of RT and neutron therapy in the head and neck include osteosarcoma of the mandible, malignant fibrous histiocytoma, synovial fistula of the temporo-mandibular joint, and osteo-necrosis of the temporal bone [92, 93].

Conclusions on indications of RT are thus hard to outline. Furthermore, it is unclear after which recurrent event is RT beneficial and should be recommended. Also, since patients usually present tumors at an early age, the side effects of RT need to be considered, and whether RT can induce the growth of other nodules in the future. Based on the results of Aro et al. [53] from their series and the current literature, postoperative RT seems warranted in multifocal recurrent disease and in patients for whom additional surgery would most likely cause significant morbidity.

13.9 Conclusions

A recurrence rate in surgery for PA of <1% is considered acceptable.

Recurrences may present 15–20 years after initial surgery. Recurrent PA is encountered much less frequently nowadays because of correct primary surgical procedure is being performed initially.

Recurrences are most commonly due to poor surgical technique rather than tumor biology.

Recurrence of PAs seems to be increased in the myxoid PA subtype in which the capsule is more often thinner and incomplete. Recurrences seem also more frequent in larger tumors, which not only exhibit incomplete capsules but are also associated with more numerous satellite nodules. Surgical variables related to recurrence include positive margins and tumor spillage [31].

The original histopathology should be reviewed and FNAC performed before starting further treatment.

Management of recurrent PA is currently "further surgery," aiming at complete local excision with preservation of neurological structures, with consideration to adding adjunctive RT postoperatively.

There remains a risk of further recurrence even after apparent successful revision surgery, and even after postoperative RT.

Radiotherapy should currently be reserved for patients who refuse surgery if the facial nerve is likely to be excised and resultant paralysis is unacceptable in an adjunctive setting following resection of a CEPA.

Frequent or persistent PA recurrences may proceed to the metastasizing PA with a potential fatal outcome.

A persistent risk of malignant degeneration remains in patients who have PA. Repeated recurrences, whether the patient has had adjunctive radiotherapy or not, carry a lifelong risk of malignant degeneration, which may result in a fatal outcome.

Future research is required to develop new follow-up methods and management options for recurrent PA in order to avoid further recurrences [53].

References

1. Quer M, Guntinas-Lichius O, Marchal F, Vander Poorten V, Chevalier D, Leon X, et al. Classification of parotidectomies: a proposal of the European Salivary Gland Society. Eur Arch Otorhinolaryngol. 2016;273(10):3307–12.
2. Witt RL. The significance of the margin in parotid surgery for pleomorphic adenoma. Laryngoscope. 2002;112(12):2141–54.
3. Benedict EG, Meigs JV. Tumors of the parotid gland. A study of 225 cases with complete end-results in 80 cases. Surg Gynecol Obstet. 1930;51:626–47.
4. McFarland J. Three hundred mixed tumors of the salivary glands, of which sixty-nine recurred. Surg Gynecol Obstet. 1936;63:457–68.
5. Colella G, Cannavale R, Chiodini P. Meta-analysis of surgical approaches to the treatment of parotid pleomorphic adenomas and recurrence rates. J Craniomaxillofac Surg. 2015;43:738–45.
6. Andreasen S, Therkildsen MH, Bjorndal K, Homoe P. Pleomorphic adenoma of the parotid gland 1985-2010: a Danish nationwide study of incidence, recurrence rate, and malignant transformation. Head Neck. 2016;38(Suppl. 1):E1364–9.
7. Seifert G, Langrock I, Donath K. Pathomorphologische Subklassifikation der pleomorphen Speicheldrusenadenome. Analyse von 310 pleomorphen Parotisadenomen. HNO. 1976;24(12):415–26.
8. Naeim F, Forsberg MI, Waisman J, Coulson WF. Mixed tumors of the salivary glands. Growth pattern and recurrence. Arch Pathol Lab Med. 1976;100(5):271–5.
9. Krolls SO, Boyers RC. Mixed tumors of salivary glands. Long-term follow-up. Cancer. 1972;30(1):276–81.
10. Stennert E, Wittekindt C, Klussmann JP, Arnold G, Guntinas-Lichius O. Recurrent pleomorphic adenoma of the parotid gland: a prospective histopathological and immunohistochemical study. Laryngoscope. 2004;114(1):158–63.
11. Wittekindt C, Streubel K, Arnold G, Stennert E, Guntinas-Lichius O. Recurrent pleomorphic adenoma of the parotid gland: analysis of 108 consecutive patients. Head Neck. 2007;29(9):822–8.
12. Hamada T, Matsukita S, Goto M, Kitajima S, Batra SK, Irimura T, et al. Mucin expression in pleomorphic adenoma of salivary gland: a potential role for MUC1 as a marker to predict recurrence. J Clin Pathol. 2004;57(8):813–21.
13. Park GC, Cho KJ, Kang J, Roh JL, Choi SH, Kim SY, et al. Relationship between histopathology of pleomorphic adenoma in the parotid gland and recurrence after superficial parotidectomy. J Surg Oncol. 2012;106(8):942–6.
14. Goudot P, Auriol M, Chomette G, Vaillant JM, Guilbert F. Pleomorphic adenoma of the salivary glands. Impact of the myxoid component on the prognosis. Rev Stomatol Chir Maxillofac. 1989;90(2):119–22.
15. Bankamp DG, Bierhoff E. Proliferative activity in recurrent and nonrecurrent pleomorphic adenoma of the salivary glands. Laryngorhinootologie. 1999;78(2):77–80.
16. Patey DH, Thackray AC. The treatment of parotid tumours in the light of a pathological study of parotidectomy material. Br J Surg. 1958;45(193):477–87.
17. Eneroth CM. Mixed tumors of major salivary glands: prognostic role of capsular structure. Ann Otol Rhinol Laryngol. 1965;174(4):944–53.
18. Stennert E, Guntinas-Lichius O, Klussmann JP, Arnold G. Histopathology of pleomorphic adenoma in the parotid gland: a prospective unselected series of 100 cases. Laryngoscope. 2001;111(12):2195–200.

19. Webb AJ, Eveson JW. Pleomorphic adenomas of the major salivary glands: a study of the capsular form in relation to surgical management. Clin Otolaryngol Allied Sci. 2001;26(2):134–42.
20. Zbären P, Stauffer E. Pleomorphic adenoma of the parotid gland: histopathologic analysis of the capsular characteristics of 218 tumors. Head Neck. 2007;29(8):751–7.
21. Li C, Xu Y, Zhang C, Sun C, Chen Y, Zhao H, et al. Modified partial superficial parotidectomy versus conventional superficial parotidectomy improves treatment of pleomorphic adenoma of the parotid gland. Am J Surg. 2014;208(1):112–8.
22. Chen RL, Wang CM, Wen YM. Study of the relative factors of the biological behaviour of pleomorphic adenoma of parotid. Zhonghua Kou Qiang Yi Xue Za Zhi. 2004;39:277–9.
23. Hendrikisson HH, Westrin KM, Carlsoo B, Silfverswärd C. Recurrent primary pleomorphic adenomas of salivary origin. Cancer. 1998;82:617–20.
24. Lawson HH. Capsular penetration and perforation in pleomorphic adenoma of the parotid salivary gland. Br J Surg. 1989;76:594–6.
25. McGregor AD, Burgoyne M, Tan KC. Recurrent pleomorphic adenoma salivary adenoma: the relevance of age at first presentation. Br J Plast Surg. 1988;41:177–81.
26. Orita Y, Hamaya K, Miki K, Sugaya A, Hirai M, Nakai K, et al. Satellite tumors surrounding primary pleomorphic adenomas of the parotid gland. Eur Arch Otorhinolaryngol. 2010;267(5):801–6.
27. Riad MA, Abdel-Rahman H, Ezzat WF, Adly A, Dessouky O, Shehata M. Variables related to recurrence of pleomorphic adenomas: outcome of parotid surgery in 182 cases. Laryngoscope. 2011;121(7):1467–72.
28. Ghosh S, Panarese A, Bull PD, Lee JA. Marginally excised parotid pleomorphic salivary adenomas: risk factors for recurrence and management. A 12.5-year mean follow-up study of histologically marginal excisions. Clin Otolaryngol Allied Sci. 2003;28(3):262–6.
29. Glas AS, Hollema H, Nap RE, Plukker JT. Expression of estrogen receptor, progesterone receptor, and insulin-like growth factor receptor-1 and of MIB-1 in patients with recurrent pleomorphic adenoma of the parotid gland. Cancer. 2002;94(8):2211–6.
30. Gao P, Zhou GY, Song XR, Hou JX, Zhang CJ, Ma C. The relationship of abnormal expression of cell glucoprotein with recurrence of pleomorphic adenoma in salivary gland. Hua Xi Kou Qiang Yi Xue Za Zhi. 2005;23(2):164–6.
31. Soares AB, Demasi AP, Altemani A, de Araujo VC. Increased mucin 1 expression in recurrence and malignant transformation of salivary gland pleomorphic adenoma. Histopathology. 2011;58(3):377–82.
32. Dawson AK. Radiation therapy in recurrent pleomorphic adenoma of the parotid gland. Int J Radiat Oncol Biol Phys. 1989;16:819–21.
33. Dawson AK, Orr LA. Long-term results of local excision and radiotherapy in pleomorphic adenoma of the parotid gland. Int J Radiat Oncol Biol Phys. 1985;11:451–5.
34. McGurk M. Benign parotid tumors. BMJ. 2004;329:1299–300.
35. McGurk M, Thomas BL, Renehan AG. Extracapsular dissection for clinically benign parotid lumps: reduced morbidity without oncological compromise. Br J Cancer. 2003;89:1610–3.
36. Paris J, Facon F, Chrestian MA, Giovanni A, Zanaret M. Recurrences of pleomorphic adenomas of the parotid: changing attitudes. Rev Laryngol Otol Rhinol (Bord). 2003;124:229–34.
37. Piekarski J, Nejc D, Szymczak W, Wronski K, Jeziorski A. Results of Extracapsular dissection of pleomorphic adenoma of parotid gland. J Oral MaxilloFac Surg. 2004;62:1198–202.
38. Witt RL. The significance of the margin in parotid surgery for pleomorphic adenoma. Laryngoscope. 2002;112:2141–54.
39. Armitstead PR, Smiddy FG, Frank HG. Simple enucleation and radiotherapy in the treatment of pleomorphic adenoma of the parotid gland. Br J Surg. 1979;66:716–7.
40. Clairmont AA, Richardson GS, Hanna DC. The pseudocapsule of pleomorphic adenoma (benign mixed tumors). Am J Surg. 1977;134:242–3.
41. McEvedy BV, Ross WM. The treatment of mixed parotid tumors by enucleation and radiotherapy. Br J Surg. 1976;63:341–2.
42. Buchman C, Stringer SP, Mendenhall WM, Parsons JT, Jordan JR, Cassisi NJ. Pleomorphic adenoma: effect of tumor spill and inadequate resection on tumor recurrence. Laryngoscope. 1994;104(10):1231–4.

43. Maran AGD, MacKenzie IJ, Stanley RE. Recurrent pleomorphic adenoma of the parotid gland. Arch Otolaryngol. 1984;110:167–71.
44. Rabinov CR, Canalis RF, Alavi S, Lee EJ. Recurrent pleomorphic adenoma of the parotid gland involving the osseous external auditory canal. Ann Otol Rhinol Laryngol. 1997;106:589–93.
45. Natvig K, Soberg R. Relationship of intraoperative rupture of pleomorphic adenoma to recurrence: 11-25 year follow up study. Head Neck. 1994;16:213–7.
46. McGurk M, Hussain K. Role of fine needle aspiration cytology in the management of the discrete parotid lump. Ann R Coll Surg Engl. 1997;79:198–202.
47. Touquet R, McKenzie IJ, Carrouth JAS. Management of the parotid pleomorphic adenoma: the problem of exposing tumor tissue at operation: the logical pursuit of treatment policies. Br J Oral Maxillofac Surg. 1990;28:404–8.
48. McGregor AD, Burgoyne M, Tan KC. Recurrent pleomorphic salivary adenoma—the relevance of age at first presentation. Br J Plast Surg. 1988;41(2):177–81.
49. Laskawi R, Schott T, Schroder M. Recurrent pleomorphic adenomas of the parotid gland: clinical evaluation and long-term follow-up. Br J Oral Maxillofac Surg. 1998;36(1):48–51.
50. Abu-Ghanem Y, Mizrachi A, Popovtzer A, Abu-Ghanem N, Feinmesser R. Recurrent pleomorphic adenoma of the parotid gland: institutional experience and review of the literature. J Surg Oncol. 2016;114(6):714–8.
51. Valstar MH, de Ridder M, van den Broek EC, Tuiver MM, van Dijk BAC, van Velthuysen MLF, et al. Salivary gland pleomorphic adenoma in the Netherlands: a nationwide observational study of primary tumor incidence, malignant transformation, recurrence, and risk factors for recurrence. Oral Oncol. 2017;66:93–9.
52. Espinosa CA, Fernandez-Valle A, Lequerica-Fernandez P, de Villalaín L, de Vicente JC. Clinicopathologic and surgical study of pleomorphic adenoma of the parotid gland: analysis of risk factors for recurrence and facial nerve dysfunction. J Oral Maxillofac Surg. 2018;76:347–54.
53. Aro K, Valle J, Tarkkanen J, Mäkitie A, Atula T. Repeatedly recurring pleomorphic adenoma: a therapeutic challenge. Acta Otorhinolaryngol Ital. 2019;39(3):156–61.
54. Fee WE Jr, Goffinet DR, Calcaterra TC. Recurrent mixed tumors of the parotid gland: results of surgical therapy. Laryngoscope. 1987;88:265–73.
55. Mann W, Beck C, Karatay MC. Recurrent benign tumors of the parotid gland and their tendency for becoming malignant. Laryngol Rhinol Otol (Stuttg). 1985;64(3):133–5.
56. Chang EZ, Lee WC. Surgical treatment of pleomorphic adenoma of the parotid gland: report of 110 cases. J Oral Maxillofac Surg. 1985;43(9):680–2.
57. Witt RL, Eisele DW, Morton RP, Nicolai P, Poorten VV, Zbären P. Etiology and management of recurrent parotid pleomorphic adenoma. Laryngoscope. 2015;125:888–93.
58. Christensen RK, Bjorndal K, Godballe C, Krogdahl A. Value of fine-needle aspiration biopsy of salivary gland lesions. Head Neck. 2010;32:104–8.
59. Heaton CM, Chazen JL, van Zante A, Glastonbury CM, Kezirian EJ, Eisele DW. Pleomorphic adenoma of the major salivary glands: diagnostic utility of FNAB and MRI. Laryngoscope. 2013;123:3056–60.
60. Atula T, Panigrahi J, Tarkkanen J, Mäkitie A, Aro K. Preoperative evaluation and surgical planning of submandibular gland tumors. Head Neck. 2017;39:1071–7.
61. Zbaren P, Zbaren S, Caversaccio MD, Stauffer E. Carcinoma ex pleomorphic adenoma: diagnostic difficulty and outcome. Otolaryngol Head Neck Surg. 2008;138:601–5.
62. Glikson E, Sagiv D, Mansour J, Bedrin L, Talmi YP, Alon EE. Recurrent pleomorphic adenoma: is treatment considerably delayed thus affecting surgical morbidity? Acta Otolaryngol. 2018;138:407–10.
63. Myssiorek D, Ruah GB, Hybels RL. Recurrent pleomorphic adenomas of the parotid gland. Head Neck. 1990;12:332–6.
64. Carew JF, Spiro RH, Singh B, Shah JP. Treatment of recurrent pleomorphic adenoma of the parotid gland. Otolaryngol Head Neck Surg. 1999;121:539–42.
65. Laskawi R, Schott T, Schroder M. Recurrent pleomorphic adenoma of the parotid gland: clinician evaluation and long-term follow up. Br J Oral Maxillofac Surg. 1998;36:48–51.

66. Leonetti JP, Marzo SJ, Petruzzelli GJ, Herr B. Recurrent pleomorphic adenoma of the parotid gland. Otolaryngol Head Neck Surg. 2005;133:319–22.
67. Phillips PP, Olsen KD. Recurrent pleomorphic adenoma of the parotid gland: report of 126 cases and a review of the literature. Ann Otol Rhinol Laryngol. 1995;104:100–4.
68. Leverstein H, Tiwari RM, Snow GB, van der Wal JE, van der Waal I. The surgical management of recurrent or residual pleomorphic adenoma of the parotid gland: analysis and results of 40 patients. Eur Arch Otorhinolaryngol. 1997;254:313–7.
69. Liu F-F, Rotstein L, Davison AJ, Pintilie M, O'Sullivan B, Payne DG, et al. Benign parotid adenomas: a review of the Princess Margaret Hospital Experience. Head Neck. 1995;17:177–83.
70. Fleming WB. Recurrent pleomorphic adenoma of the parotid gland. Aust N Z J Surg. 1987;57:173–6.
71. Glas AS, Vermey A, Hollema H, Robinson PH, Roodenburg JL, Nap RE, et al. Surgical treatment of recurrent pleomorphic adenoma of the parotid gland: a clinical analysis of 52 patients. Head Neck. 2001;23:311–6.
72. Vaughan ED, Richardson D. Facial nerve reconstruction following ablative parotid surgery. Br J Oral Maxillofac Surg. 1993;31:274–80.
73. Dulguerov P, Marchal F, Lehmann W. Post parotidectomy facial nerve paralysis: possible aetiological factors and results with routine facial nerve monitoring. Laryngoscope. 1999;109:754–62.
74. Olsen KD, Daube JR. Intra-operative monitoring of the facial nerve: an aid in the management of parotid gland pleomorphic adenomas. Laryngoscope. 1994;104:232–9.
75. Makeieff M, Venail F, Cartier C, Garrel R, Crampette L, Guerrier B. Continuous facial nerve monitoring during pleomorphic adenoma recurrence surgery. Laryngoscope. 2005;115:1310–4.
76. Zabren P, Tschumi I, Nuyens M, Stauffer E. Recurrent pleomorphic adenoma of the parotid gland. Am J Surg. 2005;189:203–7.
77. Jackson SR, Roland NJ, Clarke RW, Jones AS. Recurrent pleomorphic adenoma. J Laryngol Otol. 1993;103:546–9.
78. Maxwell EL, Hall FT, Freeman JL. Recurrent pleomorphic adenoma of the parotid gland. J Otolaryngol. 2004;33:181–4.
79. Mann W, Beck C, Karatay MC. Recurrent benign tumors of the parotid gland and their tendency for becoming malignant. Laryngol Rhinol Otol (Stuttg). 1985;64:133–5.
80. Suh MW, Hah JH, Kwon SK, Jung YH, Kwon TK, Kim KH, et al. Clinical manifestations of recurrent parotid pleomorphic adenoma. Clin Exp Otorhinolaryngol. 2009;2:193–7.
81. Barton J, Slevin NJ, Gleaves EN. Radiotherapy for pleomorphic adenoma of the parotid gland. Int J Radiat Oncol Biol Phys. 1992;22:925–8.
82. Renehan A, Gleaves EN, McGurk M. An analysis of the treatment of 114 patients with recurrent pleomorphic adenoma of the parotid gland. Am J Surg. 1996;172:710–4.
83. Gnepp DR. Malignant mixed tumors of the salivary glands: a review. Pathol Ann. 1993;28:279–328.
84. Olsen KD, Lewis JE. Carcinoma ex-pleomorphic adenoma: a clinicopathologic review. Head Neck. 2001;23:705–12.
85. Hoorweg JJ, Hilgers FJM, Keus RB, Zoetmulder FA, Loftus BM. Metastasising pleomorphic adenoma: a report of three cases. Eur J Surg Oncol. 1998;24:452–5.
86. Bradley PJ. Metastasizing pleomorphic salivary adenoma should now be considered a low-grade malignancy with a lethal potential. Curr Opin Otolaryngol Head Neck Surg. 2005;13:123–6.
87. Nouraei SAR, Fergusin MS, Clarke PM, Sandison A, Sandhu GS, Michaels L, et al. Metastasizing pleomorphic salivary adenoma. Arch Otolaryngol Head Neck Surg. 2006;132:788–93.
88. Hodge CW, Morris CG, Werning JW, Mendenhall WM. Role of radiotherapy for pleomorphic adenoma. Am J Clin Oncol. 2005;28:148–51.
89. Samson MJ, Metson R, Wang CC, Montgomery WW. Preservation of the facial nerve in the management of recurrent pleomorphic adenomas of the parotid gland. Laryngoscope. 1991;101:1060–2.

90. Buchholz TA, Laramore GE, Griffin TW. Fast neutron radiation for recurrent pleomorphic adenoma of the parotid gland. Am J Clin Oncol. 1992;15:441–115.
91. Douglas JG, Einck J, Austin-Seymour M, Koh WJ, Laramore GE. Neutron radiotherapy for recurrent pleomorphic adenomas of major salivary glands. Head Neck. 2001;23:1037–42.
92. Patel SG, See ACH, Williamson PA, Williamson PA, Archer DJ, Evans PH. Radiation induced sarcoma of the head and neck. Head Neck. 1999;21:346–9.
93. van der Laan BFAM, Baris G, Gregor RT, Hilgers FJ, Balm AJ. Radiation induced tumors of the head and neck. J Laryngol Otol. 1995;109:346–9.

Malignant Epithelial Tumors of the Parotid Gland

14

14.1 Introduction

Cancer of the parotid gland represents <1% of all body cancer and about 20% of all parotid tumors. It either occurs "de novo" or "on top of pleomorphic adenoma." There is no gender predilection, though some authors reported that males are slightly more affected than females. The age of developing this cancer is usually >50 years.

Malignant tumors are as varied as their benign counterparts. Certain tumors are almost always low grade (polymorphous low-grade adenocarcinoma, acinic cell carcinoma, and epithelial–myoepithelial carcinoma), while others are high grade (salivary duct carcinoma, large cell carcinoma, and small cell carcinoma).

Signs of malignant transformation in a preexisting benign tumor include rapid rate of growth, harder consistency, or fixation to the underlying muscles or the overlying skin, which may be severe enough to show fungation.

The patient may develop pain and tenderness that are usually due infiltration of the auriculo-temporal nerve (ATN) with the pain being referred to the ipsilateral ear. Trismus due to invasion of the masseter or pterygoid muscles, or due to restricted movements of the temporo-mandibular joint (TMJ), is another finding.

In approximately 10–15% of cases, the facial nerve will be paralyzed. Unequal pulsations of superficial temporal artery may as well be noticed. Manifestations of metastases to regional lymph nodes or distant organs such as the lungs or the liver may ensue. On the first suspicion of any change in the behavior of the preexisting tumor, fine-needle aspiration cytology (FNAC) should be done immediately after magnetic resonance imaging (MRI) preferably with a diffusion-weighted and perfusion sequences.

Spread of parotid malignancy occurs through the well-established routes of metastases, where the first echelon lymph node (LN) is the intra- and

© The Author(s), under exclusive license to Springer Nature Switzerland AG 2024
M. Sakr, *Surgery of the Salivary Glands*,
https://doi.org/10.1007/978-3-031-82069-4_14

peri-glandular nodes. The next echelon is level II LNs. Local spread can affect any of the critical nearby organs. Hematogenous spread occurs very late and is mainly to the lungs and bones, particularly the vertebral column. However, adenoid cystic carcinoma (AdCC) tends to grow through perineural lymphatics with increased risk of nerve involvement and intracranial extension, as well as increased rate of recurrence.

14.2 Epidemiology

Salivary gland malignancies make up 0.5–1.2% of all cancers in the body and 5% of head and neck cancers. They more commonly affect women with a male-to-female ratio of 1:1.5 [1–3]. Malignant lesions are found in approximately 21.7% of all salivary gland neoplasms [4, 5]. The majority of malignant cases occur in the parotid gland, followed by the submandibular, sublingual, and minor salivary glands. The probability of malignancy in a parotid mass ranges from 15% to 32%, compared to 41–50% in a submandibular mass; 70–90% in minor salivary gland masses; and almost 100% in sublingual masses [6].

The parotid gland harbors 60–75% of all salivary gland tumors [7]. The most common malignant tumors are MEC, AdCC, carcinoma ex-pleomorphic adenoma (CEPA), adenocarcinoma, and squamous cell carcinoma (SCC) [8, 9].

Salivary gland tumors in children are more likely to be malignant. In children under 10 years old, malignant tumors tend to be of a higher grade with poorer prognosis [10]. While those in children older than 10 years were found to be benign in 85% of cases, similar to that of the adult population [11]. The most common pediatric malignant salivary gland tumors include mucoepidermoid carcinoma (MEC), adenocarcinoma, and acinic cell carcinoma (ACC) [1, 3].

14.3 Etiology/Pathophysiology

The exact etiology of salivary gland cancer is unknown, but various mechanisms have been proposed, including radiation exposure, viruses such as Ebstein-Barr virus (EBV) and human immunodeficiency virus (HIV), immunosuppression, ultraviolet (UV) light exposure, occupational exposure hazards in rubber or nickel industries, prior diagnosis of medulloblastoma, prior diagnosis of basal cell carcinoma, androgen receptor expression, and genetics [12–18]. The most common salivary gland malignancy associated with radiation exposure appears to be MEC [19, 20].

Compared to other head and neck cancers, the risk of developing malignant salivary gland tumors from exposure to tobacco and alcohol has been controversial, with several studies noting positive association and others reporting no appreciable association. Some authors reported no significant association between cigarette smoking and MEC, contrary to other malignant salivary histologies [21,

22]. Chronic inflammation of the salivary glands has not been established as a risk factor although autoimmune conditions such as Sjogren's syndrome may predispose an individual to develop a salivary gland malignancy such as lymphoma [23–26].

Although SCC of the head and neck has been linked to tobacco, alcohol, and UV exposure, the presence of primary SCC (PSCC) in the salivary glands is rare and does not retain the same risk factors [27]. The most significant risk factor of PSCC of the salivary glands appears to be prior radiation of the gland [28, 29].

The presence of biological receptors in salivary gland malignancies has recently come under investigation. Tyrosine kinase receptors such as the epidermal growth factor receptor (EGFR) are present in up to 71% of all salivary gland cancers [30]. Human epidermal growth factor receptor 2 (HER2) is present in cancers derived from excretory ducts such as salivary duct carcinoma (SDC) [31]. C-kit is expressed in malignancies derived from the intercalated ducts of salivary glands such as adenoid cystic carcinoma (AdCC) [32].

14.4 Clinical Presentation

14.4.1 History-Taking

Patients with a malignant parotid neoplasm often present with a "history" of a palpable mass in the parotid region. A detailed history including pain symptoms, onset and duration of the mass, growth rate, associated dysphagia, and occurrence of facial weakness should be obtained. Past medical history, including a history of previous skin cancers of the head and neck, surgical history, family history of malignancies, and social risk factors such as smoking, past radiation exposure, and occupational exposures, should also be elicited.

14.4.2 Physical Examination

Clinical examination should include a comprehensive head and neck examination with a focus directed to the involved parotid gland and other salivary glands, cranial nerves, and cervical lymph nodes (LNs). Malignant tumors may present as a painless, fixed, or mobile mass, which is difficult to distinguish from benign tumors. Advanced malignancies may present with pain, palatal fullness, para-pharyngeal fullness, trismus, overlying skin ulceration, or fistulas [33]. Rapid growth, pain, facial nerve paresis, and cervical lymphadenopathy are concerning signs of malignancy [7].

Parotid malignancies presenting as large, fixed preauricular masses (Fig. 14.1 a–d) may be associated with erythema, fungation, and cervical LN metastasis. Facial nerve paralysis can be seen in up to 12–15% of cases and is often associated with AdCC, MEC, and SDC [34].

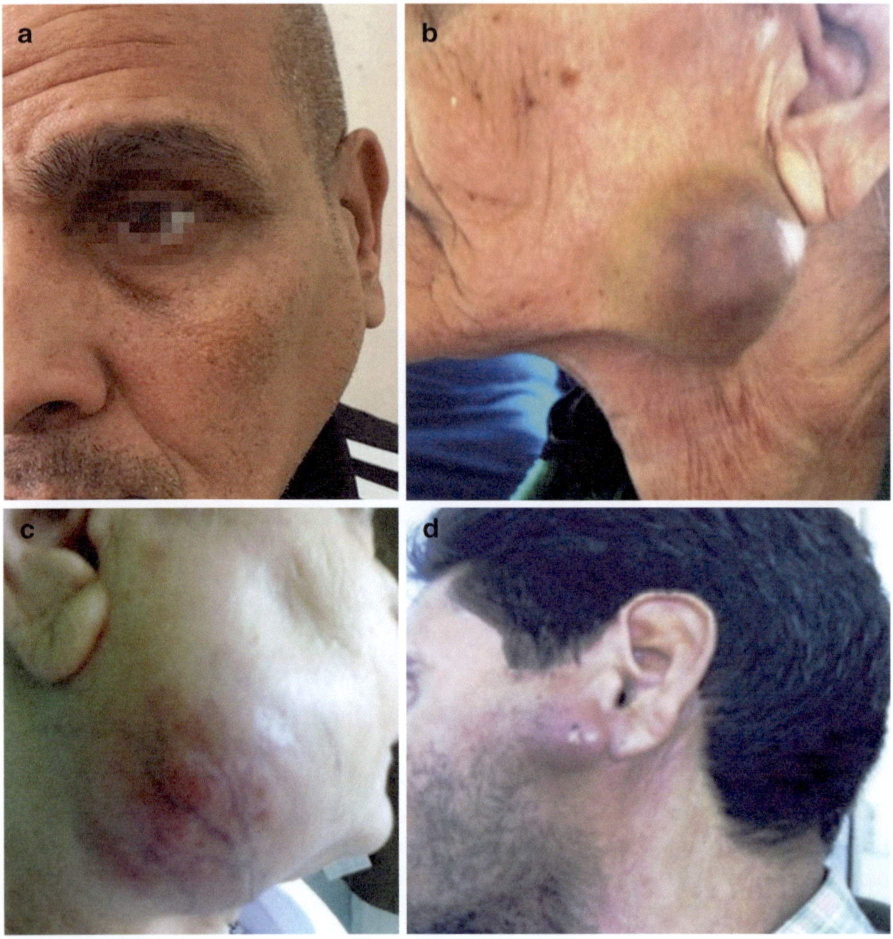

Fig. 14.1 Malignant tumors of the parotid gland present with a hard, rapidly growing mass (**a**), which may become fixed to the overlying skin (**b**), with erythema and increased vascularity (**c**) miming an abscess, and may be severe enough to show fungation (**d**)

14.5 Evaluation

14.5.1 Imaging Studies

14.5.1.1 Ultrasonography (US)

Ultrasonography (US) is the first noninvasive option for evaluating parotid gland tumors, especially superficial parotid lesions. It can help localize tumors, distinguish solid from cystic masses, and help guide fine-needle aspiration biopsy (FNAB). Sonographic signs of malignancy include heterogenous echogenicity, local invasion, poorly defined margins, and lymphadenopathy [35, 36].

14.5.1.2 Computerized Tomography (CT) Scan

Conventional CT scan can evaluate the tumor extent, bony infiltration, and lymphadenopathy. However, it is limited by the dental artifact and has a poor soft-tissue resolution, especially for MEC, AdCC, and acinic cell carcinoma (ACC), leading to underestimating the lesion [3].

14.5.1.3 Magnetic Resonance Imaging (MRI)

For lesions in the deep parotid lobe (sublingual glands and minor salivary glands), MRI is recommended to assess the tumor extent, soft tissue invasion, and nerve involvement. It can be performed to detect the facial nerve branches and their interface with surrounding soft tissue for surgical planning. It has a higher sensitivity and specificity than CT scan in detecting perineural spread, especially in case of AdCC [37]. Characteristics of malignancy on MRI include heterogenous contrast enhancement, local soft tissue invasion, poorly defined margins, hypo-intensity on T2-weighted imaging, and lymphadenopathy [35, 38]. Diffusion-weighted (DW) MRI can quantify the diffusion properties of water in tumor tissue into the apparent diffusion coefficient (ADC) that can help distinguish malignant from benign tumors. Salivary gland malignancies have significantly smaller ADC than benign tumors, although the ADC of Warthin's tumor is even smaller than that of malignant tumors owing to the excessive lymphoid tissue resembling lymphoma [39, 40].

14.5.1.4 Positron Emission Tomography (PET)

The role of PET in malignant parotid tumors is to detect locoregional and distant metastasis. Compared with conventional CT scan, PET is more accurate in demonstrating tumor extension, nodal involvement, local recurrence, and distant metastasis due to the tissues' higher levels of standardized uptake values (SUV) [41, 42]. However, PET cannot differentiate between benign (such as pleomorphic adenoma (PA) and Warthin's tumor) and malignant tumors since both exhibit high glucose uptake values due to the presence of cells with high mitochondrial content [43, 44].

14.5.1.5 Cytology/Histopathology

Imaging alone is unable to distinguish between benign and malignant lesions of the parotid gland. Therefore, obtaining histological samples is the key to determining the final diagnosis and planning the next steps of management. Although an "incisional" biopsy can be used for intraoral minor salivary glands, it is not recommended for parotid lesions due to the risk of facial nerve injury, and the possibility of tumor-seeding. Hence, US-guided FNA is preferred [45]. The sensitivity and specificity of FNA in differentiating between benign and malignant lesions are 80% and 97%, respectively [46]. However, FNA may not have the ability to determine the specific malignant subtype and tumor grade [47].

An US-guided core-needle biopsy can obtain larger tissue specimens for demonstrating the histological architecture of the tumor, which improves recognition of the tumor grade to allow further subtyping [48]. Compared to FNA, disadvantages of core biopsy include more pain, increased risk of facial nerve injury, and hematoma formation [49]. Intraoperative frozen-section biopsy has a sensitivity and specificity of 90% each, for distinguishing between benign and malignant parotid lesions [50].

14.6 Differential Diagnosis

Malignant parotid neoplasms should be differentiated form the following:

Benign salivary lesions (pleomorphic adenoma [PA], myoepithelioma, basal cell adenoma [BCA], Warthin's tumor, oncocytoma, canalicular adenoma, sebaceous adenoma, lymphadenoma, inverted ductal papilloma, intraductal papilloma, and cystadenoma).

Benign salivary cysts (benign lymphoepithelial cyst [BLEC], sialocele, epidermal/epidermoid cyst, dermoid cyst, and hydatid cyst).

Sialadenitis.

Sialoliths.

Lymphadenopathy (from infectious or inflammatory causes).

Tuberculosis (TB).

Infectious mononucleosis (IMN).

Chronic sclerosing sialadenitis (Küttner tumor, which is more common in the submandibular gland).

First branchial cleft cysts.

Lymphoepithelial cysts (in Immunocompromised patients such as HIV patients).

Metastases from tumors of other body sites.

14.7 Clinical Staging

Major salivary gland carcinomas are staged according to the TNM system of the American Joint Committee on Cancer (AJCC) eighth edition (Table 14.1) [33, 51, 52].

Table 14.1 Staging of parotid malignancy according to TNM system of AJCC

T	Tumor size and characteristics
Tx	Primary tumor cannot be assessed
Tis	Carcinoma in situ
T0	No evidence of primary
T1	Tumor <2 cm without extra-parenchymal extension
T2	Tumor 2–4 cm without extra-parenchymal extension
T3	Tumor >4 cm and or tumor has an extra-parenchymal extension
T4a	Tumor invades skin, mandible, external auditory canal, and/or facial nerve
T4b	Tumor invades the skull base, pterygoid plates, or encases the carotid artery
N	**Node criteria**
cNx	Regional LN cannot be assessed
cN0	No regional LN metastasis
cN1	Ipsilateral single metastatic LN <3 cm and ENE-negative
cN2a	Ipsilateral single metastatic node >3 cm but <6 cm, ENE-negative
cN2b	Metastatic multiple ipsilateral nodes >6 cm, ENE-negative
cN2c	Metastatic bilateral or contralateral LNs <6 cm, ENE negative
cN3a	Metastatic LN <6 cm, ENE-negative
cN3b	Metastasis in any LN with ENE-positive
M	**Metastasis criteria**
Mx	Metastasis cannot be assessed
M0	No distant metastasis
M1	Distant metastasis identified

LN lymph node, *ENE* extra-nodal extension

14.8 Treatment

14.8.1 Treatment Options/Indications

Surgical excision with negative (free) margins is the mainstay of treatment of all salivary gland malignancies. Despite preoperative attempts to obtain a diagnosis through a FNAB, histological diagnosis may sometimes not be available until at the time of surgery when frozen-section specimens can be obtained for histopathological examination. The extent of surgery and the need for neck dissection or adjuvant radiotherapy (RT) will be dependent on the subtype, grade, and stage of the tumor [3].

Adjuvant RT is indicated after surgical excision to improve locoregional control in cases with positive margins, cervical metastases, advanced cancer stage, aggressive histology or grade, perineural invasion, lympho-vascular invasion, or extra-glandular extension [53–57]. On the other hand, primary RT is usually reserved for patients with unresectable disease, metastatic disease, or poor surgical candidacy [58, 59].

Chemotherapy and biological targeted therapy are the standard treatment of lymphoma, but have limited roles in the other malignancies; often utilized in the palliative setting with partial response [60, 61]. More prospective research and clinical trials are needed before chemotherapy and targeted therapies become routine clinical tools in the management of epithelial malignant tumors of the salivary glands [33, 61].

14.8.2 Surgical Treatment

Wide local excision is the first-line treatment for all malignant parotid gland tumors; "superficial parotidectomy" is the standard treatment of choice with preservation of the facial nerve [7]. The procedure involves elevating a skin flap over the parotid capsule, identifying the facial nerve trunk and dissecting along all its branches, with preservation of the facial nerve branches that are uninvolved by malignancy, and subsequent removal of the superficial lobe of the parotid while maintaining the integrity of the tumor pseudo-capsule [7]. A "total parotidectomy" is required for advanced or deep lobe lesions. If the facial nerve is infiltrated, a "radical total parotidectomy" with facial nerve sacrifice and reconstruction is then required [62]. For tumors abutting the facial nerve, the tumor can be peeled off and followed with adjuvant RT to clear microscopic disease [62, 63].

Disadvantages of superficial parotidectomy include excessive resection of parotid tissue leading to loss of parotid function, and risk of facial nerve injury due to complete facial nerve dissection. For low-grade or smaller lesions located in the lateral or latero-inferior part of the superficial lobe, "partial superficial parotidectomy" has been proposed. In this procedure, the tumor is resected with a normal margin of parotid tissue and the facial nerve is dissected only in the vicinity of the tumor [64, 65]. A comparison of the two techniques was studied, in a controlled randomized trial (CRT), by Roh et al. (2007) who reported that partial superficial parotidectomy had better cosmesis, improved sensory and salivary functions, less facial nerve weakness, but no difference in recurrence rate (RR) [66].

Cervical metastases in parotid gland malignancies range from 10% to 40% depending on tumor grade, location, histological subtype, and size of the tumor [67, 68]. Cervical metastasis is present in 35–62% of high-grade tumors and 0–15% of low-grade tumors [69]. Histological subtypes such as salivary duct carcinoma, adenocarcinoma, or high-grade MEC have a rate of neck metastasis ranging from 40% to 80% [67, 70–72]. In patients with a clinically negative neck, occult metastasis has been identified in 12–50% of cases [68, 73]. The presence of occult metastasis has been associated with tumor grade, advanced patient age, lymphatic invasion, and extra-parotid tumor extension [74]. In malignant tumors with clinically negative neck disease, elective neck dissection is recommended for high-grade, T3/T4 tumors, facial nerve paralysis, age > 54 years, extra-glandular extension, and lymphatic invasion [75, 76].

14.8.3 Radiation Therapy (Radiotherapy—RT)

Radiation therapy (RT) to the primary site is recommended in the post-operative or adjuvant setting to improve locoregional control and survival, especially in high-grade tumors, advanced stage, positive or close margins, perineural invasion, lympho-vascular invasion, cervical LN metastases, or extra-glandular extension [53–57]. A total dose of 60–66 Gy divided into daily fractions of 2 Gy over 6 weeks has been recommended. Elective neck radiation for clinically negative neck disease is optional. Positive neck disease can be irradiated with 50–60 Gy [33]. Several authors reported that combining surgery and adjuvant RT in advanced-stage disease resulted in 10-year local control rates of 83–91% [55, 77, 78].

Primary RT is advised only in selected cases, including unresectable disease, poor surgical candidacy, unacceptable functional and cosmetic comorbidities from surgery, and for palliation [55, 59]. Mendenhall et al. (2005) reported 10-year locoregional control rate with primary RT was dependent on the disease stage, ranging from 70% for stage I–III down to 24% for stage IV.

Back in 1993, Laramore et al. reported that neutron therapy had better locoregional control rates than photon therapy in unresectable tumors, albeit with no difference in long-term survival [79].

14.8.4 Chemotherapy/Targeted Therapy

Although chemotherapy is the mainstay of treatment of salivary gland lymphoma [48], its benefit is limited for other salivary gland malignancies. Combining chemotherapeutic agents (e.g., carboplatin, paclitaxel, fluorouracil, and hydroxyurea) with adjuvant RT has been reported in some studies to yield a moderate benefit with 5-year locoregional control rates of 90–95%. However, there was no overall survival benefit compared with non-responding patients [80–82]. However, other studies have failed to demonstrate any significant locoregional control or survival benefit in incorporating chemotherapy to primary or adjuvant RT [61, 83, 84]. In patients who are not surgical or radiation candidates, palliative chemotherapy involving cisplatin, paclitaxel, and gemcitabine has been shown to have a partial response in 20–25% of non-AdCC cases and in <10% of AdCC cases [85, 86].

Targeted therapy against C-Kit (Imatinib), HER2 (Trastuzumab), EGFR (Cetuximab), and mTOR (Temsirolimus) have gained popularity due to the expression of biological receptors in several malignant salivary tumors. However, response rates have not been superior, probably due to a discrepancy between protein overexpression and gene mutation, as well as loss of tumor suppressor PTEN that interferes with target therapy responsiveness [87–92].

Table 14.2 Five-year survival of salivary gland cancer

Stage	5-year survival rate
I	91%
II	75%
III	39–65%
IV	39–65%

14.9 Prognosis

The prognosis of salivary gland malignancies has a wide spectrum due to the heterogeneous array of histologies. In general, the prognosis of salivary malignant tumors is better for children and adolescents than that for adults due to lower frequencies of cervical metastasis, absence of local soft tissue invasion, and more differentiated histologies. The 5-year overall survival for children after surgical treatment is 85% compared with 60% for adults [93, 94].

Regardless of malignant subtype, negative prognostic factors for survival include advanced age, high-stage disease, high-grade histology, cervical metastasis, male gender, presence of pain, facial nerve involvement, perineural invasion, local soft tissue invasion, positive or close margins, distant metastasis, and comorbidities [59, 95–101]. Smoking and alcohol consumption were controversial; some studies showed no significant difference in overall survival or disease-free survival [102, 103], whereas other studies found them to be poor prognostic factors [3, 21]. Distant metastasis most commonly involves the lungs (40–91%) followed by bone (13–40%), liver (4–19%), soft tissue (9%), distant nodal basins (8%), and brain (4–7%) [104]. Distant metastasis is the main cause of mortality from malignant salivary glands [33].

Overexpression of epidermal growth factor receptor (EGFR) and human epidermal growth factor receptor 2 (HER2) has been identified in several salivary gland malignancies, such as salivary duct carcinoma. They tend to predict a higher incidence of cervical metastasis and worse survival [3]. The absence of c-kit expression in AdCC is correlated with poorer prognosis [71].

The overall 5-year survival rate (SR) of salivary gland cancer is 72%. The 5-year SR by stage is shown in Table 14.2.

14.10 Complications

The incidence of temporary facial nerve palsy after parotidectomy ranges from 10% to 65%, with permanent paralysis seen in <5% [64, 105, 106]. The incidence of Frey's syndrome after parotidectomy varies widely from 2% to 80% due to the time interval since surgery and the surveillance criteria by the surgeons [107]. Treatment of Frey's syndrome includes antiperspirant ointment, botulinum toxin A injections, and barrier flaps such as superficial musculoaponeurotic system (SMAS) flap, temporoparietal flap, sternocleidomastoid flap, anterolateral thigh flap, or thick skin flaps [107–110]. Additional complications from surgical resection include sialocele, salivary fistula, neuromas of the great auricular nerve (GAN), and preauricular skin anesthesia [33].

Complications of RT include sensorineural hearing loss, chronic otitis media/externa, otalgia, skin erythema, mucositis, dysphagia, dysgeusia, xerostomia, soft tissue fibrosis, osteoradionecrosis, and radiation-induced malignancy [33, 61].

14.11 Characteristics of Individual Malignant Parotid Tumors

14.11.1 Mucoepidermoid Carcinoma (MEC)

14.11.1.1 Epidemiology

Mucoepidermoid carcinoma (MEC) is the most common salivary gland malignancy in adults and children [10]. Approximately, 80–89% of cases are found in the parotid gland, followed by the submandibular gland (8–13%) in the sublingual gland (1.5%) [111]. Parotid MEC is less aggressive than that of the submandibular gland and has a better prognosis. In some series, MEC is more common in women by a ratio of 3:2, while in others there is no gender predominance [112]. It mostly occurs in adults around the fourth to fifth decades of life, but still, it is the commonest salivary malignancy of the pediatric age group [44].

14.11.1.2 Pathophysiology

Mucoepidermoid carcinoma (MEC) arises from the epithelium of the interlobular and intralobular salivary ducts. The most common genetic finding is the chromosomal translocation t(11;19)(q21:p13), leading to the fusion of MECT1 and MAML2 genes, which is responsible for disrupting the NOTCH signaling pathway [113, 114]. This translocation is found in 50–70% of patients with MEC, and is more often seen in low-grade tumors associated with a better prognosis [115, 116].

14.11.1.3 Histopathology

Histopathologically, MEC is a nonencapsulated, poorly circumscribed mass with cystic components that can often be mistaken for mucoceles [117]. It may be composed of up to six different types of cells: maternal, intermediate, epidermoid, clear, columnar, and mucous cells. Maternal cells are the progenitors for the other cell types and have small, round nuclei with a scanty, basophilic cytoplasm. Intermediate cells can develop into either glandular or epidermoid cells. Epidermoid cells present with homogenous cytoplasm and occasional keratin pearls and intracellular bridges. Clear cells have watery cytoplasm with small, central nuclei. Columnar cells resemble the secretory duct cells of the salivary gland and transform into mucous cells. Mucous cells have small nuclei at the periphery with foamy, reticular cytoplasm and can occasionally develop a signet-ring appearance [117, 118].

The tumor can occur as low-, intermediate-, or high-grade lesion depending on the quantity of aggressive, epidermoid tissue. Low-grade MEC has well-formed cystic spaces with high glandular composition (Fig. 14.2). Intermediate grade tends to have more solid nests of epidermoid and intermediate cells with less prominent

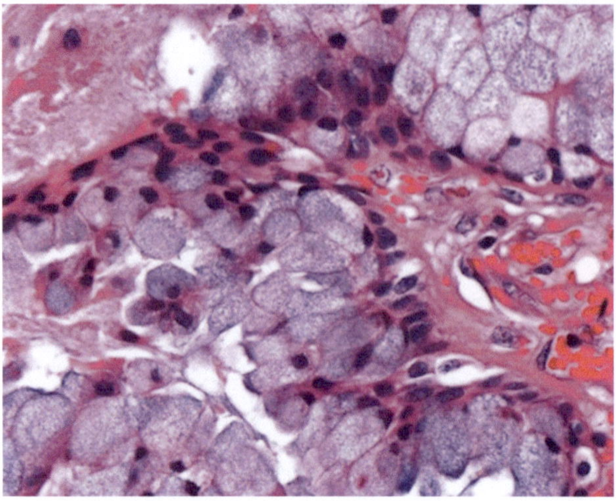

Fig. 14.2 Low-grade mucoepidermoid carcinoma (MEC) shown as composed predominantly of mucinous cells lining cystic and glandular spaces. The tumor cells have abundant, basophilic foamy cytoplasm and small hyperchromatic basally located nuclei. There is no cytological atypia. H&E stain

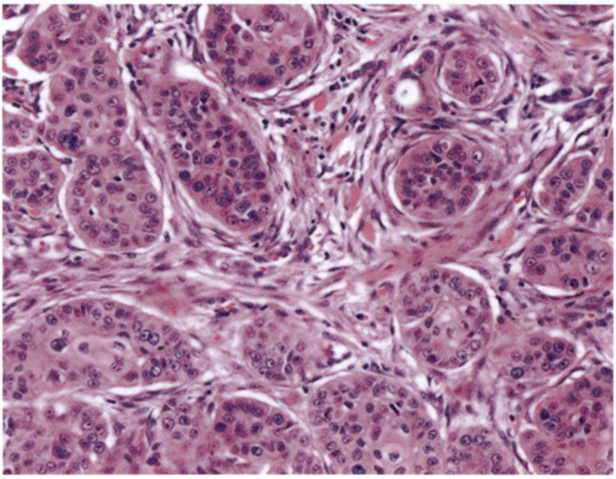

Fig. 14.3 High-grade mucoepidermoid carcinoma (MEC) shown as solid tumor with no cyst formation, composed predominantly of solid sheets and clusters of epidermoid and intermediate cells with prominent nucleoli and cytological atypia. H&E stain

cystic spaces, while high-grade MEC has limited mucous cells with large amounts of solid, squamous cells that can often be misdiagnosed as squamous cell carcinoma (SCC) (Fig. 14.3) [119, 120].

14.11.1.4 Clinical Presentation

Mucoepidermoid carcinoma (MEC) usually presents as a slowly growing painless (asymptomatic), firm mass; however, rapid growth, pain and tenderness may be seen with the high-grade variant [121, 122] (Fig. 14.4) as well as facial paralysis [10]. It often presents as an asymptomatic, firm mass with occasional pain and "First-bite syndrome" (FBS): a condition that classically presents as severe pain in the preauricular region, initiated on the first bite of a meal, has been associated with MEC [34]. Low-grade and high-grade variants are recognized to metastases

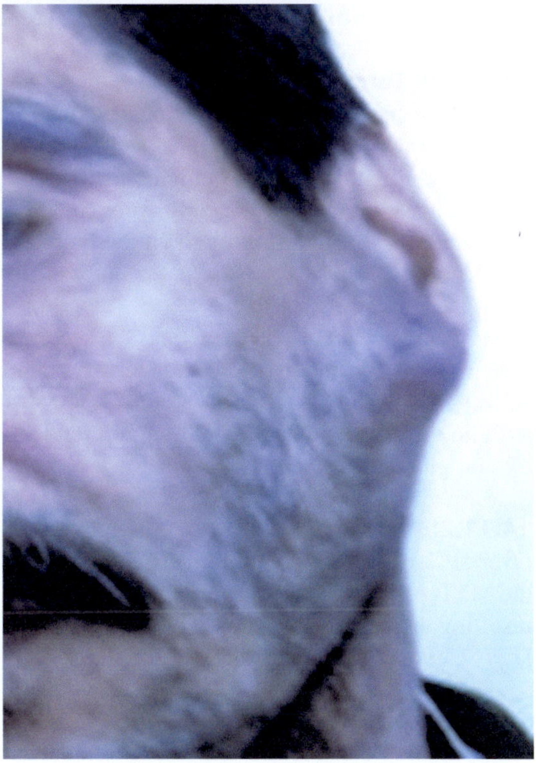

Fig. 14.4 A rapidly growing (high-grade) mucoepidermoid carcinoma (MEC) in a 51-year-old gentleman that became fixed to the overlying skin within 2 weeks

to LNs, lungs, and bones [123], where the low-grade one very rarely metastasizes [124–126].

14.11.1.5 Treatment

Treatment of MEC is surgical resection with neck dissection being reserved for high-grade variants [124].

14.11.1.6 Prognosis

Prognosis is influenced by the grade and stage of the tumor, as well as patient's age (above 45 years is associated with poor prognosis) and gender. Histological grade is considered one of the most important factors in prognosis. Low-grade MEC, especially cases with the MECT1–MAML2 gene fusion, have a good prognosis with a 5-year survival rate (SR) of >90%. However, the high-grade squamous variant of MEC has a high tendency for recurrence, cervical metastasis, and distant metastasis with a 5-year survival as low as 30–41.6% [97, 127]. Brandwein et al. (2001) reported that approximately 33% of patients with MEC were found to have regional metastasis, of which 85% exhibited a high-grade primary tumor [128]. The 5-year SR has been shown to range from 75% to 96% [129–131], and the overall 10-year SR for MEC is about 53% [132].

14.11.2 Adenoid Cystic Carcinoma (AdCC)

14.11.2.1 Terminology

This tumor has been given many names since it was first described by Robin and colleagues in 1853. From these names, "cylindroma" was particularly discouraged to avoid confusion with the benign cutaneous appendage tumor carrying the same name. This tumor arises not only from major and minor salivary glands but also from seromucous glands throughout the body [133, 134].

14.11.2.2 Epidemiology

Adenoid cystic carcinoma (AdCC) is the second most common salivary malignancy and accounts for about 10% of all salivary gland neoplasms and 30% of all minor salivary gland tumors. It has a predilection for patients in the fifth to sixth decade with no difference in gender, although it tends to be more common in the submandibular gland in women [10, 135, 136].

14.11.2.3 Pathophysiology

Over 50% of AdCCs contain the t(6;9)(q22–23;p23–24) translocation, which fuses the MYB proto-oncogene on chromosome 6q to the NFIB gene on chromosome 9p, resulting in an overexpression of MYB-NFIB fusion oncogene and worse prognosis [137–139].

14.11.2.4 Histopathology

Histopathologically, AdCC appears as a nonencapsulated, well-circumscribed mass with biphasic ductal and myoepithelial components and three distinct patterns: tubular, cribriform, and solid [3, 10]. The cribriform variant presents with a "Swiss-cheese" appearance containing cylindrical pseudo-cysts lined with epithelial cells and filled with hyaline material (Fig. 14.5). The tubular variant consists of ducts lined by one to two layers of myoepithelial-like cells. The solid variant has solid

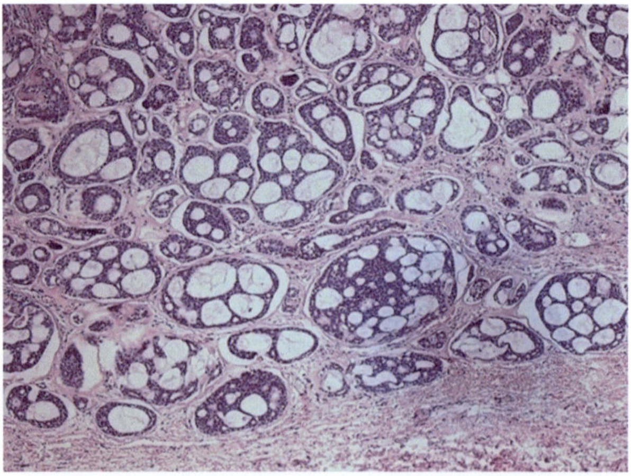

Fig. 14.5 Low-grade adenoid cystic carcinoma (AdCC) with a notable cribriform pattern ("Swiss-cheese" appearance) (H&E × 100)

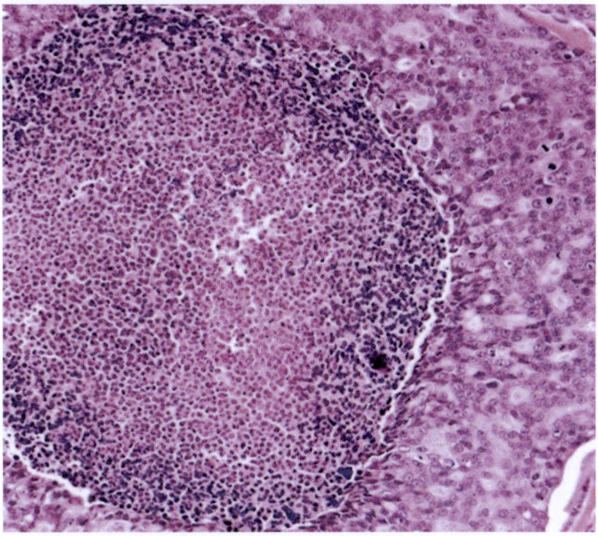

Fig. 14.6 High-grade adenoid cystic carcinoma (AdCC) with a predominant (>70%) solid pattern showing necrosis, nuclear pleomorphism, and increased mitotic activity (H&E × 100)

epithelial islands with central areas of necrosis (Fig. 14.6) [1, 140]. The solid variant is the most aggressive and has a tendency for hematogenous metastasis in 40–60% of cases with perineural invasion along the palatine branches through which it can extend into the pterygopalatine fossa and cavernous sinus [140–142].

14.11.2.5 Clinical Presentation

Clinically, AdCC presents as a slow-growing, solid mass with pain secondary to perineural and extra-parenchymal invasion. It frequently presents as a painless mass giving a false sense of security. Cervical LN metastases are uncommon (approximately 20% at presentation) [10]. First-bite syndrome has also been associated with AdCC [143].

Distant metastases occur in up to 60% of the cases, mainly to the liver, lung, bones, and brain [134, 144]. It has a high affinity to perineural invasion, which results in paresthesia or paralysis of the nerve affected.

14.11.2.6 Treatment

Best results of treatment are obtained through radical surgery and postoperative RT. The tumor is radiosensitive, but not radio-curable. Although controversial, neck dissection may be reserved for patients with clinically positive LNs [144–146].

14.11.2.7 Prognosis

Distant metastasis in AdCC takes a prolonged course and is often more common than cervical metastasis [147]. The rate of distant metastasis ranges from 25% to 60%, whereas the local recurrence rate ranges from 15% to 85%. The 5-year survival rate cited in the literature is as high as 60–90%; however, patients with stage III and IV diseases have a poorer prognosis with low survival rates: as low as 15–50% at 10 years. Due to the prolonged, indolent growth pattern of AdCC, it can ultimately result in poor disease-free survival of 10–20% at 10–15 years. The solid pattern histology has the worst prognosis [10, 132, 148, 149]. Some studies showed that age over 45 years, advanced clinical stage, paresthesia, as well as increased expression of p53 are associated with poor prognosis [134, 144]. The prognostic significance of perineural invasion and DNA ploidy remain controversial.

14.11.3 Carcinoma Ex-pleomorphic Adenoma (CEPA)

14.11.3.1 Epidemiology

Carcinoma ex-pleomorphic adenoma (CEPA) is by definition the malignant transformation of a long-standing PA, which occurs in about 25% of such cases [146, 150, 151] accounting for 5–15% of all salivary gland malignancies [152]. Malignant transformation is often seen in recurrent PA with the risk of transformation ranging from 5% to 10% for untreated PAs over a 15-year period [147]. Approximately, 82% of cases occur in the parotid and submandibular glands, followed by 18% in the intraoral minor salivary glands [147].

The average age at diagnosis is 50–60 years, which is approximately 10 years older than most individuals with PA. It is extremely uncommon in individuals below the age of 20 years [146, 153]. Female-to-male ratio is 1.2:1–3:1.

14.11.3.2 Pathophysiology

Epigenetic mutations involving DNA promoter methylation of tumor suppressor genes can lead to transcriptional inactivation and increase both the risk of salivary duct carcinoma and the transformation of pleomorphic adenoma into CEPA [154, 155].

14.11.3.3 Histopathology

Histologically, CEPA arises from an existing PA. The presence of hyalinized stroma is the most predictive parameter for malignant transformation [156]. The carcinoma is usually a high-grade adenocarcinoma or an undifferentiated carcinoma although numerous other types including SCC, MEC, AdCC, myoepithelial carcinoma, clear cell carcinoma, papillary carcinoma, and terminal duct carcinoma have been reported [152, 157]. It can microscopically present with varying extents of invasion, including intracapsular, minor extracapsular (<5 mm beyond the capsule), and wide extracapsular (>5 mm beyond the capsule). The wide extracapsular variant presents with a high risk of recurrence and distant metastasis [3, 152, 157].

14.11.3.4 Clinical Presentation

Clinically, CEPA commonly presents in a patient with a history of a long-standing parotid mass characterized by a sudden increase in size. It can be associated with pain and facial nerve palsy in 12–30% of cases [158] as well as fixation to the surrounding soft tissues [159]. Clinical features predictive of malignant transformation are age, tumor size, long history, and submandibular location.

14.11.3.5 Treatment

Treatment of CEPA is surgical resection usually with neck dissection. In situ variant is that tumor which did not invade the capsule of a PA and thence was diagnosed postoperatively. In this case, the performed standard resection of a PA is curative.

14.11.3.6 Prognosis

CEPA can display a wide range of recurrence and survival rates depending on the extent of differentiation and invasion. Tumors with wide extracapsular invasion beyond 5 mm of the capsule present with a high risk of recurrence and distant metastasis in up to 70% of cases rather than regionally, with special affinity to the lungs and vertebral column [3, 152, 157]. The presence of regional metastasis in CEPA reduces the 5-year survival rate from 67% to 16% [160]. Clinical neck metastasis is present in 33% of patients with CEPA and occult neck metastasis in 16% of patients [161]. The 5-year SR is 30–96% depending on the histology variant [152, 162]. The overall 10-year SR of CEPA is 62% [132].

14.11.3.7 True Malignant Mixed Tumor (TMMT)

True malignant mixed tumor is a very rare neoplasm that may be regarded as carcinosarcoma since both epithelial and stromal components are histologically malignant, and both can metastasize. Such metastases are more commonly via a hematogenous rather than lymphatic route, with the lungs and bones being the most frequent sites [163, 164].

There is a wide range of age involvement (14–87 years) and there is no gender predilection [164, 165]. Clinical presentation is similar to that of CEPA. Treatment is surgical resection, combined with radiation and chemotherapy. Even with such radical treatment, most patients die within 5 years [153].

14.11.4 Acinic Cell Carcinoma

14.11.4.1 Epidemiology

Acinic cell carcinoma (ACC) is the third most common cancer of the parotid gland. It is located in the parotid gland in more than 80% of all cases, followed by the intraoral minor salivary glands (16%) and the submandibular gland (4%). Bilateral parotid involvement is seen in 3–5% of cases [166], being second to Warthin's tumor in bilateral incidence [167]. It is also second to MEC in pediatric age group involvement [168]. Acinic cell carcinoma has a predilection for women and more commonly occurs in the fifth decade [10, 112, 136].

14.11.4.2 Pathophysiology

ACC develops from tumorigenesis of cells responsible for acinar development, namely the reserve cells of the intercalated ducts and terminal tubule. In experimental studies on mice, inactivation of PTEN and Apc led to an upregulation of mTOR and Wnt signaling, which increased the incidence of acinic cell carcinoma [169]. In humans, ACC has also been found to have a higher expression of mTOR compared to other salivary malignancies [18].

14.11.4.3 Histopathology

Histologically, ACC presents with several growth patterns, including solid (most common), papillary-cystic, follicular, and microcystic [170]. It appears well-circumscribed by a lymphoid stroma or a capsule. Individual cells can be granulated serous-type cells, primitive tubule cells, or undifferentiated polymorphous cells [170, 171]. Although ACC is usually considered a low-grade malignancy (Fig. 14.7), it can undergo high-grade transformation into high-grade adenocarcinoma or undifferentiated carcinoma and present with complete loss of acinar differentiation, desmoplasia, tumor necrosis, frequent mitosis, and cervical or distant metastasis [172–174].

14.11.4.4 Clinical Presentation

Patients with ACC typically present with a slowly enlarging, painless mass that is not fixed to the surrounding soft tissue or skin, and usually do not spread to local LNs. Clinically, it is indistinguishable from benign parotid neoplasms being of low-grade malignancy [172, 175]. Yet, it can rarely dedifferentiate into an aggressive high-grade tumor. Pain occurs in approximately 22% of patients and facial nerve palsy in nearly 3–8% [10, 172, 176].

14.11.4.5 Treatment

Treatment of ACC is complete surgical resection. Neck dissection is usually not recommended because of the relatively low incidence of metastases to regional LNs [172]. It is usually radioresistant; however, RT is resorted to when complete resection is not achieved, in case of perineural invasion, and if LNs are involved [177, 178].

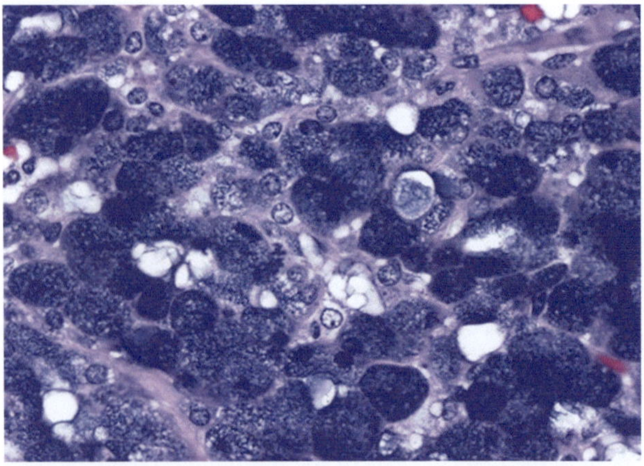

Fig. 14.7 Histopathology of acinic cell carcinoma shows acinar cells with deeply basophilic cytoplasm arranged in solid sheets. Intercalated duct-like cells with eosinophilic cytoplasm and vacuolated cells are also seen. The basophilic appearance of the acinar cells is due to zymogen-like granules, which can be easily discerned at this magnification

14.11.4.6 Prognosis

Overall survival of ACC is influenced by male gender, age > 45 years, tumor size >3 cm, and distant metastasis [179]. Cervical neck metastasis occurs in 6–10% and distant metastasis in 12–16% of cases [167, 172, 177, 180–182]. The overall survival rate at 5-years is 75–96% [183, 184], which drops to 56% at 20 years [171, 185, 186]. The recurrence rate averages 10–35% and the distant metastatic rate 13–16%. The 5-year survival rate ranges from 78% to 90%.

14.11.5 Basal Cell Adenocarcinoma (BCAC)

14.11.5.1 Epidemiology

Basal cell adenocarcinoma is the malignant counterpart of basal cell adenoma (BCA). It is an uncommon low-grade malignancy that accounts for approximately 1.5% of all salivary gland tumors and 3% of all salivary gland malignancies [187]. BCAC is more common in Caucasians, does not have a gender predilection [188], and most patients are in their sixth or seventh decade, though cases have been reported in patients as young as 2 months and as old as 92 years [187–192].

14.11.5.2 Etiology/Pathophysiology

Most of BCACs occur de novo. Origin in a preexisting BCA has been reported in approximately 25% of cases and usually involves the membranous subtype [188, 189, 192]. Nearly 90% of tumors arise in the major salivary glands, mostly parotid (>80%) [193]. It is rare in other salivary glands and minor salivary gland tissue.

14.11.5.3 Cytology/Histopathology

Cytological diagnosis is exceedingly difficult due to morphological overlap with other more common biphasic salivary gland neoplasms, including pleomorphic adenoma (PA) and adenoid cystic carcinoma (AdCC).

Histological features are similar to BCA, but with evidence of invasive growth pattern (Fig. 14.8). Characteristic features thus include: (1) uncapsulated tumor, with circumscribed to infiltrative edges with infiltration into salivary gland parenchyma, fat, nerve (Fig. 14.9), or lympho-vascular spaces, (2) solid, trabecular, tubular, and membranous growth patterns; (3) biphasic tumors with central ductal cells and luminal basal cells; (4) ductal cells that appear cuboidal, with moderate amounts of eosinophilic cytoplasm and round to ovoid nuclei; (5) basal cells with scanty cytoplasm and hyperchromatic ovoid nuclei; (6) nuclear palisading of the peripheral basal cells (Fig. 14.10); (7) squamous and sebaceous differentiation may be seen; and (8) necrosis may also be seen in 45% of tumors, with an increase in mitoses [194]. Diagnosis is based on the demonstration of a dual cell population of centrally located ductal cells and luminal basal cells with peripheral palisading of nuclei.

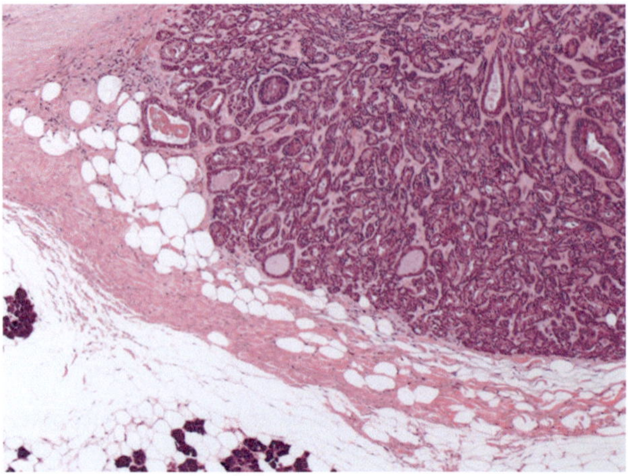

Fig. 14.8 Histopathology of basal cell adenocarcinoma showing tubules with an angulated appearance can be seen infiltrating through the fibrous stroma. H&E stain

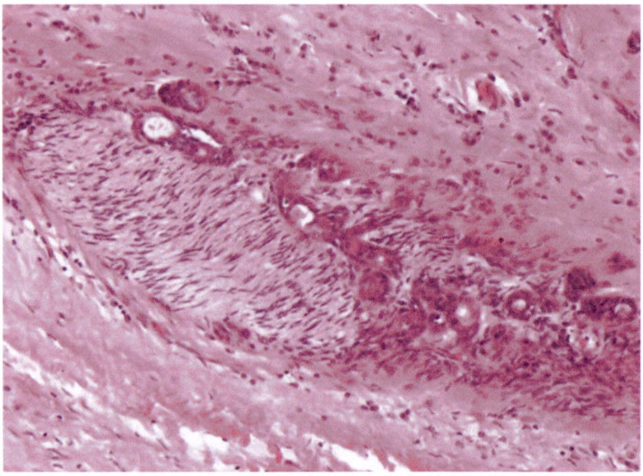

Fig. 14.9 Histopathology of basal cell adenocarcinoma showing neoplastic cells arranged in tubules are seen invading nerves. H&E stain

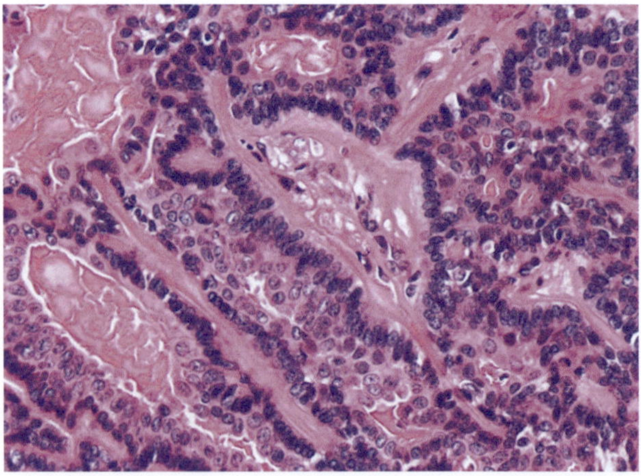

Fig. 14.10 Histopathology of basal cell adenocarcinoma showing tumor cells typically show peripheral palisading of basal cells. H&E stain

14.11.5.4 Clinical Presentation

Patients with BCAC usually present with a slowly growing, asymptomatic mass, often present for many years; pain and tenderness are uncommon [195]. In 10–15% of cases, it may occur in the context of familial cylindromatosis syndromes (e.g., such as Brooke-Spiegler syndrome), in conjunction with dermal cylindromas and trichoepitheliomas, as compared to 40% of BCA [196, 197]. Metastasis may occur in the LNs in approximately 15% of cases, and rarely to the lungs.

14.11.5.5 Differential Diagnosis

Basal cell adenoma (BCA).

Well-circumscribed, no invasion/infiltration into adjacent tissues.

Multifocal or membranous type can simulate invasion.

Nuclear β-catenin-positive.

Pleomorphic adenoma (PA).

Presence of myxoid/chondro-myxoid matrix.

Frequent plasmacytoid and spindled cells.

Epithelial/myoepithelial cells blend into stroma; BCAC has abrupt border with matrix.

Multi-nodular growth may simulate invasion.

Canalicular adenoma.

May be multifocal, but nearly always involves upper lip/minor salivary gland.

Beaded chains of short columnar cells.

No basement membrane material.

S100-positive, SOX10-positive, GFAP-positive (only at periphery).

P63-negative, actin-negative.

14.11.5.6 Adenoid Cystic Carcinoma (AdCC)

Cribriform patterns and punched out spaces surrounded by small cells with minimal cytoplasm.

Palisading not prominent.

Lacks large pale and small dark cells common in BCAC.

Coarse nuclear chromatin, high mitotic rate.

Basaloid squamous cell carcinoma (SCC).

High-grade neoplasm, usually in the oral or sino-nasal tract rather than salivary glands.

Basaloid, comedo-necrosis, and hyaline type material seen in both.

Abrupt squamous differentiation.

Skin basal cell carcinoma (BCC).

Skin tumors may metastasize to intra-parotid LNs or directly invade the parotid gland.

Palisading, basaloid architecture, necrosis, and increased mitotic figures.

Lacks biphasic appearance and myoepithelial cells.

BerEP4-positive.

14.11.5.7 Treatment

Treatment is complete surgical excision with clear margins; neck dissection is reserved for patients with clinically positive LNs [198–200].

14.11.5.8 Prognosis

Basal cell adenocarcinoma is a low-grade malignant tumor with good long-term prognosis; death from the disease is rarely reported [201]. It may be locally destructive, and local recurrences are seen in nearly 50% of cases, up to 10 years later, highlighting the importance of a long-term follow-up. Poorer prognostic features include location in minor salivary glands, advanced stage, incomplete excision, and recurrence [197].

14.11.6 Myoepithelial Carcinoma (Malignant Myo-epithelioma)

14.11.6.1 Epidemiology

Myoepithelial carcinoma is the malignant counterpart of myoepithelioma. It is a rare tumor accounting for only 1–2% of all salivary gland tumors [198], and involving the parotid glands in 70–75%% of cases, the submandibular glands in 12%, and lastly minor salivary glands in the palate and upper aerodigestive tract [196, 198, 199]. Myoepithelial carcinoma is most common in the sixth and seventh decades of life and occurs with no gender predilection, though a male-to-female ratio of 1:1.6 has been reported [198].

14.11.6.2 Pathophysiology

Myoepithelial carcinoma may arise de novo, but approximately 50% of cases arise in a preexisting benign tumor, usually a myoepithelioma or a PA [202]. It is presumed to be of intercalated duct origin. Up to 85% of epithelial myoepithelial carcinomas carry an *HRAS* mutation [203].

14.11.6.3 Histopathology

By definition, myoepithelial carcinoma is composed of myoepithelial cells with an infiltrative growth pattern (Fig. 14.11).

Characteristic features include: (1) bilayered arrangement of small luminal cells with eosinophilic cytoplasm and outer myoepithelial cells with clear cytoplasm rich in glycogen; (2) a few morphological types may be seen (classic, epithelial dominant, and myoepithelial dominant) depending on the proportion of epithelial and myoepithelial cells present; (3) tubular, glandular, and solid growth patterns; (4) papillary and cystic areas may also be present—tumor necrosis can be seen within the hypercellular central zone of a tumor nodule [203]; (5) basement membrane-like hyalinized matrix may be present; (6) the myoepithelial component can often be spindled (Fig. 14.12) or have clear cells (Fig. 14.13); (7) high-grade transformation (20%) showing sheets and solid nests of markedly atypical cells with increased mitoses and necrosis and usually involving the epithelial component; and (8) the presence of pre-existing/residual pleomorphic adenoma component can be seen in myoepithelial carcinoma ex-PA.

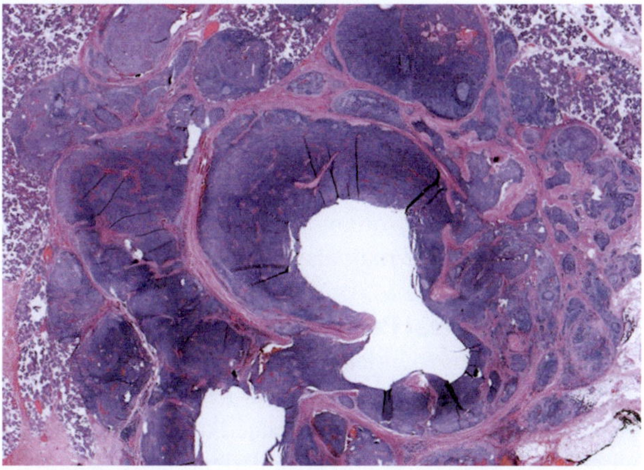

Fig. 14.11 Histopathology of myoepithelial carcinoma showing a multinodular invasive growth without desmoplastic reaction. Tumor-associated lymphoid stroma is seen at the periphery of the tumor. H&E stain

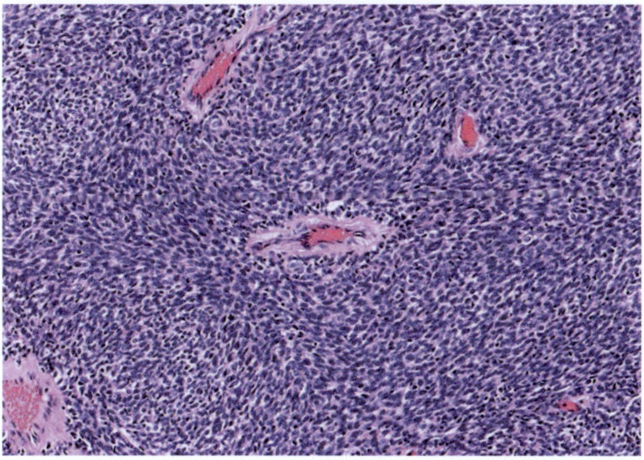

Fig. 14.12 Histopathology of myoepithelial carcinoma with the myoepithelial component showing spindle cell morphology arranged as loose fascicles. H&E stain

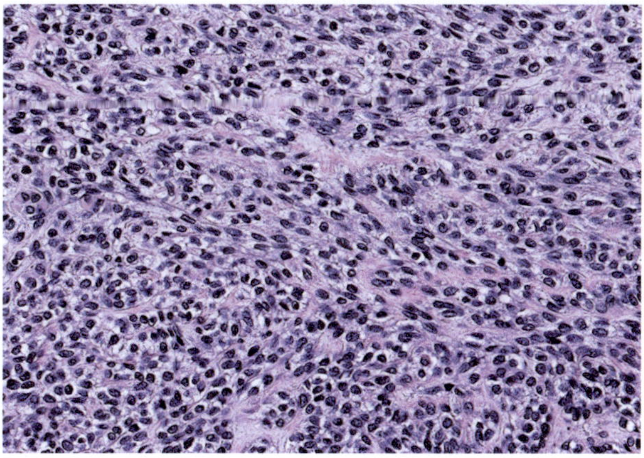

Fig. 14.13 Histopathology of myoepithelial carcinoma showing myoepithelial cells with clear cell features containing vacuolated to clear cytoplasm. H&E stain

Other morphological variants include: (1) oncocytic variant, which usually presents in older patients and shows papillary growth pattern with calcifications and luminal cells that contain densely granular cytoplasm; and (2) apocrine variant, which shows cribriform to solid growth patterns, and brightly eosinophilic ductal cells with apical snouts and luminal secretions: it is positive for androgen receptor and GCDFP-15 [204].

Rare findings of squamous, sebaceous differentiation, as well as ancient and Verocay-like change may also be seen [204].

14.11.6.4 Clinical Presentation

A slowly growing, painless mass is usually the only clinical complaint. Myoepithelial carcinoma of the parotid gland is usually unilateral. The clinical behavior of this tumor is unpredictable and unrelated to histological features [200]. It rarely presents with facial nerve palsy and lymphadenopathy, which may indicate high-grade transformation [205].

14.11.6.5 Differential Diagnosis

Pleomorphic adenoma (PA).
Multinodular with bosselated growth.
Chondro-myxoid matrix.
Can have adipose tissue as a stromal element imparting a permeative appearance.
Can show pseudopodia extending into the adjacent tissues.
Adenoid cystic carcinoma (AdCC).
Cribriform growth pattern (less common in epithelial myoepithelial carcinoma).
MYB rearrangement.
Basal cell adenoma (BCA).
Prominent stromal hyalinization.
Lacks invasive growth and nuclear pleomorphism.
Nuclear β-catenin-positive.
Mucoepidermoid carcinoma (MEC)—clear cell variant.
Presence of mucocytes and cyst formation.
MAML2 translocation.

14.11.6.6 Treatment

Treatment of myoepithelial carcinoma is complete surgical excision with clear margins. Adjuvant radiotherapy (RT) provides no survival benefit but reduces locoregional recurrence.

14.11.6.7 Prognosis

Generally, myoepithelial carcinoma has a good prognosis mean survival up to 165 months; another group found up to 81% of patients to be disease free at 15 years [206].

Univariate tumor-related predictors of lower disease-free survival include margin status, lympho-vascular invasion, tumor necrosis, myoepithelial anaplasia (greater than threefold variation in size, irregular nuclear membranes, coarse chromatin, macro-nucleoli) [207]. Multivariate patient-related predictors of lower disease-free survival include >80 years at time of diagnosis, worse in African American population, nonsurgical treatment [208].

Poorer prognosis is associated with minor salivary gland location, large tumor (>4 cm), high proliferation index, margin status, and high-grade transformation [209].

14.11.6.8 Cystadenocarcinoma

Cystadenocarcinoma is the malignant counterpart of cystadenoma. It was first described in 1991 by World Health Organization (WHO) as a separate entity and cystadenocarcinoma with or without papillary component in the Armed Forces Institute of Pathology (AFIP) classification [210]. Cystadenocarcinomas of the salivary glands are low-grade cystic neoplasms, which are twice as common in the major salivary glands as in the minor salivary glands, and most frequently occur in the parotid gland. They account for about 2% of all salivary gland tumors [211]. The majority of patients (75%) are over the age of 50 years [211].

The malignant nature of this tumor is confirmed by nuclear pleomorphism, mitosis, and infiltrative growth pattern. Perineural invasion is not a feature of this neoplasm. Complete surgical excision is usually curative as these tumors are of low-grade malignancy [212].

14.11.7 Salivary Duct Carcinoma (SDC)

14.11.7.1 Epidemiology

Salivary duct carcinoma (SDC) is a very aggressive malignant tumor that accounts for 6–10% of all carcinomas of the parotid [213]. It occurs most commonly in the parotid gland (78%) followed by the submandibular gland (12%) and the minor salivary glands (10%) [214]. The peak incidence of this tumor occurs in the sixth and seventh decades. It is more common in men than women with a ratio of 2.5:1 [3, 10, 215].

14.11.7.2 Pathophysiology

Salivary duct carcinoma is thought to arise from the large excretory ducts [216]. Androgen receptor expression has been found in salivary duct carcinoma and adenocarcinoma [217]. Gonadal hormone receptors such as the estrogen and progesterone receptors have been found in SDC [218]. Salivary duct carcinoma tends to overexpress erb-B2, which has been associated with a worse prognosis [219, 220].

14.11.7.3 Histopathology

Salivary duct carcinoma (Fig. 14.14) is similar in histology to high-grade duct carcinoma of the breast [221]. It can present with cribriform, solid (Fig. 14.15), cystic, or papillary growth patterns [3]. It should be differentiated from metastatic adenocarcinoma of the prostate and metastatic ductal carcinoma of the breast. Immuno-peroxidase staining for prostate-specific antigen aids in ruling out

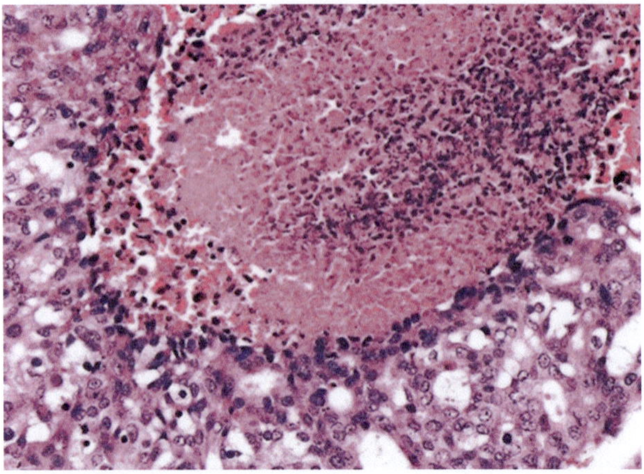

Fig. 14.14 Histologically, salivary duct carcinoma resembles ductal carcinoma of breast. Tumor cells are large polygonal with hyperchromatic nuclei, prominent nucleoli, and abundant eosinophilic cytoplasm. Increased mitotic activity and marked nuclear pleomorphism are usually present. H&E stain

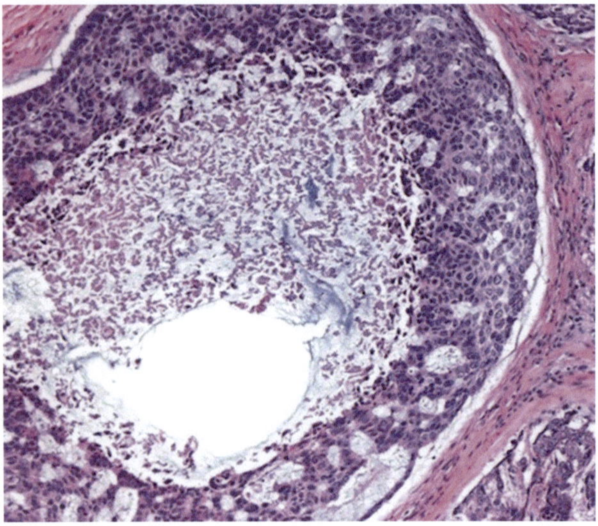

Fig. 14.15 Histopathology of salivary duct carcinoma showing solid nests with central comedo-necrosis. H&E stain

metastatic prostate carcinoma [222]. Identifying areas of intraductal (in situ) tumor would serve to distinguish SDC from both metastatic prostate and breast carcinoma [214].

14.11.7.4 Clinical Presentation

Salivary duct carcinoma usually presents as a firm, poorly defined mass with invasion of the surrounding glandular and soft tissue resulting in associated pain and facial nerve palsy. In the series by Hosal et al., approximately two-thirds of patients presented with T3 or T4 tumors [214]. The presence of calcifications has been reported to be seen on CT scans in one-third of the patients with salivary duct carcinoma [223–229]. More than 50% of patients display cervical metastasis at initial presentation [10].

14.11.7.5 Treatment

Because of the aggressive clinical behavior, SDC is treated by complete surgical excision of the primary tumor combined with neck dissection and adjuvant RT.

14.11.7.6 Prognosis

Salivary duct carcinoma presents with perineural and lympho-vascular invasion in 60% and 30% of cases, respectively [3]. Cervical LN metastasis is seen in 33–60% of cases, with 50% of patients already having distant metastasis at the time of presentation [71, 230]. The 5-year overall survival ranges from 20% to 50% [33, 215, 230, 231]. Approximately, two-thirds of patients die of their disease within 4 years of treatment, usually from distant metastases, which occur most commonly to the lungs and bone [232, 233].

14.11.8 Primary Squamous Cell Carcinoma (PSCC)

14.11.8.1 Epidemiology

They are thought to be rare due to the infrequent occurrence of squamous metaplasia of ductal epithelium that is thought to be responsible for the malignant transformation [234]. High-grade MEC and extension from an extra-parotid source are often misdiagnosed as primary SCC of the parotid. The true incidence of PSCC of the parotid is unknown due to its rarity and its frequency of being a misclassification of metastatic SCC. Evidence from the literature suggests the true incidence, may be around 0.75–1% [235]. In a review of 2807 salivary gland tumors, PSSC accounted for only 1.9% [236, 237]. Although a range of 0.3–4.3% has also been cited, these higher frequencies are thought to be due to misrepresentations or misclassification of these tumors [234, 238].

The parotid gland is involved in over two-thirds of cases and the remaining involves the submandibular gland [236]. Primary SCC (PSCC) is twice as common in men as women [239]. Although it has been reported in all decades of life, it is most common in the seventh decade. It is extremely uncommon in individuals below the age of 20 years [240].

14.11.8.2 Etiology/Pathophysiology

The specific etiology of the malignant transformation is not known, although there is evidence implicating high-risk HPV viruses [241]. About 9% of patients have a history of prior radiation exposure [236–238, 242–244]. The presence of SCC in the salivary glands is suspected to arise from several sources including: (1) malignant squamous portion of MEC, (2) metastasis from a cutaneous or mucosal head and neck source, (3) metastasis from distant primary carcinoma, or (4) primary SCC [27].

14.11.8.3 Histopathology

Squamous cell carcinoma (SCC) presents with intracellular keratinization, intercellular bridging, and keratin-pearl formation without any intracellular mucin (Fig. 14.16) [118]. Differential diagnosis includes squamous metaplasia,

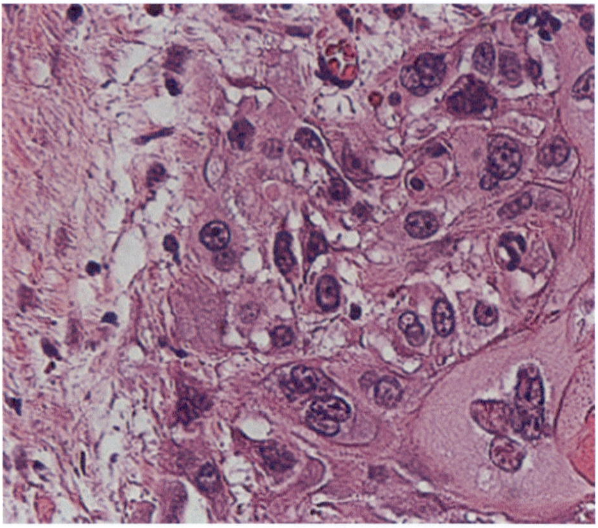

Fig. 14.16 Histopathology of primary squamous cell carcinoma (PSCC) showing keratinization, keratin pearls, and intercellular bridges. H&E × 100

necrotizing sialo-metaplasia, terato-cystoma, high-grade MEC, and metastatic SCC. Metastatic SCC to salivary glands is more common than PSSC, particularly in the parotid gland with its rich supply of both peri- and intraglandular LNs [245]. The presence of a focus of SCC in situ distinguishes PSSC of the parotid from metastatic SCC, which usually originates from skin lesions of the head and neck. The skin of the frontal and temporal areas, the periorbital region, the cheek, the pinna, the external ear canal, and the pre- and postauricular areas are favored primary sites that metastasize to the parotid gland.

14.11.8.4 Clinical Presentation

Primary SCCs of the salivary glands are extremely aggressive neoplasms with the majority of patients presenting with advanced disease due early extracapsular extension [236, 246]. It can present as a long-standing mass with sudden-onset of rapid growth, pain, facial nerve palsy, or overlying skin ulceration [247], although up to 50% of patients may present with an asymptomatic mass [236, 238, 248–250].

14.11.8.5 Treatment

In the parotid gland, extracapsular extension of PSCC may threaten the surrounding local structures and so prompt surgical intervention is required. A few weeks' delays can make a significant difference to the complexity of the planned surgery, with tumors readily invading the skin and surrounding structures. Since it is such an aggressive tumor, radical resection with neck dissection is usually indicated even in an N0 neck. Up to 75% of patients have histologically positive cervical LNs. The facial nerve may be spared if not directly infiltrated by tumor. There is a significant incidence of local–regional recurrence, which has led to the use of postoperative radiation therapy in many instances.

14.11.8.6 Prognosis

Distant metastases occur in 20–30% of patients. The overall 5-year survival of PSCC of the salivary glands is approximately 25%. It is influenced by the tumor stage and ranges from 50% to 80% for early-stage tumors and 15% for advanced staged tumors [28, 29, 238]. Advanced age, facial palsy, and regional nodal metastasis are poor prognostic factors [238, 249].

References

1. Batsakis JG, Regezi JA. The pathology of head and neck tumors: salivary glands, part 1. Head Neck Surg. 1978;1(1):59–68.
2. Speight PM, Barrett AW. Salivary gland tumours. Oral Dis. 2002;8(5):229–40.
3. Ettl T, Schwarz-Furlan S, Gosau M, Reichert TE. Salivary gland carcinomas. Oral Maxillofac Surg. 2012;16(3):267–83.
4. de Oliveira FA, Duarte EC, Taveira CT, Máximo AA, de Aquino EC, Alencar Rde C, et al. Salivary gland tumor: a review of 599 cases in a Brazilian population. Head Neck Pathol. 2009;3(4):271–5.
5. Satko I, Stanko P, Longauerová I. Salivary gland tumours treated in the stomatological clinics in Bratislava. J Craniomaxillofac Surg. 2000;28(1):56–61.
6. Spiro RH. Management of malignant tumors of the salivary glands. Oncology (Williston Park). 1998;12(5):671–80.
7. Carlson ER, McCoy JM. Margins for benign salivary gland neoplasms of the head and neck. Oral Maxillofac Surg Clin North Am. 2017;29(3):325–40.
8. Spiro RH. Salivary neoplasms: overview of a 35-year experience with 2807 patients. Head Neck Surg. 1986;8(3):177–84.
9. Gallo O, Franchi A, Bottai GV, Fini-Storchi I, Tesi G, Boddi V. Risk factors for distant metastases from carcinoma of the parotid gland. Cancer. 1997;80(5):844–51.
10. Bradley PJ. Frequency and histopathology by site, major pathologies, symptoms and signs of salivary gland neoplasms. Adv Otorhinolaryngol. 2016;78:9–16.
11. Stevens E, Andreasen S, Bjørndal K, Homøe P. Tumors in the parotid are not relatively more often malignant in children than in adults. Int J Pediatr Otorhinolaryngol. 2015;79(8):1192–5.
12. Goldstein AM, Yuen J, Tucker MA. Second cancers after medulloblastoma: population-based results from the United States and Sweden. Cancer Causes Control. 1997;8(6):865–71.
13. Horn-Ross PL, Ljung BM, Morrow M. Environmental factors and the risk of salivary gland cancer. Epidemiology. 1997;8(4):414–9.
14. Milán T, Pukkala E, Verkasalo PK, Kaprio J, Jansén CT, Koskenvuo M, et al. Subsequent primary cancers after basal-cell carcinoma: a nationwide study in Finland from 1953 to 1995. Int J Cancer. 2000;87(2):283–8.
15. Fan CY, Wang J, Barnes EL. Expression of androgen receptor and prostatic specific markers in salivary duct carcinoma: an immunohistochemical analysis of 13 cases and review of the literature. Am J Surg Pathol. 2000;24(4):579–86.
16. Nasser SM, Faquin WC, Dayal Y. Expression of androgen, estrogen, and progesterone receptors in salivary gland tumors. Frequent expression of androgen receptor in a subset of malignant salivary gland tumors. Am J Clin Pathol. 2003;119(6):801–6.
17. Schwarz-Furlan S, Brase C, Stockmann P, Furlan I, Hartmann A. Hereditary head and neck tumors. Pathologe. 2010;31(6):477–84.
18. Ettl T, Schwarz-Furlan S, Haubner F, Müller S, Zenk J, Gosau M, et al. The PI3K/AKT/mTOR signalling pathway is active in salivary gland cancer and implies different functions and prognoses depending on cell localisation. Oral Oncol. 2012;48(9):822–30.
19. Rice DH, Batsakis JG, McClatchey KD. Postirradiation malignant salivary gland tumor. Arch Otolaryngol. 1976;102(11):699–701.

20. Boukheris H, Ron E, Dores GM, Stovall M, Smith SA, Curtis RE. Risk of radiation-related salivary gland carcinomas among survivors of Hodgkin lymphoma: a population-based analysis. Cancer. 2008;113(11):3153–9.
21. Hayes RB, Bravo-Otero E, Kleinman DV, Brown LM, Fraumeni JF, Harty LC, et al. Tobacco and alcohol use and oral cancer in Puerto Rico. Cancer Causes Control. 1999;10(1):27–33.
22. Sadetzki S, Oberman B, Mandelzweig L, Chetrit A, Ben-Tal T, Jarus-Hakak A, Duvdevani S, Cardis E, Wolf M. Smoking and risk of parotid gland tumors: a nationwide case-control study. Cancer. 2008;112(9):1974–82.
23. Licitra L, Grandi C, Prott FJ, Schornagel JH, Bruzzi P, Molinari R. Major and minor salivary glands tumours. Crit Rev Oncol Hematol. 2003;45(2):215–25.
24. Spitz MR, Tilley BC, Batsakis JG, Gibeau JM, Newell GR. Risk factors for major salivary gland carcinoma. A case-comparison study. Cancer. 1984;54(9):1854–9.
25. Muscat JE, Wynder EL. A case/control study of risk factors for major salivary gland cancer. Otolaryngol Head Neck Surg. 1998;118(2):195–8.
26. Spitz MR, Fueger JJ, Goepfert H, Newell GR. Salivary gland cancer. A case-control investigation of risk factors. Arch Otolaryngol Head Neck Surg. 1990;116(10):1163–6.
27. Taxy JB. Squamous carcinoma in a major salivary gland: a review of the diagnostic considerations. Arch Pathol Lab Med. 2001;125(6):740–5.
28. Shemen LJ, Huvos AG, Spiro RH. Squamous cell carcinoma of salivary gland origin. Head Neck Surg. 1987;9(4):235–40.
29. Spitz MR, Batsakis JG. Major salivary gland carcinoma. Descriptive epidemiology and survival of 498 patients. Arch Otolaryngol. 1984;110(1):45–9.
30. Locati LD, Perrone F, Losa M, Mela M, Casieri P, Orsenigo M, Cortelazzi B, Negri T, Tamborini E, Quattrone P, Bossi P, Rinaldi G, Bergamini C, Calderone RG, Liberatoscioli C, Licitra L. Treatment relevant target immunophenotyping of 139 salivary gland carcinomas (SGCs). Oral Oncol. 2009;45(11):986–90.
31. Skálová A, Stárek I, Vanecek T, Kucerová V, Plank L, Szépe P, et al. Expression of HER-2/neu gene and protein in salivary duct carcinomas of parotid gland as revealed by fluorescence in-situ hybridization and immunohistochemistry. Histopathology. 2003;42(4):348–56.
32. Andreadis D, Epivatianos A, Poulopoulos A, Nomikos A, Papazoglou G, Antoniades D, Barbatis C. Detection of C-KIT (CD117) molecule in benign and malignant salivary gland tumours. Oral Oncol. 2006;42(1):57–65.
33. Guzzo M, Locati LD, Prott FJ, Gatta G, McGurk M, Licitra L. Major and minor salivary gland tumors. Crit Rev Oncol Hematol. 2010;74(2):134–48.
34. Wierzbicka M, Kopeć T, Szyfter W, Kereiakes T, Bem G. The presence of facial nerve weakness on diagnosis of a parotid gland malignant process. Eur Arch Otorrinolaringol. 2012;269(4):1177–82.
35. Lee YY, Wong KT, King AD, Ahuja AT. Imaging of salivary gland tumours. Eur J Radiol. 2008;66(3):419–36.
36. Kovacević DO, Fabijanić I. Sonographic diagnosis of parotid gland lesions: correlation with the results of sonographically guided fine-needle aspiration biopsy. J Clin Ultrasound. 2010;38(6):294–8.
37. Hanna E, Vural E, Prokopakis E, Carrau R, Snyderman C, Weissman J. The sensitivity and specificity of high-resolution imaging in evaluating perineural spread of adenoid cystic carcinoma to the skull base. Arch Otolaryngol Head Neck Surg. 2007;133(6):541–5.
38. Burke CJ, Thomas RH, Howlett D. Imaging the major salivary glands. Br J Oral Maxillofac Surg. 2011;49(4):261–9.
39. Wittekindt C, Burmeister HP, Guntinas-Lichius O. Diagnostic and therapy of salivary gland diseases: relevant aspects for the pathologist from the clinical perspective. Pathologe. 2009;30(6):424–31.
40. Habermann CR, Arndt C, Graessner J, Diestel L, Petersen KU, Reitmeier F, Ussmueller JO, et al. Diffusion-weighted echo-planar MR imaging of primary parotid gland tumors: is a prediction of different histologic subtypes possible? AJNR Am J Neuroradiol. 2009;30(3):591–6.

41. Roh JL, Ryu CH, Choi SH, Kim JS, Lee JH, Cho KJ, et al. Clinical utility of 18F-FDG PET for patients with salivary gland malignancies. J Nucl Med. 2007;48(2):240–6.
42. Jeong HS, Chung MK, Son YI, Choi JY, Kim HJ, Ko YH, et al. Role of 18F-FDG PET/CT in management of high-grade salivary gland malignancies. J Nucl Med. 2007;48(8):1237–44.
43. Uchida Y, Minoshima S, Kawata T, Motoori K, Nakano K, Kazama T, et al. Diagnostic value of FDG PET and salivary gland scintigraphy for parotid tumors. Clin Nucl Med. 2005;30(3):170–6.
44. Keyes JW, Harkness BA, Greven KM, Williams DW, Watson NE, McGuirt WF. Salivary gland tumors: pretherapy evaluation with PET. Radiology. 1994;192(1):99–102.
45. Kechagias N, Ntomouchtsis A, Valeri R, Patrikidou A, Kitikidou K, Xirou P, et al. Fine-needle aspiration cytology of salivary gland tumours: a 10-year retrospective analysis. Oral Maxillofac Surg. 2012;16(1):35–40.
46. Schmidt RL, Hall BJ, Wilson AR, Layfield LJ. A systematic review and meta-analysis of the diagnostic accuracy of fine-needle aspiration cytology for parotid gland lesions. Am J Clin Pathol. 2011;136(1):45–59.
47. Colella G, Cannavale R, Flamminio F, Foschini MP. Fine-needle aspiration cytology of salivary gland lesions: a systematic review. J Oral Maxillofac Surg. 2010;68(9):2146–53.
48. Routsias JG, Goules JD, Charalampakis G, Tzima S, Papageorgiou A, Voulgarelis M. Malignant lymphoma in primary Sjögren's syndrome: an update on the pathogenesis and treatment. Semin Arthritis Rheum. 2013;43(2):178–86.
49. Schmidt RL, Hall BJ, Layfield LJ. A systematic review and meta-analysis of the diagnostic accuracy of ultrasound-guided core needle biopsy for salivary gland lesions. Am J Clin Pathol. 2011;136(4):516–26.
50. Schmidt RL, Hunt JP, Hall BJ, Wilson AR, Layfield LJ. A systematic review and meta-analysis of the diagnostic accuracy of frozen section for parotid gland lesions. Am J Clin Pathol. 2011;136(5):729–38.
51. Edge SB, Compton CC. The American Joint Committee on Cancer: the 7th edition of the AJCC cancer staging manual and the future of TNM. Ann Surg Oncol. 2010;17(6):1471–4.
52. Lydiatt WM, Patel SG, O'Sullivan B, Brandwein MS, Ridge JA, Migliacci JC, et al. Head and neck cancers-major changes in the American Joint Committee on cancer eighth edition cancer staging manual. CA Cancer J Clin. 2017;67(2):122–37.
53. Fu KK, Leibel SA, Levine ML, Friedlander LM, Boles R, Phillips TL. Carcinoma of the major and minor salivary glands: analysis of treatment results and sites and causes of failures. Cancer. 1977;40(6):2882–90.
54. Armstrong JG, Harrison LB, Spiro RH, Fass DE, Strong EW, Fuks ZY. Malignant tumors of major salivary gland origin. A matched-pair analysis of the role of combined surgery and postoperative radiotherapy. Arch Otolaryngol Head Neck Surg. 1990;116(3):290–3.
55. Terhaard CH, Lubsen H, Rasch CR, Levendag PC, Kaanders HH, Tjho-Heslinga RE, et al. The role of radiotherapy in the treatment of malignant salivary gland tumors. Int J Radiat Oncol Biol Phys. 2005;61(1):103–11.
56. Lewis AG, Tong T, Maghami E. Diagnosis and management of malignant salivary gland tumors of the parotid gland. Otolaryngol Clin N Am. 2016;49(2):343–80.
57. Lin HH, Limesand KH, Ann DK. Current state of knowledge on salivary gland cancers. Crit Rev Oncol. 2018;23(3–4):139–51.
58. Terhaard CH. Postoperative and primary radiotherapy for salivary gland carcinomas: indications, techniques, and results. Int J Radiat Oncol Biol Phys. 2007;69(2 Suppl):S52–5.
59. Mendenhall WM, Morris CG, Amdur RJ, Werning JW, Villaret DB. Radiotherapy alone or combined with surgery for salivary gland carcinoma. Cancer. 2005;103(12):2544–50.
60. Turner MD. Salivary gland disease in Sjögren's syndrome: sialoadenitis to lymphoma. Oral Maxillofac Surg Clin North Am. 2014;26(1):75–81.
61. Thomson DJ, Slevin NJ, Mendenhall WM. Indications for salivary gland radiotherapy. Adv Otorhinolaryngol. 2016;78:141–7.
62. Spiro JD, Spiro RH. Cancer of the parotid gland: role of 7th nerve preservation. World J Surg. 2003;27(7):863–7.

63. Harish K. Management of primary malignant epithelial parotid tumors. Surg Oncol. 2004;13(1):7–16.
64. Lim YC, Lee SY, Kim K, Lee JS, Koo BS, Shin HA, et al. Conservative parotidectomy for the treatment of parotid cancers. Oral Oncol. 2005;41(10):1021–7.
65. Domenick NA, Johnson JT. Parotid tumor size predicts proximity to the facial nerve. Laryngoscope. 2011;121(11):2366–70.
66. Roh JL, Kim HS, Park CI. Randomized clinical trial comparing partial parotidectomy versus superficial or total parotidectomy. Br J Surg. 2007;94(9):1081–7.
67. Spiro RH, Armstrong J, Harrison L, Geller NL, Lin SY, Strong EW. Carcinoma of major salivary glands. Recent trends. Arch Otolaryngol Head Neck Surg. 1989;115(3):316–21.
68. Armstrong JG, Harrison LB, Thaler HT, Friedlander-Klar H, Fass DE, Zelefsky MJ, et al. The indications for elective treatment of the neck in cancer of the major salivary glands. Cancer. 1992;69(3):615–9.
69. Rodríguez-Cuevas S, Labastida S, Baena L, Gallegos F. Risk of nodal metastases from malignant salivary gland tumors related to tumor size and grade of malignancy. Eur Arch Otorrinolaringol. 1995;252(3):139–42.
70. Lloyd S, Yu JB, Ross DA, Wilson LD, Decker RH. A prognostic index for predicting lymph node metastasis in minor salivary gland cancer. Int J Radiat Oncol Biol Phys. 2010;76(1):169–75.
71. Ettl T, Schwarz S, Kleinsasser N, Hartmann A, Reichert TE, Driemel O. Overexpression of EGFR and absence of C-KIT expression correlate with poor prognosis in salivary gland carcinomas. Histopathology. 2008;53(5):567–77.
72. Jaehne M, Roeser K, Jaekel T, Schepers JD, Albert N, Löning T. Clinical and immunohistologic typing of salivary duct carcinoma: a report of 50 cases. Cancer. 2005;103(12):2526–33.
73. Stennert E, Kisner D, Jungehuelsing M, Guntinas-Lichius O, Schröder U, Eckel HE, et al. High incidence of lymph node metastasis in major salivary gland cancer. Arch Otolaryngol Head Neck Surg. 2003;129(7):720–3.
74. Frankenthaler RA, Byers RM, Luna MA, Callender DL, Wolf P, Goepfert H. Predicting occult lymph node metastasis in parotid cancer. Arch Otolaryngol Head Neck Surg. 1993;119(5):517–20.
75. Bell RB, Dierks EJ, Homer L, Potter BE. Management and outcome of patients with malignant salivary gland tumors. J Oral Maxillofac Surg. 2005;63(7):917–28.
76. Medina JE. Neck dissection in the treatment of cancer of major salivary glands. Otolaryngol Clin N Am. 1998;31(5):815–22.
77. Salgado LR, Spratt DE, Riaz N, Romesser PB, Wolden S, Rao S, et al. Radiation therapy in the treatment of minor salivary gland tumors. Am J Clin Oncol. 2014;37(5):492–7.
78. Garden AS, el-Naggar AK, Morrison WH, Callender DL, Ang KK, Peters LJ. Postoperative radiotherapy for malignant tumors of the parotid gland. Int J Radiat Oncol Biol Phys. 1997;37(1):79–85.
79. Laramore GE, Krall JM, Griffin TW, Duncan W, Richter MP, Saroja KR, et al. Neutron versus photon irradiation for unresectable salivary gland tumors: final report of an RTOG-MRC randomized clinical trial. Radiation Therapy Oncology Group. Medical Research Council. Int J Radiat Oncol Biol Phys. 1993;27(2):235–40.
80. Schoenfeld JD, Sher DJ, Norris CM, Haddad RI, Posner MR, Balboni TA, et al. Salivary gland tumors treated with adjuvant intensity-modulated radiotherapy with or without concurrent chemotherapy. Int J Radiat Oncol Biol Phys. 2012;82(1):308–14.
81. Cooper JS, Pajak TF, Forastiere AA, Jacobs J, Campbell BH, Saxman SB, et al. Postoperative concurrent radiotherapy and chemotherapy for high-risk squamous-cell carcinoma of the head and neck. N Engl J Med. 2004;350(19):1937–44.
82. Pederson AW, Salama JK, Haraf DJ, Witt ME, Stenson KM, Portugal L, et al. Adjuvant chemoradiotherapy for locoregionally advanced and high-risk salivary gland malignancies. Head Neck Oncol. 2011;3:31.
83. Cerda T, Sun XS, Vignot S, Marcy PY, Baujat B, Baglin AC, et al. A rationale for chemoradiation (vs radiotherapy) in salivary gland cancers? On behalf of the REFCOR (French rare head and neck cancer network). Crit Rev Oncol Hematol. 2014;91(2):142–58.

84. Nakano K, Sato Y, Sasaki T, Shimbashi W, Fukushima H, Yonekawa H, et al. Combination chemotherapy of carboplatin and paclitaxel for advanced/metastatic salivary gland carcinoma patients: differences in responses by different pathological diagnoses. Acta Otolaryngol. 2016;136(9):948–51.
85. Papaspyrou G, Hoch S, Rinaldo A, Rodrigo JP, Takes RP, van Herpen C, et al. Chemotherapy and targeted therapy in adenoid cystic carcinoma of the head and neck: a review. Head Neck. 2011;33(6):905–11.
86. Laurie SA, Siu LL, Winquist E, Maksymiuk A, Harnett EL, Walsh W, et al. A phase 2 study of platinum and gemcitabine in patients with advanced salivary gland cancer: a trial of the NCIC Clinical Trials Group. Cancer. 2010;116(2):362–8.
87. Williams MD, Roberts DB, Kies MS, Mao L, Weber RS, El-Naggar AK. Genetic and expression analysis of HER-2 and EGFR genes in salivary duct carcinoma: empirical and therapeutic significance. Clin Cancer Res. 2010;16(8):2266–74.
88. Holst VA, Marshall CE, Moskaluk CA, Frierson HF. KIT protein expression and analysis of c-kit gene mutation in adenoid cystic carcinoma. Mod Pathol. 1999;12(10):956–60.
89. Frattini M, Saletti P, Romagnani E, Martin V, Molinari F, Ghisletta M, et al. PTEN loss of expression predicts cetuximab efficacy in metastatic colorectal cancer patients. Br J Cancer. 2007;97(8):1139–45.
90. Haddad R, Colevas AD, Krane JF, Cooper D, Glisson B, Amrein PC, et al. Herceptin in patients with advanced or metastatic salivary gland carcinomas. A phase II study. Oral Oncol. 2003;39(7):724–7.
91. Vidal L, Tsao MS, Pond GR, Cohen EE, Cohen RB, Chen EX, et al. Fluorescence in situ hybridization gene amplification analysis of EGFR and HER2 in patients with malignant salivary gland tumors treated with lapatinib. Head Neck. 2009;31(8):1006–12.
92. Ciardiello F, Tortora G. EGFR antagonists in cancer treatment. N Engl J Med. 2008;358(11):1160–74.
93. Sultan I, Rodriguez-Galindo C, Al-Sharabati S, Guzzo M, Casanova M, Ferrari A. Salivary gland carcinomas in children and adolescents: a population-based study, with comparison to adult cases. Head Neck. 2011;33(10):1476–81.
94. Kupferman ME, de la Garza GO, Santillan AA, Williams MD, Varghese BT, Huh W, et al. Outcomes of pediatric patients with malignancies of the major salivary glands. Ann Surg Oncol. 2010;17(12):3301–7.
95. Renehan AG, Gleave EN, Slevin NJ, McGurk M. Clinico-pathological and treatment-related factors influencing survival in parotid cancer. Br J Cancer. 1999;80(8):1296–300.
96. Therkildsen MH, Christensen M, Andersen LJ, Schiødt T, Hansen HS. Salivary gland carcinomas--prognostic factors. Acta Oncol. 1998;37(7–8):701–13.
97. Schwarz S, Stiegler C, Müller M, Ettl T, Brockhoff G, Zenk J, et al. Salivary gland mucoepidermoid carcinoma is a clinically, morphologically and genetically heterogeneous entity: a clinicopathological study of 40 cases with emphasis on grading, histological variants and presence of the t(11;19) translocation. Histopathology. 2011;58(4):557–70.
98. Bhattacharyya N, Fried MP. Determinants of survival in parotid gland carcinoma: a population-based study. Am J Otolaryngol. 2005;26(1):39–44.
99. Speight PM, Barrett AW. Prognostic factors in malignant tumours of the salivary glands. Br J Oral Maxillofac Surg. 2009;47(8):587–93.
100. Hocwald E, Korkmaz H, Yoo GH, Adsay V, Shibuya TY, Abrams J, et al. Prognostic factors in major salivary gland cancer. Laryngoscope. 2001;111(8):1434–9.
101. Kelley DJ, Spiro RH. Management of the neck in parotid carcinoma. Am J Surg. 1996;172(6):695–7.
102. Oliveira LR, Soave DF, Oliveira-Costa JP, Zorgetto VA, Ribeiro-Silva A. Prognostic factors in patients with malignant salivary gland neoplasms in a Brazilian population. Asian Pac J Cancer Prev. 2011;12(2):363–8.
103. Becker C, Dahlem KKK, Pfeiffer J. Prognostic value of comorbidities in patients with carcinoma of the major salivary glands. Eur Arch Otorrinolaringol. 2017;274(3):1651–7.
104. Glazer TA, Shuman AG. Distant metastases and palliative care. Adv Otorhinolaryngol. 2016;78:182–8.

105. Guntinas-Lichius O, Klussmann JP, Schroeder U, Quante G, Jungehuelsing M, Stennert E. Primary parotid malignoma surgery in patients with normal preoperative facial nerve function: outcome and long-term postoperative facial nerve function. Laryngoscope. 2004;114(5):949–56.
106. Eisele DW, Wang SJ, Orloff LA. Electrophysiologic facial nerve monitoring during parotidectomy. Head Neck. 2010;32(3):399–405.
107. Sanabria A, Kowalski LP, Bradley PJ, Hartl DM, Bradford CR, de Bree R, et al. Sternocleidomastoid muscle flap in preventing Frey's syndrome after parotidectomy: a systematic review. Head Neck. 2012;34(4):589–98.
108. Curry JM, Fisher KW, Heffelfinger RN, Rosen MR, Keane WM, Pribitkin EA. Superficial musculoaponeurotic system elevation and fat graft reconstruction after superficial parotidectomy. Laryngoscope. 2008;118(2):210–5.
109. Filho WQ, Dedivitis RA, Rapoport A, Guimarães AV. Sternocleidomastoid muscle flap preventing Frey syndrome following parotidectomy. World J Surg. 2004;28(4):361–4.
110. de Bree R, van der Waal I, Leemans CR. Management of Frey syndrome. Head Neck. 2007;29(8):773–8.
111. Eversole LR. Mucoepidermoid carcinoma: review of 815 reported cases. J Oral Surg. 1970;28(7):490–4.
112. Krolls SO, Trodahl JN, Boyers RC. Salivary gland lesions in children. A survey of 430 cases. Cancer. 1972;30(2):459–69.
113. O'Neill ID. t(11;19) translocation and CRTC1-MAML2 fusion oncogene in mucoepidermoid carcinoma. Oral Oncol. 2009;45(1):2–9.
114. Tonon G, Modi S, Wu L, Kubo A, Coxon AB, Komiya T, et al. t(11;19)(q21;p13) translocation in mucoepidermoid carcinoma creates a novel fusion product that disrupts a Notch signaling pathway. Nat Genet. 2003;33(2):208–13.
115. Quyen HD, Duc NM, Tuan HX, Tu NT, Khoi NA, Dung PX. Acinic cell carcinoma of parotid gland. Radiol Case Rep. 2023;18(6):194–2198.
116. El-Naggar AK, Lovell M, Killary AM, Clayman GL, Batsakis JG. A mucoepidermoid carcinoma of minor salivary gland with t(11;19)(q21;p13.1) as the only karyotypic abnormality. Cancer Genet Cytogenet. 1996;87(1):29–33.
117. Jakobsson PA, Blanck C, Eneroth CM. Mucoepidermoid carcinoma of the parotid gland. Cancer. 1968;22(1):111–24.
118. Batsakis JG, Chinn E, Regezi JA, Repola DA. The pathology of head and neck tumors: salivary glands, part 2. Head Neck Surg. 1978;1(2):167–80.
119. Foote FW, Frazell EL. Tumors of the major salivary glands. Cancer. 1953;6(6):1065–133.
120. Healey WV, Perzin KH, Smith L. Mucoepidermoid carcinoma of salivary gland origin. Classification, clinical-pathologic correlation, and results of treatment. Cancer. 1970;26(2):368–88.
121. Ogawa I, Nikai H, Takata T, Yasui R. Clear-cell variant of mucoepidermoid carcinoma: report of a case with immunohistochemical and ultrastructural observations. J Oral Maxillofac Surg. 1992;50(8):906–10.
122. Terada T, Ikeuchi S, Inomoto C, Shimamura K. Mucoepidermoid carcinoma of the palate composed exclusively of clear cells (clear cell variant). Virchows Arch. 2004;445(5):541–3.
123. Waldron CA, Koh ML. Central mucoepidermoid carcinoma of the jaws: report of four cases with analysis of the literature and discussion of the relationship to mucoepidermoid, sialodontogenic, and glandular odontogenic cysts. J Oral Maxillofac Surg. 1990;48(8):871–7.
124. Boahene DK, Olsen KD, Lewis JE, Pinheiro AD, Pankratz VS, Bagniewski SM. Mucoepidermoid carcinoma of the parotid gland: the Mayo clinic experience. Arch Otolaryngol Head Neck Surg. 2004;130(7):849–56.
125. Gustafsson H, Dahlqvist A, Anniko M, Carlsoo B. Mucoepidermoid carcinoma in a minor salivary gland in childhood. J Laryngol Otol. 1987;101(12):1320–3.
126. Loy TS, McLaughlin R, Odom LF, Dehner LP. Mucoepidermoid carcinoma of the parotid as a second malignant neoplasm in children. Cancer. 1989;64(10):2174–7.

127. Thorvaldsson SE, Beahrs OH, Woolner LB, Simons JN. Mucoepidermoid tumors of the major salivary glands. Am J Surg. 1970;120(4):432–8.
128. Brandwein MS, Ivanov K, Wallace DI, Hille JJ, Wang B, Fahmy A, et al. Mucoepidermoid carcinoma: a clinicopathologic study of 80 patients with special reference to histological grading. Am J Surg Pathol. 2001;25(7):835–45.
129. Guzzo M, Andreola S, Sirizzotti G, Cantu G. Mucoepidermoid carcinoma of the salivary glands: clinicopathologic review of 108 patients treated at the National Cancer Institute of Milan. Ann Surg Oncol. 2002;9(7):688–95.
130. Clode AL, Fonseca I, Santos JR, Soares J. Mucoepidermoid carcinoma of the salivary glands: a reappraisal of the influence of tumor differentiation on prognosis. J Surg Oncol. 1991;46(2):100–6.
131. Witt RL. Major salivary gland cancer. Surg Oncol Clin N Am. 2004;13(1):113–27.
132. Rinaldo A, Ferlito A, Pellitteri PK, Robbins KT, Shaha AR, Bradley PJ, et al. Management of malignant submandibular gland tumors. Acta Otolaryngol. 2003;123(8):896–904.
133. Lee DJ, Smith RR, Spaziani JT, Rostock R, Holliday M, Moses H. Adenoid cystic carcinoma of the nasopharynx. Case reports and literature review. Ann Otol Rhinol Laryngol. 1985;94(3):269–72.
134. Bradley PJ. Adenoid cystic carcinoma of the head and neck: a review. Curr Opin Otolaryngol Head Neck Surg. 2004;12(2):127–32.
135. Martínez-Rodríguez N, Leco-Berrocal I, Rubio-Alonso L, Arias-Irimia O, Martínez-González JM. Epidemiology and treatment of adenoid cystic carcinoma of the minor salivary glands: a meta-analytic study. Med Oral Patol Oral Cir Bucal. 2011;16(7):e884–9.
136. Bishop JA, Yonescu R, Batista D, Eisele DW, Westra WH. Most nonparotid "acinic cell carcinomas" represent mammary analog secretory carcinomas. Am J Surg Pathol. 2013;37(7):1053–7.
137. Mitani Y, Li J, Rao PH, Zhao YJ, Bell D, Lippman SM, et al. Comprehensive analysis of the MYB-NFIB gene fusion in salivary adenoid cystic carcinoma: incidence, variability, and clinicopathologic significance. Clin Cancer Res. 2010;16(19):4722–31.
138. Brill LB, Kanner WA, Fehr A, Andrén Y, Moskaluk CA, Löning T. Analysis of MYB expression and MYB-NFIB gene fusions in adenoid cystic carcinoma and other salivary neoplasms. Mod Pathol. 2011;24(9):1169–76.
139. Brayer KJ, Frerich CA, Kang H, Ness SA. Recurrent fusions in MYB and MYBL1 define a common, transcription factor-driven oncogenic pathway in salivary gland adenoid cystic carcinoma. Cancer Discov. 2016;6(2):176–87.
140. Yaga US, Gollamudi N, Mengji AK, Besta R, Panta P, Prakash B, et al. Adenoid cystic carcinoma of the palate: case report and review of literature. Pan Afr Med J. 2016;24:106.
141. DeAngelis AF, Tsui A, Wiesenfeld D, Chandu A. Outcomes of patients with adenoid cystic carcinoma of the minor salivary glands. Int J Oral Maxillofac Surg. 2011;40(7):710–4.
142. Shimamoto H, Chindasombatjaroen J, Kakimoto N, Kishino M, Murakami S, Furukawa S. Perineural spread of adenoid cystic carcinoma in the oral and maxillofacial regions: evaluation with contrast-enhanced CT and MRI. Dentomaxillofac Radiol. 2012;41(2):143–51.
143. Diercks GR, Rosow DE, Prasad M, Kuhel WI. A case of preoperative "first-bite syndrome" associated with mucoepidermoid carcinoma of the parotid gland. Laryngoscope. 2011;121(4):760–2.
144. Gurney TA, Eisele DW, Weinberg V, Shin E, Lee N. Adenoid cystic carcinoma of the major salivary glands treated with surgery and radiation. Laryngoscope. 2005;115(7):1278–82.
145. Rapidis AD, Givalos N, Gakiopoulou H, Faratzis G, Stavrianos SD, Vilos GA, et al. Adenoid cystic carcinoma of the head and neck. Clinicopathological analysis of 23 patients and review of the literature. Oral Oncol. 2005;41(3):328–35.
146. Gerughty RM, Scofield HH, Brown FM, Hennigar GR. Malignant mixed tumors of salivary gland origin. Cancer. 1969;24(3):471–86.
147. Ord RA, Ghazali N. Margin analysis: malignant salivary gland neoplasms of the head and neck. Oral Maxillofac Surg Clin North Am. 2017;29(3):315–24.

148. Hamper K, Lazar F, Dietel M, Caselitz J, Berger J, Arps H, Falkmer U, Auer G, Seifert G. Prognostic factors for adenoid cystic carcinoma of the head and neck: a retrospective evaluation of 96 cases. J Oral Pathol Med. 1990;19(3):101–7.
149. Perzin KH, Gullane P, Clairmont AC. Adenoid cystic carcinomas arising in salivary glands: a correlation of histologic features and clinical course. Cancer. 1978;42(1):265–82.
150. LiVolsi VA, Perzin KH. Malignant mixed tumors arising in salivary glands. I. Carcinomas arising in benign mixed tumors: a clinicopathologic study. Cancer. 1977;39(5):2209–30.
151. Milford CA, Mugliston TA, O'Flynn P, McCarthy K. Carcinoma arising in a pleomorphic adenoma of the epiglottis. J Laryngol Otol. 1989;103(3):324–7.
152. Lewis JE, Olsen KD, Sebo TJ. Carcinoma ex pleomorphic adenoma: pathologic analysis of 73 cases. Hum Pathol. 2001;32(6):596–604.
153. Gnepp DR. Malignant mixed tumors of the salivary glands: a review. Pathol Annu. 1993;28(1):279–328.
154. Durr ML, Mydlarz WK, Shao C, Zahurak ML, Chuang AY, Hoque MO, Westra WH, Liegeois NJ, Califano JA, Sidransky D, Ha PK. Quantitative methylation profiles for multiple tumor suppressor gene promoters in salivary gland tumors. PLoS One. 2010;5(5):e10828.
155. Schache AG, Hall G, Woolgar JA, Nikolaidis G, Triantafyllou A, Lowe D, et al. Quantitative promoter methylation differentiates carcinoma ex pleomorphic adenoma from pleomorphic salivary adenoma. Br J Cancer. 2010;103(12):1846–51.
156. Zarbo RJ. Salivary gland neoplasia: a review for the practicing pathologist. Mod Pathol. 2002;15(3):298–323.
157. Weiler C, Zengel P, van der Wal JE, Guntinas-Lichius O, Schwarz S, Harrison JD, Kirchner T, Ihrler S. Carcinoma ex pleomorphic adenoma with special reference to the prognostic significance of histological progression: a clinicopathological investigation of 41 cases. Histopathology. 2011;59(4):741–50.
158. Eneroth CM, Zetterberg A. A cytochemical method of grading the malignancy of salivary gland tumours preoperatively. Acta Otolaryngol. 1976;81(5–6):489–95.
159. Eneroth CM, Zetterberg A. Malignancy in pleomorphic adenoma. A clinical and microspectrophotometric study. Acta Otolaryngol. 1974;77(6):426–32.
160. Chen AM, Garcia J, Bucci MK, Quivey JM, Eisele DW. The role of postoperative radiation therapy in carcinoma ex pleomorphic adenoma of the parotid gland. Int J Radiat Oncol Biol Phys. 2007;67(1):138–43.
161. Olsen KD, Lewis JE. Carcinoma ex pleomorphic adenoma: a clinicopathologic review. Head Neck. 2001;23(9):705–12.
162. Tortoledo ME, Luna MA, Batsakis JG. Carcinomas ex pleomorphic adenoma and malignant mixed tumors. Histomorphologic indexes. Arch Otolaryngol. 1984;110(3):172–6.
163. Barnes L, Appel BN, Perez H, El-Attar AM. Myoepithelioma of the head and neck: case report and review. J Surg Oncol. 1985;28(1):21–8.
164. Kwon MY, Gu M. True malignant mixed tumor (carcinosarcoma) of parotid gland with unusual mesenchymal component: a case report and review of the literature. Arch Pathol Lab Med. 2001;125(6):812–5.
165. Fowler MH, Fowler J, Ducatman B, Barnes L, Hunt JL. Malignant mixed tumors of the salivary gland: a study of loss of heterozygosity in tumor suppressor genes. Mod Pathol. 2006;19(3):350–5.
166. Tuffin JR, Daniel F, Davies AS, Tyrrell CJ. Acinic cell carcinoma—Plymouth's experience with postoperative radical radiotherapy. Br J Oral Maxillofac Surg. 1989;27(3):186–91.
167. Miki H, Masuda E, Ohata S, Komaki K, Hirokawa M, Uehara H, et al. Late recurrence of acinic cell carcinoma of the parotid gland. J Med Investig. 1999;46(3–4):213–6.
168. Ellis G, Simpson R. Acinic cell carcinoma. In: Barnes L, Eveson J, Reichart P, Sidransky D, editors. Pathology and genetics head and neck tumours. Lyon, France: IARC Press; 2005. p. 216–8.
169. Diegel CR, Cho KR, El-Naggar AK, Williams BO, Lindvall C. Mammalian target of rapamycin-dependent acinar cell neoplasia after inactivation of Apc and Pten in the mouse salivary gland: implications for human acinic cell carcinoma. Cancer Res. 2010;70(22):9143–52.

170. Abrams AM, Cornyn J, Scofield HH, Hansen LS. Acinic cell adenocarcinoma of the major salivary glands. A clinicopathologic study of 77 cases. Cancer. 1965;18:1145–62.
171. Eneroth CM, Jakobsson PA, Blanck C. Acinic cell carcinoma of the parotid gland. Cancer. 1966;19(12):1761–72.
172. Lewis JE, Olsen KD, Weiland LH. Acinic cell carcinoma. Clinicopathologic review. Cancer. 1991;67(1):172–9.
173. Gomez DR, Katabi N, Zhung J, Wolden SL, Zelefsky MJ, Kraus DH, et al. Clinical and pathologic prognostic features in acinic cell carcinoma of the parotid gland. Cancer. 2009;115(10):2128–37.
174. Skálová A, Sima R, Vanecek T, Muller S, Korabecna M, Nemcova J, et al. Acinic cell carcinoma with high-grade transformation: a report of 9 cases with immunohistochemical study and analysis of TP53 and HER-2/neu genes. Am J Surg Pathol. 2009;33(8):1137–45.
175. Mehta RP, Faquin WC, Deschler DG. Pathology quizcase 1. Acinic cell carcinoma of the parotid gland with ductal extension. Arch Otolaryngol Head Neck Surg. 2004;130(6):790–3.
176. Hanson TA. Acinic cell carcinoma of the parotid salivary gland presenting as a cyst. Report of two cases. Cancer. 1975;36(2):570–5.
177. Chong GC, Beahrs OH, Woolner LB. Surgical management of acinic cell carcinoma of the parotid gland. Surg Gynecol Obstet. 1974;138(1):65–8.
178. Neto AG, Pineda-Daboin K, Spencer ML, Luna MA. Sinonasal acinic cell carcinoma: a clinicopathologic study of four cases. Head Neck. 2005;27(7):603–7.
179. Neskey DM, Klein JD, Hicks S, Garden AS, Bell DM, El-Naggar AK, Kies MS, Weber RS, Kupferman ME. Prognostic factors associated with decreased survival in patients with acinic cell carcinoma. JAMA Otolaryngol Head Neck Surg. 2013;139(11):1195–202.
180. Spiro RH, Huvos AG, Strong EW. Cancer of the parotid gland. A clinicopathologic study of 288 primary cases. Am J Surg. 1975;130(4):452–9.
181. Moon P, Tusty M, Divi V, Megwalu UC. Significance of nodal metastasis in parotid gland acinar cell carcinoma. Laryngoscope. 2021;131(4):E1125–9.
182. Wang Y, Wang S, Zhou X, Zhou H, Cui Y, Li Q, Zhang L. Acinar cell carcinoma: a report of 19 cases with a brief review of the literature. World J Surg Oncol. 2016;14(1):172.
183. El-Naggar AK, Batsakis JG, Luna MA, McLemore D, Byers RM. DNA flow cytometry of acinic cell carcinomas of major salivary glands. J Laryngol Otol. 1990;104(5):410–6.
184. Skalova A, Leivo I, Von Boguslawsky K, Saksela E. Cell proliferation correlates with prognosis in acinic cell carcinomas of salivary gland origin. Immunohistochemical study of 30 cases using the MIB 1 antibody in formalin-fixed paraffin sections. J Pathol. 1994;173(1):13–21.
185. Vidyadhara S, Shetty AP, Rajasekaran S. Widespread metastases from acinic cell carcinoma of parotid gland. Singapore Med J. 2007;48:e13–5.
186. Hickman RE, Cawson RA, Duffy SW. The prognosis of specific types of salivary gland tumors. Cancer. 1984;54(8):1620–4.
187. Muller S, Barnes L. Basal cell adenocarcinoma of the salivary glands. Report of seven cases and review of the literature. Cancer. 1996;78(12):2471–7.
188. Gross M, Maly B, Goldfarb A, Eliashar R. Basal cell adenocarcinoma in a buccal minor salivary gland. Acta Otolaryngol. 2004;124(2):213–6.
189. Jayakrishnan A, Elmalah I, Hussain K, Odell EW. Basal cell adenocarcinoma in minor salivary glands. Histopathology. 2003;42(6):610–4.
190. Nagao T, Sugano I, Ishida Y, Hasegawa M, Matsuzaki O, Konno A, et al. Basal cell adenocarcinoma of the salivary glands: comparison with basal cell adenoma through assessment of cell proliferation, apoptosis, and expression of p53 and bcl-2. Cancer. 1998;82(3):439–47.
191. Warrick PD, Irish JC, Mancer K, Dardick I, Pynn BR, Gullane P. Basal cell adenocarcinoma: a rare malignancy of the salivary glands. J Otolaryngol. 2000;29(2):102–9.
192. de Sousa SO, Schwarzschild M, de Araujo NS, de Araujo VC. Basal cell adenocarcinoma of the palate with squamous metaplasia. J Clin Pathol. 2000;53(2):153–6.
193. Ellis GL, Wiscovitch JG. Basal cell adenocarcinomas of the major salivary glands. Oral Surg Oral Med Oral Pathol. 1990;69(4):461–9.

194. Thompson LDR, Wenig BM. Diagnostic pathology: head and neck. 2nd ed. Amsterdam, Netherlands: Elsevier; 2015.
195. Seifert G. Classification and differential diagnosis of clear and basal cell tumors of the salivary glands. Semin Diagn Pathol. 1996;13(2):95–103.
196. Chhieng DC, Paulino AF. Cytology of myoepithelial carcinoma of the salivary gland. Cancer. 2002;96(1):32–6.
197. Robinson RA. Basal cell adenoma and basal cell adenocarcinoma. Surg Pathol Clin. 2021;14(1):25–42.
198. Savera AT, Sloman A, Huvos AG, Klimstra DS. Myoepithelial carcinoma of the salivary glands: a clinicopathologic study of 25 patients. Am J Surg Pathol. 2000;24(6):761–74.
199. Said S, Campana J. Myoepithelial carcinoma ex pleomorphic adenoma of salivary glands: a problematic diagnosis. Oral Surg Oral Med Oral Pathol Oral Radiol Endod. 2005;99(2):196–201.
200. Foss RD, Ellis GL, Auclair PL. Salivary gland cystadenocarcinomas. A clinicopathologic study of 57 cases. Am J Surg Pathol. 1996;20(12):1440–7.
201. Vitorinoa M, Tinocob J, Chaves AF. Basal cell adenocarcinoma arising from the parotid gland. Biomed Hub. 2022;7:173–8.
202. El Hallani S, Udager AM, Bell D, Fonseca I, Thompson LDR, Assaad A, Agaimy A, et al. Epithelial-myoepithelial carcinoma: frequent morphologic and molecular evidence of preexisting pleomorphic adenoma, common HRAS mutations in PLAG1-intact and HMGA2-intact cases, and occasional TP53, FBXW7, and SMARCB1 alterations in high-grade cases. Am J Surg Pathol. 2018;42(1):18–27.
203. Urano M, Nakaguro M, Yamamoto Y, Hirai H, Tanigawa M, Saigusa N, et al. Diagnostic significance of HRAS mutations in epithelial-myoepithelial carcinomas exhibiting a broad histopathologic spectrum. Am J Surg Pathol. 2019;43(7):984–94.
204. Seethala RR, Richmond JA, Hoschar AP, Barnes EL. New variants of epithelial-myoepithelial carcinoma: oncocytic-sebaceous and apocrine. Arch Pathol Lab Med. 2009;133(6):950–9.
205. Li B, Yang H, Hong X, Wang Y, Wang F. Epithelial-myoepithelial carcinoma with high-grade transformation of parotid gland: a case report and literature review. Medicine (Baltimore). 2017;96(49):e8988.
206. Vázquez A, Patel TD, D'Aguillo CM, Abdou RY, Farver W, Baredes S, et al. Epithelial-myoepithelial carcinoma of the salivary glands: an analysis of 246 cases. Otolaryngol Head Neck Surg. 2015;153(4):569–74.
207. Seethala RR, Barnes EL, Hunt JL. Epithelial-myoepithelial carcinoma: a review of the clinicopathologic spectrum and immunophenotypic characteristics in 61 tumors of the salivary glands and upper aerodigestive tract. Am J Surg Pathol. 2007;31(1):44–57.
208. Gore MR. Epithelial-myoepithelial carcinoma: a population-based survival analysis. BMC Ear Nose Throat Disord. 2018;18:15.
209. Roy P, Bullock MJ, Perez-Ordoñez B, Dardick I, Weinreb I. Epithelial-myoepithelial carcinoma with high grade transformation. Am J Surg Pathol. 2010;34(9):1258–65.
210. Ellis GL, Auclair PL. Atlas of tumour pathology series 4: tumour of the salivary glands. Washington, DC: Armed Forces Institute of Pathology; 2008. p. 281–9.
211. Kleinsasser O, Klein HJ, Hubner G. Salivary duct carcinoma. A group of salivary gland tumors analogous to mammary duct carcinoma. Arch Klin Exp Ohren Nasen Kehlkopfheilkd. 1968;192(1):100–5.
212. Hosal AS, Fan C, Barnes L, Myers EN. Salivary duct carcinoma. Otolaryngol Head Neck Surg. 2003;129(6):720–5.
213. Anderson C, Muller R, Piorkowski R, et al. Intraductal carcinoma of major salivary gland. Cancer. 1992;69:609–14.
214. Hosal AS, Fan C, Barnes L, et al. Salivary duct carcinoma. Otolaryngol Head Neck Surg. 2003;129:720–5.
215. Gilbert MR, Sharma A, Schmitt NC, Johnson JT, Ferris RL, Duvvuri U, Kim S. A 20-year review of 75 cases of salivary duct carcinoma. JAMA Otolaryngol Head Neck Surg. 2016;142(5):489–95.

216. Jaehne M, Roeser K, Jaekel T, et al. Clinical and immunohistologic typing of salivary duct carcinoma: a report of 50 cases. Cancer. 2005;103:2526–33.
217. Williams L, Thompson LD, Seethala RR, Weinreb I, Assaad AM, Tuluc M, et al. Salivary duct carcinoma: the predominance of apocrine morphology, prevalence of histologic variants, and androgen receptor expression. Am J Surg Pathol. 2015;39(5):705–13.
218. Glas AS, Hollema H, Nap RE, Plukker JT. Expression of estrogen receptor, progesterone receptor, and insulin-like growth factor receptor-1 and of MIB-1 in patients with recurrent pleomorphic adenoma of the parotid gland. Cancer. 2002;94(8):2211–6.
219. Sugano S, Mukai K, Tsuda H, Hirohashi S, Furuya S, Shimosato Y, Ebihara S, Takeyama I. Immunohistochemical study of c-erbB-2 oncoprotein overexpression in human major salivary gland carcinoma: an indicator of aggressiveness. Laryngoscope. 1992;102(8):923–7.
220. Felix A, El-Naggar AK, Press MF, Ordonez NG, Fonseca I, Tucker SL, et al. Prognostic significance of biomarkers (c-erbB-2, p53, proliferating cell nuclear antigen, and DNA content) in salivary duct carcinoma. Hum Pathol. 1996;27(6):561–6.
221. Huang AT, Tang C, Bell D, Yener M, Izquierdo L, Frank SJ, El-Naggar AK, Hanna EY, Weber RS, Kupferman ME. Prognostic factors in adenocarcinoma of the salivary glands. Oral Oncol. 2015;51(6):610–5.
222. Barnes L, Rao U, Krause J, et al. Salivary duct carcinoma. Part I. A clinicopathologic evaluation and DNA image analysis of 13 cases with review of the literature. Oral Surg Oral Med Oral Pathol. 1994;78:64–73.
223. Brandwein MS, Jagirdar J, Patil J, et al. Salivary duct carcinoma (cribriform salivary carcinoma of excretory ducts). A clinicopathologic and immunohistochemical study of 12 cases. Cancer. 1990;65:2307–14.
224. Delgado R, Vuitch F, Albores-Saavedra J. High grade salivary duct carcinoma. Mod Pathol. 1992;5:71A.
225. Haines K, Murad T. Infiltrating salivary duct carcinoma of the parotid. Lab Investig. 1989;60:36A.
226. Lewis JE, McKinney BC, Weiland LH, Ferreiro JA, Olsen KD. Salivary duct carcinoma. Clinicopathologic and immunohistochemical review of 26 cases. Cancer. 1996;77:223–30.
227. Murrah VA, Batsakis JG. Salivary duct carcinoma. Ann Otol Rhinol Laryngol. 1994;103:244–7.
228. Ockner DM, Mills SE, Swanson PE, et al. Salivary duct carcinoma: an immunohistologic comparison with invasive ductal carcinoma of the breast. Lab Investig. 1994;70:100A.
229. Smith JA, Warhol MJ, Brodsky GL. An immunohistochemical study of a carcinoma of the parotid gland exhibiting both ductal and acinic cell differentiation. Oral Surg Oral Med Oral Pathol. 1983;55:267–73.
230. Barnes L, Rao U, Krause J, Contis L, Schwartz A, Scalamogna P. Salivary duct carcinoma. Part I. A clinicopathologic evaluation and DNA image analysis of 13 cases with review of the literature. Oral Surg Oral Med Oral Pathol. 1994;78(1):64–73.
231. Guzzo M, Di Palma S, Grandi C, Molinari R. Salivary duct carcinoma: clinical characteristics and treatment strategies. Head Neck. 1997;19(2):126–33.
232. Brandwein-Gensler M, Hille J, Wang BY, Urken M, Gordon R, Wang LJ, et al. Low-grade salivary duct carcinoma: description of 16 cases. Am J Surg Pathol. 2004;28:1040–4.
233. Delgado R, Klimstra D, Albores-Saavedra J. Low grade salivary duct carcinoma. A distinctive variant with a low-grade histology and a predominant intraductal growth pattern. Cancer. 1996;78:958–67.
234. Edafe O, Hughes B, Tsirevelou P, Goswamy J, Kumar R. Understanding primary parotid squamous cell carcinoma—a systematic review. Surgeon. 2020;18(1):44–8.
235. Batsakis JG, McClatchey KD, Johns M, Regazi J. Primary squamous cell carcinoma of the parotid gland. Arch Otolaryngol. 1976;102(6):355–7.
236. Shemen LJ, Huvos AG, Spiro RH. Squamous cell carcinoma of salivary gland origin. Head Neck Surg. 1987;9:235–40.

237. Auclair PL, Ellis GL. Primary squamous cell carcinoma. In: Ellis GL, Auclair PL, Gnepp DR, editors. Surgical pathology of the salivary glands. Philadelphia, PA: WB Saunders Co.; 1991. p. 369–78.
238. Gaughan RK, Olsen KD, Lewis JE. Primary squamous cell carcinoma of the parotid gland. Arch Otolaryngol Head Neck Surg. 1992;118(8):798–801.
239. Li S, Baloch ZW, Tomaszewski JE, LiVolsi VA. Worrisome histologic alterations following fine-needle aspiration of benign parotid lesions. Arch Pathol Lab Med. 2000;124:87–91.
240. Nagao T, Serizawa H, Iwaya K, Shimizu T, Sugano I, Ishida Y, et al. Keratocystoma of the parotid gland: a report of two cases of an unusual pathologic entity. Mod Pathol. 2002;15(9):1005–10.
241. Xu B, Wang L, Borsu L, Ghossein R, Katabi N, Ganly I, Dogan S. A proportion of primary squamous cell carcinomas of the parotid gland harbour high-risk human papillomavirus. Histopathology. 2016;69(6):921–9.
242. Cornog JL. Surgical and clinical pathology of salivary gland tumors. In: Rankow R, Polayes I, editors. Diseases of salivary glands. Philadelphia, PA: WB Saunders Co.; 1970. p. 92–142.
243. Lee S, Kim GE, Park CS, Choi EC, Yang WI, Lee CG, et al. Primary squamous cell carcinoma of the parotid gland. Am J Otolaryngol. 2001;22:400–6.
244. Marks MW, Ryan RF, Litwin MS, Sonntag BV. Squamous cell carcinoma of the parotid gland. Plast Reconstr Surg. 1987;79:550–4.
245. Lewis JE, Olsen KD. Tumors of salivary glands. In: Barnes EL, Eveson J, Reichart P, Sidransky D, editors. Pathology and genetics head and neck tumors. Lyon, France: IARC; 2005. p. 245–6.
246. Marciani RD, Trodahl JN, Dauchess VG, Canlas MS. Squamous cell carcinoma of the submandibular gland. J Oral Surg. 1976;34:646–50.
247. Magaki SD, Bhuta S, Abemayor E, Nabili V, Sepahdari AR, Lai CK. Carcinoma ex-pleomorphic adenoma of the parotid gland consisting of high-grade salivary duct carcinoma and keratinizing squamous cell carcinoma. Oral Surg Oral Med Oral Pathol Oral Radiol. 2015;120(3):e169–73.
248. Batsakis JG. Primary squamous cell carcinomas of major salivary glands. Ann Otol Rhinol Laryngol. 1983;92:97–8.
249. Lee S, Kim GE, Park CS, et al. Primary squamous cell carcinoma of the parotid gland. Am J Otolaryngol. 2001;22(6):400–6.
250. Marks MW, Ryan RF, Litwin MS, et al. Squamous cell carcinoma of the parotid gland. Plast Reconstr Surg. 1987;79:550–4.

Parotid Gland Lymphoma

15

15.1 Background

There are two types of lymphoma: Hodgkin lymphoma (HL) and non-Hodgkin lymphoma (NHL). Parotid lymphoma may be primary (less common) or secondary (far more common). Primary lymphoma first involves the parotid gland and later can involve other parts of the body including lymph nodes (LNs) and bone marrow. Secondary lymphoma, on the other hand, involves other parts of the body first, such as peripheral blood, LNs, bone marrow, and other organs; salivary gland involvement occurs later.

Lymphoma accounts for approximately 12% of all malignant salivary gland tumors. The parotid gland is the most commonly affected salivary gland (80%). It is generally seen in older men and women. It can occur worldwide and all races and ethnic groups may be affected. It is associated with human immunodeficiency virus (HIV) infection and approximately 4–6% of patients with Sjogrin's syndrome develop lymphoma of the parotid gland. Treatment of parotid lymphoma depends upon the stage, overall health, age, and subtype of lymphoma.

15.2 Epidemiology

The prevalence of extra-nodal NHL is most common in the gastrointestinal tract, whereas the head and neck region serves as the second most frequent anatomic site of extra-nodal lymphomas [1, 2]. Lymphoma is the second most common neoplasm of the head and the neck region after squamous cell carcinoma [3]. The salivary glands serve as the site for nearly 12% of extra-nodal lymphomas of the head and neck region, which accounts for 2–5% of salivary gland neoplasms [4–6]. The parotid gland is the most common site for salivary gland lymphomas, whereas nearly 20% of salivary gland lymphomas affect the submandibular and minor salivary glands [1, 2, 7–9].

© The Author(s), under exclusive license to Springer Nature Switzerland AG 2024
M. Sakr, *Surgery of the Salivary Glands*,
https://doi.org/10.1007/978-3-031-82069-4_15

Parotid lymphoma preferentially occurs in women and patients over 50 years old. The most common variant of lymphoma associated with Sjogren's syndrome is mucosa-associated lymphoid tissue lymphoma (MALT), with 48–75% of all cases followed by diffuse large B-cell lymphoma (DLBCL) and follicular lymphoma [4, 10, 11].

15.3 Etiology/Risk Factors

15.3.1 Risk (Predisposing) Factors

The exact cause of the parotid lymphoma is generally unknown. No specific risk factors have been identified. However, the condition is known to be associated with the following risk factors:

Autoimmune/inflammatory disorders such as Sjögren's syndrome. Studies have shown that 4.3% of patients with Sjogren's syndrome develop NHL within 5–10 years [10].

Lymphoepithelial sialadenitis.
Hepatitis C virus (HCV) infection.
Advanced age.
Immunodeficiency as in acquired immunodeficiency syndrome (AIDS).
Family history of immune disease.
Smoking.
Exposure to radiation and industrial chemicals.
Chemotherapy.
Viruses (rare), e.g., Epstein-Barr virus (EBV) infection.
Professions involving radiation exposure, which may include nuclear plant workers, pilots, astronauts, etc.
Certain medications and drugs.

15.3.2 International Prognostic Index (IPI)

According to some scientists, the IPI may not be very helpful in evaluating lymphoma of salivary gland. However, some scientists believe that it is helpful in some cases to determine prognosis. The IPI for aggressive NHL lists a few factors that determine the overall risk:

Age over 60 years.
Elevated level of serum lactate dehydrogenase (LDH).
Performance status, which could range from being fully active (low risk) to being completely disabled (very high risk).
Individuals who have already suffered from lymphoma or other types of blood cancers may have a relapse or a recurrence.

Presence of an immunodeficiency syndrome such as AIDS is a high-risk factor. Individuals infected with EBV.

15.4 Pathogenesis/Pathophysiology

It is believed that the abnormal development of lymphocytes gives rise to cancerous cells leading to the formation of lymphoma. Nevertheless, how this occurs and the factors that cause it remain under investigation.

There may be certain genetic defects, such as translocation, which is a juxtaposition of regions of the chromosomes. This may result in (1) change of the regulatory elements of certain cancer-causing genes (oncogenes), which can lead to increased production of their mRNA (over-expression), thus increasing their protein levels, and (2) exchange of protein coding regions of the gene, giving rise to new proteins that can stimulate the inappropriate growth of cells.

The development of lymphoma from Sjogren's syndrome (SS) is theorized to be due to prolonged B-cell activity and survival. Sjogren's syndrome is associated with excessive expression of cytokines, chemokines, and inflammatory factors such as interferon (IFN) and B-cell activating factor (BAFF) [12, 13]. BAFF induces the migration of T- and B-lymphocytes into the salivary glands to create an autoimmune reaction. The B-cells start producing SS-A and SS-B antibodies, which are used to diagnose Sjogren's syndrome [10]. Although the exact pathway is unknown, the constant activity of these B-cells is believed to be the inciting event of lymphoma genesis in Sjogren's syndrome [14].

15.5 Pathology

Parotid lymphoma can either be a B-cell lymphoma (far more common) or a T-cell lymphoma. There is increased number of intra-parotid lymph nodes with infiltrative characteristics. There are various (histological) subtypes of parotid gland lymphomas and some of these include (1) MALT (mucosa-associated lymphoid tissue) lymphoma of the salivary gland (most common subtype), (2) diffuse large B-cell lymphoma (rare subtype), and (3) follicular lymphoma (rare subtype) [15].

In parotid lymphoma (NHL), fine needle aspiration cytology (FNAC) may reveal heterogeneous population of atypical lymphoid cells consisting of small- and intermediate-sized lymphocytes with round-to-irregular nuclear borders, finely granular chromatin, prominent nucleoli, and brisk mitoses. Plasmacytoid cells with abundant cytoplasm and eccentric nucleus, large monocytoid cells with pale staining cytoplasm, and indented nucleus with prominent 1–3 nucleoli may be noted (Fig. 15.1).

Histopathologically, NHL of the major salivary gland presents with atypical lymphocytes with invasion into the adjacent ductal epithelium, lymphoepithelial lesions, and lymphoid follicles or germinal centers (Fig. 15.2) [11].

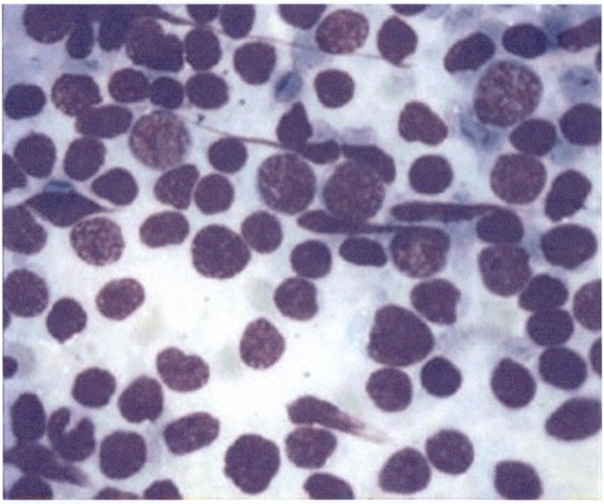

Fig. 15.1 Fine needle aspiration cytology (FNAC) of parotid lymphoma showing plasmacytoid cells with abundant cytoplasm and eccentric nucleus, large monocytoid cells with pale staining cytoplasm, and indented nucleus with prominent nucleoli (Giemsa stain ×200)

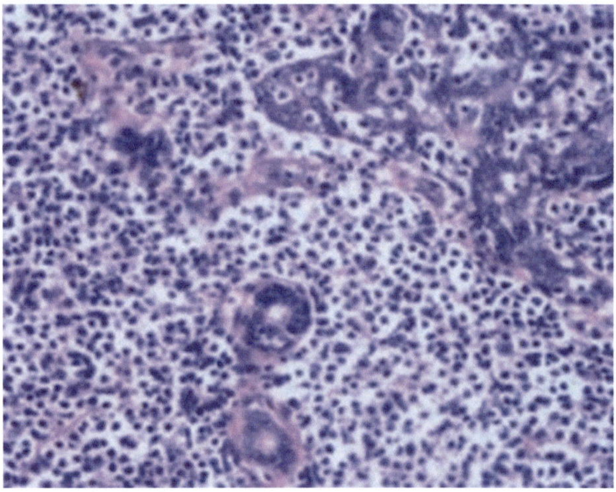

Fig. 15.2 Histological features of lymphoma of the mucosa-associated lymphoid tissue (MALT) of the parotid gland showing the normal structure of the parotid gland destroyed by the diffuse hyperplasia of lymphoid tissue, forming lymphoepithelial lesions (H&E stain ×400)

Immunohistochemistry (IHC) shows that lymphoid cells are immunoreactive for CD20 and focally immunoreactive for B-cell lymphoma 6 protein (Bcl-6), but immuno-negative for cluster of differentiation (CD) 3, CD5, CD10, and MUM1.

15.6 Clinical Presentation

The signs and symptoms of parotid lymphoma depend on whether it is a primary or a secondary condition. In the early stages of primary parotid lymphoma, if the tumor is small, it is usually asymptomatic and the individuals will not have any significant symptoms, but patients may then develop facial symptoms including facial pain, facial paralysis, and growth acceleration of a painless mass [16]. Symptoms, in general, depend upon the extent of lymphoma involvement in other parts of the body.

The signs and symptoms of lymphoma of the parotid gland may include the following [10]:

Presence of a lump in the face, which may be unilateral or bilateral and may be accompanied by pain.
Cervical lymphadenopathy.
Swelling of the face.
Facial palsy (usually by large tumors).
Difficulty during eating, drinking, or even opening the mouth.
Dryness of mouth.
Foul taste or smell from the mouth.
Unintentional weight loss; changes in appetite.
Fatigue and weakness, headache.
Anemia.
Frequent infections.
Hypotension.

When organs other than the parotid gland are involved, then the signs and symptoms may be based on the specific organs that are affected such as splenomegaly, vasculitis, and palpable purpura.

15.7 Complications

Complications due to parotid lymphoma include:

Involvement of local and distant organs; it can lead to systemic or disseminated disease in some cases.
Loss of function of the organ/area to which cancer has spread due to systemic involvement.
Acute difficulty while eating, swallowing, or speaking.
Immunosuppression, which can become more severe during treatment. Consequently, patients are more vulnerable to infections.
Occasionally, the tumor can transform into a more aggressive form or subtype of lymphoma.

Complications related to chemotherapy used for treatment may include dizziness, vomiting, loss of appetite, mouth ulcers, hair loss, infertility (in men and women), secondary infections, and secondary cancers such as skin cancer.

15.8 Diagnosis/Investigations

At present, there is no unified standard for the definitions of primary and secondary parotid lymphoma. However, it is suggested that the diagnosis of primary parotid lymphoma should meet the following criteria: (1) the first site or symptom of the tumor was found in the parotid gland and the tumor was shown to be involved in the parenchyma of the parotid gland using pathology; (2) there is no superficial lymphadenopathy (except in the regional LNs); (3) there is no hepatosplenomegaly or mediastinal lymphadenopathy; (4) the peripheral hemogram and the myelogram are normal; and (5) it was 6 months after the first malignant lymphoma appeared that malignant lymphoma appeared in other parts [17].

In addition to obtaining a complete medical history and performing a thorough physical examination, the definitive diagnosis of parotid lymphoma is generally reached by pathological examination of the surgical specimens. There are other tests and procedures that could help in the diagnosis and these include the following.

15.8.1 Laboratory Tests

Blood tests that may include complete blood cell count (CBC), absolute lymphocyte count on peripheral blood, liver function tests (LFTs), and specifically, lactate dehydrogenase (LDH) enzyme

15.8.2 Imaging Studies

Imaging may be performed specific to location of the involved organ, as well as to determine the extent of lymphoma in the body. It includes plain X-ray, ultrasonography (US), computed tomography (CT) scan of the neck (Fig. 15.3), whole body bone scan, whole body CT-PET (positron emission tomography) scans to determine how far the lymphoma has spread, and brain MRI (if neurological symptoms are present).

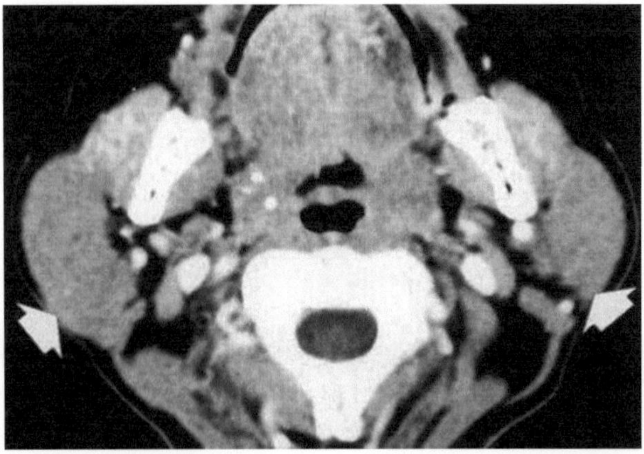

Fig. 15.3 Computed tomography (CT) scan of the neck showing bilateral lymphoma of the parotid glands (arrows)

15.8.3 Tissue Biopsy

Tissue biopsy from the affected salivary gland is considered to be the "gold standard" in arriving at a conclusive diagnosis, either through a fine needle aspiration biopsy (FNAB) or core-needle biopsy [18]. Biopsy specimens are studied initially using Hematoxylin and Eosin (H&E) staining. Sometimes, the pathologist may perform special studies, which may include immunohistochemical (IHC) stains, molecular testing, flow cytometric analysis, and very rarely, electron microscopic studies, to assist in the diagnosis.

IHC proved to be useful in obtaining a correct diagnosis, and it is also suitable for diagnosing adenolymphoma, pleomorphic adenoma, carcinoma of the parotid gland, and metastatic tumors. The majority of primary lymphoma of the parotid gland is B-cell NHL, accounting for 84–97%, and the minority is T-cell NHL or HL [19].

15.8.4 Bone Marrow Aspiration and Biopsy

Bone marrow aspiration and biopsy may be needed to determine if the bone marrow is involved. However, a bone marrow biopsy is not needed in the early stages of the condition.

15.8.5 Flow Cytometry

Flow cytometry measures the number and percentage of cells in a blood sample, as well as cell characteristics such as size, shape, and the presence of biomarkers on the cell surface. This method helps to subclassify the condition and also to detect residual levels of disease after treatment. This tool can help in diagnosing relapse and restart treatment as needed.

15.8.6 Fluorescence In Situ Hybridization (FISH)

Fluorescence in situ hybridization (FISH) is a cytogenetic analysis test performed on blood or bone marrow cells to detect chromosome changes (genetic abnormalities) in blood malignant cells.

15.8.7 Immunophenotyping

Immunophenotyping may be resorted in order to identify a specific type of cell in a sample, which can help determine the best treatment course to be prescribed to the patient.

Table 15.1 Staging of non-Hodgkin lymphoma (NHL) of the parotid gland

Stage	Nodal involvement	Extra-nodal involvement
Stage 1	One LN or group of adjacent LNs	Single extra-nodal lesion without nodal involvement
Stage 2	Two or more nodal groups on the same side of the diaphragm	Stage 1 or 2 with limited contiguous extra-nodal spread
Stage 3	LNs on both sides of the diaphragm, nodes above diaphragm with spleen involvement	N/A
Stage 4	Wide noncontiguous spread beyond lymph system to bone, liver, and lung	N/A

LN lymph node, *N/A* not applicable

15.8.8 Polymerase Chain Reaction (PCR)

Polymerase chain reaction (PCR) is used to measure the presence of certain biomarkers in blood or bone marrow cells. The test is ultrasensitive and detects extremely low amounts of biomarkers remaining in blood, which can be missed by cytogenetic methods, such as FISH, karyotype, or flow cytometry. Thus, PCR allows a more sensitive follow-up of patients in remission and can help determine whether additional treatment is necessary.

15.8.9 Exploratory (Diagnostic) Laparoscopy

Exploratory laparoscopy (diagnostic laparoscopy) may be required, if gastrointestinal symptoms are present. A diagnostic laparoscopy is also helpful in staging of the tumor. Nevertheless, this procedure is not very much used anymore.

15.9 Staging

The WHO Classification of Tumors of Hematopoietic and Lymphoid Tissue staging system is usually used for tumor staging before surgery [20]. The staging standard used by most hematologists in extra-nodal lymphoma cases is the Ann Arbor staging system [21, 22].

Staging of non-Hodgkin lymphoma (NHL) of the parotid gland based on the Lugano classification [23] is summarized in Table 15.1. It comprises four stages, each describing nodal and extra-nodal involvement.

15.10 Prevention

Currently, it is not possible to prevent lymphoma of the salivary glands. However, controlling certain factors may help lower one's risk for the condition as follows:

Healthy diet and exercise, as well as avoidance of unnecessary exposure to chemicals, may help decrease its risk.

Avoiding smoking.

Undertaking appropriate and early treatment of any condition affecting the salivary gland.

Using appropriate protective gear while working with X-rays and other radioactive source.

In order to avoid a relapse, or be prepared for a recurrence, the entire diagnosis, treatment, drugs administered, and so on should be well-documented and follow-up measures initiated.

Regular medical screening at periodic intervals with blood tests, scans, and physical examinations are mandatory. Often several years of active vigilance are necessary.

15.11 Treatment

There is no unified plan for treatment of parotid lymphoma [24]. Treatment depends upon the stage, overall health, age, and subtype of lymphoma. It includes the following.

15.11.1 Chemotherapy

Chemotherapy is the mainstay of treatment for lymphoma of the salivary gland. This approach uses a combination of drugs or target therapy that achieved remarkable results, and can be used for all stages of the tumor [25]. Postoperative chemotherapy was carried out according to the pathological type and molecular phenotype of the tumor. Many lymphomas, however, can be resistant to chemotherapy and there can be severe side-effects including infertility, immunosuppression, secondary infections, and secondary cancers.

Patients with MALT lymphoma are commonly treated with rituximab, 2-chlorodeoxyadenosine, fludarabine, and chlorambucil-cyclophosphamide [26]. Rituximab is a chimeric monoclonal antibody that binds to the surface CD20 proteins of B-cells, triggering cellular death [10]. For cases of DLBCL transformation, the standard chemotherapeutic regimen is cyclophosphamide, doxorubicin, vincristine, and prednisone (CHOP) with rituximab [27].

15.11.2 Surgical Treatment

The treatment for MALT lymphoma of the parotid gland is different from the treatment for other NHLs. Because most parotid MALT lymphoma cases involve localized masses and have a low malignancy and less systemic metastasis, its treatment is mainly surgical resection with adjuvant radiotherapy (RT) and chemotherapy after the operation, and the prognosis is good. Although surgery is a common treatment, some scholars do not recommend it as the first-line treatment for parotid lymphoma [28]. Surgical excision of the lymphoma of the parotid gland entails total parotidectomy or radical (nonconservative) parotidectomy if the facial nerve cannot be preserved.

15.11.3 Radiotherapy (RT)

Radiation therapy is generally used for early stage lymphomas. One study found that adjuvant local radiotherapy (RT) can control tumor development [29]. It is most commonly used in combination with chemotherapy. The side-effects of radiation therapy include nausea, vomiting, fatigue, pain, risk of cancer later in life, and risk of heart disease.

15.11.4 Supportive Treatment

Steroids, blood transfusions, anti-nausea medications, and antibiotics may be used as supportive therapy. In combination with other treatment measures, these can help combat the symptoms of immunodeficiency. Undertaking treatment of underlying infection/disorder should be done as warranted [30].

15.11.5 Transplantation

If salivary gland lymphoma is not fully responsive to treatment, or if the chance of recurrence is high, then bone marrow transplantation or stem cell transplantation can be considered.

15.12 Prognosis (Outcomes/Resolutions)

Parotid lymphoma is a slow-growing malignancy that has a generally good prognosis with early diagnosis and treatment. Prognosis depends on many factors including the subtype and stage of lymphoma, progression of the condition, response to treatment, and overall health of the individual [31].

Patients with MALT have a 3-year overall survival of 80% [26]. Patients with more aggressive DLBCL transformation have a 3-year overall survival ranging from 37% to 100% [27]. Poor prognostic factors include age > 60, elevated serum LDH level, more than 1 extra-nodal site, and stage III or IV disease [32].

Prognosis of parotid lymphoma depends on the factors given in Table 15.2.

Table 15.2 Prognostic factors and their impact in parotid lymphoma

Factor	Impact on prognosis
Histopathology	Absence of a tumor capsule indicates a poor prognosis
Stage of the tumor	With lower-stage tumors, when the tumor is confined to site of origin, the prognosis is usually excellent with appropriate therapy. In higher-stage tumors, such as tumors with metastasis, the prognosis is poor
Overall health	Individuals with overall excellent health have better prognosis compared with those with poor health
Age	Older patients generally have poorer prognosis than younger ones
Size of the tumor	Individuals with small-sized tumors fare better than those with large-sized ones. Individuals with bulky disease have a poorer prognosis
Involvement of vital organs	May complicate the condition and worsen prognosis
Surgical respectability	Surgically respectable tumors have better prognosis
Recurrence	Recurrent tumors have worse prognosis compared to tumors that do not recur
Response to treatment	Tumors that respond to treatment have better prognosis compared to those that do not. Tolerance to chemotherapy sessions is a positive influencing factor
Disease progression	Progression of the condition makes the outcome worse (progressive salivary gland lymphoma). Progression to "bone marrow failure" is usually associated with short survival

References

1. Hart S, Horsman JM, Radstone CR, Hancock H, Goepel JR, Hancock BW. Localised extranodal lymphoma of the head and neck: the Sheffield Lymphoma Group experience (1971–2000). Clin Oncol (R Coll Radiol). 2004;16:186–92.
2. Vega F, Lin P, Medeiros LJ. Extranodal lymphomas of the head and neck. Ann Diagn Pathol. 2005;9:340–50.
3. Nassie DI, Berkowitz M, Wolf M, Kronenberg J, Talmi YP. Parotid mass as presenting symptom of lymphoma. Isr Med Assoc J. 2010;12:416–8.
4. Travaglino A, Giordano C, Pace M, Varricchio S, Picardi M, Pane F, et al. Sjögren syndrome in primary salivary gland lymphoma. Am J Clin Pathol. 2020;153(6):719–24.
5. Takahashi H, Cheng J, Fujita S, Tsuda N, Tezuka F, Liu AR, et al. Primary malignant lymphoma of the salivary gland: a tumor of mucosa-associated lymphoid tissue. J Oral Pathol Med. 1992;21(7):318–25.
6. Zucca E, Roggero E, Bertoni F, Conconi A, Cavalli F. Primary extranodal non-Hodgkin's lymphomas. Part 2: Head and neck, central nervous system and other less common sites. Ann Oncol. 1999;10(9):1023–33.
7. Wolvius EB, van der Valk P, van der Wal JE, van Diest PJ, Huijgens PC, van der Waal I, et al. Primary non-Hodgkin's lymphoma of the salivary glands. An analysis of 22 cases. J Oral Pathol Med. 1996;25:177–81.
8. Dunn P, Kuo TT, Shih LY, Lin TL, Wang PN, Kuo MC, et al. Primary salivary gland lymphoma: a clinicopathologic study of 23 cases in Taiwan. Acta Haematol. 2004;112:203–8.
9. Weber AL, Rahemtullah A, Ferry JA. Hodgkin and non-Hodgkin lymphoma of the head and neck: clinical, pathologic, and imaging evaluation. Neuroimaging Clin N Am. 2003;13:371–92.

10. Turner MD. Salivary gland disease in Sjögren's syndrome: sialoadenitis to lymphoma. Oral Maxillofac Surg Clin North Am. 2014;26(1):75–81.
11. Delli K, Vissink A, Spijkervet FK. Salivary gland biopsy for Sjögren's syndrome. Oral Maxillofac Surg Clin North Am. 2014;26(1):23–33.
12. Wildenberg ME, van Helden-Meeuwsen CG, van de Merwe JP, Drexhage HA, Versnel MA. Systemic increase in type I interferon activity in Sjögren's syndrome: a putative role for plasmacytoid dendritic cells. Eur J Immunol. 2008;38(7):2024–33.
13. Gottenberg JE, Cagnard N, Lucchesi C, Letourneur F, Mistou S, Lazure T, et al. Activation of IFN pathways and plasmacytoid dendritic cell recruitment in target organs of primary Sjögren's syndrome. Proc Natl Acad Sci USA. 2006;103(8):2770–5.
14. Mariette X. Lymphomas complicating Sjögren's syndrome and hepatitis C virus infection may share a common pathogenesis: chronic stimulation of rheumatoid factor B cells. Ann Rheum Dis. 2001;60(11):1007–10.
15. Lennert K. Histopathology of non-Hodgkin's lymphomas: based on the Kiel classification. Amsterdam, Dutchlans: Springer-Verlag; 2013.
16. Thielker J, Grosheva M, Ihrer S, Witting A, Guntinas-Lichius O. Contemporary management of benign and malignant parotid tumors. Front Surg. 2018;39:1–17.
17. Gu WD, Feng Y. Treatment of primary parotid non-Hodgkin's lymphoma: an analysis of 29 patients. Chin J Radiat Oncol. 2003;12:172–4.
18. Manson SD. Mucosa-associated lymphoid tissue (MALT) lymphoma. Semin Oncol Nurs. 2006;22:73–9.
19. Zhu L, Wang P, Yang J. Non-Hodgkin lymphoma involving the parotid gland: CT and MR imaging findings. Dentomaxillofac Radiol. 2013;42:20130046.
20. Swerdlow SH, Campo E, Pileri SA, Harris NL, Stein H, Siebert R, et al. The 2016 revision of the World Health Organization classification of lymphoid neoplasms. Blood. 2016;127:2375–90.
21. Carbone PP, Kaplan HS, Musshoff K, Smithers DW, Tubiana M. Report of the committee on Hodgkin's disease staging classification. Cancer Res. 1971;31:1860–1.
22. Skarin AT, Dorfma DM. Non-Hodgkin's lymphomas: current classification and management. CA Cancer J Clin. 1997;47:351–72.
23. Cheson BD, Fisher RI, Barrington SF, Cavalli F, Schwartz LH, Zucca E. Recommendations for initial evaluation, staging, and response assessment of Hodgkin and non-Hodgkin lymphoma: the Lugano classification. J Clin Oncol. 2014;32(27):3059–68.
24. Wang J, Li R, Wang Q, Chen Y, Gao T, Han R, et al. The clinicopathological features of parotid lymphoma. Int J Clin Exp Pathol. 2020;13(8):2050–7.
25. Jackson AE, Mian M, Kalpadakis C, Pangalis GA, Stathis A, Porro E, et al. Extranodal marginal zone lymphoma of mucosa-associated lymphoid tissue of the salivary glands: a multicenter, international experience of 248 patients. Oncologist. 2015;20:1149–53.
26. Routsias JG, Goules JD, Charalampakis G, Tzima S, Papageorgiou A, Voulgarelis M. Malignant lymphoma in primary Sjögren's syndrome: an update on the pathogenesis and treatment. Semin Arthritis Rheum. 2013;43(2):178–86.
27. Voulgarelis M, Ziakas PD, Papageorgiou A, Baimpa E, Tzioufas AG, Moutsopoulos HM. Prognosis and outcome of non-Hodgkin lymphoma in primary Sjögren syndrome. Medicine (Baltimore). 2012;91(1):1–9.
28. Raderer M, Kiesewetter B, Ferreri AJ. Clinicopathologic characteristics and treatment of marginal zone lymphoma of mucosa-associated lymphoid tissue (MALT lymphoma). CA Cancer J Clin. 2016;66:153–71.
29. Olszewski AJ, Desai A. Radiation therapy administration and survival in stage I/II extranodal marginal zone B-cell lymphoma of mucosa-associated lymphoid tissue. Int J Radiat Oncol Biol Phys. 2014;88:642–9.
30. Adler EM. Living with lymphoma: a patient's guide. Maryland, MD: Johns Hopkins University Press; 2005.
31. Adler NE, Page AE, editors. Cancer care for the whole patient: meeting psychosocial health needs. Washington, DC: National Academies Press; 2008.
32. International Non-Hodgkin's Lymphoma Prognostic Factors Project. A predictive model for aggressive non-Hodgkin's lymphoma. N Engl J Med. 1993;329(14):987–94.

Primary Melanoma of the Parotid Gland 16

16.1 Epidemiology

Malignant melanomas (MMs) of the parotid gland are an uncommon condition and are generally metastatic with primaries usually originating in the skin of the head and neck [1]. Primary malignant melanoma (PMM) of the parotid gland is estimated to be very rare, accounting for <0.7% of all malignant tumors of the parotid gland and the recognition of their features is based mainly on sporadic case reports [1–6].

Amelanotic MM, which accounts for 1.8–8.1% of all MMs [7, 8], is a melanoma subtype with little or no pigmentation and, because of this lack of pigmentation and its wide-ranging clinical appearance, it often defies clinical diagnosis. A high level of vigilance is, therefore, necessary in diagnosing such a tumor in the parotid gland. Gao et al. (2008) in their study reported a primary "amelanotic" melanoma of the parotid gland [2].

16.2 Pathogenesis

The entity of PMM of the parotid gland is characterized by a difficult late diagnosis, poor prognosis, and controversial pathogenesis. Multiple hypotheses regarding its pathogenesis have been postulated; however, the exact etiology remains unclear [9]. According to these hypotheses, melanocytes are derived embryologically from the neural crest and do not usually form part of the salivary tissue. While Greene and Bernier [3] reasoned that melanoblasts would become a part of the parotid gland with the down-growth of oral epithelium during the development of the parotid, they also found that some cells in the normal human parotid gland tested positive for melanin when stained using the L-DOPA (3,4-dihydroxy-L-phenylalanine) method. Roberts and Jayaramachandren (1992) found that melanin is also present in the ductal and acinar cells of parotid [10].

© The Author(s), under exclusive license to Springer Nature Switzerland AG 2024
M. Sakr, *Surgery of the Salivary Glands*,
https://doi.org/10.1007/978-3-031-82069-4_16

Moreover, Takeda (1997) reported the presence of melanocytes in the interlobular ducts of the parotid gland during an autopsy performed on a Japanese male. Melanocytes with long cytoplasmic processes were distributed in the basal and supra-basal layers of hyperplastic duct epithelium, and melanin granules were sparsely scattered in the duct epithelial cells [11]. These findings demonstrate that the occurrence of malignant melanoma in the parotid gland as a primary lesion is possible.

The parotid gland contains three groups of LNs formed during embryological development, involving the parotid parenchyma, parotid fascia, and preauricular extraglandular soft tissue [12]. Rarely, melanoma is diagnosed in the parotid parenchyma or parotid LNs without an identifiable primary site; this could result from either a regressed cutaneous head and neck melanoma with parotid metastases, or from a PMM derived from ectopic melanocytes within the parotid parenchyma [3, 4, 11]. Nevertheless, the PMMs of the parotid gland are considered a "diagnosis by exclusion."

16.3 Diagnosis

16.3.1 Diagnostic Criteria

In 1961, Greene and Bernier have published [3] several criteria for the diagnosis of PMM of the parotid gland, and in 1993, Woodwards et al. has established the following criteria (Table 16.1) to assert the intraglandular PMM characters [4].

16.3.2 Clinical Examination

Patients with PMM of the parotid gland classically present with an indolent and firm parotid mass that tends to extend slowly to surrounding tissues, making clinical distinction from other malignancies very difficult. Dermal changes such as erythema and ulceration or pain and facial nerve palsy caused by local tumor compression or infiltration of advancing process may be observed [1].

A thorough physical examination should include a diligent search of the eyes, skin, nose, pharynx, mouth, esophagus, anogenital region, meninges, and panendoscopy for evidence of MM.

Table 16.1 Criteria proposed by Woodwards et al. [4]

Criteria	Description
Tumor site	The predominant tumor mass should be in the parotid gland
Lymph nodes	The tumor does not contain any identifiable lymph node tissue
Other site involvement	There should be no evidence of malignant melanoma elsewhere in the body
History of previous excision	There should be no evidence of previous excision of a malignant melanoma or progressing (suspicious) pigmented lesion

16.3.3 Imaging Studies

Imaging studies should include ultrasound (US)/computed tomography (CT) scan of the abdomen, a positron emission tomography (PET), and a CT scan of the chest and brain [5]. Some authors suggest that there will still be doubt about the primary origin of MM even with normal results; they believe that the location of the PMM is in an internal organ that is difficult to explore [1].

Generally, on CT scan, the mass is in the parotid gland, infiltrative, either homogeneous or heterogeneous, and central necrosis is found in some cases. The majority of malignant melanomas are associated with local or regional LN metastases [13]. Although CT scan of the chest and abdomen is still considered indispensable in the conventional staging investigation of melanoma, limitations of CT scan have been recognized in detection of small pulmonary or liver metastases <1 cm [14]. Currently, whole-body 18 fluoro-deoxyglucose (18F-FDG) PET imaging has been shown to be superior to CT scan in the assessment of pulmonary and LN metastases and can also detect primary melanoma up to 6 months earlier than conventional imaging [15]. However, 18F-FDG is not tumor-specific; the isotope being also taken up by benign masses such as Warthin's tumor and inflammatory cells [15]. Because of the physiological uptake of FDG by the brain, 18F-FDG PET has limited utility for brain metastases screening.

During the last decades, combined 18F-FDG PET/CT has fundamentally changed the approach of images interpretation in oncology indications and now plays key roles in detection, staging, and monitoring of therapy as well as differentiation of benign from malignant lesions [16]. According to American College of Radiology (ACR), Society of Nuclear Medicine (SNM), Society of Computed Body Tomography (SCBT) and MR, 18F-FDG PET/CT including both upper and lower extremities and head for patients with MM allows early diagnosis of primary tumor, lymph nodes involvement, distant metastases, as well as recurrent disease [17].

Although, the CT scan or 18F-FDG PET/CT appearance of PMM of the parotid may be nonspecific, placing the morphological and metabolic findings in clinical context and assessment of immunohistological findings is helpful for establishing the diagnosis. Integrated 18F-FDG PET/CT helps to determine the presence of parotid PMM or in the other surrounding soft tissue of the neck and head and subsequent LN metastases and therefore helps in pre- and postsurgical management. Darouichi (2016) reported a 54-year-old man with PMM of the parotid gland confirmed by immunohistochemical findings and integrated 18F-fluoro-deoxy-glucose positron emission tomography/computed tomography (18F-FDG PET/CT) to exclude primary melanoma elsewhere in the body [9].

16.3.4 Histopathology

Fine needle aspiration biopsy (FNAB) is a helpful adjunctive test for diagnosis, but its utility remains controversial [18]. Only histological and immunochemical findings can establish the diagnosis of PMM. Histologically (Fig. 16.1), tumor cells are large, mostly noncohesive with abundant eosinophilic cytoplasm, a marked pleomorphic

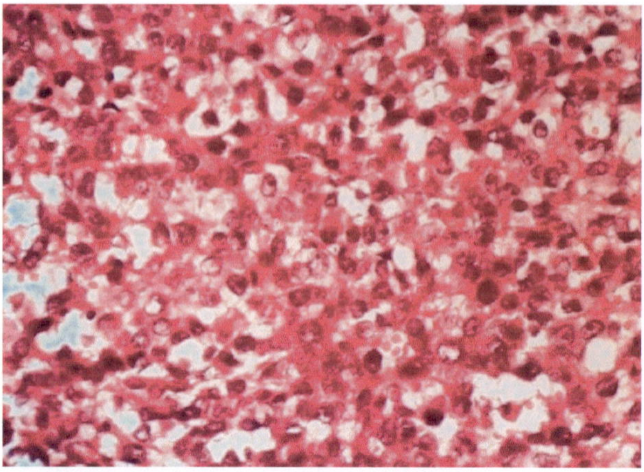

Fig. 16.1 Histopathology of primary malignant melanoma (PMM) of the parotid gland showing intraglandular melanoma whose cells were melanin A-positive and HMB-45 positive and absence of lymph node metastasis. H&E stain

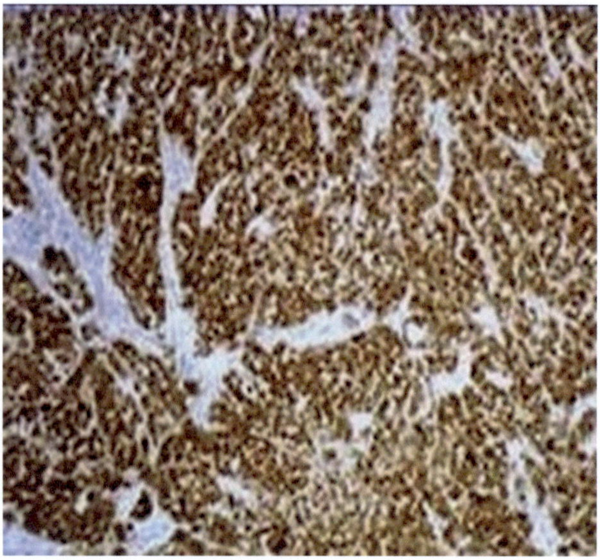

Fig. 16.2 Immunohistochemistry (IHC) of primary malignant melanoma (PMM) of the parotid gland positive for S100 protein establishing diagnosis

nucleus and prominent nucleoli. The core is composed of enlarged nucleoli and often pushes the periphery. The presence of intracellular melanin pigmentation represents the gold diagnostic criterion for MM, which is only found in 40–60% of cases [19].

16.3.5 Immunohistochemistry (IHC)

Immunohistochemically, cells are diffusely positive for S100 protein (Fig. 16.2) and HMB45 [20]. Melan A is positive in 80% and MiTF in the 90% of melanoma [21].

16.4 Differential Diagnosis

Primary malignant melanoma (PMM) of the parotid gland must be differentiated clinically, radiologically and immunohistochemically from other malignancies, especially adenosarcomas, squamous cell carcinoma, parotid lymphoma, and sarcoma of the parotid. Additional differentiation must be made with melanoma metastases arising in another site of the body [10].

16.5 Treatment

The standard treatment of a parotid malignancy is surgical, and a total parotidectomy should be performed [1]; however, radical parotidectomy should be avoided if possible, as this does not improve life expectancy, and the resulting facial palsy considerably worsens the quality of life of the patient [22, 23].

Due to the high incidence of occult LN metastases, at least a selective neck dissection should always be carried out in the N0 neck [24]. This can significantly reduce the incidence of cervical recurrences [25]. In the case of clinically manifest cervical LN metastases, a functional, and, in exceptional cases, a radical neck dissection is recommended [1]. Facial nerve palsy is the most common complication of the surgical management of parotid malignancies [26].

Postoperative irradiation, chemotherapy, and/or immunotherapy are controversial [1, 27–29] and difficult to evaluate due to the limited number of cases of parotid PMM. So far, there are no studies that could provide clear evidence for the positive influence of adjuvant therapy on survival rate and quality of life. However, in this type of tumor, adjuvant radiotherapy (RT) is recommended for high-risk patients, based on grade, stage, and margin of excision to improve local control even if it is not part of a regular treatment protocol [26].

16.6 Prognosis

Patients with PMM of the parotid gland have a poor prognosis even with the best treatment efforts [19]. Nevertheless, the prognosis of patients with MM in parotid or an intra-parotid LN without other detectable melanoma manifestations at diagnosis seems to be better in comparison to patients with known cutaneous or mucocutaneous primary tumor. Santini et al. (1985) reported that patients with melanoma metastases in the parotid gland or cervical LNs with an unknown primary tumor have a 5-year survival rate of 38.5% compared to only 22.6% with a known primary tumor [30].

Following the surgical case report (SCARE) guidelines [31], Chaouki et al. described in 2020 a PMM of the parotid gland in a 27-year-old woman who presented with a voluminous, round, painless, mass about 5 cm in size, located in the left parotid compartment. Positivity for HMB45 and Melan-A by immunohistochemistry (IHC) confirmed the diagnosis. The patient died 11 months later with generalized visceral metastases [32].

References

1. Barbieri M, Gentile R, Cordone MP, Mora R, Mora F. Primitive malignant melanoma of the parotid gland. ORL (Oto-Rhino-Laryngol) (Basel). 2002;64:297–9.
2. Gao N, Li LJ, Li Y, Wang L. Primary amelanotic malignant melanoma of the parotid gland: a case report. J Int Med Res. 2008;36(6):1435–9.
3. Greene GW, Bernier JL. Primary malignant melanomas of the parotid gland. Oral Surg Oral Med Oral Pathol. 1961;14:108–16.
4. Woodwards RT, Shepherd NA, Hensher R. Malignant melanoma of the parotid gland: a case report and literature review. Br J Oral Maxillofac Surg. 1993;31:313–5.
5. Bussi M, Cardarelli L, Riontino E, Valente G. Primary malignant melanoma arising in the parotid gland: case report and literature review. Tumori. 1999;85:523–5.
6. Bahar M, Anavi Y, Abraham A, et al. Primary malignant melanoma in the parotid gland. Oral Surg Oral Med Oral Pathol. 1990;70:627–30.
7. Koch SE, Lange JR. Amelanotic melanoma: the great masquerader. J Am Acad Dermatol. 2000;42:731–4.
8. Adler MJ, White CR Jr. Amelanotic malignant melanoma. Semin Cutan Med Surg. 1997;16:122–30.
9. Darouichi M. Primary malignant melanoma of the parotid gland combined 18F-FDGPET/CT and immunochemical diagnosis with literature review. J Digest Disord Diagn. 2016;1(2):1–7.
10. Roberts C, Jayaramachandren S. Malignant melanoma of the parotid gland. Br J Clin Pathol. 1992;46:217–8.
11. Takeda V. Melanocytes in the human parotid gland. Pathol Int. 1997;47:581–3.
12. Nuyens M, Schüpbach J, Stauffer E, Zbären P. Metastatic disease to the parotid gland. Otolaryngol Head Neck Surg. 2006;135(6):844–8.
13. Shah JP, Kraus DH, Dubner S, Sarkar S. Patterns of regional lymph node metastases from cutaneous melanomas of the head and neck. Am J Surg. 1991;162(4):320–3.
14. Reinhardt MJ, Wiethoelter N, Matthies A. PET recognition of pulmonary metastases on PET/CT imaging: impact of attenuation-corrected and non-attenuation corrected PET images. Eur J Nuc Med Mol Imaging. 2006;33:134–9.
15. Tyler DS, Onaitis M, Kherani A. Positron emission tomography scanning in malignant melanoma: clinical utility in patients with stage III disease. Cancer. 2000;89:1019–25.
16. Krug B, Dietlein M, Groth W. Fluor-18-fluorodeoxyglucose positron emission tomography (FDG-PET) in malignant melanoma: diagnostic comparison with conventional imaging methods. Acta Radiol. 2000;41:446–52.
17. Rinne D, Baum RP, Hor G. Primary staging and follow-up of high risk melanoma patients with whole-body 18F-fluorodeoxyglucose positron emission tomography: results of a prospective study of 100 patients. Cancer. 1998;82:1664–71.
18. Wang BY, Lawson W, Robinson RA, Perez-Ordonez B, Brandwein M. Malignant melanoma of the parotid. Arch Otolaryngol Head Neck Surg. 1999;125:635–9.
19. Bron LP, Traynor SJ, McNeil EB, O'Brien CJ. Primary and metastatic cancer of the parotid: comparison of clinical behavior in 232 cases. Laryngoscope. 2003;113(6):1070–5.
20. Saqi A, McGrath CM, Skovronsky D, Yu GH. Cytomorphologic features of fine-needle aspiration of metastatic and recurrent melanoma. Diagn Cytopathol. 2002;27(5):286–90.
21. Patel SG, Prasad ML, Escrig M, Singh B, Shaha AR, Kraus DH, et al. Primary mucosal malignant melanoma of the head and neck. Head Neck. 2002;24(3):247–57.
22. Ball AB, Thomas JM. Management of parotid metastases from cutaneous melanoma of the head and neck. J Laryngol Otol. 1990;104(4):350–1.
23. Jecker P, Hartwein J. Metastasis to the parotid gland: is a radical surgical approach justified? Am J Otolaryngol. 1996;17(2):102–5.
24. Vaglini M, Belli F, Santinami M, Cascinelli N. The role of parotidectomy in the treatment of nodal metastases from cutaneous melanoma of the head and neck. Eur J Surg Oncol. 1990;16(1):28–32.

25. O'Brien CJ, McNeil EB, McMahon JD, Pathak I, Lauer CS. Incidence of cervical node involvement in metastatic cutaneous malignancy involving the parotid gland. Head Neck. 2001;23(9):744–8.
26. Villarreal IM, Arellano B, Sáenz J, Martin L, Castello JR, García-Berrocal JR. Primary malignant parotid melanoma: searching for a rare entity. Int J Otolaryngol Head Neck Surg. 2014;3(5):228.
27. Balm AJ, Kroon BB, Hilgers FJ, Jonk A, Mooi WJ. Lymph node metastases in the neck and parotid gland from an unknown primary melanoma. Clin Otolaryngol Allied Sci. 1994;19(2):161–5.
28. Nasri S, Namazie A, Dulguerov P, Mickel R. Malignant melanoma of cervical and parotid lymph nodes with an unknown primary site. Laryngoscope. 1994;104(10):1194–8.
29. O'Brien CJ, Petersen-Schaefer K, Stevens GN, Bass PC, Tew P, Gebski VJ, et al. Adjuvant radiotherapy following neck dissection and parotidectomy for metastatic malignant melanoma. Head Neck. 1997;19(7):589–94.
30. Santini H, Byers RM, Wolf PF. Melanoma metastatic to cervical and parotid nodes from an unknown primary site. Am J Surg. 1985;150:510–2.
31. Agha RA, Borrelli MR, Farwana R, Koshy K, Fowler A, Orgill DP. The SCARE 2018 statement: updating consensus Surgical CAse REport (SCARE) guidelines. Int J Surg. 2018;60:132–6.
32. Chaouki A, Berrada O, Najib Z, Oukessou Y, Abada RA, Rouadi S, et al. Primary malignant melanoma of the parotid gland: a case report and review of literature. Ann Med Surg. 2020;60:660–3.

Cancer Metastatic to the Parotid Gland 17

17.1 Epidemiology

Carcinoma metastatic to the parotid gland is a region-specific disorder where the relative incidence of the various histopathological types is dependent on geographical location. In Australia, metastatic cutaneous squamous cell carcinoma (SCC) is the most common malignancy seen in the parotid, including primary cancer of the parotid gland [1]. This contrasts with North America and Europe where primary cancer of the parotid gland is more frequent [2]. Although metastatic cancer to the parotid is relatively infrequent worldwide, in 40% of patients with this disease it will be the first manifestation of skin cancer [3]. Variable proportion of metastatic parotid malignancies has been reported, including 25% in the United States, 45% in Germany, and the highest (78%) in Australia [4].

Franzen et al. (2017) retrospectively examined 772 consecutive cases of parotid surgery in a university hospital between 1975 and 2015 and assessed changes in incidence and management over four decades. They diagnosed 683 parotid tumors of which 15.8% (n = 108) were malignant; 44% (n = 48) of all malignant lesions were metastases. The incidence of malignant tumors rose from 8% in the first decade to 14% in the second, 17% in the third, and 21% in the fourth. Most frequent tumors were metastases of SCC (79%), and the majority of these lesions (87%) arose from above the clavicle, with 30 primary tumors in the skin [5].

Between January 2003 and December 2018, 90 patients were reported by He et al. (2023) to have parotid metastases, including 60 men and 30 women (2:1), and the mean age of the patients was 65 ± 14 years (range: 27–96 years) [4].

© The Author(s), under exclusive license to Springer Nature Switzerland AG 2024

M. Sakr, *Surgery of the Salivary Glands*,
https://doi.org/10.1007/978-3-031-82069-4_17

17.2 Pathology of Cancer Metastatic to the Parotid Gland

Various histopathological types of primary malignant tumors have been implicated in the development of metastases to the parotid gland (Table 17.1). The most common is head and neck cutaneous and mucosal SCC and malignant melanoma (MM), followed by other primaries in solid organs such as the kidneys and breasts, as well as lymphoproliferative disorders (lymphoma). In 2023, He et al. reported the clinical and pathological data of 90 patients with parotid gland metastases. These originated from the head and neck in 86 patients (95.6%), and from non-head and neck primaries via hematogenous spread in only 4 (4.4%). Oral cavity primary malignancies were the cause in 30 patients and the eyelid in 21 [4].

17.2.1 Squamous Cell Carcinoma (SCC)

It is estimated that 5% of cutaneous SCCs metastasize to regional lymph node (LN) basins, including the parotid [6]. Current evidence suggests that between 25% and 50% of patients with nodal metastases to the parotid from SCC will also have cervical nodal disease [6]. Clinicopathological features that increase the risk of nodal metastases are listed in Table 17.2. In high-risk SCC, the associated risk of nodal metastases is up to 20% [7]. Overall mortality of cutaneous SCC is low at 3.4%, but increases substantially in patients with regional metastatic disease [8]. In a

Table 17.1 Pathology of metastatic cancer to the parotid gland

Cutaneous and mucosal primary	Solid organ	Lymphoproliferative
Squamous cell carcinoma	Renal cell carcinoma	Lymphoma
Melanoma	Lung cancer	
Merkel cell carcinoma	Other rare malignancies	
Sino-nasal carcinoma		
Nasopharyngeal carcinoma		
Other rare cancers (dermatofibrosarcoma, metastatic basal cell carcinoma)		

Table 17.2 Clinicopathological features that increase risk of nodal metastases

High-risk squamous cell carcinoma
Size >2 cm
Invasion into subcutaneous fat
Depth > 5 mm
Poorly differentiated tumors
Perineural invasion
Lympho-vascular invasion
Site: ear or lip
Incomplete excision
Local recurrence
Immunosuppression

multicenter study of 325 patients with metastatic SCC to the parotid, there was a 27% rate of synchronous neck disease and overall survival was 72% at 5 years [8]. Locoregional control in metastatic SCC of the parotid is high with the exception of patients with highly invasive disease (bone or other deep structures) or extensive perineural invasion. Cutaneous SCC has a high predilection for perineural invasion, which may affect both motor (facial) and sensory (auriculotemporal nerve [ATN], CN-V) nerve within the parotid and surrounding tissue.

17.2.2 Malignant Melanoma (MM)

"Primary" MMs of the parotid gland are extremely rare. Some melanomas may exhibit no or low pigmentation, known as "amelanotic melanomas." Malignant melanomas of the parotid gland are largely "metastatic," with primaries usually originating in the skin of the head and neck [9]. Nevertheless, some cutaneous MMs may metastasize and subsequently regress. Therefore, it may not be possible to observe a metastatic MM and its primary melanoma simultaneously. The investigation of a patient's old photographs may help in the detection of preexisting and regressed pigmented lesions in the facial and neck regions.

About 10–20% of cutaneous MMs arise in the head and neck [10] and nearly 20% of patients develop regional metastases [11]. Patients with clinically palpable metastatic MM in the parotid have a high rate of occult neck disease, ranging from 28% to 58% [6, 12, 13]. Metastasis from head and neck MM to the parotid results in areas of lymphatic drainage of parotid LN, which include forehead, anterior frontal and temporal regions, eyelids, conjunctiva, lacrimal gland, anterior ear, cranial vault, and posterior cheek regions [14]. The overall mortality of cutaneous head and neck MM is high, with 10-year survival rates ranging from 45% to 72%. This falls to 34% for patients with proven nodal metastases and further decreases with increasing number of positive nodes [15, 16]. The clinicopathological features predictive of nodal disease and mortality from malignant melanoma are listed in Table 17.3.

17.2.3 Other Primacy Malignancies

Merkel cell carcinoma is a rare, aggressive neuroendocrine cutaneous malignancy. The largest reported series of head and neck Merkel cell carcinoma showed nodal metastases in 43.6% of patients (48/110). Locoregional control is most effective

Table 17.3 Clinicopathological features that predict nodal disease and metastases

High-risk cutaneous melanoma
Tumor thickness (>1 mm)
Tumor ulceration
Site (scalp)
Level of invasion (Clark level IV)
Gender (male)
Age (increasing age)

when surgery is combined with radiotherapy (RT) [17, 18]. There is no evidence to support routine use of adjuvant chemotherapy [19].

Mucosal cancer, including SCC, infrequently metastasizes to the parotid gland. Nasopharyngeal cancer has been reported as a primary site [20] and extensive sinonasal cancers involving the subcutaneous tissue of the cheek and orbit may disseminate to the parotid gland. Advanced oropharyngeal cancers may also invade directly through the parapharyngeal space to involve the parotid gland. Renal cell carcinoma is the most common solid organ cancer to metastasize to the parotid [21].

17.3 Pathophysiology

The parotid tissue is an uncommon location for metastases. Most metastases to the parotid region originate from the head and neck cutaneous SCC and malignant melanoma (MM) [22–24]. This can be attributed to the rich intercommunicating lymphatic vessels that drain from the scalp and face to the parotid, and make the parotid tail work as the "basin" for head and neck lymphatic system [25]. Cancer cells migrate to the parotid and peri-parotid lymph nodes (LNs) via the adjacent lymphatic system and form metastatic lesions in the parotid. More than 75% of parotid metastases are believed to spread into the intra-parotid LNs of a nearby malignancy. The parotid gland is known to function as a filtering center for lymphatic drainage in the head and neck region [26]. Some studies have reported facial melanomas with metastasis to the parotids and ipsilateral levels I–IV [27].

Meanwhile, malignancies from the non-head and neck region, such as the breast, prostate, and kidney, can also "hematogenously" metastasize to the parotid gland either via the thoracic duct to the LNs or via Batson's paraspinal venous plexus to the parenchymal gland [28].

17.4 Clinical Assessment

17.4.1 History-Taking

For patients with cancer metastatic to the parotid, a thorough history of previous cutaneous surgery is essential. Pathology reports should be obtained and the original pathology slides may need to be reviewed by an experienced pathologist to confirm unusual primary lesions such as poorly differentiated SCC, Merkel cell carcinoma, spindle cell tumors, and even melanoma. Intra-parotid metastases usually occur 1–3 years after surgical removal of the primary skin SCC [5, 29, 30], while concomitant parotid metastases are present in approximately 20% of subjects [31].

Approximately, 10–35% of MMs show regression and may even disappear completely. Regressed melanomas can be categorized into two groups: lentigo maligna melanoma and superficial spreading melanoma. Some studies suggest that regressed malignant melanomas are more likely to metastasize [32].

17.4.2 Physical Examination

All potential cutaneous and mucosal sites need examination. This includes fiber-optic examination of the nasopharynx and oropharynx (panendoscopy). Particular care is necessary when inspecting potential cutaneous sites since cutaneous malignancies may be small relative to the bulk of regional disease. In conspicuous lesions hiding in the hair, behind the ear, nasal vestibule, and in the external auditory canal are easily overlooked. "Nonpigmented" nodular lesions are difficult to diagnose and may represent amelanotic melanoma or Merkel cell cancer.

Physical examination should include assessment of fixation, parapharyngeal extension, synchronous cervical disease, and facial nerve grading as standard. The great auricular nerve (GAN) may be involved directly causing ear lobule/angle of mandible dysesthesia and the trigeminal nerve may be involved via branches of the auriculotemporal nerve (ATN). Hence, sensation in the distribution of both these nerves should also be assessed.

Patients with secondary parotid cancer are usually older and most frequently male as compared to those with primary parotid cancer [23, 33]. The prevalence of males is due to the higher incidence of skin SCC in this gender [34]. Likewise, in 2023, Pecorari et al. [31] who reported that all secondary tumors in their study were intra-parotid metastases from cutaneous SCC found that subjects with secondary tumors were older than those with primary parotid cancer (mean age 80.60 ± 6.77 years versus 61.17 ± 17.32 years, respectively, $p < 0.001$). No statistically significant difference was observed for other clinical features. Maximum dimension of the parotid lesion was lower for primary tumors (2.12 ± 1.33 cm and 3.79 ± 1.19 cm, respectively, $p < 0.001$).

17.5 Work-Up (Investigations)

17.5.1 Imaging

17.5.1.1 Computed Tomography (CT) Scan

Imaging with high resolution multi-slice computed tomography (CT) scanning with intravenous contrast is recommended in patients with and without fixed disease. This allows assessment of the parotid and surrounding structures, including the parapharyngeal space. Bone windows are used to determine cranial or mandibular invasion. The CT scan examines both potential mucosal sites and the neck to detect subclinical synchronous nodal disease. A dedicated temporal bone CT is obtained where there is fixation or facial nerve deficit.

17.5.1.2 Magnetic Resonance Imaging (MRI)

Magnetic resonance imaging (MRI) can be substituted for CT scan and is particularly useful in patients with parapharyngeal extension and neurotrophic cancers and is equivalent to CT scan in cervical LN assessment. However, it is more expensive: less readily obtained, poorly tolerated by patients, and provides poor cortical bone definition.

17.5.1.3 Ultrasonography (US)

Ultrasonography (US) has been reported to be highly specific and sensitive for cervical node disease in selected series [35] and can be combined with US-guided fine needle aspiration (FNA). However, it is inferior to CT scan or MRI in patients with extensive parotid disease, in particular those with facial paresis.

17.5.1.4 Positron Emission Tomography (PET)

There are few data examining the role of positron emission tomography (PET) in metastatic cancer to the parotid gland. PET or PET-CT is being used more frequently as a standard investigation and has a role in the assessment of regional and distant metastatic disease. PET is more likely to be positive in patients with melanoma where distant disease is common. 18F-FDGPET is superior to other modalities in the detection of distant metastases and in patients with recurrent disease where the sensitivity and specificity ranges from 70% to 100% [36]. However, PET is relatively insensitive (0–40%) in the detection of regional metastases in patients with early-stage disease when compared to sentinel node biopsy.

Detection of distant metastases has both prognostic and therapeutic value, since isolated distant disease is amenable to surgical resection [37]. Regardless of distant disease status, locoregional control is of value for symptomatic relief since the rate of disease progression is unpredictable.

17.5.1.5 Biopsy

Fine needle aspiration biopsy (FNAB) is recommended for all parotid tumors and is useful for planning the extent of surgery and stratifying urgency for intervention [38]. All clinically malignant parotid tumors need cytological confirmation, and FNA is reliable in the detection of metastatic SCC [39].

A study by Pytynia et al. (2008) proposed that an accurate method of determining the lymphatic drainage pattern of the cutaneous melanoma is sentinel node biopsy. The first echelon of drainage for cutaneous malignant melanoma of the scalp or face is to intra-parotid LNs. Sentinel node biopsy is the proposed procedure for identification of these first echelon nodes, through a combination of lymphoscintigraphy and injection of methylene blue dye. The direction of drainage is determined by dynamic imaging and mapped by lymphoscintigraphy [40].

17.6 Staging

17.6.1 Staging of Cutaneous Metastatic SCC

The current staging system stages all patients with cutaneous squamous cell carcinoma (SCC) and nodal metastases to the parotid as N1 regardless of the extent or volume of disease [41]. O'Brien [42] has proposed a revised staging system for parotid involvement (Table 17.4) to achieve a cancer stage that was more related to prognosis.

Table 17.4 Revised staging of metastatic squamous cell carcinoma [42]

Parotid		Neck	
P0	No clinical parotid disease	N0	No clinical neck disease
P1	Metastatic node <3 cm	N1	Single ipsilateral neck node <3 cm
P2	Metastatic node >3 cm but <6 cm Multiple parotid nodes	N2	Single node >3 cm Multiple or contralateral neck nodes
P3	Metastatic node >6 cm Multiple or contralateral neck nodes		

Table 17.5 AJCC staging of cutaneous melanoma

Tumor		Node		Metastasis	
T1	<1 mm thick	N1	Single nodal or parotid metastases	M1a	Distant skin, SC, or distant nodal mets
T2	1–2 mm thick	N2	2–3 nodal metastases	M1b	Lung metastases
T3	2–4 mm thick	N3	>3 nodal metastases	M1c	Other visceral mets or any distant mets with ↑ LDH
T4	>4 mm thick				
a	No ulceration	a	Micro-nodal metastases		
b	Ulceration	b	Macro-nodal metastases		

SC subcutaneous, *LDH* lactic dehydrogenase

This system classified metastatic SSC according to the number and size of the parotid (P) and cervical (N) metastases, and the facial nerve/skull base involvement.

17.6.2 Staging of Melanoma

Breslow thickness (in millimeters) is the most important prognostic indicator of MM. Currently, Breslow depth is included in the AJCC staging guidelines of melanoma [43]. Staging of melanoma is listed in Table 17.5. Parotid metastases are included as regional nodal disease. There is no separate staging for parotid disease.

17.7 Surgery for Cancer Metastatic to the Parotid Gland

17.7.1 Ablative Surgery

The extent of surgery in both the parotid and the neck is an ongoing area of controversy as shown in Table 17.6. Current evidence does not indicate that more extensive surgery is associated with either improved disease control or survival [44]. This may reflect the frequent use of adjuvant radiotherapy (RT) [45], which is effective

Table 17.6 Ablative surgery for metastatic cancer to the parotid gland

Parotidectomy	Neck dissection (elective and therapeutic)
Limited parotidectomy	Selective neck dissection
Superficial parotidectomy	Comprehensive neck dissection
Total parotidectomy with nerve preservation	Extended neck dissection
Radical parotidectomy	
Extended parotidectomy	
Skin resection	
Mandibulectomy	
Lateral temporal bone resection	

for control of microscopic nodal disease in both the parotid and neck. This is applicable for both SCC and MM, although melanoma traditionally is considered to be radioresistant [46].

17.7.2 Superficial Parotidectomy

Superficial parotidectomy is the standard procedure. There is no evidence that a limited or more aggressive approach is preferable. Parotid lymphatics and LNs are present throughout the parotid substance, both superficial and deep. However, superficial LNs are more numerous and more likely to harbor metastatic disease. McKean et al. [47] reported up to 22 nodes in the superficial lobe compared with <5 in the deep lobe.

17.7.3 Total Parotidectomy/Radical Parotidectomy

Total parotidectomy with facial nerve sacrifice (radical parotidectomy) is highly morbid with aesthetic and functional consequences (Table 17.7) and current trends are toward more conservative surgery where possible [48]. However, the deep lobe should be removed (total parotidectomy) if the tumor is located or involved in the deep lobe or if the tumor has spread to superficial intra-parotid or cervical LNs and in case of high-grade cancer [49]. More extensive dissection is indicated in invasive parotid metastases or recurrent disease, and may necessitate facial nerve sacrifice with or without temporal bone resection and resection of adjacent structures involved by the cancer such as skin, mandible, and skull base.

17.7.4 Resection of Skin

Resection of skin is relatively simple and can be restored using a number of standard techniques such as a cervicofacial rotation flap [50] or free flap where indicated. In more advanced disease, the likelihood of local control needs to be balanced against the morbidity of surgery. As more radical procedures are undertaken, the

Table 17.7 Functional and aesthetic consequences of radical parotidectomy

Functional consequences	Aesthetic consequences
Visual disturbance (brow ptosis—frontalis)	Contour defect
Corneal exposure and ulceration (orbicularis oculi)	Brow ptosis
Oral incompetence (orbicularis oris, depressor anguli oris, depressor labii inferioris)	Eyelid paralysis
	Ectropion
Speech impairment (buccinator, orbicularis oris)	Nasal collapse
	Upper lip asymmetry
	Lower lip asymmetry

rate of positive surgical margins also increases [51]. Hence, more radical surgery does not necessarily confer disease control. An argument can be made for more radical parotid surgery where RT is contraindicated, such as recurrent disease, or where RT may be avoided by adequate surgery, such as single small nodal metastasis with no extracapsular extension or neck disease.

17.7.5 Neck Dissection

Neck dissection may be combined with parotidectomy as an elective or therapeutic procedure. Therapeutic neck dissection is appropriate to maximize disease control [51] and should incorporate all at risk nodal basins. This depends on the location of the primary and the extent of nodal metastasis. In general, neck dissection of levels I–V is standard; however, in low volume neck disease, a selective dissection of levels II–V is appropriate for posterior primaries or levels I–IV for anterior lesions [42]. Resection of non-lymphatic structures, such as the sternocleidomastoid muscle (SCM) and internal jugular vein (IJV), is indicated where disease is suspected to involve them directly.

Consideration needs to be given to nodal groups that are not traditionally encompassed in neck dissection for mucosal SCC. This includes external jugular LNs, which are at high risk for any malignancy involving the parotid and should be included routinely [12]. Level IIb should be routinely dissected. Occipital and retroauricular LNs are at high risk in posterior scalp malignancy and lesions involving the pinna. Peri-facial LNs are at high risk in cheek, lip, and nasal primaries.

Elective neck dissection has not been shown to confer improved disease control or survival despite the substantial rate of occult neck disease. Presumably, this is due to the frequent use of adjuvant RT [6, 52]. Selective neck dissection of levels II and III may be appropriate as a staging procedure in selected patients; however, this depends on the location of the primary. In patients where adjuvant RT is not possible, a more comprehensive neck dissection should be combined with parotidectomy.

Elective neck dissection in patients with cervical disease is not generally employed. However parotid nodes are frequently involved in patients with cervical disease from primary cutaneous malignancy, in particular primary melanoma and

Table 17.8 Complications of parotid surgery for metastatic malignancy

Facial nerve paralysis or paresis—increased in malignancy
Lip depressor weakness—increased when combined with neck dissection
Great auricular neuroma or dysesthesia
Frey's syndrome
Sialocele
Salivary fistula
Wound infection or necrosis

SCC of the ear, face, and anterior scalp. Shah et al. [53] reported that 33 of 57 elective parotidectomies for neck disease had melanoma involving the parotid and adjacent nodes. This is supported by the high rate of sentinel nodes biopsies occurring in the peri-parotid region [54]; however, other series have not replicated this high rate of positive metastases to the parotid [55]. There may be a role for lymphoscintigraphy to determine whether the parotid contains any sentinel nodes for the primary. Complications of parotid surgery for metastatic malignancy are summarized in Table 17.8.

17.7.6 Reconstructive Surgery

Reconstruction following radical parotid surgery is frequently required. The most common structure sacrificed is the "skin" followed by the "facial nerve." Cutaneous reconstruction depends on the extent of cutaneous defect, type of neck dissection, other structures sacrificed, and whether RT has been given previously. In moderate-sized defects, a cervicofacial rotation flap [56] is an excellent method, particularly for elderly patients not concerned about the contour deformity that arises from extensive parotid surgery. The cervicofacial flap [56] is favored in patients where the facial artery is preserved due to its reliability and lesser dissection. The submental island flap is also very useful due to the excellent color match with the cheek [57]; however, it requires planning with regards to incisions and the pedicle needs to be carefully dissected.

Many patients are best managed with free tissue reconstruction, in particular, those with prior irradiation or extensive cutaneous defects where a cervicofacial flap is insufficient or likely to fail. This is important in patients with exposed bone and where postoperative RT or chemoradiation is planned and marginal flap necrosis will delay the onset of RT, which should be commenced within 6 weeks after surgery. Reliable free flaps such as the radial forearm flap have a low failure rate of <1% [58, 59]. However, morbidity of this donor site is substantial if large flaps are harvested, and the color match with the head and neck is poor. Color match is important in the face and is best obtained by using flaps located in proximity of the head and neck.

Following radical parotidectomy, there are several components to optimal reconstruction, which can be performed primarily (ideally) or secondarily. These include the cutaneous defect (if present), contour defect, bone defect, facial nerve, brow ptosis, eyelid paralysis, ectropion, and lip paralysis. There are many options in reconstructing these complex problems depending on individual or institutional expertise.

17.7.7 Facial Nerve

Where the proximal facial nerve can be accessed in the temporal bone without disease, a cable nerve graft can be performed using sural, saphenous, or antebrachial cutaneous nerve. Facial nerve function following neurorrhaphy is unlikely to be better than a House–Brackmann grade-III (moderate dysfunction) and some synkines is unavoidable.

17.7.8 Contour

The contour defect is well corrected using a de-epithelialized fascio-cutaneous free flap such as para-scapular or anterolateral thigh. A temporoparietal flap can be used as a pedicled flap for small defects. Muscle flaps should be avoided since the ultimate volume is unpredictable.

17.7.9 Static Reconstruction

The upper eyelid is managed using a gold weight and the lower eyelid using a tendon sling to prevent ectropion with or without canthoplasty. Using this combination a lateral tarsorrhaphy, which is aesthetically inferior, is usually unnecessary. The oral commissure is lateralized using a woven tendon sling (plantaris or palmaris). This is favored over fascia lata, which tends to stretch over time. The commissure and lip is suspended from the zygomatic arch using multiple passes to recreate the appropriate vectors. The lip is overcorrected initially (lateralized) to create a more natural lip position in the long-term. The lower lip can be everted and depressed using the anterior belly of digastric as a semi-dynamic reconstruction [60].

All of the above-mentioned components are undertaken primarily. Other minor corrections can be performed secondarily such as a brow lift, revision canthoplasty, or tarsorrhaphy and flap revision to remove excess bulk.

17.7.10 Complications to Avoid

17.7.10.1 Wound-Related

Skin flap necrosis due to inappropriate incision design or flap elevation.

Unreliable local or regional skin flaps in patients who require timely adjuvant RT.

17.7.10.2 Tumor-Related

Inappropriate surgery due to inadequate preoperative investigation (e.g., excision biopsy by neglecting to perform an FNA or omitting neck dissection in patients with concomitant neck disease who did not undergo imaging).

Tumor rupture due to dissection of tumor on facial nerve or excessive retraction.

Local tumor recurrence due to not performing a lateral temporal bone resection where indicated.

17.7.10.3 Gland-Related

Salivary fistula and sialocele due to preserving parotid tissue when the parotid duct is ligated.

17.7.10.4 Nerve-Related

Facial nerve injury.

Frey's syndrome (gustatory sweating).

Great auricular nerve neuroma.

17.8 Adjuvant Therapy for Cancer Metastatic to the Parotid Gland

17.8.1 Squamous Cell Carcinoma (SCC)

Adjuvant therapy for metastatic SCC to the parotid includes radiotherapy (RT) and concurrent chemotherapy.

17.8.2 Radiotherapy (RT)

Traditionally, the parotid was regarded as "radioresistant" and there is limited data regarding "primary" RT treatment for metastases to the parotid. One such study [61] reported a 2-year local control rate of 50% in 14 patients. After 5 years the figure dropped to 20%. The sole use of RT should be restricted to those in whom surgery is not possible. In patients with bulky disease, RT is likely to be palliative only.

Currently, in patients with metastatic SCC to the parotid, the vast majority will undergo "adjuvant" RT. Local failure rates with combined therapy are approximately one-third of those with surgery alone. Guillamondegui et al. [62] showed a reduction in local recurrence from 30% to 9% and Taylor et al. [63] from 27% to 11%. Various radiation schedules have been used for metastatic cancer to the parotid; however, standard fractionation has been advocated [64] as described in Table 17.9.

Data from M.D. Anderson demonstrated that for high-risk SCC of the head and neck, increasing the postoperative dose beyond a biologically effective dose of

Table 17.9 Standard radiation therapy for metastatic SCC to the parotid gland

Fractionation	Radiation schedule
Clinical target volume (CTV)	The volume including the site of resected gross disease, surgical bed/scar, and next echelon of draining lymph nodes with a minimum of a 0.5-cm margin in all dimensions
Planning target volume	Defined as CTV 1 with a minimum of a 1.0-cm margin in all dimensions
Radiation dose	50–60 Gy in 25–30 fractions, 2 Gy per fraction, 5 fractions per week

60 Gy increased the risk of late complications, with no increased benefit in locoregional control [65]. Where parotid metastases have occurred 12 months or more following definitive treatment to the index lesion, consideration should be given to including the primary site and intervening dermal lymphatics in the treatment volume.

17.8.3 Concurrent Chemoradiotherapy

Concurrent chemoradiotherapy is superior over RT alone for advanced mucosal SCC. Recent data have also demonstrated improved locoregional control and survival with concurrent chemoradiation in the postoperative setting [44] for high-risk mucosal cancer, albeit at the cost of a substantial increase in both early and late adverse effects. At present, there is no compelling data to suggest that the same benefit is present in cutaneous SCC and this is the subject of several trials [66].

Current therapeutic agents have included cisplatin and fluorouracil in conjunction with RT. Brizel et al. [67] reported on hyper-fractionated irradiation with or without concurrent chemotherapy. For mucosal cancer, cisplatin was given for 5 days at a dose of 12 mg/m^2 of body surface area/day and 600 mg/m^2 of fluorouracil/day during weeks 1 and 6 of irradiation. Two cycles of cisplatin and fluorouracil were given after the completion of RT. Locoregional control at 3 years was 70% in the combined group and 44% with RT alone. There was no statistically significant difference in overall complications of the two groups, although the rates of nasogastric feeding or gastrostomy feeding tubes were higher in the combined treatment group.

More recently, trials using carboplatin rather than cisplatin have been used in an attempt to minimize the toxicity, particularly for elderly patients who are most commonly affected by advanced cutaneous disease. For the PostOperative Skin Trial (POST) trial, carboplatin is given once per week for 6 weeks, 30 min prior to RT. The dose is calculated according to Calvert formula and based on glomerular filtration rate (GFR). Hermann and Christiansen (2018) reported that carboplatin does not increase the effectiveness of adjuvant RT in advanced cutaneous squamous cell carcinoma of the head and neck region [68].

17.8.4 Malignant Melanoma (MM)

Adjuvant therapy for metastatic melanoma includes radiotherapy (RT) and chemo-immunotherapy.

17.8.5 Radiotherapy (RT)

After parotidectomy, postoperative RT is indicated for patients with MM that has metastasized to cervical LNs and to the parotid gland [69]. Patients receiving RT have improved locoregional control, but not overall survival [70]. Despite the high incidence of distant metastases, locoregional control is a vital component in the management plan. Parotid metastases fall into the high-risk group for regional relapse; these include >1 parotid node, >2 neck or axillary nodes, and >3 groin nodes.

Hypo-fractionated schedules are thought to improve the therapeutic ratio for melanoma [71]. In one such study [35], indications for RT included microscopically involved or close surgically resected margins, neurotrophic desmoplastic histopathology, perineural spread, or tumor satellites. With a starting date for the majority of patients <6 weeks post-surgery, they received 30–36 Gy in 6 fractions over 18 days. Parotid and neck LN fields were treated with direct electron fields or photon wedge pair fields. In-field recurrence was the only significant predictor of survival.

A randomized clinical trial [72] proposed a schedule of 48 Gy delivered in 20 fractions over 30 days. Outcome measures included regional metastasis, as well as morbidity, patterns of relapse, and overall survival.

On the other hand, Bron et al. [73] and Tsutsumida et al. [74] reported that RT and chemotherapy are considered to be of low value and recommended that adjuvant RT is not part of a regular treatment protocol, but it is recommended for only high-risk patients, based on grade, stage, and margin of excision; the aim is to improve local control of the disease.

17.8.6 Chemo-Immunotherapy

The role of chemotherapeutic agents and immunotherapy has yet to be established in the treatment of locally advanced or metastatic melanoma. It is proposed that interferon-alfa (IFN-α) may interfere with the growth of tumor cells [68].

Whether there may be a synergistic role with IFN-α and interleukin-2 (IL-2) in combination has been investigated. IL-2 is thought to stimulate white blood cells to mount a response to melanoma cells. It is hoped that colony-stimulating factors such as sargramostim may result in increased immune cells in bone marrow and peripheral blood, and also the use of vaccines has been postulated.

17.9 Prognosis

Because of the rarity and heterogeneity of parotid tumors, the prognosis is difficult to assess [31]. Compared to primary malignancy, metastatic parotid disease is associated with a higher rate of local recurrence and poorer overall survival. Patients with oral SCC and meibomian adenocarcinoma with parotid metastatic disease have poorer overall survival than other primaries [4, 5, 31].

Recently, Jering et al. (2022) reported a 5-year cancer-specific survival of 87.3% among patients with primary parotid cancer and 54.5% among patients with metastatic parotid cancer from cutaneous SCC [75]. Likewise, Meyer et al. (2021) found a higher 5-year overall survival in subjects with primary parotid cancer as compared to metastatic disease (77.2% vs. 32.6%) [23]. However, all patients with intraparotid metastases from cutaneous SCC included in such a study had neck node involvement. Including subjects without neck metastases can allow us to perform a more realistic survival analysis. Girardi et al. (2021) showed that patients presenting with "isolated" parotid metastasis during follow-up had better disease-specific survival than those with neck metastasis or both [76]. Indeed, prognostic factors in secondary parotid cancer include immunodepression, age, positive margins, facial nerve involvement, and neck nodes [77, 78].

References

1. Bron L, Traynor MD, McNeil E, O'Brien CJ. Primary and metastatic cancer of the parotid: comparison of clinical behavior in 232 cases. Laryngoscope. 2003;113:1070–5.
2. Woods JE, Chong GC, Beahrs OH. Experience with 1360 primary parotid tumors. Am J Surg. 1975;130:460–2.
3. Malata C, Camilleri I, McLean N, Piggott T, Soames J. Metastatic tumors of the parotid gland. Br J Oral Maxillofac Surg. 1998;36:190–5.
4. He A, Lei H, Li H, Li X, Yang Y, Wang Y, et al. Metastatic parotid gland malignancy: a preliminary study in an eastern Chinese population. J Stomatol Oral Maaxillofac Surg. 2023;124(2):101309.
5. Franzen A, Buchali A, Lieder A. The rising incidence of parotid metastases: our experience from four decades of parotid gland surgery. Acta Otorhinolaryngol Ital. 2017;37(4):264–9.
6. O'Brien CJ, McNeil ED, McMahon JD. Incidence of cervical node involvement in metastatic cutaneous malignancy involving the parotid gland. Head Neck. 2001;23(9):744–8.
7. Audet N, Palme C, Gullane P, Gilbert R, Brown D, Irish J, Neligan P. Cutaneous metastatic squamous cell carcinoma to the parotid gland: analysis and outcome. Head Neck. 2004;26:727–32.
8. Joseph MG, Zulueta WP, Kennedy PJ. Squamous cell carcinoma of the skin of the trunk and limbs: the incidence of metastases and their outcome. Aust N Z J Surg. 1992;62(9):697–701.
9. Gao N, Li L-J, Li Y, Wang L. Primary amelanotic malignant melanoma of the parotid gland: a case report. J Int Med Res. 2008;36(6):1435–9.
10. Myers JN. Value of neck dissection in the treatment of patients with intermediate–thickness cutaneous malignant melanoma of the head and neck. Arch Otolaryngol Head Neck Surg. 1999;125:110–5.
11. Mack L, McKinnon G. Controversies in the management of metastatic melanoma to regional lymphatic basins. J Surg Oncol. 2004;86:189–99.
12. Barr LC, Skene AI, Fish S, Thomas JM. Superficial parotidectomy in the treatment of cutaneous melanoma of the head and neck. Br J Surg. 1994;81:64–5.

13. Caldwell CB, Spiro RH. The role of parotidectomy in the treatment of cutaneous head and neck melanoma. Am J Surg. 1988;156:318–22.
14. Storm FK, Eilber FR, Sparks FC, Morton DL. A prospective study of parotid metastases from head and neck cancer. Am J Surg. 1977;134:115–9.
15. O'Brien CJ, Petersen-Schaefer K, Ruark D, Menzie SJ, Harrison RI. Radical, modified and selective neck dissection for cutaneous malignant melanoma. Head Neck. 1995;17:232–41.
16. O'Brien CJ, Coates AS, Petersen-Schaefer K, Shannon K, Thompson JF, et al. Experience with 998 cutaneous melanomas of the head and neck. Cancer. 1993;71:751–8.
17. Clark JR, Veness MJ, Gilbert R, O'Brien CJ, Gullane PJ. Merkel cell carcinoma of the head and neck: is adjuvant radiotherapy necessary? Head Neck. 2007;29(3):249–57.
18. Veness MJ, Morgan GJ, Gebski V. Adjuvant locoregional radiotherapy as best practice in patients with Merkel cell carcinoma of the head and neck. Head Neck. 2005;27(3):208–16.
19. Poulsen M. Merkel-cell carcinoma of the skin. Lancet Oncol. 2004;5:593–9.
20. King AD, Ahuja AT, Leung SF, Lam WW, Teo P, Chan YL, et al. Neck node metastases from nasopharyngeal carcinoma: MR imaging patterns of disease. Head Neck. 2000;22(3):275–81.
21. Coppa GF, Oszczakiewicz M. Parotid gland metastasis from renal carcinoma. Int Surg. 1990;75(3):198–202.
22. Xiao M, Song H, You Y, Liu M, Yang X, Wang Y. Metastasis of oral squamous cell carcinoma to the parotid lymph nodes. Int J Oral Maxillofac Surg. 2021;50(4):437–43.
23. Mayer M, Thoelken R, Jering M, Märkl B, Zenk J. Metastases of cutaneous squamous cell carcinoma seem to be the most frequent malignancies in the parotid gland: a hospital-based study from a Salivary Gland Center. Head Neck Pathol. 2021;15(3):843–51.
24. Liang ZP, Xu SE, Jiang L, Zhao C, Sun XQ, Qin G. Scalp junctional nevus with malignant transformation (melanoma) metastatic to parotid lymph node region, cervical lymph nodes and the back: a case report and review of literature. Int J Clin Exp Pathol. 2015;8(1):954–9.
25. O'Brien CJ. The parotid gland as a metastatic basin for cutaneous cancer. Arch Otolaryngol Head Neck Surg. 2005;131(7):551–5.
26. Elshenawy Y, Youngberg G, Al-Abbadi MA. Unusual clinical presentation of cutaneous malignant melanoma metastatic to the parotid gland; initially discovered by fine needle aspiration: case report and review of literature. Diagn Cytopathol. 2011;39(5):373–6.
27. Ettl T, Irga S, Müller S, Rohrmeier C, Reichert TE, Schreml S, et al. Value of anatomic site, histology and clinicopathological parameters for prediction of lymph node metastasis and overall survival in head and neck melanomas. J Craniofac Surg. 2014;42(5):e252–8.
28. Rocca BJ, Gini A, Calandra C, Ginori A, Crivelli F. Parotid metastasis of renal cell carcinoma, mimicking primary clear cell oncocytoma: report of a case and brief review of the literature. Pathologica. 2017;109(4):384–8.
29. Barzilai G, Greenberg E, Cohen-Kerem R, Doweck I. Pattern of regional metastases from cutaneous squamous cell carcinoma of the head and neck. Otolaryngol Head Neck Surg. 2005;132:852–6.
30. Czerwonka L, De Santis RJ, Horowitz G, Hong M, Orsini M, Enepekides D, et al. Staging cutaneous squamous cell carcinoma metastases to the parotid gland. Laryngoscope. 2017;127:2063–9.
31. Pecorari G, Pizzo C, Briguglio M, Cravero E, Riva G. Primary and secondary tumors of the parotid gland: clinical features and prognosis. Cancers (Basel). 2023;15(4):1293.
32. Botella-Estrada R, Traves V, Requena C, Guillen-Barona C, Nagore E. Correlation of histologic regression in primary melanoma with sentinel node status. JAMA Dermatol. 2014;150(8):828–35.
33. Meyer MF, Wolber P, Arolt C, Wessel M, Quaas A, Lang S, et al. Survival after parotid gland metastases of cutaneous squamous cell carcinoma of the head and neck. Oral Maxillofac Surg. 2021;25:383–8.
34. O'Hara J, Ferlito A, Takes RP, Rinaldo A, Strojan P, Shaha AR, et al. Cutaneous squamous cell carcinoma of the head and neck metastasizing to the parotid gland—a review of current recommendations. Head Neck. 2011;33:1789–95.

35. Stuckensen T, Kovacs AF, Adams S, Baum RP. Staging of the neck in patients with oral cavity squamous cell carcinomas: a prospective comparison of PET, ultrasound, CT and MRI. J Craniomaxillofac Surg. 2000;28(6):319–24.
36. Belhocine TZ, Scott AM, Even-Sapir E, Urbain JL, Essner R. Role of nuclear medicine in the management of cutaneous malignant melanoma. J Nucl Med. 2006;47:957–67.
37. Essner R. Surgical treatment of malignant melanoma. Surg Clin North Am. 2003;83(1):109–56.
38. Seethala RR, LiVolsi VA, Baloch ZW. Relative accuracy of fine-needle aspiration and frozen section in the diagnosis of the parotid gland. Head Neck. 2005;27(3):217–23.
39. Alphs HH, Eisele DW, Westra WH. The role of fine needle aspiration in the evaluation of parotid masses. Curr Opin Otolaryngol Head Neck Surg. 2006;14(2):62–6.
40. Pytynia K, Warso M. Treatment of the parotid gland in cutaneous melanoma. Oper Tech Otolaryngol. 2008;19(4):230–3.
41. Greene FL. TNM staging for malignancies of the digestive tract: 2003 changes and beyond. Semin Surg Oncol. 2003;21(1):23–9.
42. O'Brien CJ. The parotid gland as a metastatic basin for cutaneous cancer. Arch Otolaryngol Head Neck Surg. 2006;131:551.
43. Agrawal G, Gupto A, Chaudary V, Qureshi F. Metastatic malignant melanoma: a case report and review of literature. Otolaryngol Case Rep. 2017;3:1–3.
44. Eicher S, Clayman G, Myers J, Gillenwater A. A prospective study of intraoperative lymphatic mapping for head and neck cutaneous melanoma. Arch Otolaryngol Head Neck Surg. 2002;128:241–6.
45. O'Brien CJ, Peterson-Schaefer K, McCarthy W, Bass PC, Tew P, Gebski VJ, et al. Adjuvant radiotherapy following neck dissection and parotidectomy for metastatic malignant melanoma. Head Neck. 1997;19:589–94.
46. Ballo MT, Ang KK. Radiation therapy for malignant melanoma. Surg Clin North Am. 2003;83:323–42.
47. McKean ME, Lee K, McGregor IA. The distribution of lymph nodes in and around the parotid gland: an anatomical study. Br J Plast Surg. 1985;38:1–5.
48. Veness M, Morgan G, Palme C, Gebski V. Surgery and Adjuvant radiotherapy in patients with cutaneous head and neck squamous cell carcinoma metastatic to lymph nodes: combined treatment should be considered best practice. Laryngoscope. 2005;115:870–5.
49. Thielker J, Grosheva M, Ihrler S, Wittig A, Guntinas-Lichius O. Contemporary management of benign and malignant parotid tumors. Front Surg. 2018;5:39.
50. Moore BA, Wine T, Netterville JL. Cervicofacial and cervicothoracic rotation flaps in head and neck reconstruction. Head Neck. 2005;27(12):1092–101.
51. Khurana VG, Mentis DH, O'Brien CJ, Hurst TL, Stevens GN, Packham NA. Parotid and neck metastases from cutaneous squamous cell carcinoma of the head and neck. Am J Surg. 1995;170:446–50.
52. Pedraza V, Guerrero MR, Luna del Castillo JD. Time-dose-response relationship in postoperatively irradiated patients with head and neck squamous cell carcinomas. Radiother Oncol. 2001;60:137–45.
53. Shah JP, Kraus DH, Dubner S, Sarkar S. Patterns of regional lymph node metastases from cutaneous melanomas of the head and neck. Am J Surg. 1991;162:32–323.
54. Chao C, Wong SL, Edwards MJ, Ross MI, Reintgen DS, Noyes RD, et al. Sentinel lymph node biopsy for head and neck melanomas. Ann Surg Oncol. 2003;10:21–6.
55. Vaglini M, Belli F, Santinami M, Cascinelli N. The role of parotidectomy in the treatment of nodal metastases from cutaneous melanoma of the head and neck. Eur J Surg Oncol. 1990;16:28–32.
56. Tan ST, MacKinnon CA. Deep plane cervicofacial flap: a useful and versatile technique in head and neck surgery. Head Neck. 2006;28(1):46–55.
57. Pistre V, Pelissier P, Martin D, Lim A, Baudet J. Ten years experience with the submental flap. Plast Reconstr Surg. 2001;108(6):1576–81.

58. Bae YC, Zuker RM, Manktelow RT, Wade S. A comparison of commissure excursion following gracilis muscle transplantation for facial paralysis using a cross face nerve graft versus the motor nerve to the masseter nerve. Plast Reconstr Surg. 2006;117(7):2407–13.
59. Disa JJ, Pusic AL, Hidlago DH, Cordeiro PG. Simplifying microvascular reconstruction: a rational approach to donor site selection. Ann Plast Surg. 2001;47(4):385–9.
60. Tulley P, Webb A, Chana JS, Grobbelaar AO, et al. Paralysis of the marginal mandibular branch of the facial nerve: treatment options. Br J Plast Surg. 2000;53(5):378–85.
61. Krengli M, Pisani P, Pia F. Exclusive radiotherapy of parotid metastases. Results in 14 cases. Radiol Med. 1993;86(5):684–6.
62. Guillamondegui OM, Byers RM, Luna MA. Aggressive surgery in treatment for parotid cancer; the role of adjuvant postoperative radiotherapy. Am J Roentgentol. 1975;123:49–53.
63. Taylor BW, Brant TA, Mendenhall NP, Mendenhall WM. Carcinoma of the skin metastatic to parotid area lymph nodes. Head Neck. 1991;13:427–33.
64. Trans-Tasman Radiation Oncology Group. TROG 05.01. Post-operative concurrent chemoradiotherapy versus post-operative radiotherapy in high-risk cutaneous squamous cell carcinoma of the head and neck. Version 1: 11 March 2005.
65. Peters LJ, Goepfert H, Ang KK, Byers RM, Maor MH, Guillamondegui O, et al. Evaluation of the dose for post-operative radiation therapy of head and neck cancer: first report of a prospective randomized trial. Int J Radiat Oncol Biol Phys. 1993;26:3–11.
66. Cooper J, Pajak T, Forastiere A, Jacobs J, Jacobs J, Campbell BH, Saxman SB, et al. Postoperative concurrent radiotherapy and chemotherapy for high risk squamous cell carcinoma of the head and neck. N Engl J Med. 2004;350(19):1937–44.
67. Brizel D, Albers M, Fisher S, Scher R, Scher RL, Richtsmeier WJ, Hars V, et al. Hyperfractionated irradiation with or without concurrent chemotherapy for locally advanced head and neck cancer. N Engl J Med. 1998;338:1798–804.
68. Hermann RM, Christiansen H. Carboplatin does not increase the effectiveness of adjuvant radiotherapy in advanced cutaneous squamous cell carcinoma of the head and neck region. Strahlenther Onkol. 2018;194(12):1180–2.
69. Wang BY, Lawson W, Robinson RA, Perez-Ordonez B, Brandwein M. Malignant melanoma of the parotid. Comp Surviv Patients Metastases Known verses Unkn Prim Tumor Sites Arch Otolaryngol Head Neck Surg. 1999;125(6):635–9.
70. Overgaard J. The role of radiotherapy in recurrent and metastatic malignant melanoma: a clinical radiobiological study. Int J Radiat Oncol Biol Phys. 1986;12:867–72.
71. Bentzen SM, Overgaard J, Thames HD, Overgaard M, Hansen PV, von der Maase H, Meder J. Clinical radiobiology of malignant melanoma. Radiother Oncol. 1989;16:169–82.
72. Trans-Tasman Radiation Oncology Group Inc. Australia and New Zealand melanoma trials group. A randomized clinical trial of surgery versus surgery plus adjuvant radiotherapy for regional control in patients with completed resected macroscopic nodal metastatic melanoma TROG 02.01 ANZMTG Trial 1–02 July 2003.
73. Bron LP, Traynor SJ, McNeil EB, O'Brien CJ. Primary and metastatic cancer of the parotid: comparison of clinical behavior in 232 cases. Laryngoscope. 2003;113(6):1070–5.
74. Tsutsumida A, Yamamoto Y, Sekido M, Itoh T. Suspected case of primary malignant melanoma of the parotid gland. Scand J Plast Reconstr Surg Hand Surg. 2008;42(2):105–7.
75. Jering M, Mayer M, Thölken R, Schiele S, Müller G, Zenk J. Cancer-specific and overall survival of patients with primary and metastatic malignancies of the parotid gland—a retrospective study. J Craniomaxillofac Surg. 2022;50:456–61.
76. Girardi FM, Wagner VP, Martins MD, Abentroth AL, Hauth LA. Better outcome for parotid versus neck metastasis of head and neck cutaneous squamous cell carcinoma: a new report on reemerging data. Braz J Otorhinolaryngol. 2021;87:389–95.
77. Bobin C, Ingrand P, Dréno B, Rio E, Malard O, Espitalier F. Prognostic factors for parotid metastasis of cutaneous squamous cell carcinoma of the head and neck. Eur Ann Otorhinolaryngol Head Neck Dis. 2018;135:99–103.
78. Mooney CP, Clark JR, Shannon K, Palme CE, Ebrahimi A, Gao K, et al. The significance of regional metastasis location in head and neck cutaneous squamous cell carcinoma. Head Neck. 2021;43:2705–11.

Parotidectomy

18

18.1 Introduction

Parotidectomy is the partial or complete removal of the parotid gland, and it may be indicated for a variety of reasons that can include inflammatory conditions, certain infectious processes, congenital malformations, and benign or malignant neoplasms. Regardless of the indication for surgery, parotidectomy is a meticulous procedure requiring experienced surgeons, particularly due to the relationship of the gland to the facial nerve. Therefore, identification and preservation of the facial nerve are the most crucial steps during the procedure (second only to oncologic safety in the case of known malignancy). Emphasis is on identification because, in the vast majority of cases, preoperative prediction of the relationship of the tumor to the nerve is not possible with much accuracy unless facial paralysis is already present prior to intervention [1–4].

Before the 1940s, "enucleation" of benign neoplastic processes such as pleomorphic adenoma (PA) was the most common extirpative procedure; however, it was associated with high a recurrence rate (RR) reaching up to 43%. This high RR was attributed at that time to "multicentricity" of the tumor. The reason to perform enucleation rather than removal of the gland was concern regarding injury to the facial nerve. Hamilton Bailey (1941) performed "superficial parotidectomy" and reported a lower RR than enucleation albeit at the expense of increased facial nerve complications [5].

In 1951, Shucksmith et al. [6] described the resection of superficial parotid initially exposing the main branch of facial nerve that was localized right after its emergence by the stylomastoid foramen and, from there on, perform dissection of its nervous branches. This was one of the main techniques used at that time and that is still used nowadays. In 1952, Hayes Martin [7] reported that the reason for recurrence after enucleation was the incomplete capsule of the lesion (tumor satellites).

In 1958, Beahrs and Adson [8] eloquently described the relevant anatomy and surgical technique of current parotid gland surgery. They stressed the importance of

© The Author(s), under exclusive license to Springer Nature Switzerland AG 2024
M. Sakr, *Surgery of the Salivary Glands*,
https://doi.org/10.1007/978-3-031-82069-4_18

surgical landmarks for avoiding injury to the facial nerve and advocated complete removal of the superficial portion of the parotid gland for noninvasive lesions confined to that location.

Recently, the introduction of bipolar diathermy, magnifying loups, and nerve stimulator in parotid surgery resulted in better results and allowed limited resections such as partial superficial parotidectomy (PSP) and extracapsular dissection (ECD) with low RRs and less facial nerve complications.

18.2 Relevant Surgical Anatomy

The parotid gland is the largest major salivary gland. It is bounded by the masseter muscle anteriorly, zygomatic arch superiorly, anteromedial aspect of the sternocleidomastoid (SCM) muscle inferiorly, and the external auditory canal (EAC) posteriorly. The gland is divided "virtually" into superficial and deep lobes (pars superficialis and pars profunda, respectively) by the facial nerve. The superficial lobe is lateral while the facial nerve and the deep lobe extend medially into the parapharyngeal space. The deep cervical fascia divides into a deep and superficial layer to surround the gland. The superficial fascia extends from the masseter and SCM to the zygomatic arch. The superficial musculoaponeurotic system (SMAS) extends from the platysma to the superficial temporal fascia superiorly. It lies superficial to the parotid fascia and should not be confused with it [1, 4, 9].

The parotid gland drains its serous secretions through the long (~7 cm) Stensen's duct that arises from the most anterior superficial part of the gland, travels parallel to and 1 cm below the zygoma, running on the lateral surface of masseter, then it finally dives at an angle of 90° at the anterior border of masseter to pierce the buccal pad of fat, buccopharyngeal fascia, then buccinator muscle, and opens in the oral (gingivo-buccal) vestibule opposite the second maxillary molar tooth over the summit of a papilla [9–11].

After leaving the stylomastoid foramen, the main trunk of the facial nerve divides into two divisions: the temporofacial, branching into frontal, zygomatic, and buccal branches; and the cervicofacial, giving rise to the marginal mandibular nerve (MMN) and cervical branches. The course of the temporal branch can be predicted using surface landmarks as described by Pitanguy and Ramos (1966): a line starting from a point 0.5 cm below the tragus in the direction of the eyebrow, passing 1.5 cm above the lateral extremity of the eyebrow. The middle branch of the facial nerve (zygomatic/buccal) can be identified at Zuker's point, which lies midway on a line drawn from the root of the helix and the lateral commissure of the mouth. The buccal branch accompanies Stensen's duct over the masseter muscle. The MMN is located immediately in a plane deep to the platysma in close proximity to the inferior border of the mandible. Along its course, it runs superficial to the facial vessels. The retromandibular vein travels through the parotid gland just deep to the facial nerve [4, 9, 12–15].

The greater auricular nerve (GAN) travels parallel to the external jugular vein (EJV) and splits into anterior and posterior branches at the level of the tail of the parotid gland. Injury to this nerve leads to loss of sensation in the skin at the angle of the mandible, the side of the upper neck, and the inferior half of the external ear. Preservation of the anterior branch is often impossible as it frequently overlies the tail of the parotid and physically hampers exposure of the tail of the gland while raising the skin flap. The GAN can also be used as a nerve graft in case of facial nerve injury [16].

The parotid gland contains lymph nodes (LNs) in the superficial and deep lobes with a 90% to 10% distribution, respectively. The superficial group drains the pinna, scalp, eyelids, and lacrimal glands. The deep group drains the gland, middle ear, nasopharynx, and soft palate. The EAC drains into both groups. This is important in the setting of sentinel LN biopsy for melanoma or other epithelial tumors, which may necessitate superficial or total parotidectomy [9].

18.3 Types of Parotid Procedures

Throughout history, many different types and techniques have been developed in order to complete a parotidectomy and consequently, many different names have been associated with each type. However, there are really only two main distinctions to be made in parotidectomies [17]: (1) specific nerve(s) to be dissected or not, and (2) the amount of gland excised/recurrence. The main techniques associated with parotid surgery are summarized in Table 18.1.

In all cases, the patient needs to be counseled before surgery about the risk of temporary or permanent facial nerve paralysis, the need for a suction drain, compressive dressing, and the possibility of an aesthetic contour deformity at the site of surgery.

18.3.1 Superficial (Lateral) Parotidectomy

Superficial (lateral) parotidectomy entails excising the superficial lobe of the gland lateral to the facial nerve. These are of two types, formal and partial:

Formal superficial parotidectomy: Superficial parotidectomy where the main trunk of the facial nerve and its two divisions (cervicofacial and temporofacial) and their branches are dissected [18].

Partial superficial parotidectomy (PSP): It is similar to superficial parotidectomy, but only the portion of the gland surrounding the tumor is excised. The main

Table 18.1 Parotid surgery techniques

Parotidectomy	Limited surgery	Enucleation
Superficial (lateral) parotidectomy Total parotidectomy Radical parotidectomy Extended total parotidectomy	Partial superficial parotidectomy (PSP) Extracapsular dissection (ECD)	Extracapsular enucleation Intracapsular enucleation

trunk of the facial nerve and only one division with its branches are dissected during this procedure [18]. It is usually used for benign lesions and LN metastasis into the superficial lobe of the parotid.

18.3.2 Total Parotidectomy

Total parotidectomy entails total removal of both lobes of the parotid gland. The surgeon removes the gland with identification and preservation of the facial nerve and its all branches [19]. It is typically performed for aggressive malignant tumors, deep lobe tumors, sentinel LN excision when located in the deep lobe, vascular malformations, or in large tumors where the distinction between superficial and deep lobes is unclear [18].

18.3.3 Radical (Nonconservative) Parotidectomy

Radical or nonconservative parotidectomy is typically performed if the malignant neoplasm is impinging on the facial nerve, which is excised in addition to the parotid gland, i.e., in addition to total parotidectomy [20]. Thus, it is usually used when preoperative facial paralysis is well-established, or circumferential involvement of the nerve by malignant tumor is encountered. Simultaneous nerve grafting or other facial reanimation procedures can be employed in this situation [18].

18.3.4 Extended Total (Radical) Parotidectomy

Extended total parotidectomy means total parotidectomy plus excision of adjacent structures such as the overlying skin, the underlying mandible, temporal bone and external auditory canal (EAC), or the deep musculature of the parapharyngeal space.

18.3.5 Extracapsular Dissection (ECD)

Extracapsular dissection (ECD) is a limited resection procedure in which only the tumor and a surrounding cuff of normal parotid tissue (about 2–3 mm) are excised (with the help of a facial nerve monitor). In such case, neither the main trunk of the facial nerve nor its two divisions or terminal branches are dissected (Fig. 18.1). It is usually indicated for benign lesions other than pleomorphic adenoma for fear of recurrence.

18.3.6 Enucleation

It was the most common extirpative procedure for benign neoplastic lesions (e.g., pleomorphic adenoma) before the 1940s. It is of two types:

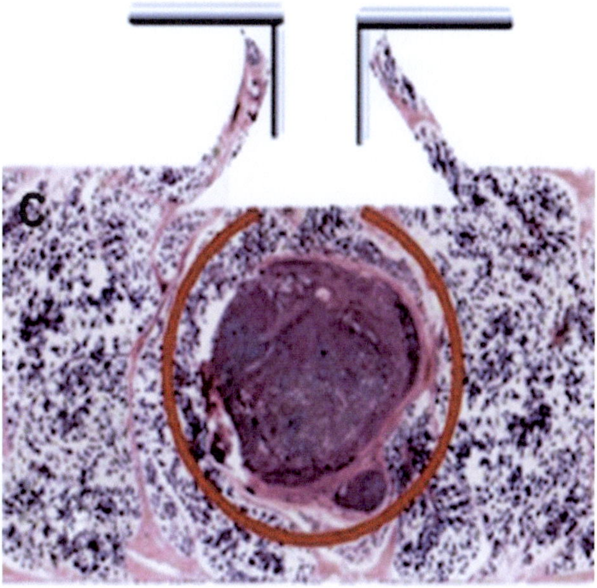

Fig. 18.1 Extracapsular dissection (ECD): the tumor and a surrounding cuff of normal parotid tissue (2–3 mm) are excised

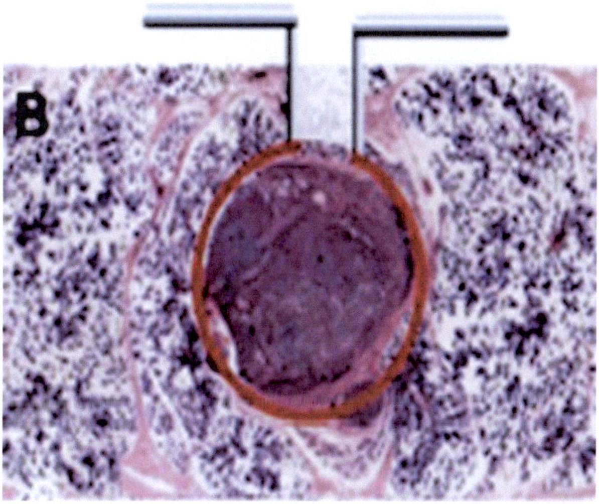

Fig. 18.2 Extracapsular enucleation: the tumor with its capsule is enucleated from the rest of the parotid tissue

Extracapsular enucleation: In this procedure, the tumor with its capsule is enucleated from the rest of the parotid tissue (Fig. 18.2).

Intracapsular enucleation: In this procedure, the tumor is enucleated from within its capsule (Fig. 18.3).

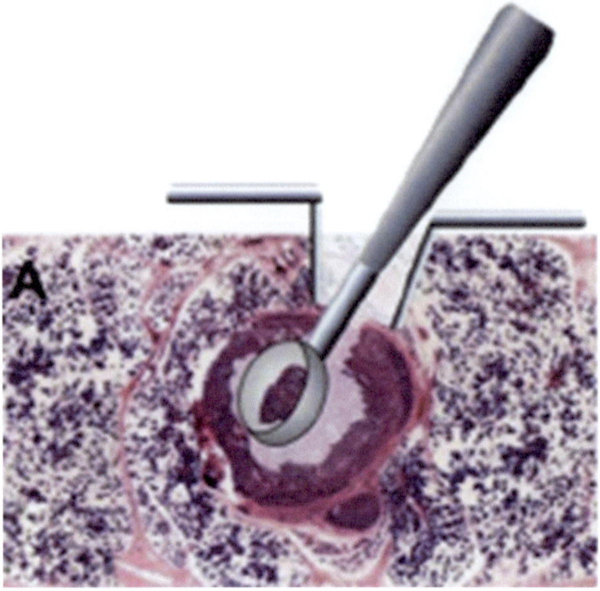

Fig. 18.3 Intracapsular enucleation: the tumor is enucleated from within its capsule

18.4 Indications of Parotidectomy

Indications of parotidectomy generally include the following.

18.4.1 Neoplasms

Neoplasms are the most common indication for parotidectomy. The vast majority of primary parotid tumors are benign, but approximately 20% are found to be malignant. Pleomorphic adenoma (PA) and Warthin's tumors represent the majority of tumors, with PA representing the most common benign parotid tumor. Of malignant tumors, mucoepidermoid carcinoma (MEC) and adenoid cystic carcinoma (AdCC) are the two most common primary parotid tumors, in that order.

In addition, regional and distant disease can metastasize to the parotid and necessitate removal for diagnosis or cure. Metastasis from a cutaneous primary such as squamous cell carcinoma (SCC) and malignant melanoma (MM) represent the most common parotid malignancy in some series, notably in Australia [21].

18.4.2 Inflammatory Processes

Inflammatory processes (e.g., chronic parotitis, deep salivary calculi, recurrent sialadenitis, or parotid abscess) are occasionally treated with total parotidectomy, with the recognition that surgery in an inflamed gland probably carries a higher risk of postoperative facial nerve dysfunction [20]. Parotidectomy is usually resorted to when medical treatment and sialoendoscopy fail or are unavailable [22–26].

18.4.3 Salivary Duct Stones

Salivary duct stones may be approached through minimal external parotid incisions, and are aided by sialoendoscopy when possible.

18.4.4 Sialorrhea

Sialorrhea (excessive salivation) is rarely treated with parotidectomy; more often, it is medically managed with anti-sialagogues or botulinum toxin or treated with duct ligation.

18.4.5 Other Indications

Other indications of parotidectomy include caseating granulomas, tuberculosis (TB), toxoplasmosis, branchial cleft cyst, and symptomatic lymphoepithelial cyst [22–26].

18.5 Contraindications of Parotidectomy

There are no contraindications for parotidectomy as long as the patient is medically fit for general anesthesia. While there are reports of this procedure being performed under local anesthesia, this is very unusual and not routinely recommended. In certain cases, intubation might be challenging, for example, a tumor extending to the deep lobe/the parapharyngeal space or an extensive lesion invading the temporomandibular joint leading to trismus. In such situations, awake nasal fiberoptic intubation or a tracheostomy is necessary to secure the airway. Patients with benign tumors who are at high anesthetic risk may be observed on a case-by-case basis.

Patients with multiple parotid cysts should be evaluated for human immunodeficiency virus (HIV) with detailed imaging and/or cytological workup before undergoing surgical excision. Benign lymphoepithelial cysts are relatively common in the HIV-positive population, but otherwise uncommon. Surgery is a last resort for this entity given the bilateral, multiple, and progressive nature of the disease, with the tendency to recur, and the higher risk of facial nerve injury. A more appropriate option in this scenario will be one of the following: observation, repeat aspiration, antiretroviral medication, sclerosing therapy, or radiation therapy [27, 28]. Because these cysts are usually bilateral and multiple and tend to recur, they are typically managed by means of repeated aspiration or sclerotherapy rather than parotidectomy; they may also respond to antiretroviral therapy.

18.6 Pre-procedural Planning and Perioperative Care

Measures that may be considered before parotidectomy include complete clinical evaluation, diagnostic imaging, fine needle aspiration (FNA), staging of malignant tumors, as well as consideration of neck dissection and adjuvant therapy.

18.6.1 Clinical Evaluation

Every patient should be clinically evaluated properly before surgery. History-taking and physical examination are essential for optimal decision-making. Most patients are asymptomatic and present with an enlarging mass that was incidentally noted. Pain, if present, is not predictive of a malignant histology [1]. A fixed mass could be malignant, inflammatory, or located in the deep lobe, though even benign masses can have limited mobility owing to the dense structure of the gland parenchyma, and so has more limited predictive utility.

Physical examination of the oral cavity is useful to rule out the involvement of the parapharyngeal space. Facial nerve function is examined and is ideally documented with photographs. Worrisome signs include facial paralysis, trismus, formication (tactile hallucination of the sensation of having insects crawling on or under the skin), and numbness [1]. The neck is palpated systematically; a parotid tail lesion might be confused with a jugulodigastric LN.

18.6.2 Preoperative Imaging

Both computed tomography (CT) scan with contrast and magnetic resonance imaging (MRI) can be helpful in operative planning, but they may not be necessary in patients with small, mobile tumors of the parotid tail. Any clinical feature suggestive of malignancy (e.g., lymphadenopathy, fixation to surrounding structures, or preoperative facial nerve weakness) warrants radiographic evaluation of the parotid gland and nodal basins in the neck.

"Static" MRI parameters can help differentiate a benign from a malignant lesion with a diagnostic accuracy of 95% when accounting for well-defined margins. "Dynamic" contrast-enhanced MRI with its resultant time signal intensity curve has a 96.5% diagnostic accuracy for differentiating benign and malignant lesions. It can also differentiate a malignant lesion from a Warthin's tumor and PA by studying the T-peak time, and this is especially useful since PA shows a cumulative malignant transformation risk of 1% per year, in contrast to a Warthin's tumor that shows only a 0.3% overall risk of malignant transformation. Studying the apparent diffusion coefficient is also useful. When the cut-off value is set at 1.3×10^{-3} mm^2/s and excluding lymphomas, the diagnostic accuracy for differentiating Warthin's tumor from a malignant tumor is 94.28%. This value reaches 97.06% for PA [29]. MRI sialography proved to be a very useful technique replacing conventional sialography in most centers; it can also help with the evaluation of Sjogren's disease by showing sialectasis clearly [30].

Imaging can provide useful clues to the relation between the tumor and the facial nerve. If the tumor lies in a plane inferior to the stylomastoid foramen, the nerve will probably lie on the superior surface of the tumor; likewise, if the tumor is high in the gland, the nerve may pass inferiorly. If the tumor occupies the most superficial portion of the gland, with a significant area of parotid tissue deep to it, the nerve is likely to be deep to the tumor; similarly, a deep tumor abutting the mandible should have the nerve on its superficial surface.

18.6.3 Fine Needle Aspiration Cytology (FNAC)/Biopsy

Fine needle aspiration cytology (FNAC) can be used to diagnose parotid tumors preoperatively with a high degree of sensitivity and specificity [31]. With small, mobile tumors of the tail of the parotid, preoperative histological diagnosis may not be required, but even in this setting, such diagnosis can contribute to patient counseling and informed consent. The British Guidelines recommend ultrasound (US)-guided FNAC for every patient [32]. It has an accuracy of 96% in distinguishing benign from malignant neoplasm [33]. If a malignant tumor is suspected on the basis of radiographic evaluation or physical examination, FNA should be done to establish the diagnosis and help guide operative planning. It is important to correlate FNAC results with clinical findings, for example, a Warthin's tumor on FNAC in a very young patient should not necessarily reassure the surgeon into advising observation; this could represent a low-grade MEC since typically benign tumors present at more advanced ages. Each patient's entire clinical picture must be used to make decisions, rather than any single test [34].

Core-biopsy is helpful when FNAC is not sufficient for diagnosis. It has 96% sensitivity and 100% specificity for the diagnosis of malignancy [35]. The role of the frozen section is not clear; however, it may be able to differentiate malignancy from benign pathology with 99% specificity reported in some studies [31]

18.6.4 Staging

The TNM staging system is frequently used for major salivary gland tumors. Aro et al. (2018) analyzed the data of 4520 patients from the United States National Cancer Database in an attempt at creating an adapted LN staging system for salivary gland tumors. Mortality increased rapidly for every LN below 4 and at a slower pattern above 4. The staging system can be criticized for encompassing all types of salivary gland tumors, while obviously, each histological subtype behaves differently. The standard of care staging system remains the AJCC eighth edition [36].

18.6.5 Neck Dissection

Removal of all palpable or radiographically suspicious lymph nodes (LNs) via selective neck dissection is appropriate in the setting of malignancy. Elective neck dissection in the N0 neck is controversial and usually is performed (levels I–III) for high-grade lesions, T3/T4 tumors, and advanced ages, since these are risk factors of locoregional recurrence only for high-grade malignancies [37, 38].

18.6.6 Adjuvant Therapy

Adjuvant RT is indicated for T3/T4 tumors, close or positive margins, and perineural/perivascular invasion. Nearly all AdCCs can benefit from adjuvant RT. Therapeutic radiation is acceptable when surgery is not feasible. On the other hand, conventional chemotherapy has demonstrated consistently poor outcomes as a primary treatment modality in salivary gland tumors, though it has been employed in ongoing trials in a palliative setting [33].

18.7 Equipment

In general, parotid surgery can be performed with the basic instruments set used in head and neck operations. Bipolar is used for hemostasis. Some surgeons use a “facial nerve monitor” to facilitate identification of the facial nerve during surgery. This device consists of electromyography (EMG) electrodes that are placed, at a minimum, in the orbicularis oris and the orbicularis oculi. Stimulation of the cervicofacial and temporofacial divisions of the facial nerve causes the respective muscles to contract. In addition to the stimulation inherent in manipulation of the nerve, a probe can be connected to the monitor to permit direct stimulation of suspected nerve branches. Some authors reported that there is no substantial evidence to suggest that continuous EMG facial nerve monitoring prevents injury to the facial nerve [39, 40]. Moreover, intraoperative abnormalities on the facial nerve monitor have not been shown to predict postoperative dysfunction [41]. Nevertheless, evidence in the literature suggests that EMG facial nerve monitoring (1) decreases the rate of immediate facial weakness in primary surgeries, (2) helps localize the facial nerve, (3) offers prognostic value regarding postoperative facial nerve function, and (4) is mandatory in extracapsular dissection (ECD) where, by definition, the facial nerve is not identified [33].

The facial nerve can also be monitored through simple observation of facial twitching, although such monitoring requires a vigilant observer during facial nerve dissection. When identification of the facial nerve is in question, the nerve can be directly stimulated with a hand-held nerve stimulator to elicit twitching.

18.8 Technical Considerations

Positive identification and preservation of the facial nerve are essential for preventing inadvertent facial nerve injury. A thorough understanding of the anatomy of the stylomastoid foramen, the facial nerve, and the parotid gland and its surrounding structures underlies identification and preservation of the nerve. Whenever possible, a normal cuff of parotid tissue should be resected around a tumor to prevent recurrence [42]. In the setting of a benign tumor, if a facial nerve branch is found directly on the tumor capsule, the nerve should be gently dissected off the tumor. In the setting of a malignancy, consideration should be given to sacrificing as opposed to preserving the nerve.

"Raw gland surface" contributes to postoperative salivary leakage (sialocele or salivary fistula). In addition, raw gland opposed to skin provides a ready pathway for postganglionic parasympathetic fibers to migrate from the salivary tissue and cross-innervate facial sweat glands, resulting in gustatory sweating (Frey's syndrome). Efforts should be made to close the parotid capsule after removal of a parotid tumor or a portion of the gland. If closure of the capsule is not feasible, consideration should be given to interposing tissue (e.g., dermal fat graft) [43] or implantable biological material (e.g., acellular dermis) between the raw gland and the skin.

Injury to the posterior branch of the greater auricular nerve (GAN), which supplies sensation to the ear, is often avoidable. If the nerve must be cut, it can be marked with a stitch to facilitate re-approximation at the conclusion of the operation. Patients should be warned to expect at least temporary earlobe numbness and should take precautions to prevent heat or cold injury to the insensate area (e.g., frostbite or curling iron burns).

Closed suction drainage is used in most cases, if not all, to prevent postoperative hematoma or seroma formation.

18.9 Patient Preparation

Patient preparation includes adequate anesthesia and appropriate positioning.

18.9.1 Anesthesia

Parotidectomy is typically performed with the patient under general anesthesia with the endotracheal tube fixed to the contralateral side. To allow adequate monitoring of the facial nerve, the anesthesia team should be advised to avoid muscle relaxants. It is important to confirm that the patient has regained full motor function (as determined by twitch monitoring) before attempting to dissect out the facial nerve and its branches.

18.9.2 Positioning

The patient is placed in the supine position with the head turned as far as possible away from the side of the operation. A shoulder roll can help with neck extension and thereby facilitate the surgical exposure.

The eye on the side to be operated on is lubricated and closed with either a transparent dressing or a fine suture that approximates the lids (tarsorrhaphy stitch). If a "nerve integrity monitor" for continuous facial nerve monitoring is to be used, four electrodes are placed in the area of the temporal, zygomatic, buccal, and marginal mandibular branches of the facial nerve. The alternative is to place the monitoring electrodes (at a minimum) in the orbicularis oris and the orbicularis oculi, and the grounding electrodes are placed outside the field.

The face may be covered in a transparent dressing or may be prepared, with particular care taken around the eyes and mouth. The remainder of the operative field is draped, including the temple, the ear, the preauricular and postauricular areas, and the neck. A cotton ball can be placed in the ear canal during prepping to prevent cleaning solution from collecting and causing postoperative irritation (if cleaning solution does get into the canal, it should be washed out with room temperature water or saline at the end of the procedure).

18.10 Superficial Parotidectomy

18.10.1 Incision

Skin incisions should be camouflaged in normal facial contours and should be placed with consideration of whether a neck dissection is necessary. The anterior skin incision can be placed either in the preauricular crease or post-tragally in the manner of a face-lift [44]. The position of the earlobe should be precisely marked for repositioning at the conclusion of the procedure.

Most surgeons prefer the modified Blair (Lazy-S) incision, which starts in the preauricular skin crease just in front of the external auditory meatus (EAM). It then courses around the ear lobule posteriorly, and is extended inferiorly into the upper cervical skin crease (Fig. 18.4). Some amount of skin should be left around the lobule to avoid pixie-ear (or satyr) deformity [45].

An alternative incision is a modified face-lift incision, which starts behind the tragus down to the lobule of the ear, then it extends posteriorly and superiorly into the retro-auricular crease to continue within the occipital hairline for a short distance as indicated. It may be extended into the hairline for cosmesis or curved down to a prominent neck crease to allow a neck dissection (Fig. 18.5) [46].

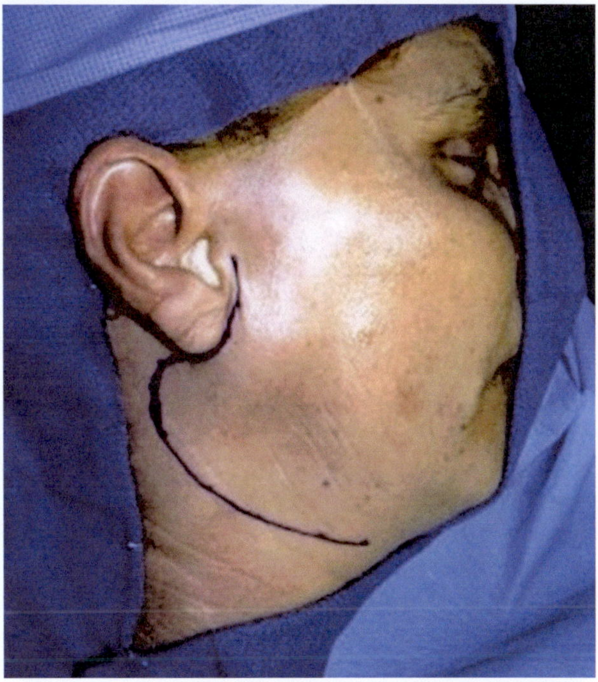

Fig. 18.4 Standard Lazy-S incision: Blair incision (intraoperative presentation)

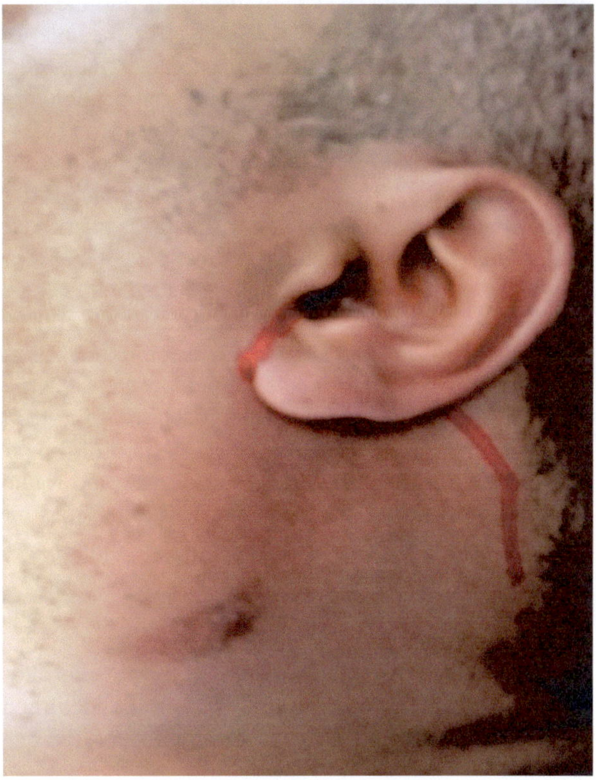

Fig. 18.5 Modified face-lift incision (intra-presentation)

18.10.2 Technique (Steps of the Procedure)

18.10.2.1 Flap Creation

The skin incision is carried down through the subcutaneous (SC) tissues and platysma muscle. An anterior subplatysmal/subsuperficial musculoaponeurotic system (SMAS) flap is made by using the natural plane on the surface of the parotid gland. This flap is advised to be as thick as possible to minimize the risk of Frey's syndrome as well as skin necrosis. Some surgeons advocate that dissection in a plane just deep the superficial parotid fascia to further decrease the risk of Frey's syndrome is elevated superficial to the GAN (which is preserved whenever possible) and the parotid fascia. Elevation of the flap is carried beyond the extent of the tumor to completely expose parotid fascia anterior to the tissue to be removed. Great caution is exercised in approaching the zygomatic arch, the anterior border of the parotid gland, and the submandibular fascia, all of which are areas where distal branches of the facial nerve emerge from the gland. Another option is to raise a supra-SMAS flap, taking care not to injure the subdermal plexus, and then raise a second SMAS flap in the style of a face-lift. This SMAS flap can then be reattached to minimize cosmetic deformity as well as Frey syndrome. Care is taken anteriorly not to damage branches of the facial nerve that become superficial at this level [1].

A posterior flap is then raised at the level of the sternocleidomastoid (SCM) fascia. At the uppermost end of the SCM, some muscle fibers are inserted into the skin and these must be transected. The great auricular nerve (GAN) branches and the external jugular vein (EJV) are identified, and the plane is developed superficial to these structures. At this point, if necessary, the anterior branch of the GAN is transected sharply and tagged for reanastomosis. The proximal end is left enveloped in SCM fascia to facilitate re-approximation at the end of the case (Fig. 18.6). It is often possible to preserve the posterior branch. This is done by careful dissection along the nerve after its identification while raising the cervical subplatysmal flap; at the level of the bifurcation, the anterior branch is divided. If the entire nerve is to be sacrificed, this should be done as distal as possible to preserve a lengthy segment in case it is needed as a cable graft for facial nerve reconstruction. It is often necessary to ligate the EJV. The flaps are retracted with silk sutures or self-retaining hooks.

The tail of the parotid gland then is elevated off the SCM until the posterior belly of the digastric muscle is seen. During this maneuver, one should watch for the small nerve branch to the posterior belly of the digastric muscle, which is not always seen but can provide a clue to the location of the facial nerve [1]. Saha et al. [47] measured the distance between the insertion of the posterior belly of the digastric over the mastoid and the facial nerve trunk and found it to be around 8 mm. The posterior belly of the digastric inserts into the mastoid tip, so tissue superficial to this structure can be divided with relative impunity once the distal marginal mandibular branch has been located. Dissection cephalad to the digastric muscle might injure the facial nerve as it exits the stylomastoid foramen between the mastoid and styloid processes. It is important in this area is to avoid the cervical and marginal branches, which usually pass over the facial veins and in the submandibular fascia. If the main trunk of the facial nerve is to be identified, the posterior gland is then separated from the cartilage of the tragus and the external auditory canal (EAC),

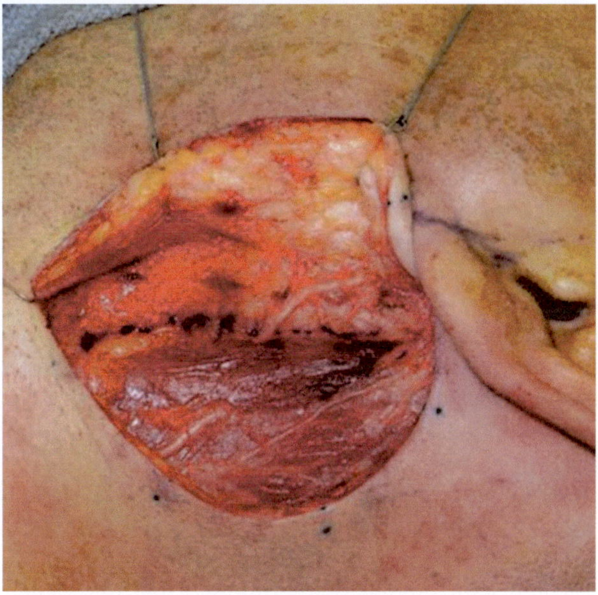

Fig. 18.6 Greater auricular nerve (GAN) has been transected near junction of parotid gland and sternocleidomastoid (SCM). Junction is marked with dotted line. The proximal nerve is left enveloped in fascia of SCM to aid in re-approximation at the end of case. Posterior branch of the GAN can be seen crossing SCM more superiorly and was left intact

with care taken to preserve the perichondrium. This elevation is continued deep to the bony–cartilaginous junction. Once this step is accomplished, attention is turned to identification of the facial nerve.

18.10.2.2 Identification and Dissection of the Facial Nerve

The basic principle of facial nerve dissection is to avoid any unnecessary stimulation of the nerve. Specific tools used in dissection vary from surgeon to surgeon and include cold, bipolar electrocauterization, and ultrasonic dissection. Most surgeons advise against the use of a monopolar cautery in close proximity to the facial nerve.

The facial nerve can be identified in any of the following six ways:

1. The "tympano-mastoid suture line" can be palpated and followed to the stylomastoid foramen. Emphasis is on palpation since it is often difficult to visualize the suture properly. It is considered the most consistent and reliable landmark for the main trunk of the facial nerve, which emerges a few millimeters deep to its lateral edge. Bushey et al. (2011) reported a mean distance between the facial nerve and the tympano-mastoid suture of 4.9 mm [48].
2. The so-called "tragal pointer" is a triangular extension of cartilage inferiorly off the tragus and suggests the location of the facial nerve in the direction of its infero-anterior point. It is important to note that the pointer is a cartilaginous structure that can be fractured or dislocated during the dissection; this factor needs to be taken into consideration when used as a landmark for the facial nerve.
3. The "posterior belly of the digastric muscle" crosses the SCM approximately 1 cm inferior and 1 cm superficial to the location of the nerve; it is highly useful as a marker of the depth of the facial nerve.

4. Any "peripheral branch," including the branch to the digastric muscle, can be followed back to the main trunk, which is then dissected in the usual fashion.
5. The "styloid process" can be exposed bluntly from a superior approach, and the nerve is found infero-lateral to it. This is an especially useful approach in the setting of revision surgery, because the plane superior to the styloid process is typically not previously dissected.
6. The mastoid can be drilled to allow identification of the facial nerve in settings of severely abnormal anatomy, complicated revision surgery, or large tumors abutting the stylomastoid foramen.

If complete dissection of the nerve is planned, once the main trunk is identified, it is traced to the "pes anserinus," the structure marking the separation of the cervicofacial (lower) and temporofacial (upper) divisions (Fig. 18.7). It is important to dissect directly atop the nerve to visualize it the entire time directly. The parotid tissue overlying the area of the facial nerve that has been dissected is divided, never beyond that area. This can be done with fine scissors or a non-locking, smooth-jawed, right-angle dissector (McCabe facial nerve dissector), while the glandular tissue is splayed with the hemostat. Hemostasis at this step is ensured with bipolar diathermy and fine ties (when tightening the knots, care must be taken not to apply pressure on the facial nerve and its branches with the tightening finger).

Smaller branches are then followed carefully with the aim of mapping their relation to the tumor. The typical approach is to start at the uppermost branch of the upper division or the lowermost branch of the lower division, as appropriate, and follows the branch out to a point where it is well clear of the tumor. The next branch

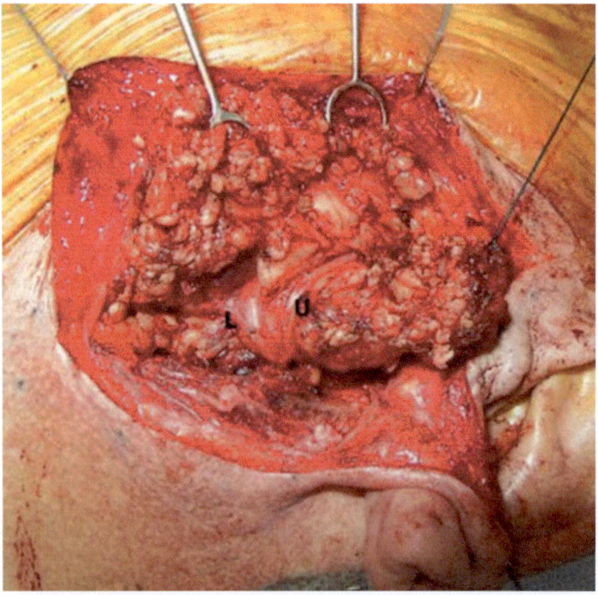

Fig. 18.7 Main trunk of facial nerve (asterisk) has been exposed to pes anserinus, branch point of upper (U) and lower (L) divisions

is then followed, and so forth, until all branches in the area of the tumor are dissected free and the tumor is mobilized for removal.

In the setting of malignancy, especially if preoperative facial nerve dysfunction is present, consideration is given to severing the nerves involved with the tumor and tagging them with nonabsorbable sutures for immediate re-approximation, interposition, or other grafting as appropriate either at the conclusion of the tumor removal or at a later time. Isolated midfacial branches might not need to be repaired because the resulting deformity is often unnoticed [49, 50].

18.10.2.3 Removal of Parotid Tissue

If the whole superficial lobe of the parotid gland is to be removed (formal superficial parotidectomy) and not just the cuff of gland around the tumor, all of the facial nerve branches are dissected and mobilized (Fig. 18.8). Any bleeding that occurs related to division of the gland is carefully controlled under vision. When removing the superior part of the gland, the superficial temporal artery may need to be ligated; if so, this is performed just anterior to the auricle. When dissection continues anteriorly, the parotid duct is reached and divided if necessary. It is necessary to remember that the buccal branch of the facial nerve is adjacent to the duct.

Before closure and once tissue removal is complete, the facial nerve can be tested with a hand-held stimulator or monitor probe to confirm that it is unharmed. Repeated unnecessary stimulation of the nerve, however, is to be avoided out of concern for potential injury.

18.10.2.4 Reconstruction and Closure

Once the resection is complete and any necessary repair or grafting of the facial nerve has been performed, attention is turned to closure. The primary goals of reconstruction are (1) to cover any raw gland surface remaining, (2) to restore normal facial contours, and (3) to provide coverage of the facial nerve and a reliable plane of dissection in the event that reoperation proves necessary.

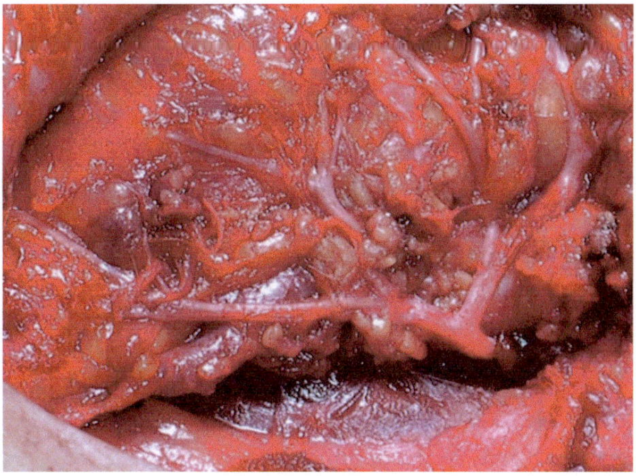

Fig. 18.8 The facial trunk is dissected and followed peripherally to expose and preserve the two divisions and terminal branches before removing the specimen

Many techniques are used for reconstruction. In small resections, the parotid capsule can often be closed primarily. In larger resections, the defect can be filled with autologous buccal or abdominal fat [43] or acellular dermis.

The digastric muscle can be cut at the intermediate tendon and the posterior belly rotated into the defect, or a superiorly based flap that includes a portion of the SCM can be used in a similar manner. However, muscle reconstruction tends to lose volume over time. In massive resections involving removal of mandible or skin, the options include skin (e.g., cervicofacial), myocutaneous (e.g., pectoralis major), and free flaps.

To reconstruct the GAN, the fascia next to the opposing ends of the cut nerve are sutured together to allow tension-free neurorrhaphy. Interrupted 8-0 or 9-0 nylon sutures are then placed in the perineurium to re-approximate the nerve. If the nerve cannot be re-approximated, some authors advocate clipping or burying the proximal end to prevent neuroma formation, although evidence for the effectiveness of these techniques is lacking.

Once reconstruction is complete, closed suction drains are placed through stab incisions in the posterior neck or hairline. The skin is then closed in layers in an interrupted fashion. To prevent a pixie-ear deformity, care is taken not to put excessive tension on the earlobe.

In the recovery room, facial nerve function should be assessed as soon as possible. After the patient is gently awakened and has recovered from anesthesia, the face is examined for motor nerve function. If the facial nerve was not identified as intact and the patient wakes up with a dense paralysis that persists beyond the effects of any local anesthetic, reexploration should be considered. If the nerve is known to be intact, the patient can be reassured that mild postoperative facial nerve weakness will usually resolve completely though full recovery can take many months.

18.10.2.5 Postoperative Care and Follow-Up

The drain is left in place until the output is <15–50 mL in 24 h. It is usually removed on the first postoperative day, and the skin sutures are removed within 1 week.

Duration of postoperative hospitalization is subject to change from patient to patient, with most patients being discharged within 24 h after surgery. For benign tumors and slow growing cancers, surgery typically provides a complete cure or remission with no evidence of disease [50].

Long-term follow-up depends on the results of pathology. Most patients with benign tumors are followed every 3–6 months for 2 years and yearly thereafter. Patients with malignant tumors may be followed every 2–3 months for 2 years, and then every 6 months for 5 years after procedure [50].

Mild facial numbness and weakness are normal immediately after a parotidectomy, with symptoms usually subsiding within a few months. Most patients regain full facial function within 1 year of the procedure [50]. Patients with facial nerve weakness should thus be regularly monitored and watched for improvement or stabilization; plans should be made for reanimation as necessary.

If a mass develops lateral to the SCM in the location of the GAN, a greater auricular neuroma should be considered. Such masses tend to be painful with manipulation. In the setting of benign disease, reassurance and treatment are both reasonable. Confirmation of this diagnosis with FNA or excision should be considered in the setting of a previous malignancy.

18.10.2.6 Main Complications of the Procedure

Early and late complications of superficial parotidectomy may occur. There is a reported 25–50% risk of facial nerve palsy directly after parotidectomy and a 1–2% risk of permanent weakness [51]. Frey's syndrome may occur in up to 90% of patients [51]. Risk of mortality is very low in reference to the surgery [19]. Survival rates due to malignancy depend on the patient and extent of disease [19]. A 10-year survival ranges from 32% to 83% [51].

18.11 Partial Superficial Parotidectomy (PSP)

18.11.1 Technique

Partial superficial parotidectomy (PSP) is started as superficial parotidectomy by identification of the main trunk of facial nerve and its bifurcation. The branch related to the tumor is then completely identified and dissected depending on the tumor site whether in the lower part (Fig. 18.9) or in the upper part of the gland. A small part of the superficial parotid lobe containing the tumor with at least 1 cm of healthy tissue around the tumor is stripped out from the branch of the facial nerve, related to the tumor. The procedure is completed in a similar fashion to formal superficial parotidectomy.

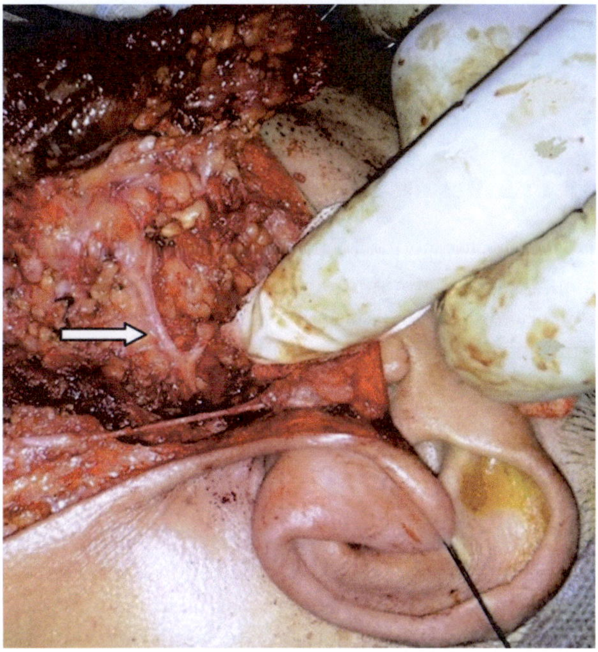

Fig. 18.9 Partial superficial parotidectomy (PSP) is started as superficial parotidectomy by identification of the main trunk of facial nerve and its bifurcation. The branch related to the tumor is then completely identified and dissected (arrow)

18.11.2 Why Perform Partial Superficial Parotidectomy?

Partial superficial parotidectomy has been proposed as an alternative to formal superficial parotidectomy in certain situations for the following reasons: (1) about 50–60% of parotid tumors are in contact with only one division of the facial nerve, (2) the facial nerve can be preserved (protected) by minimal dissection at the interface between nerve branches and the tumor, and (3) the rate of recurrence can be minimized by dissection away from the parotid tumor (at least 1 cm margin).

18.11.3 Tumors Amenable to PSP (Indications)

Not all parotid tumors are amenable to PSP. Only benign parotid tumors located in the superficial lobe in relation to the upper or lower division of the facial nerve and/or its branches can be excised using this technique.

18.11.4 Contraindications

Partial superficial parotidectomy is contraindicated in the following conditions:

Large tumors (>3 cm) involving most of the parotid gland.
Centrally located tumors irrespective of size.
Malignant tumors and suspicious tumors by the FNAC.
Previous parotid surgery.
Deep lobe tumors.
Facial nerve palsy.
Scarring in or irradiation to the parotid area.

18.11.5 Results

Partial superficial parotidectomy is an adequate and safe procedure for treatment of small benign parotid tumors located in the superficial lobe and related to only one division of the facial nerve. With PSP, there is a considerable reduction of operative time and blood loss; at the same time, there is no increase in postoperative morbidity.

18.12 Total Parotidectomy

While superficial parotidectomy entails removal of the lateral (superficial) lobe of the parotid gland with preservation of the facial nerve, total parotidectomy entails complete removal of the superficial and deep lobes of the parotid. In such cases, all of the facial nerve branches are dissected and mobilized, and the deep parotid tissue is then removed from between the branches with blunt and sharp dissection. The tumor can also be removed by retracting the mass inferiorly. If this proves to be difficult or inadequate, the transcervical approach with the division of the stylomandibular ligament provides excellent exposure of the parapharyngeal space, which includes the deep lobe of the parotid. If a tumor must be removed from the deep lobe via a lateral approach (as with a tumor invading between nerve branches from the superficial lobe), some authors advocate selective division of some nerve branches with immediate reanastomosis after tumor removal to avoid stretching branches and causing permanent dysfunction.

Of note, when performing total parotidectomy for chronic parotitis, Stensen's duct needs to be followed-up to the oral mucosa to avoid retention of any stones within a distal stump, which might lead to subsequent infection.

Total parotidectomy is typically performed if the benign tumor is involving the deep part of parotid gland [52]. It should be performed for malignant tumors in the following situations: (1) metastasis to a superficial parotid LNs from a primary parotid tumor or an extra-parotid malignancy, (2) any parotid malignancy with metastatic involvement of cervical LNs, (3) any high-grade parotid malignant tumor with a high risk of metastasis, (4) primary parotid malignant tumors originating in the deep lobe, and (5) primary malignancies that extend outside the parotid gland. Total parotidectomy is also performed for multifocal tumors, such as oncocytomas, to ensure complete resection. The operation may involve sparing or sacrificing the facial nerve branches or trunk depending on tumor extent to the nerve.

18.13 Radical (Nonconservative) Parotidectomy

Radical or nonconservative parotidectomy is typically performed if the malignant tumor is impinging on or infiltrating the facial nerve. In such cases, the facial nerve is excised in addition to the parotid gland, i.e., in addition to total parotidectomy [19].

In 2021, Yesensky et al. reported that out of 53 patients with parotid metastasis (from cutaneous squamous cell carcinoma [SCC]) and normal preoperative facial nerve function, 13% required sacrifice of the main trunk of the facial nerve and 27% required sacrifice of a branch of the facial nerve. The likelihood of nerve sacrifice is highest for tumors with extracapsular spread, perineural invasion, and metastatic disease within the body of the parotid [53].

The parotid lymph nodes (LNs) are the most common first echelon site of metastatic spread for CSCC of the head and neck. Metastatic involvement of intra-parotid LNs poses a therapeutic challenge. Surgical resection via comprehensive parotidectomy is recommended with the goals of complete removal of tumor and preservation of nerve function. However, the involved nodal disease is often in close proximity or directly involving the facial nerve, and nerve sacrifice is sometimes necessary to achieve microscopic or gross total resection [54]. On the other hand, Iyer et al. (2009) reported no decline in local control or survival in patients in whom a positive margin was tolerated to preserve facial nerve function when patients were treated with adjuvant radiotherapy (RT) for eradication of residual, microscopic disease. Still, however, more data are necessary to determine the appropriate extent of surgery in patients with metastatic disease to the parotid [55].

18.14 Extended Total (Radical) Parotidectomy

In the case of malignant tumors of the parotid gland extending to the temporal bone or to the mandibular bone or to the skin, an extended radical parotidectomy is performed Extended parotidectomy involves complete removal of the entire parotid gland, including also excision of the facial nerve, sectioned at the level of extracranial emergence, associated with resection of the adjacent structures (skin, temporal bone and external auditory canal, mandibular bone and mandibular joint, blood vessels, and nerves, or the deep musculature of the parapharyngeal space) invaded by the neoplasm; the choice depends on each individual case and is dictated by tumor growth and behavior [46].

Patients with extensive parotid malignancies should be counseled regarding the possibility of extended resections and the resulting functional and cosmetic morbidity. A neck dissection is performed for clinically positive LNs. For the clinically negative neck, the first echelon nodes are inspected. Enlarged or suspicious LNs are examined and a neck dissection is performed if metastatic disease is confirmed by frozen-section biopsy. Reconstruction of the loss of substance is usually carried out with a myocutaneous pectoralis major flap or with adjacent flaps. In conclusion, for particularly widespread neoplasms, extended radical parotidectomy, associated with postoperative RT, is the treatment of choice, which provides a positive benefit to the life expectancy of these patients [56].

18.15 Complications of Parotidectomy

Early and late complications of parotidectomy procedures are summarized in Table 18.2.

18.15.1 Early Complications

18.15.1.1 Facial Nerve Injury

Unintentional injury to the facial nerve is the most devastating complication of parotid surgery. In a study of surgery for benign disease by Koch et al. (2010), temporary postoperative weakness was reported in 18–65% and permanent weakness in 0–19% [57]. This risk must be explicitly discussed with every patient undergoing parotid surgery. Even with ostensibly perfect technique, facial nerve injury can occur for unknown reasons.

The nerve at most risk for injury during surgery is the marginal mandibular nerve (MMN), resulting in deviation of the angle of the mouth toward the normal (sound) side (Fig. 18.10) [58–60]. The ability to close the eye without any corneal exposure

Table 18.2 Complications following parotidectomy

Early complications	Late complications
Facial nerve palsy	Frey's syndrome
Hematoma/seroma	Hypertrophic scar/keloid
Surgical site infection	Unsightly scar
Skin flap necrosis	Facial asymmetry/soft tissue defect
Salivary fistula/sialocele	Tumor recurrence
External otitis	
Trismus	
Hyposthesia/numbness around the ear	
First bite syndrome (FBS)	

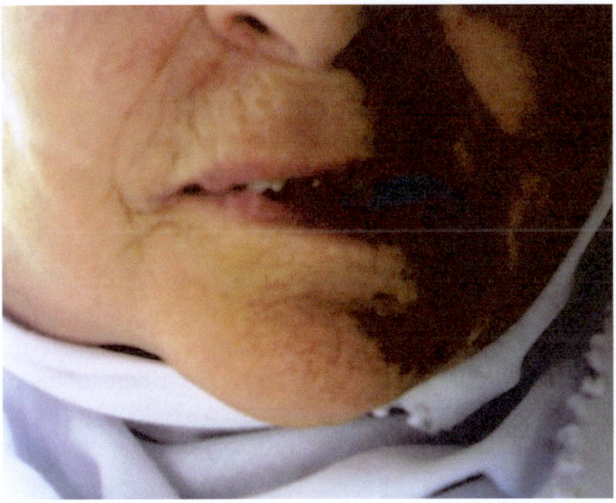

Fig. 18.10 Deviation of the angle of the mouth toward the sound side (left side) due to injury of the right marginal mandibular branch of the facial nerve

needs to be assessed and preventive measures should be taken to prevent exposure keratitis. Thus, if the motor supply to the orbicularis oculi is weak or absent, aggressive eye care must be instituted to prevent corneal drying and injury. Such care includes the use of lubricants, taping the eye shut at night, and moisture chambers during the day [61, 62]. If long-term paralysis occurs, static facial rehabilitation techniques may be used, including brow lift, gold weight insertion and canthoplasty, and facial slings. Dynamic techniques or nerve repair may also be appropriate.

When the facial nerve is anatomically identified and its branches are known to be intact, the most probable cause of the paralysis is stretching. This is also supported by the significantly more common incidence of paresis/paralysis in total parotidectomy when compared to superficial parotidectomy. The incidence of "transient" paralysis or temporary paresis is somewhere between 16.6% and 34%, and 90% will recover within 1 month; however, it could last as long as 18 months postoperatively.

To achieve the best functional results of the facial nerve, nerve transection during surgery requires immediate microsurgical repair.

18.15.1.2 Hematoma/Seroma

Hemorrhage or hematoma is uncommon after parotidectomy (0.9%) and is usually related to incomplete hemostasis during the procedure. Meticulous hemostasis is thus the key to prevention. Treatment consists of hematoma evacuation and surgical re-intervention to control any identified bleeding vessels under general anesthesia [63]. Seroma is managed by needle aspiration and compression dressing [62].

18.15.1.3 Surgical Site Infection

Surgical site infection is also an uncommon complication after parotidectomy due to the rich vascular supply to the parotid region. It is avoided by the use of aseptic techniques and careful handling of tissues. Perioperative prophylactic antibiotics are generally not used. Treatment of infection consists of appropriate antibiotics. Extensive procedures with neck dissection with or without free flap reconstruction are at higher risk of infection and benefit from perioperative antibiotics. In more standard parotidectomy, intraoperative antibiotics are sufficient in most patients.

Abscess formation is rare and requires surgical incision and drainage together with the appropriate antibiotics.

18.15.1.4 Skin-Flap Necrosis

Skin-flap necrosis is an uncommon complication after parotidectomy. The distal tip of the postauricular skin flap is the most common location of flap necrosis. Appropriate design of skin incisions can minimize distal flap necrosis. Smoking, diabetes mellitus, and prior RT may contribute to this complication by impairing the blood supply to the flap. If flap necrosis does occur, treatment entails conservative debridement of necrotic tissue and appropriate local wound care.

18.15.1.5 Salivary Leakage (Salivary Sialocele or Fistula)

Raw gland surface can result in a collection of saliva below the skin (sialocele) or leakage of saliva from the wound (salivary fistula) in 1–14% of patients [57, 64]. Salivary leakage is usually mild and self-limited.

A sialocele is usually treated with repeated needle aspirations or drainage plus pressure dressings. Salivary fistula can be treated with local wound revision if low-flow leakage is present. Sometimes decreasing oral intake is necessary; even completion parotidectomy has been suggested. Botulinum toxin injection, by blocking the release of acetylcholine from postganglionic parasympathetic fibers, results in decreased salivary flow and has been reported to be remarkably effective in several small series [63, 65, 66]. A chronic salivary fistula is rare following superficial parotidectomy. Recalcitrant salivary leakage may necessitate surgical reexploration.

18.15.1.6 External Otitis

External otitis may occur postoperatively and may be related to intraoperative blood collection in the external auditory canal (EAC). Treatment consists of just cleaning the EAC and instillation of antibiotic ear drops.

18.15.1.7 Mild Trismus

Mild trismus may occur following parotidectomy and may be related to inflammation and fibrosis of the masseter muscle. It is transient and mild and usually resolves with range of motion exercises of the jaw [62].

18.15.1.8 Ear Numbness/Hyposthesia

Hyposthesia in the distribution of the great auricular nerve (GAN), around the ear, especially the lobule, occurs in almost all patients undergoing parotid surgery. The numbness lessens over time in some patients; significant but incomplete improvement is expected within 1 year. Its incidence may be reduced by making efforts to preserve the GAN [42]. Preservation of the posterior branch of the GAN will hasten recovery [62]. When it must be sacrificed, neurorrhaphy at the conclusion of the case should be performed (tried).

18.15.1.9 First Bite Syndrome (FBS)

First bite syndrome may occur days, weeks, or even years after parotid surgery. It presents as a painful spasm in the parotid region at the first bite during mastication and decreasing afterward. This pain accompanies each meal usually. It is a unique complication of surgeries targeting the deep lobe of the parotid gland, the parapharyngeal space, and the infratemporal fossa. The presumed etiology is loss of sympathetic innervation of the parotid gland, which leads to relative parasympathetic overstimulation, resulting in the contraction of parotid myoepithelial cells. This complication is exceedingly rare, and is only encountered in extensive parotidectomy and extended neck dissections that violate the deep fascia of the floor of the neck, traumatizing the superior cervical ganglion. Treatment is often challenging and begins with carbamazepine, which must be titrated. Most patients report improvement with time, but never complete recovery [67].

18.15.2 Late Complications

18.15.2.1 Frey's Syndrome (Gustatory Sweating)

Gustatory sweating results from aberrant reinnervation of cholinergic sympathetic sweat glands in the skin with postganglionic fibers from the auriculotemporal nerve (ATN) that have been exposed following parotidectomy [68]. Thus, a stimulus intended for saliva stimulation evokes hypersthesia and sweating. The patient complains of facial sweating and hotness on smell or taste of food, which might sometimes be associated with pain. Diagnosis can be confirmed with iodine-starch test (Minor test), where iodine starch placed on the affected area turns blue signaling sweat secretion.

Frey's syndrome is now considered an inevitable long-term complication following parotidectomy unless preventive measures are taken [69]. It has been reported in 2–80% of patients, depending on the method of diagnosis [57]; an acceptable incidence would be the lower end of this range when efforts are made to close the parotid capsule or reconstruct the parotid defect [70]. The incidence of Frey's syndrome may be correlated with the amount of gland removed. It has been suggested that the greater the quantity of parotid tissue removed, the greater the amount of raw surface available to provide aberrant innervation to the skin. With modern surgical techniques and the use of SMAS flaps and thicker skin flaps at the time of initial flap elevation, the incidence of gustatory sweating has been greatly reduced and is now considered quite rare.

Preventive measures include SCM flap, temporalis fascial flap, and insertion of an artificial membrane or autologous tissue between the skin and the parotid bed. If Frey's syndrome develops, treatment options include topical application of antiperspirant or topical anticholinergics (1% glycopyrolate), surgical interposition of tissue (e.g., temporoparietal fascia or SCM), or implantable material (e.g., acellular dermis). Surgical approaches carry the risks associated with reoperative surgery, but are usually effective in minimizing or eliminating Frey's syndrome. Recently, local intradermal injection of botulinum toxin has yielded good results. Botulinum toxin blocks the release of acetylcholine from presynaptic neurons. It is postulated to provide long-term results due to poor reinnervation of the skin's cholinergic sweat glands; relief of symptoms is obtained for 6–36 months. It is performed as an out-patient [62, 71].

18.15.2.2 Facial Asymmetry/Surgical Site Depression

The significance of the defect and the resulting facial asymmetry after parotidectomy is related to the amount of gland removed and thinness of the patient. Those with more subcutaneous fat may be better able to hide small defects than thin patients are and therefore may not require reconstruction.

Acellular dermis rolled and implanted in the defect can both reconstruct normal facial contours and serve to close the parotid capsule and cover raw gland surface. Local rotation of the posterior belly of the digastric muscle can fill moderate defects and does not result in significant morbidity. Reconstruction with an SCM flap is helpful, but it has the drawback of creating a defect in the neck. An autologous abdominal fat graft can be used to fill large defects and maintains volume over the long term if carefully and atraumatically harvested [43, 62].

18.15.2.3 Tumor Recurrence

Parotid tumors can recur as a result of positive margins, microsatellite disease, or unrecognized nerve invasion. A few basic principles should be followed to ensure adequate extirpation and minimize recurrence.

If the facial nerve or branch is grossly invaded, sacrifice of the nerve should be considered to ensure complete removal.

Every effort should be made to keep tumor capsules intact in both benign and malignant disease. If tumor spillage occurs, then copious irrigation is wise.

Capsular dissection can lead to incomplete excision as a result of failure to recognize microscopic extensions of tumor; therefore, a cuff of healthy gland should be removed with these tumors.

Capsular dissection of pleomorphic adenomas is controversial; classic teaching is to remove a cuff of healthy tissue around the tumor, but modern data suggest that capsular dissection may not increase recurrence rates; a balance must be made between taking a cuff of healthy tissue and minimizing dissection of facial nerve branches. The cuff of normal parotid does not need to be large and wide margins are not needed for benign disease [42].

Large-bore needle or incisional biopsies should not be performed; if they have been performed, the biopsy tract should be removed in continuity with the surgical specimen whenever possible.

References

1. Wang SJ, Eisele DW. Parotidectomy—anatomical considerations. Clin Anat. 2012;25(1):12–8.
2. Mutlu V, Kaya Z. Which surgical method is superior for the treatment of parotid tumor? Is it classical? Is it new? Eurasian J Med. 2019;51(3):273–6.
3. Jin H, Kim BY, Kim H, Lee E, Park W, Choi S, et al. Incidence of postoperative facial weakness in parotid tumor surgery: a tumor subsite analysis of 794 parotidectomies. BMC Surg. 2019;19(1):199.
4. Laing MR, McKerrow WS. Intraparotid anatomy of the facial nerve and retromandibular vein. Br J Surg. 1988;75(4):310–2.
5. Bailey H. The treatment of tumours of the parotid gland with special reference to total parotidectomy. Br J Surg. 1941;28(11):337–46.
6. Shucksmith HS, Boyle TM, Walls WK. The surgery of parotid tumours; exposure of main trunk of facial nerve. Br Med J. 1951;2(4735):830–1.
7. Martin H. The operative removal of tumors of the parotid salivary gland. Surgery. 1952;31(5):670–82.
8. Beahrs OH, Adson MA. The surgical anatomy and technic of parotidectomy. Am J Surg. 1958;95(6):885–96.
9. Kochhar A, Larian B, Azizzadeh B. Facial nerve and parotid gland anatomy. Otolaryngol Clin N Am. 2016;49(2):273–84.
10. Bialek EJ, Jakubowski W, Zajkowski P, Szopinski KT, Osmolski A. US of the major salivary glands: anatomy and spatial relationships, pathologic conditions, and pitfalls. Radiographics. 2006;26(3):745–63.
11. Porcheri C, Mitsiadis TA. Physiology, pathology and regeneration of salivary glands. Cells. 2019;8(9):976.
12. Pitanguy I, Ramos AS. The frontal branch of the facial nerve: the importance of its variations in face lifting. Plast Reconstr Surg. 1966;38(4):352–6.
13. Dorafshar AH, Borsuk DE, Bojovic B, Brown EN, Manktelow RT, Zuker RM, Rodriguez ED, Redett RJ. Surface anatomy of the middle division of the facial nerve: Zuker's point. Plast Reconstr Surg. 2013;131(2):253–7.
14. Bag AK, Curé JK, Chapman PR, Pettibon KD, Gaddamanugu S. Practical imaging of the parotid gland. Curr Probl Diagn Radiol. 2015;44(2):167–92.
15. Chu J, Zhou Z, Hong G, Guan J, Li S, Rao L, Meng Q, Yang Z. High-resolution MRI of the intraparotid facial nerve based on a microsurface coil and a 3D reversed fast imaging with steady-state precession DWI sequence at 3T. AJNR Am J Neuroradiol. 2013;34(8):1643–8.
16. Iwai H, Konishi M. Parotidectomy combined with identification and preservation procedures of the great auricular nerve. Acta Otolaryngol. 2015;135(9):937–41.
17. McGurk M, Combes J, editors. Controversies in the management of salivary gland disease. Oxford, Oxfordshire, England: Oxford University Press; 2013. ISBN 978-0-19-957820-7
18. Wierzbicka M, Piwowarczyk K, Nogala H, Błaszczyńska M, Kosiedrowski M, Mazurek C. Do we need a new classification of parotid gland surgery? Otolaryngol Pol. 2016;70(3):9–14.
19. To VS, Chan JY, Tsang RK, Wei WI. Review of salivary gland neoplasms. ISRN Otolaryngol. 2012;2012:872982.

20. Motamed M, Laugharne D, Bradley PJ. Management of chronic parotitis: a review. J Laryngol Otol. 2003;117(7):521–6.
21. Mooney CP, Clark JR, Shannon K, Palme CE, Ebrahimi A, Gao K, et al. The significance of regional metastasis location in head and neck cutaneous squamous cell carcinoma. Head Neck. 2021;43(9):2705–11.
22. Spiro RH. Salivary neoplasms: overview of a 35-year experience with 2,807 patients. Head Neck Surg. 1986;8(3):177–84.
23. Donovan DT, Conley JJ. Capsular significance in parotid tumor surgery: reality and myths of lateral lobectomy. Laryngoscope. 1984;94(3):324–9.
24. Gandolfi MM, Slattery W. Parotid gland tumors and the facial nerve. Otolaryngol Clin N Am. 2016;49(2):425–34.
25. van der Lans RJL, Lohuis PJFM, van Gorp JMHH, Quak JJ. Surgical treatment of chronic parotitis. Int Arch Otorhinolaryngol. 2019;23(1):83–7.
26. Gallia LJ, Johnson JT. The incidence of neoplastic versus inflammatory disease in major salivary gland masses diagnosed by surgery. Laryngoscope. 1981;91(4):512–6.
27. Dave SP, Pernas FG, Roy S. The benign lymphoepithelial cyst and a classification system for lymphocytic parotid gland enlargement in the pediatric HIV population. Laryngoscope. 2007;117(1):106–13.
28. Shanti RM, Aziz SR. HIV-associated salivary gland disease. Oral Maxillofac Surg Clin North Am. 2009;21(3):339–43.
29. Elmokadem AH, Abdel Khalek AM, Abdel Wahab RM, Tharwat N, Gaballa GM, Elata MA, Amer T. Diagnostic Accuracy of multiparametric magnetic resonance imaging for differentiation between parotid neoplasms. Can Assoc Radiol J. 2019;70(3):264–72.
30. Abu-Taleb NSM, Abdel-Wahed N, Amer ME. The role of magnetic resonance imaging and magnetic resonance sialography in the diagnosis of various salivary gland disorders: an interobserver agreement. J Med Imaging Radiat Sci. 2014;45(3):299–306.
31. Seethala RR, LiVolsi VA, Baloch ZW. Relative accuracy of fine-needle aspiration and frozen section in the diagnosis of lesions of the parotid gland. Head Neck. 2005;27(3):217–23.
32. Sood S, McGurk M, Vaz F. Management of salivary gland tumours: United Kingdom National Multidisciplinary Guidelines. J Laryngol Otol. 2016;130(S2):S142–9.
33. Thielker J, Grosheva M, Ihrler S, Wittig A, Guntinas-Lichius O. Contemporary management of benign and malignant parotid tumors. Front Surg. 2018;5:39.
34. So T, Sahovaler A, Nichols A, Fung K, Yoo J, Weir MM, MacNeil SD. Utility of clinical features with fine needle aspiration biopsy for diagnosis of Warthin tumor. J Otolaryngol Head Neck Surg. 2019;48(1):41.
35. Witt BL, Schmidt RL. Ultrasound-guided core needle biopsy of salivary gland lesions: a systematic review and meta-analysis. Laryngoscope. 2014;124(3):695–700.
36. Aro K, Ho AS, Luu M, Kim S, Tighiouart M, Clair JM, et al. Development of a novel salivary gland cancer lymph node staging system. Cancer. 2018;124(15):3171–80.
37. Kawata R, Koutetsu L, Yoshimura K, Nishikawa S, Takenaka H. Indication for elective neck dissection for N0 carcinoma of the parotid gland: a single institution's 20-year experience. Acta Otolaryngol. 2010;130(2):286–92.
38. Emerick KS, Fabian RL, Deschler DG. Clinical presentation, management, and outcome of high-grade mucoepidermoid carcinoma of the parotid gland. Otolaryngol Head Neck Surg. 2007;136(5):783–7.
39. Grosheva M, Klussmann JP, Grimminger C, Wittekindt C, Beutner D, Pantel M, et al. Electromyographic facial nerve monitoring during parotidectomy for benign lesions does not improve the outcome of postoperative facial nerve function: a prospective two-center trial. Laryngoscope. 2009;119(12):2299–305.
40. Sood AJ, Houlton JJ, Nguyen SA, Gillespie MB. Facial nerve monitoring during parotidectomy: a systematic review and meta-analysis. Otolaryngol Head Neck Surg. 2015;152(4):631–7.
41. Meier JD, Wenig BL, Manders EC, Nenonene EK. Continuous intraoperative facial nerve monitoring in predicting postoperative injury during parotidectomy. Laryngoscope. 2006;116(9):1569–72.

42. Witt RL. The significance of the margin in parotid surgery for pleomorphic adenoma. Laryngoscope. 2002;112:2141–54.
43. Honeybrook A, Athavale SM, Rangarajan SV, Rohde SL, Netterville JL. Free dermal fat graft reconstruction of the head and neck: an alternate reconstructive option. Am J Otolaryngol. 2017;38:291–6.
44. Bianchi B, Ferri A, Ferrari S, Copelli C, Sesenna E. Improving esthetic results in benign parotid surgery: statistical evaluation of facelift approach, sternocleidomastoid flap, and superficial musculoaponeurotic system flap application. J Oral Maxillofac Surg. 2011;69(4):1235–41.
45. Maithani T, Pandey AK, Agrahari AK. An overview of parotidectomy for benign parotid lesions with special reference to perioperative techniques to avoid complications: our experience. Indian J Otolaryngol Head Neck Surg. 2019;71(Suppl 1):258–64.
46. Terris DJ, Tuffo KM, Fee WE. Modified facelift incision for parotidectomy. J Laryngol Otol. 1994;108(7):574–8.
47. Saha S, Pal S, Sengupta M, Chowdhury K, Saha VP, Mondal L. Identification of facial nerve during parotidectomy: a combined anatomical & surgical study. Indian J Otolaryngol Head Neck Surg. 2014;66(1):63–8.
48. Bushey A, Quereshy F, Boice JG, Landers MA, Baur DA. Utilization of the tympanomastoid fissure for intraoperative identification of the facial nerve: a cadaver study. J Oral Maxillofac Surg. 2011;69(9):2473–6.
49. Cracchiolo JR, Shaha AR. Parotidectomy for parotid cancer. Otolaryngol Clin N Am. 2016;49(2):415–24.
50. Davidson B, Robind S. Parotidectomy. Washington, DC: MedStar Georgetown University Hospital; 2013.
51. Parotidectomy SM. Diagnostic techniques and therapeutic strategies for parotid gland disorders. Hershey, PA: IGI Global. Medical Information Science Refence; 2021. p. 265–95.
52. Abd-El-Hafez T, Khalil Y, El Noaman M, Zayan A, El-Demerdash A. Total conservative parotidectomy for management of benign parotid neoplasms. Egypt J Otolaryngol. 2020;36:42.
53. Yesensky J, Solis RN, Bewley A. Facial nerve sacrifice during parotidectomy for metastatic cutaneous squamous cell carcinoma. OTO Open. 2021;5(1):2473974.
54. O'Brien CJ, McNeil EB, McMahon JD, Pathak I, Lauer CS, Jackson MA. Significance of clinical stage, extent of surgery, and pathologic findings in metastatic cutaneous squamous carcinoma of the parotid gland. Head Neck. 2002;24(5):417–22.
55. Iyer NG, Clark JR, Murali R, Gao K, O'Brien CJ. Outcomes following parotidectomy for metastatic squamous cell carcinoma with microscopic residual disease: implications for facial nerve preservation. Head Neck. 2009;31(1):21–7.
56. De Vincentiis M, Magliulo G, Soldo P, Manciocco V, Pagliuca G, Del Gaizo R, et al. Extended parotidectomy. Acta Otorhinolaryngol Ital. 2005;25(3):169–73.
57. Koch M, Zenk J, Iro H. Long-term results of morbidity after parotid gland surgery in benign disease. Laryngoscope. 2010;120(4):724–30.
58. Reilly J, Myssiorek D. Facial nerve stimulation and postparotidectomy facial paresis. Otolaryngol Head Neck Surg. 2003;128(4):530–3.
59. Witt RL. Facial nerve function after partial superficial parotidectomy: an 11-year review (1987-1997). Otolaryngol Head Neck Surg. 1999;121(3):210–3.
60. Dulguerov P, Marchal F, Lehmann W. Postparotidectomy facial nerve paralysis: possible etiologic factors and results with routine facial nerve monitoring. Laryngoscope. 1999;109(5):754–62.
61. Siddiqui AH, Shakil S, Rahim DU, Shaikh IA. Post parotidectomy facial nerve palsy: a retrospective analysis. Pak J Med Sci. 2020;36(2):126–30.
62. Marchese-Ragona R, Marioni G, Restivo DA, Staffieri A. The role of botulinum toxin in postparotidectomy fistula treatment. A technical note Am J Otolaryngol. 2006;27(3):221–4.
63. Bovenzi CD, Ciolek P, Crippen M, Curry JM, Krein H, Heffelfinger R. Reconstructive trends and complications following parotidectomy: incidence and predictors in 11,057 cases. J Otolaryngol Head Neck Surg. 2019;48(1):64.
64. Wax M, Tarshis L. Post-parotidectomy fistula. J Otolaryngol. 1991;20(1):10–3.

65. Vargas H, Galati LT, Parnes SM. A pilot study evaluating the treatment of postparotidectomy sialoceles with botulinum toxin type A. Arch Otolaryngol Head Neck Surg. 2000;126(3):421–4.
66. Ellies M, Gottstein U, Rohrbach-Volland S, Arglebe C, Laskawi R. Reduction of salivary flow with botulinum toxin: extended report on 33 patients with drooling, salivary fistulas, and sialadenitis. Laryngoscope. 2004;114(10):1856–60.
67. Linkov G, Morris LG, Shah JP, Kraus DH. First bite syndrome: incidence, risk factors, treatment, and outcomes. Laryngoscope. 2012;122(8):1773–8.
68. Mantelakis A, Lafford G, Lee CW, Spencer H, Deval JL, Joshi A. Frey's syndrome: a review of aetiology and treatment. Cureus. 2021;13(12):e20107.
69. Eisele DW. Simple method for the assessment of Frey's syndrome. Laryngoscope. 1992;102(5):583–4.
70. Curry JM, King N, Reiter D, Fisher K, Heffelfinger RN, Pribitkin EA. Meta-analysis of surgical techniques for preventing parotidectomy sequelae. Arch Facial Plast Surg. 2009;11(5):327–31.
71. Gualberto GV, Sampaio FMS, Madureira NAB. Use of botulinum toxin type A in Frey's syndrome. Ann Bras Dermatol. 2017;92(6):891–2.

Frey's Syndrome 19

19.1 Background

Frey's syndrome, also known as Baillarger's syndrome, Frey–Baillarger syndrome, auriculotemporal syndrome, Dupuy's syndrome, gustatory hyperhidrosis, gustatory sweating, or flushing syndrome, represents aberrant reinnervation following injury of the auriculotemporal nerve (ATN). The ATN, a branch of the trigeminal nerve, consists of parasympathetic fibers that signal the parotid gland to produce saliva, and sympathetic fibers that innervate the sweat glands of the face and scalp. When an insult to the parasympathetic and sympathetic nerve fibers of the ATN in the parotid region occurs, the resulting aberrant regeneration of postganglionic parasympathetic nerve fibers (responsible for salivary secretion) along the preexisting sympathetic pathways to the vessels and sweat glands of the skin leads to the development of Frey's syndrome [1, 2].

Frey's syndrome is characterized clinically by facial warmth, sweating and flushing of the lateral aspect of the face and upper neck, usually around the parotid region, during meals with no direct relation with chewing [3]. Symptoms occur during meals, especially with spicy and sour foods [4]. Once present, gustatory sweating and flushing remain unchanged; there is no spontaneous resolution, even after numerous years [5].

Frey's syndrome most commonly arises as a complication of parotidectomy, but can also be associated with submandibular gland surgery, repair of mandibular fractures, temporomandibular joint (TMJ) injury, neck lymph node (LN) dissection, infection, and trauma to the parotid region [6–8].

Despite the fact that similar cases were already reported by Baillarger in 1853, it was not until 1923 that the first accurate description of this phenomenon was provided by Dr. Lucja Frey–Gottesman, a Polish physician at the University of Warsaw and one of the first female academic neurologists in Europe. She described a 25-year-old female who sustained a gunshot wound to the parotid region and subsequently developed facial flushing and sweating 5 months afterward. She accurately

© The Author(s), under exclusive license to Springer Nature Switzerland AG 2024
M. Sakr, *Surgery of the Salivary Glands*,
https://doi.org/10.1007/978-3-031-82069-4_19

identified the autonomic innervation of the parotid gland and the ATN as the link between gustatory stimulation and facial sweat production [2]. Dr. Frey published a landmark paper entitled "syndrome du nerf auriculotemporal" in 1923 and called it "auriculotemporal nerve syndrome" [3].

In 1927, Dr. Andre Thomas theorized that the pathophysiology of the disease involved aberrant nerve regeneration [2]. Five years later, Dr. Peter Bassoe reported the first case of Frey's syndrome after a parotidectomy, which has since become the most common cause of the condition [2].

19.2 Epidemiology

Laage-Hellmann in the late 1950s studied seriously this problem. A group of 123 patients who underwent a parotidectomy was evaluated retrospectively with a questionnaire and clinical testing. On questioning, 62% of the patients complained of problems during eating, 22% had both sweating and flushing, 26% had sweating only, and 14% had only flushing. When a gustatory stimulus was used, flushing was observed in 92% of patients, and 98% of patients exhibited a positive Minor sweat test [9–12]. The author concluded that gustatory sweating is an unavoidable sequel of parotidectomy that is not overtly symptomatic in all patients [9–12].

The reported incidence of gustatory sweating after parotidectomy is highly variable [13], varying between 4% and 96% [14–24]. The wide range of rates reported in the literature reflects the great heterogeneity of symptom severity, reporting, and diagnosis [7]. The incidence of Frey's syndrome approaches 80% in parotidectomy patients based on Minor's starch-iodine test, but ranges from 30% to 60% based on subjective patient reports, indicating that there is likely a population of patients with non-bothersome symptoms or asymptomatic Frey's syndrome patients [16]. There do not appear to be age or gender predilections for the development of Frey's syndrome in adults; it is less common in children.

The severity of the gustatory sweating was judged moderate by 58% of patients, important by 15%, and embarrassing by 27% [5]. Clinical severity has been correlated to the surface involved [12, 25] and extent of parotid surgery (superficial versus total) [18, 25, 26]. Laage-Hellman [12] reported that the minimal delay between parotidectomy and the appearance of gustatory sweating as examined by sequential Minor tests was 5 weeks and the median delay was approximately 8 weeks. In some patients, the test became positive at 9 months and in <1% of patients after 1 year. Clinical gustatory sweating has also been reported to appear up to 8.5 years after parotidectomy [27].

19.3 Anatomy and Physiology

The ATN (branch) of the mandibular division of the trigeminal nerve (CN-V) carries parasympathetic fibers to the parotid salivary gland and sympathetic fibers to the sweat glands of the face and scalp. During eating, a reflex arc is stimulated leading to increased salivary secretion of minor and major salivary glands, including the parotid gland. The origin of the afferent limb is at the level of the gustatory papillae of the oral cavity and oropharynx. The afferent neurons terminate in the "nucleus solitaries" and project to the inferior salivary nucleus.

Preganglionic parasympathetic efferent fibers leave the inferior salivary nucleus and the brain stem with the glossopharyngeal nerve (CN-IX). After passing through the jugular foramen and the superior and inferior glossopharyngeal ganglions, the parasympathetic fibers follow the tympanic (Jacobson's) nerve, which enters the temporal bone on its inferior aspect and travels in the inferior tympanic canaliculus toward the middle ear cavity. A plexus is formed on the promontory, but the parasympathetic fibers not supplying the middle ear unite to form the lesser superficial petrosal nerve. This nerve exits the temporal bone and travels on the floor of the middle cranial fossa.

The fibers then exit the skull through the foramen ovale and reach the otic ganglion where they synapse with postganglionic parasympathetic fibers, which then join the ATN and reach the parotid gland through its medial aspect in the parapharyngeal space. The neuro-transmitter of these fibers is acetylcholine. The muscarinic receptors of the parotid gland are of the M3 subtype. Secretion of the parotid gland is controlled predominantly by the parasympathetic system [28].

The sympathetic fibers for the cutaneous vessels and sweat glands follow the cervical sympathetic chain and a synaptic relay is found in the sympathetic cervical ganglions. The fibers then follow the periarterial plexuses of the internal carotid artery (ICA) and external carotid artery (ECA) and their branches before joining and following the branches of the trigeminal nerve supplying the cutaneous sensation of the skin [29, 30]. Thus, for the "preauricular" skin, these sympathetic fibers also travel within the ATN. The result of sympathetic activation is increased secretion from sweat glands [31] and vasoconstriction [30]. A vasodilatation role of the parasympathetic facial system [32] has been demonstrated [33] and found to follow the facial nerve and then the greater superficial petrosal branch [34]. Fibers probably synapse in the sphenopalatine ganglion before joining the corresponding branches of the trigeminal nerve [34], in this case, the ATN.

Contrary to other postganglionic sympathetic fibers, which are adrenergic, sweat glands have acetylcholine as the main neurotransmitter [35, 36]. The cholinergic receptors on sweat glands are muscarinic, predominantly of the M3 subtype [37], similar to that of parasympathetic salivary gland nerves.

19.4 Histopathology

There are few histopathological reports regarding Frey's syndrome in the literature. An interesting example was published in 1993 by Redleaf and McCabe who described a rare case of Frey's syndrome of the external auditory canal (EAC) [38]. A 36-year-old patient had presented with a 6-month history of left watery otorrhea, eventually determined to be perspiration that occurred only with eating. Resection of the canal skin with split-thickness skin graft reconstruction led to resolution of symptoms. Histopathological analysis of the canal skin revealed marked thickening (4.2 mm compared to 0.8 mm for normal) with hyperplasia and hypertrophy of sweat glands, which are not normal. This finding was postulated to be a result of aberrant parasympathetic influence.

19.5 Etiology

The ATN consists of two roots. The "superior somatosensory root" arises from the mandibular branch of the trigeminal nerve, providing innervation to the auricle, EAC, TMJ, lateral tympanic membrane, and the temporal scalp. The "inferior parasympathetic root" arises from the postganglionic fibers at the otic ganglion, originating from the glossopharyngeal nerve; it is responsible for the visceral secretomotor actions of the parotid gland [39]. After the two roots join, the ATN travels posterior to the mandible and parotid, where it gives off the secretomotor parotid branch before coursing across the superior border of the mandibular condyle, below the TMJ, and terminating in the temporal region. Frey's syndrome can occur if the ATN is proximal to the parotid branch or the parotid branch itself is injured [39, 40]. More recently, a rare variant characterized by symptoms distal to the parotid region in the temporoparietal scalp even when the injury occurs in the parotid region has been described by Wood and Netterville [8].

Although parotidectomy is the most frequent etiology of Frey's syndrome in adults [16, 41–43], the syndrome has been described with other surgical procedures such as mandibular surgery [44, 45] drainage of parotid or other local abscesses [46–51] and neck dissection [20]; together with regional trauma such as mandibular fractures [52–54] or penetrating wounds [55, 56] and with surgery or lesions of the cervical sympathetic chain [29, 54, 57–59] (Table 19.1).

Table 19.1 Causes of gustatory flushing and sweating

Typical Frey's syndrome etiologies	Atypical variants of gustatory sweating
Trauma in parotid region Parotidectomy Other procedures in the parotid region (mandibular surgery, drainage of parotid abscess, neck dissection) Penetrating trauma in the parotid region Closed mandibular fractures	Physiological Pediatric gustatory flushing syndrome Gustatory neuralgia
Trauma to the cervical sympathetic chain Endoscopic thoracic sympathectomy	
Other aberrant regeneration locations Cerebellopontine angle Middle ear Otic ganglion	
Autonomic neuropathies Diabetic neuropathy	

Rare causes of facial gustatory sweating, in single case reports, include herpes simplex (HS) of the mandibular division of the trigeminal nerve [60], large cerebellopontine angle tumor [61], and "gustatory otorrhea" [62]. These cases could also be explained by the aberrant regeneration theory, with the locus of cross-fiber regeneration being at the level of the maxillary division [61], at the level of the middle ear [62], or in the "deep" portion of the ATN instead of the "parotid space" portion of ATN [60]. A similar explanation, i.e., peripheral parasympathetic sprouting to degenerated sympathetic fibers, has been offered for the observed facial, and often neck and upper chest, gustatory sweating seen in patients with severe diabetic neuropathy [63–68].

"Physiological" gustatory sweating and flushing can be induced by certain spicy foods [36]. A variation of the threshold of individual cutaneous regions appears to be present, since only certain head and neck areas are found to respond in a given individual [36]. Opposite to Frey's syndrome, physiological gustatory sweating and flushing is bilateral and usually symmetrical [36], similar to physiologic thermal sweating [36, 69].

Frey's syndrome is less common in children and may occur during early infancy without a history of trauma or surgery. Few cases of gustatory sweating in the "pediatric" age group have been described [70–76]. The majority are normal children with unilateral [70–72, 74–76] or bilateral [71, 73] gustatory facial flushing, without any sweating, a hallmark of Frey's syndrome (atypical variant). The term "gustatory flushing syndrome," as proposed by Kozma and Gabriel [74], might be more appropriate.

In addition, a "gustatory otorrhea" in two patients without any previous pathology has been reported [77, 78]. Bilateral symptoms are more likely "idiopathic" in origin. Familial bilateral Frey's syndrome has been described in patients without a history of trauma, leading to the hypothesis that congenital dysfunction of the ATN is the culprit [79].

Recently, several cases of facial pain in the territory of the ATN nerve have been described [80–83] and the name "gustatory neuralgia" proposed [81]. Other specific characteristics of gustatory neuralgia include an electric, burning (neuralgic) pain, pain distribution in the territory of the ATN, triggering of the pain by eating, numbness in the ATN because of surgery, and lack of response to anticonvulsant medication [81]. Gustatory neuralgia should be differentiated from the classical Frey's syndrome because of the absence of sweating and flushing and because pain is not a symptom in patients with Frey's syndrome [84, 85].

19.6 Pathophysiology

Andre Thomas [86] and later Ford and Woodhall [87] postulated that the severed parasympathetic fibers to the parotid gland regenerate along the wrong neurolemmal sheaths of the sectioned cutaneous sympathetic fibers, the so-called "aberrant regeneration theory" (Fig. 19.1), which is supported by several experimental and clinical observations: (1) ATN block by local anesthetics induces a local anesthesia

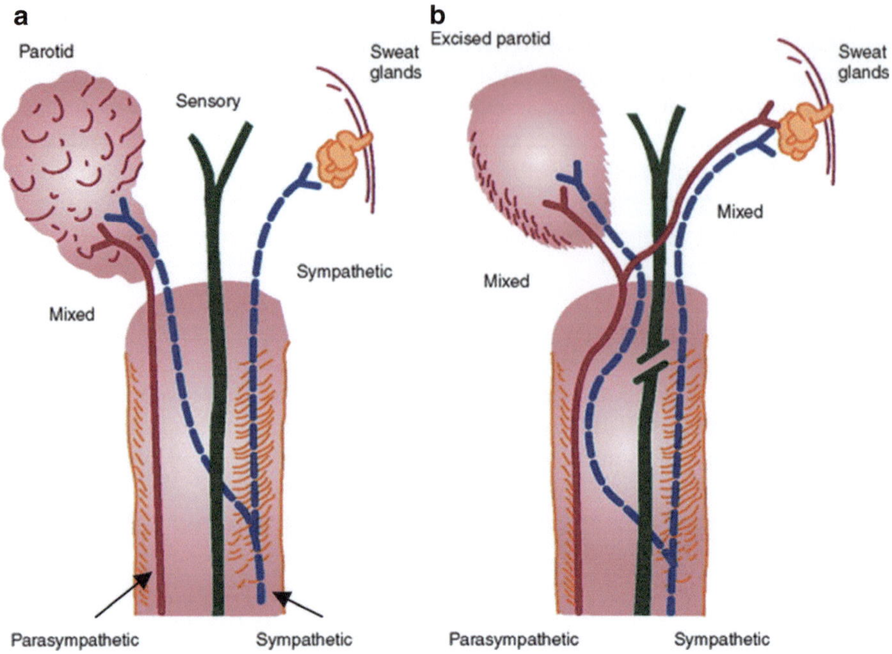

Fig. 19.1 The proposed "aberrant regeneration mechanism" of Frey's syndrome. (**a**) Normal parotid gland and sweat gland parasympathetic and sympathetic innervation; (**b**) aberrant regeneration of severed parotid postganglionic parasympathetic nerve fibers to severed sweat gland postganglionic sympathetic fibers

and cessation of gustatory sweating of similar cutaneous distribution [87, 88]; (2) stimulation of the tympanic plexus results in sweating in the involved skin area [89]; (3) symptoms are unaffected by anesthesia of the stellate ganglion, despite the appearance of a temporary Horner syndrome [84, 87–89]; (4) in the involved area, there is an impairment of the normal sympathetic function, such as reduced thermoregulatory sweating [29, 57, 87, 88, 90] and absence of emotional flushing [29, 57, 87, 90]; (5) a latent period (minimum 1–2 months [12]) is present between the initial injury and the appearance of gustatory flushing and sweating [21, 29, 57, 58, 88]; (6) sequential follow-up of patients showed that positivity of the sweat test increases and the involved area progressively increases in size [12, 21]; (7) symptoms can be abolished by local injection of anticholinergic substances such as atropine [87, 88] and botulinum toxin (8), a localized hypersensitivity to cholinergic drugs is described with mecholine [58] acetylcholine [87, 88] and pilocarpine [58, 88]; and (9) the syndrome appears after various lesions or resections of the homolateral cervical sympathetic chain [29, 58, 59, 90].

The postulated etiology is an aberrant regeneration of the sectioned parasympathetic fibers normally innervating the parotid gland. The traumatized fibers lose their parotid targets and regenerate to innervate the vessels and sweat glands of the overlying skin. In order for this aberrant regeneration to occur, the sympathetic fibers to these vessels and sweat glands have to be damaged, a frequent event in either parotid surgery or penetrating parotid trauma. The regular function of the parotid parasympathetic fibers is to increase salivary secretion during eating. The activation following aberrant regeneration produces an activation of the "new targets" during meals, resulting in a local vasodilatation (gustatory flushing) and localized sweating (gustatory sweating). Despite all these convincing arguments, the aberrant regeneration remains a hypothesis until the demonstration of parasympathetic neurons on the reinnervated sweat glands.

Frey's syndrome can also occur after submandibular excision and neck dissection due to aberrant nerve regeneration after damage to the postganglionic parasympathetic nerve fibers to the submandibular gland, postganglionic parasympathetic fibers to the sublingual gland, or postganglionic parasympathetic fibers arising from the cervical sympathetic ganglia to innervate the sweat glands of the skin [91].

Another theory regarding the development of Frey's syndrome is that damaged sympathetic nerve fibers result in increased sweat gland sensitivity, which can then be stimulated by acetylcholine released from adjacent parasympathetic fibers. This theory may be more convincing in cases wherein gustatory sweating occurs shortly after surgery when nerve regeneration has yet to occur [91].

19.7 Clinical Presentation

19.7.1 In Adults

Patients with Frey syndrome often have a history of prior parotid surgery, neck surgery, trauma, or infection of the parotid region, although idiopathic and infantile presentations may also occur. They report unilateral sweating, flushing, neuralgia, pruritus, and warmth over the preauricular and temporal areas after gustatory stimuli, especially with sour and spicy foods [4, 92]. The severity of symptoms can range from non-bothersome to mild annoyance to social anxiety and avoidance of eating in public [93]. Symptoms can appear weeks, months, or even years after the initial insult [94–96]. Physical examination may show signs of prior surgical intervention or trauma in the parotid region.

19.7.2 In Children

In children, symptoms usually occur around the age of 5 months and can be misdiagnosed as food allergy since Frey's syndrome appears during the same period as food diversification. It can be distinguished from allergies, if there is a history of instrumented vaginal delivery, quick onset after a meal compared with allergic reactions, occurrence with specific foods (sweet and sour) not related to common food allergens, rapid recovery without treatment, consistent and persistent location, and absence of other atopic symptoms [96, 97]. During traumatic instrumentation delivery using forceps and spatula, the ATN is more liable to be crushed than severed, resulting in less aberrant nerve regeneration, absence of sweating in certain patients, and occasional possibility of recovery [96].

19.8 Evaluation

19.8.1 Composition of Sweat

Since the most troublesome symptom of Frey's syndrome is sweating, testing for Frey's syndrome has in general been limited to the evaluation of sweating. The major function of sweat glands in humans is thermoregulation [98]. Sweat is a hypotonic solution that contains mainly sodium chloride (NaCl), potassium (K^+), and bicarbonate (HCO_3^-), as well as certain inorganic compounds such as lactate, urea, and ammonia (NH_3) [31, 98].

19.8.2 Sweat Output Function

Tests of autonomic thermoregulatory function are complex [99] and the measure of "sweat output" is just one of the aspects assessed. Tests of sweat output function measure the production of sweat by a group of sweat glands and these tests could be classified as: (1) topographic, where a chemical reaction provides a view of the anatomical location of sweat secretion; (2) electric, where a change of skin impedance by the humidity of sweat is measured; and (3) thermodynamic, where the skin humidity is evaporated and a "sudometer" measures the thermal mass of the air stream [99]. Advantages of the electric and thermodynamic tests include the possibility of repeated and dynamic measures, while topographic tests give a better representation of surface and anatomical distribution.

The ideal test method for gustatory sweating should provide topographic information and quantification of the amount of sweating. While dynamic measures might be interesting in investigational studies, their use in clinical practice is of limited value. Further characteristics of the test should include: (1) simplicity (one-step); (2) sensitivity; (3) reliability; (4) adequate dynamic range, so that different sweating rates could be appreciated; (5) absence of toxicity and allergenicity of the agents used; (6) easy removal from the skin of the applied agents; and (7) low cost [100, 101].

19.8.3 Minor Test

The most frequently used method of sweat secretion assessment for gustatory sweating was originally described by Victor Minor, a Russian neurologist [102]. The original solution described contains 1.5 g iodine (I_2), 10 g castor oil, and

88.5 g of absolute alcohol and is painted on the skin to be tested. Actually, any colored I_2 solution used for disinfections, such as Betadine, will work [103]. After drying, the areas are powdered with starch (e.g., regular baking corn starch). The water in the sweat produces blue coloring by a reduction reaction of the I_2–starch mixture. With limited sweat production, the apertures of individual sweat glands are marked as small blue dots, while with larger amounts of sweat secretion the blue dots are larger and eventually become confluent. Therefore, the Minor test is seen as a topographic method, allowing accurate mapping of the involved surface.

Disadvantages of the Minor test include the application of several layers of reagents, difficulty of removing the I_2 paint, possible allergy to iodine [104], and difficulty of using the method with heavy perspiration, since sweat tends to drip down, obscuring assessment of the more dependently located skin [101]. While it could be seen as objective, it is not a quantitative test and thus might not be suited for the comparison of two treatments [16, 105].

19.8.4 Modifications of Minor Test

Several modifications of the Minor test have been proposed, but all of these share the inconveniences of the original test [100, 106]. Randall [69], noting that some papers have starch coatings, modified the method by using paper instead of starch, but continued to paint the skin with the I_2-based mixture. Dole and Thaysen [107] further simplified the process by the use of paper that was coated with I_2 (Fig. 19.2).

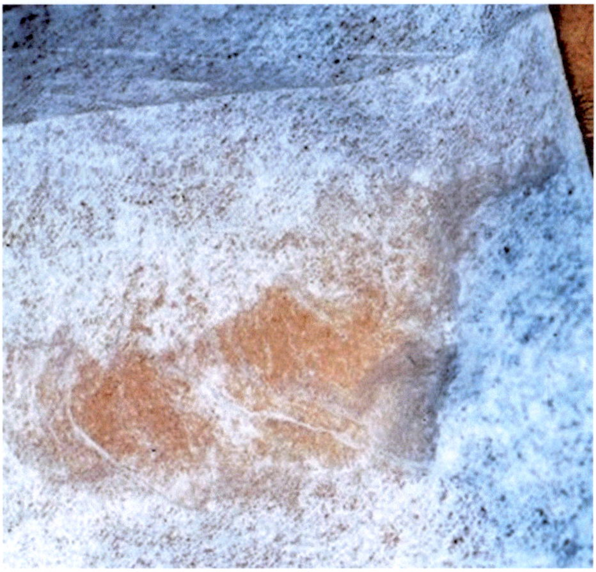

Fig. 19.2 Simple assessment of Frey's syndrome with facial tissue. The affected area is demarcated by the wet area on the tissue

19.8.5 Blotting Paper Method and Iodine-Sublimated Paper Histogram

Recently, two techniques for the evaluation of gustatory sweating have been reported [100]. The "blotting paper method" simply uses the difference in weight of a piece of blotting paper before and after gustatory stimulation. In the "iodine-sublimated paper histogram" (ISPH) method, regular office paper is sublimated with I_2 and acquires the property of changing color when wetted. The paper is then digitized and a histogram algorithm applied to measure the area of color change [100]. These tests (blotting paper and ISPH) satisfy most of the requirements of an ideal sweat test.

19.9 Differential Diagnosis

Differential diagnosis of Frey's syndrome or gustatory sweating includes the following.

19.9.1 Food Allergy

In children, Frey's syndrome can present during early infancy at the same time as food diversification and be mistaken for food allergy. It can be distinguished from allergies predominantly if there is rapid onset after a meal compared with allergic reactions, specific food triggers (sweet and sour) unrelated to common food allergens, rapid recovery without allergy treatment, symptoms localized to the parotid region, and absence of other allergic symptoms. Frey's syndrome should also be suspected if there is a history of instrumentation during delivery that may have causes traumatic injury to the ATN [94].

19.9.2 Hyperhidrosis

Primary hyperhidrosis is an autonomic disorder that affects 0.6–1% of the population [108]. Most cases are idiopathic, and patients usually younger than 25 years old and present with at least 6 months of excessive bilateral and symmetrical sweating, a positive family history, or history of cessation of sweating during sleep [109, 110]. Secondary hyperhidrosis can be induced by drugs, toxins, thyroid dysfunction, pituitary dysfunction, metabolic disorders, malignancy, central nervous system dysfunction, and congenital disorders such as Riley–Day syndrome [109, 111].

19.9.3 Emotional Sweating

Emotional sweating is activated by emotional stimuli and affects primarily the palms, soles, and sometimes the axilla. It does not occur during sleep or under sedation [111].

19.9.4 Compensatory Hyperhidrosis

Compensatory hyperhidrosis is a sequela of thoracic sympathectomy. Sympathectomy is used to treat primary hyperhidrosis, but can disrupt the thermoregulatory function of the sympathetic nervous system resulting in an uncontrolled sweating in untreated areas, usually below the level of the sympathectomy [111].

19.9.5 Gustatory Tearing

Gustatory tearing (also known as crocodile tears or Bogorad's syndrome) presents with unilateral tearing in response to gustatory stimuli. It is commonly associated with recovery from facial paralysis, Duane syndrome, and trauma. It is theorized that damage to facial and glossopharyngeal nerve fibers leads to aberrant nerve regeneration of the postganglionic parasympathetic secretomotor nerve fibers along the greater superficial petrosal nerve, which sends branches to the lacrimal gland. The treatment involves subtotal lacrimal gland excision, anticholinergics, transection of the facial or glossopharyngeal nerves, injection of alcohol to the sphenopalatine ganglion or botulinum toxin into the lacrimal gland [112, 113].

19.9.6 Gustatory Rhinorrhea

The etiology of gustatory rhinorrhea is similar to that of gustatory tearing. After trauma, the postganglionic parasympathetic secretomotor fibers that innervate the parotid gland undergo aberrant regeneration and grow along the greater superficial petrosal nerve and Vidian nerve, which innervates not only the lacrimal glands but also the glands of the nasal and palatine mucosa. This results in patients presenting with unilateral rhinorrhea in response to gustatory stimuli [114].

19.9.7 First Bite Syndrome (FBS)

First bite syndrome (FBS) is yet another nerve injury syndrome in which damaged postganglionic sympathetic fibers cannot modulate parasympathetic-mediated supramaximal myoepithelial cell contraction, which can cause pain with eating and drinking. Pain is typically most noticeable at the beginning of a meal and fades rapidly after that. This syndrome is most commonly seen following parotid and parapharyngeal surgery, but may occur in carotid endarterectomy and face-lifting procedures as well [115–117].

19.10 Prevention

The main method of preventing Frey's syndrome from developing is to create a barrier at the time of surgery that hinders aberrant nerve regeneration between the parasympathetic secretomotor fibers and the sweat glands in the parotid region. Several techniques have been described in the literature; all have associated risks and disadvantages, including creating a donor site, prolonged operative time, variable efficacy in preventing the syndrome, wound infection, and rejection, as well as postoperative complications [16, 29].

The techniques proposed for preventing Frey's syndrome reported in the literature include the following.

19.10.1 Thick Skin Flap

Increasing the thickness of the skin flap raised over the parotid gland during surgery by including fat and superficial musculoaponeurotic tissue can theoretically protect the sweat glands and their nerve fibers from being exposed. Because the sweat glands reside at the level of the hair follicles, a thickened flap reduces the chance of their exposure to aberrantly regenerating parasympathetic axons. While some recent studies have shown that increased flap thickness does not appear to lower the incidence of Frey's syndrome significantly, there was a trend toward a decrease in the total skin surface area affected and the overall severity of the symptoms [118, 119].

19.10.2 Acellular Dermal Matrix (ADM)

Acellular dermal matrix is an extracellular connective tissue graft generated via a decellularization process wherein the cellular components of the dermis are removed. This graft can function as a biological barrier between the parotid bed and the overlying skin. Zeng et al. (2012) utilized an ADM as a barrier between the skin and the operated parotid gland, resulting in a reduction of Frey's syndrome by 85% on objective starch–iodine testing and 68% on subjective assessment of symptoms [120]. However, other studies have found the effectiveness of ADM placement in reducing clinical symptoms and positive starch–iodine tests to be mixed [93, 121].

19.10.3 Autologous Fat Implantation

The autologous fat implantation technique is commonly used to ameliorate postsurgical contour defects and improve cosmesis in many parts of the body. Some studies investigating the effect of abdominal fat implantation on the prevention of Frey's syndrome have shown it to be successful, whereas others have failed to substantiate its usefulness [93, 121, 122]. Furthermore, the potential for donor site morbidity of an abdominal fat harvest such as hematoma, seroma, and infection may make it a less attractive option for Frey's syndrome prophylaxis.

19.10.4 Superficial Muscular Aponeurotic System (SMAS) Flap

The SMAS is a fascial layer that interdigitates with the facial muscles and protects the facial nerve. During a parotidectomy, the SMAS flap can be elevated separately from the underlying parotid fascia and the overlying dermis and then sutured tightly to the auricular perichondrium and sternocleidomastoid (SCM) muscle to act as a physical barrier to aberrant innervation of the sweat glands. It can also help improve contour deformities resulting from loss of parotid volume. Bonanno et al. (2000) reported that this technique is effective in preventing Frey's syndrome [123]. Although some studies using the SMAS flap have failed to reproduce these results, others have shown a significant decrease in symptom severity and total skin surface area affected [124–127].

19.10.5 Temporoparietal Fascia (TPF) Flap

The temporoparietal fascia (TPF) flap is a vascularized fascial flap supplied by branches of the superficial temporal artery. The prophylactic placement of a TPF flap between the skin and the defect aims to serve as a physical barrier to the development of Frey's syndrome. Sultan et al. (1995) reported that the use of the TPF flap reduced the contour deformity after parotid surgery and decreased the incidence of Frey's syndrome from 17% to 4% [128]. Disadvantages of this technique include an extended skin incision toward the temple, risk to the frontal branch of the facial nerve during flap harvest, and increased operative time [93].

19.10.6 Sternocleidomastoid (SCM) Muscle Flap

The SCM muscle is supplied by the occipital, superior thyroid, and suprascapular arteries [129]. Its efficacy in preventing Frey's syndrome is unclear, given the heterogeneity of results between studies [20]. Filho et al. (2004) reported that 24 parotidectomies with SCM flap reconstruction resulted in no cases of Frey's syndrome compared to 52.6% and 63.2% by clinical and starch–iodine testing, respectively, in a control group without SCM flap reconstruction [130]. A meta-analysis published by Curry et al. in 2009 concluded also that SCM flaps decrease the incidence of Frey's syndrome after parotidectomy [131]. However, other studies have shown that the SCM muscle flap is ineffective in prophylaxis against the development of Frey's syndrome after parotidectomy [132, 133].

19.11 Treatment

The treatment modalities proposed for Frey's syndrome or gustatory sweating can be categorized into three main groups: (1) external radiotherapy; (2) medical therapy (topical antiperspirants, local or systemic application of anticholinergics drugs, or botulinum toxin injection); and (3) surgical treatment (section of some portion of the efferent neural arc, and interposition of a subcutaneous barrier, as used for Frey's syndrome prevention). Considering that the symptoms are not always very troublesome, it is important that the treatment should be individualized and does not by itself result in more serious side effects.

19.11.1 Radiotherapy (RT)

Radiotherapy (RT) was first attempted by Needles [134]. In Laage-Hellman's studies [9], irradiated patients had a lower incidence of gustatory sweating with the involved surface often outside the radiotherapy fields. Similar results were obtained later from other publications [21, 135], indicating that should RT be indicated, the expected incidence and severity of gustatory sweating will be low.

19.11.2 Medical Therapy

Medical treatment of Frey's syndrome includes topical antiperspirants and local injections using alcohol, anticholinergics (atropine, scopolamine, glycopyrrolate), or botulinum toxin A (BTA) [8, 136, 137]. Since the sweat glands are innervated by postganglionic cholinergic pathways, treatment has traditionally involved anticholinergics.

19.11.3 Topical Antiperspirants

Topical antiperspirants have been shown to be ineffective in completely controlling gustatory sweating. Studies have shown that <50% of patients report any benefits, and for those who do, the duration of improvement is less than 1 day [138].

19.11.4 Alcohol Injection

Injection of alcohol to the otic ganglion has historically been employed, but can result in anesthesia to the mandibular branch of the trigeminal nerve, which can cause even more bothersome symptoms than Frey's syndrome [139].

19.11.5 Anticholinergic Medication

Systemic atropine is not effective in preventing sweating; if anhidrosis occurs with its use, it is usually a sign of atropine overdose, which can also present with other undesirable side effects such as tachycardia, blurred vision, disorientation, respiratory distress, and even coma [8, 139].

Shelley and Horvath (1951) showed that local application of anticholinergics drugs such as scopolamine could be used to reduce sweating [140]. Laage-Hellman

(1958) was the first to apply scopolamine (3% cream) for the treatment of gustatory sweating with symptom reduction in male and abolition in female patients. The difference was explained by a thinner female skin [12].

Double-blind studies have shown topical glycopyrrolate [141, 142], aluminum chloride [143–145], and diphemanil methylsulfate [146] to be superior to placebo. Few patients experienced minor side-effects such as dry mouth [141]. Despite their effectiveness, patients seem in the long run [21] to abandon the cumbersome daily application requiring skin drying with a hair dryer [13]. Moreover, skin wounds or infection, and application to the mucosa of the eyes, mouth, and nose result in an enhanced absorption and increased side-effects [27].

19.11.6 Botulinum Toxin Injection

The injection of "botulinum toxin A" (BTA) in the skin involved by gustatory sweating was recently proposed by Drobik and Laskawi [147]. Following their case report, the technique has been progressively adopted [15, 148–156]. Currently, BTA is the most widely used agent for local injection in Frey's syndrome [148, 149, 157]. Advantages include its simple and easy use in the office setting, avoiding complex procedures in the operating room, and its few reported side-effects [158]. The main disadvantage is the pain associated with the needle sticking and the secondary reluctance of some patients to be stuck, especially on the face.

19.11.7 Mechanism of Botulinum Toxin Action

Eight serotypes (A, B, Cα, Cβ, D, E, F, and G) of botulinum toxins are produced by different strains of the anaerobic bacteria *Clostridium botulinum* of which only four (A, B, E, and F) are toxic to humans [159]. The action of botulinum toxins is that of highly specific endopeptidases that cleave cytosol proteins involved in the fusion of exocytosis vesicles with the cell membrane [160], with type A toxin acting on synaptosome-associated protein (SNAP)-25 [161] and type B toxin acting on vesicle-associated membrane protein (VAMP). This action is highly specific for cholinergic synapses because the specific membrane proteins required for the internalization of botulinum toxins are found only in the presynaptic endings of cholinergic synapses [162]. By blocking the exocytosis mechanism of the presynaptic terminal, the release of acetylcholine is inhibited. The synapse remains intact, but is nonfunctional for neuromuscular junctions resulting in muscle paralysis. The recovery of function is due to collateral sprouting from the same or other axons and the formation of new synapses.

19.11.8 Practical Aspects

Botulinum toxin A (BTA) has been approved by the Food and Drug Administration (FDA) since 1989 and is commercially available as Botox (Allergan, Irvine, CA) and Dysport (Speywood Pharmaceuticals, Maidenhead, UK). A Botox vial contains 100 IU of BTA, 0.5 mg of human albumin, and 0.9 mg of NaCl as a sterile powder that can remain in a refrigerator for at least 24 months.

The practical considerations for BTA treatment in Frey's syndrome include: (1) mapping of the facial surface to be treated—the contour of the area to be injected is drawn on the patient's face [105]; (2) a grid of 1-cm squares is drawn either physically on the face or an "imaginary" one is created by the physician; (3) if anesthetic is to be used such as local anesthetic cream (EMLA, Astra, Sweden), it should be applied at this time; (4) the delimited area is injected at sites 1 cm apart, which are infiltrated with 0.1 mL (5 IU) of a solution containing BTA at a concentration of 2.5–5 IU/0.1 mL (2 cc per bottle of Botox powder) [105]; (5) the injection should be strictly intradermal, rising tiny wheals at each injection site; and (6) a light massage of the area is used for local diffusion.

19.11.9 Side-effects

Some authors reported temporary facial muscle paresis/paralysis and eyelid ptosis as a side-effect of the BTA injection [149, 150, 154]. The most plausible explanation of this rare and partial temporary paresis [149] is an injection deep to the dermis and/or diffusion to facial motor end plates.

Botulinum toxin injection may also result in localized pain, edema, erythema, and ecchymosis [163]. The pain associated with the needle injection was reported to be minimal (2/10 on an analog visual pain scale) [105, 150, 154]. The use of local anesthetic cream (EMLA, Astra, Sweden) might be tried in the few patients reluctant to undergo this procedure [150].

Allergic reaction is surprisingly low. The development of antibodies seems related to the amount of protein load injected and the shortness of the interval between injections [164]. The incidence is <1% with current Botox preparations [164, 165]. There is no overt hypersensitivity reaction, but the blocking antibodies result in decreased effectiveness of the BTA preparation. These patients could benefit from botulinum toxin B or F preparations.

19.11.10 Contraindications

Botulinum toxin injection is contraindicated in patients with motor neuron disease, myasthenia gravis, Eaton–Lambert syndrome, neuropathies, psychological instability, history of an allergic reaction to the toxin or albumin, pregnancy, and infection at the affected skin site [166].

19.11.11 Therapeutic Results

Repeat of injections several times may be needed before obtaining a complete response [105, 148]. The duration of the effect of BTA on gustatory sweating is rather long-lasting, with an average of 15 months [20, 149, 153]. An actuarial estimate puts the clinical gustatory sweating recurrence at 1, 2, and 3 years at 27%, 63%, and 92%, respectively [153]. The severity of the recurrent Frey's syndrome was found to be reduced when compared to that of the initial episode and retreatment with BTA was still effective [153]. A clear explanation for this longer time-frame relative to neuromuscular indications is lacking, but different possibilities have been suggested such as an atrophy of the sweat glands, poor sprouting of autonomic fibers, and increased scarring impeding regenerating axons [105].

19.11.12 Surgical Treatment

After its onset, surgical treatment of Frey's syndrome is rarely indicated and is reserved for refractory cases where conservative or medical therapies are no longer effective. Options for surgical management include: (1) interruption of the efferent pathway by transection of the ATN, glossopharyngeal nerve, tympanic nerve, or greater auricular nerve; and (2) surgical interposition (the placement of a barrier) and excision of the affected skin with grafting for the defect (can create an unacceptable cosmetic defect for patients) [167].

19.11.13 Interruption of the Efferent Pathway

Section of the ATN was originally described by Leriche in 1914 for the treatment of traumatic parotid fistula [168]. Debets and Munting [169] and, more recently, Coldwater [170] attempted ATN section, with only partial and temporary improvement of the symptoms [171]. Moreover, the access to this deeply located region in a previously operated field is technically challenging and carries the risk of injuring several important structures, including the facial nerve. In addition, the ATN is capable of regeneration, which may ultimately reduce any initial benefits obtained [12, 139, 172].

At the other end of the efferent pathway, a division of the intracranial portion of the glossopharyngeal nerve was done by Gardner and McCubbin (1956), with a good result lasting 5 years in one patient and a short period of relief in a second [173]. However, because of the extensive surgery, many patients and surgeons feel that the risk of an intracranial procedure to divide the glossopharyngeal nerve is not justified for a benign entity such as Frey's syndrome [51, 55, 73]. Thus, this therapy has not been pursued.

In 1960, Hemenway [139] suggested interrupting the efferent neuronal pathway at the level of the middle ear, by sectioning the tympanic nerve of Jacobson (a branch of the glossopharyngeal nerve). It can be performed by raising a tympanomeatal flap inferiorly and identifying Jacobson's nerve as it emerges from the inferior tympanic canaliculus, coursing across the promontory anterior to the round window. The nerve is sectioned, and the canaliculus is obliterated to prevent the regeneration of the nerve fibers [55, 60]. The first such procedure for gustatory sweating was carried out on three patients with apparently excellent results by Golding-Wood (1962) who named it "tympanic neurectomy" (also known as "Jacob's neurectomy") [174]. Other authors reported recurrence of symptoms with this procedure in most of their patients on long follow-up [89, 95, 171, 175]. It is believed that other parasympathetic innervation to the parotid exists and is responsible for this incomplete response. Two potential pathways were postulated including: (1) a connection between the chorda tympani and the otic ganglion or the facial nerve, and (2) a connection between the greater superficial petrosal nerve and the lesser petrosal nerve [73].

Resection of the chorda tympani, in addition to Jacobson's neurectomy, increases the rate of gustatory sweating control, but results in unilateral denervation of the major salivary glands and xerostomia as well as loss of taste sensation on the ipsilateral anterior two-thirds of the tongue. Thus, the division of the chorda tympani should only be offered to patients with debilitating, persistent gustatory sweating after Jacobson's neurectomy.

19.11.14 Surgical Interposition

Sessions et al. [176] pioneered the use of a barrier between the facial skin and the parotid bed in the treatment of established Frey's syndrome. They used the surgical interposition of a "fascia lata graft" in four patients with excellent results. This technique appeared to be effective in the small group of patients reported [176, 177]. However, disadvantages include the need for a second operation, flap failure, poor cosmesis, and risk to injure the facial nerve since it lies just under the skin after superficial or total parotidectomy.

A variation of this technique with the use of a "pedicled temporal fascia" has been reported [178] in one patient without prior facial nerve dissection. Placement of ADM, autologous fat, and TPF flaps can also be used as treatment methods and are not solely limited to prophylaxis [178, 179].

19.11.15 Treatment Strategy

Frey's syndrome usually occurs after parotid surgery. Asymptomatic patients do not require any intervention [180]. Prophylactic barriers should be employed during surgery, particularly for high-risk patients, including those with large (>4 cm) parotid tumors or extensive parotid injury [16, 180]. Patients who present with postoperative gustatory sweating should be treated initially with conservative medical management. Topical antiperspirant and anticholinergic ointments can provide symptomatic relief with minimal systemic side-effects, but require frequent applications [138, 167]. Serial botulinum toxin injections provide an extended duration of control without the need for frequent reapplications [149, 181]. If patients have persistent or refractory symptoms to medical treatment, surgical options including tympanic neurectomy, chorda tympani resection, muscle flap reconstruction, or excision of involved skin with graft reconstruction may be offered to the patient. Patients should be counseled that surgical intervention has a higher risk of complications such as xerostomia, facial nerve injury, flap rejection, and cosmetic defects [24, 167, 182].

19.12 Prognosis

Frey's syndrome is a benign condition and tends not to progress once established. Asymptomatic patients do not need treatment and are usually studied only for academic purposes [180]. The majority of symptomatic patients can be treated effectively with conservative medical management, including topical antiperspirants, anticholinergics, and BTA injection. Those with severe or refractory cases can be treated with surgery [93]. In children, spontaneous symptom regression occurs in approximately 69% of unilateral presentations. The bilateral form is usually unrelated to postnatal trauma and resolves during the first year of life in about 58% of patients [94].

Although there are no significant medical complications associated with Frey's syndrome, it can significantly reduce the patient's quality of life. Subjective perception and discomfort associated with gustatory sweating can persist beyond 5 years after surgery [183]. Quality-of-life questionnaires showed a statistically significant correlation between decreased social functioning, economic difficulties, speech defects, reduced sexuality, poor oral nutrition, and Frey's syndrome [184].

References

1. Dulguerov P, Marchal F, Gysin C. The bullet that hit a nerve: the history of Lucja Frey and her syndrome. J Laryngol Otol. 2006;120(12):1087.
2. Dulguerov P, Marchal F, Gysin C. Frey syndrome before Frey: the correct history. Laryngoscope. 1999;109:1471–3.
3. Le FL. syndrome du nerf auriculo-temporal. Rev Neurol. 1923;2:92–104.
4. Scully C, Langdon J, Evans J. Marathon of eponyms: 6 Frey syndrome (Gustatory sweating). Oral Dis. 2009;15(8):608–9.
5. Balfour HH Jr, Bloom JE. The auriculotemporal syndrome beginning in infancy. J Pediatr. 1970;77:872–4.
6. Bonanno PC, Casson PR. Frey's syndrome: a preventable phenomenon. Plast Reconstr Surg. 1992;89(3):452–6.
7. O'Neill JP, Condron C, Curran A, Walsh A. Lucja Frey--historical relevance and syndrome review. Surgeon. 2008;6(3):178–81.
8. Wood CB, Netterville JL. Temporoparietal Frey syndrome: an uncommon variant of a common syndrome. Laryngoscope. 2019;129(9):2071–5.
9. Laage-Hellman JE. Gustatory sweating and flushing after conservative parotidectomy. Acta Otolaryngol. 1957;48:234–52.
10. Laage-Hellman JE. Gustatory sweating and flushing: aetiological implications of response of separate sweat glands to various stimulli. Acta Otolaryngol. 1958;49:363–74.
11. Laage-Hellman JE. Gustatory sweating and flushing; aetiological implications of latent period and mode of development after parotidectomy. Acta Otolaryngol. 1958;49:306–14.

12. Laage-Hellman JE. Treatment of gustatory sweating and flushing. Acta Otolaryngol. 1958;49:132–43.
13. Sood S, Quraishi MS, Bradley PJ. Frey's syndrome and parotid surgery. Clin Otolaryngol. 1998;23:291–301.
14. Allison GR, Rappaport I. Prevention of Frey's syndrome with superficial musculoaponeurotic system interposition. Am J Surg. 1993;166:407–10.
15. Cavalot AL, Palonta F, Preti G, Nazionale G, Ricci E, Staffieri A, et al. Post-parotidectomy Frey's syndrome. Treatment with botulinum toxin type A. Acta Otorhinolaryngol Ital. 2000;20:187–91.
16. Dulguerov P, Quinodoz D, Cosendai G, Piletta P, Marchal F, Lehmann W. Prevention of Frey syndrome during parotidectomy. Arch Otolaryngol Head Neck Surg. 1999;125:833–9.
17. Farrell ML, Kalnins IK. Frey's syndrome following parotid surgery. Aust N Z J Surg. 1991;61:295–301.
18. Gordon AB, Fiddian RV. Frey's syndrome after parotid surgery. Am J Surg. 1976;132:54–8.
19. Kornblut AD, Westphal P, Miehlke A. The effectiveness of a sternomastoid muscle flap in preventing post-parotidectomy occurrence of the Frey syndrome. Acta Otolaryngol. 1974;77:368–73.
20. Laskawi R, Drobik C, Schonebeck C. Up-to-date report of botulinum toxin type A treatment in patients with gustatory sweating (Frey's syndrome). Laryngoscope. 1998;108:381–4.
21. Linder TE, Huber A, Schmid S. Frey's syndrome after parotidectomy: a retrospective and prospective analysis. Laryngoscope. 1997;107:1496–501.
22. Nosan DK, Ochi JW, Davidson TM. Preservation of facial contour during parotidectomy. Otolaryngol Head Neck Surg. 1991;104:293–8.
23. Yu LT, Hamilton R. Frey's syndrome: prevention with conservative parotidectomy and superficial musculoaponeurotic system preservation. Ann Plast Surg. 1992;29:217–22.
24. Guntinas-Lichius O, Gabriel B, Klussmann JP. Risk of facial palsy and severe Frey's syndrome after conservative parotidectomy for benign disease: analysis of 610 operations. Acta Otolaryngol. 2006;126(10):1104–9.
25. Laccourreye O, Bernard D, de Lacharriere O, et al. Frey's syndrome analysis with biosensor. A preliminary study. Arch Otolaryngol Head Neck Surg. 1993;119:940–4.
26. Gavric M. Aurikulotemporalni sindrom kao posledica parotidektomija. Stomatol Glas Srb. 1991;37:385–91.
27. Hays LL. The Frey syndrome: a review and double blind evaluation of the topical use of a new anticholinergics agent. Laryngoscope. 1978;88:1796–824.
28. Dai YS, Ambudkar IS, Horn VJ, et al. Evidence that M3 muscarinic receptors in rat parotid gland couple to two second messenger systems. Am J Physiol. 1991;261:1063–73.
29. List CF, Peet MM. Sweat secretion in man: IV. Sweat secretion of the face and its disturbance. Arch Neurol Psychol. 1938;40:443–70.
30. Matthews B, Robinson PP. The course of post-ganglionic sympathetic fibres distributed with the trigeminal nerve in the cat. J Physiol. 1980;303:391–401.
31. Sato K. The physiology, pharmacology, and biochemistry of the eccrine sweat gland. Rev Physiol Biochem Pharmacol. 1977;79:51–131.
32. Chorobski J, Penfield W. Cerebral vasodilatator nerves and their pathway from the medulla oblongata, with observation on the pial and intracerebral vascular plexus. Arch Neurol Psychiatr. 1932;28:1257–89.
33. Blair DA, Glover WE, Roddie JC. Cutaneous vasomotor nerves to the head and trunk. J Appl Physiol. 1961;16:119–22.
34. Lambert GA, Bogduk N, Goadsby PJ, Duckworth JW, Lance JW. Decreased carotid arterial resistance in cats in response to trigeminal stimulation. J Neurosurg. 1984;61:307–15.
35. Fox RH, Goldsmith R, Kidd DJ. Cutaneous vasomotor control in the human head, neck and upper chest. J Physiol. 1962;161:298–312.
36. Lee TS. Physiological gustatory sweating in a warm climate. J Physiol. 1954;124:528–42.
37. Vilches JJ, Navarro X, Verdu E. Functional sudomotor responses to cholinergic agonists and antagonists in the mouse. J Auton Nerv Syst. 1995;55:105–11.

38. Redleaf MI, McCabe BF. Gustatory otorrhea: Frey's syndrome of the external auditory canal. Ann Otol Rhinol Laryngol. 1993;102(6):438–40.
39. Greenberg JS, Breiner MJ. Anatomy, head and neck: auriculotemporal nerve. In: StatPearls. Treasure Island (FL): StatPearls Publishing; 2023.
40. Iwanaga J, Fisahn C, Watanabe K, Bobek SL, Ogata K, Tanoue R, et al. Parotid branches of the auriculotemporal nerve: an anatomical study with implications for Frey syndrome. J Craniofac Surg. 2017;28(1):262–4.
41. Smiddy FG. Treatment of mixed parotid tumours. Br Med J. 1956;1(4962):322–5.
42. Singh N, Kohli M, Kohli H. Innovative technique to reduce incidence of Frey's syndrome after parotid surgery. Am Surg. 2011;77(3):351–4.
43. Neumann A, Rosenberger D, Vorsprach O, Dazert S. The incidence of Frey syndrome following parotidectomy: results of a survey and follow-up. HNO. 2011;59(2):173–8.
44. Kryshtalskyj B, Weinberg S. An assessment for auriculo-temporal syndrome following temporomandibular joint surgery through the preauricular approach. J Oral Maxillofac Surg. 1989;47:3–6.
45. Tuinzing DB, van der Kwast WA, Frey's syndrome. A complication after sagittal splitting of the mandibular ramus. Int J Oral Surg. 1982;11:197–200.
46. Baillarger M. Memoire sur l'obliteration du canal de Stenon. Gaz Med Paris. 1853;23:194–7.
47. Goatcher PD. The auriculo-temporal syndrome. Br Med J. 1954;4873:1233–4.
48. Morfit HM, Kramish D. Auriculotemporal syndrome (Frey's syndrome) following surgery of parotid tumors. Am J Surg. 1961;102:777–80.
49. New GB, Bozer HE. Hyperhydrosis of the cheek associated with the parotid region. Minn Med. 1922;5:652–7.
50. Payne RT. Pneumococcal parotiditis and antecedent auriculotemporal syndrome. Lancet. 1940;i:634–6.
51. Weber FP. Clinical cases V: a case of localized sweating and blushing on eating, possibly due to temporary compression of vasomotor fibers. Trans Clin Soc Lond. 1897;31:277–80.
52. Zoller J, Herrmann A, Maier H. Frey's syndrome secondary to a subcondylar fracture. Otolaryngol Head Neck Surg. 1993;108:751–3.
53. Gerbino G, Roccia F, Grosso M, Regge D. Pseudoaneurysm of the internal maxillary artery and Frey's syndrome after blunt facial trauma. J Oral Maxillofac Surg. 1997;55:1485–90.
54. Ottomo M, Heimburger RF. Alternating Horner's syndrome and hyperhidrosis due to dural adhesions following cervical spinal cord injury: case report. J Neurosurg. 1980;53:97–100.
55. Baddour HM, Ripley JF, Cortez EA, McAnear JT, Steed DL, Tilson HB. Treatment of Frey's syndrome by an interpositional fascia graft: report of case. J Oral Surg. 1980;38:778–81.
56. Duphenix M. Observations sur les fistules du canal salivaire de Stenon. Sur une playe compliquee a la joue ou le canal salivaire fut dechire. Mem Acad R Chir. 1957;3:431–9.
57. Haxton HA. Gustatory sweating. Brain. 1948;71:16–25.
58. Wilson WC. Observations relating to the innervation of the sweat glands of the face. Clin Sci. 1936;2:273–86.
59. Nesathurai S, Harvey DT, Schatz SW. Gustatory facial sweating subsequent to upper thoracic sympathectomy. Arch Phys Med Rehabil. 1995;76:104–7.
60. Drummond PD, Boyce GM, Lance JW. Postherpetic gustatory flushing and sweating. Ann Neurol. 1987;21:559–63.
61. Schnarch A, Markitziu A. Dysgeusia, gustatory sweating, and crocodile tears syndrome induced by a cerebellopontine angle meningioma. Oral Surg Oral Med Oral Pathol. 1990;70:711–4.
62. Saito H. Gustatory otalgia and wet ear syndrome: a possible cross-innervation after ear surgery. Laryngoscope. 1999;109:569–72.
63. Freedman A. Facial sweating after food in diabetes. Br Med J. 1973;3:291.
64. Hayes PC, Tulloch JA. An unusual case of gustatory sweating. Postgrad Med J. 1982;58:656–7.
65. Janka HU, Standl E, Mehnert H. Clonidine effect on diabetic gustatory sweating. Ann Intern Med. 1979;91:130.
66. Stuart DD. Diabetic gustatory sweating. Ann Intern Med. 1978;89:223–4.

67. van der Linden J, Sinnige HA, van den Dorpel MA. Gustatory sweating and diabetes. Neth J Med. 2000;56:159–62.
68. Watkins PJ. Facial sweating after food: a new sign of diabetic autonomic neuropathy. Br Med J. 1973;1:583–7.
69. Randall WC. Sweat gland activity and changing patterns of sweat secretion on the skin surface. Am J Physiol. 1946;147:391–8.
70. Beck SA, Burks AW, Woody RC. Auriculotemporal syndrome seen clinically as food allergy. Pediatrics. 1989;83:601–3.
71. Davis RS, Strunk RC. Auriculotemporal syndrome in childhood. Am J Dis Child. 1981;135:832–3.
72. Feiwel M. Auriculotemporal syndrome. Proc R Soc Med. 1959;52:191.
73. Johnson IJ, Birchall JP. Bilatral auriculotemporal syndrome in childhood. Int J Pediatr Otorhinolaryngol. 1995;32:83–6.
74. Kozma C, Gabriel S. Gustatory flushing syndrome. A pediatric case report and review of the literature. Clin Pediatr (Phila). 1993;32:629–31.
75. Sly RM. Auriculotemporal syndrome. Cutis. 1981;28:423–5.
76. Zalzal GH. Congenital gustatory facial flushing. Otolaryngol Head Neck Surg. 1991;104:878–80.
77. Redleaf MI, McCabe BF. Gustatory otorrhea: Frey's syndrome of the external auditory canal. Ann Otol Rhinol Laryngol. 1993;102:438–40.
78. Sonsale A, Sharp JF, Johnson IJ. Gustatory sweating of the external auditory canal. J Laryngol Otol. 1999;113:1000–1.
79. Sethuraman G, Mancini AJ. Familial auriculotemporal nerve (Frey) syndrome. Pediatr Dermatol. 2009;26(3):302–5.
80. De Benedittis G. Auriculotemporal syndrome (Frey's syndrome) presenting as tic douloureux. Report of two cases. J Neurosurg. 1990;72:955–8.
81. Scrivani SJ, Keith DA, Kulich R, Mehta N, Maciewicz RJ. Posttraumatic gustatory neuralgia: a clinical model of trigeminal neuropathic pain. J Orofac Pain. 1998;12:287–92.
82. Sharav Y, Benoliel R, Schnarch A, Greenberg L. Idiopathic trigeminal pain associated with gustatory stimuli. Pain. 1991;44:171–4.
83. Truax BT. Gustatory pain: a complication of carotid endarterectomy. Neurology. 1989;39:1258–60.
84. Drummond PD. Mechanisms of physiological gustatory sweating and flushing in the face. J Auton Nerv Syst. 1995;52:117–24.
85. Eckardt A, Kuettner C. Treatment of gustatory sweating (Frey's syndrome) with botulinum toxin A. Head Neck. 2003;25:624–8.
86. Le TA. double reflexe vaso-dilatateur et sudoral de la face consecutif aux blessures de la loge parotidienne. Rev Neurol (Paris). 1927;1:447–60.
87. Ford FR, Woodhall B. Phenomena due to misdirection of regenerating fibers of cranial, spinal, and autonomic nerves: clinical observations. Arch Surg. 1938;36:480–96.
88. Glaister DH, Hearnshaw JR, Heffron PF, Peck AW, Patey DH. The mechanism of post-parotidectomy gustatory sweating (the auriculo-temporal syndrome). Br Med J. 1958;2:942–6.
89. Ross JA. The function of the tympanic plexus as related to Frey's syndrome. Laryngoscope. 1970;80:1816–33.
90. Drummond PD. Sweating and vascular responses in the face: normal regulation and dysfunction in migraine, cluster headache and harlequin syndrome. Clin Auton Res. 1994;4:273–85.
91. Myers EN, Conley J. Gustatory sweating after radical neck dissection. Arch Otolaryngol. 1970;91(6):534–42.
92. de Bree R, van der Waal I, Leemans CR. Management of Frey syndrome. Head Neck. 2007;29(8):773–8.
93. Motz KM, Kim YJ. Auriculotemporal syndrome (Frey syndrome). Otolaryngol Clin North Am. 2016;49(2):501–9.

94. Blanc S, Bourrier T, Boralevi F, Sabouraud-Leclerc D, Pham-Thi N, Couderc L, Deschildre A, Dutau G, Albertini M, Tran A, Giovannini-Chami L, Frey Syndrome Collaborators. Frey syndrome. J Pediatr. 2016;174:211–7.
95. Bakke M, Max Thorsen N, Bardow A, Dalager T, Eckhart Thomsen C, Regeur L. Treatment of gustatory sweating with low-dose botulinum toxin A: a case report. Acta Odontol Scand. 2006;64(3):129–33.
96. Wenzel GI, Draf W. Unusually long latency before the appearance of Frey's syndrome after parotidectomy. HNO. 2004;52(6):554–6.
97. Smith A, Jonas N. Frey's Syndrome. N Engl J Med. 2020;382(15):1456.
98. Sato K, Kang WH, Saga K, Sato KT. Biology of sweat glands and their disorders. II. Disorders of sweat gland function. J Am Acad Dermatol. 1989;20:713–26.
99. Low PA. Testing the autonomic nervous system. Semin Neurol. 2003;23:407–21.
100. Dulguerov P, Quinodoz D, Vaezi A, Cosendai G, Piletta P, Lehmann W. New objective and quantitative tests for gustatory sweating. Acta Otolaryngol. 1999;119:599–603.
101. Sato K, Kang WH, Saga K, Sato KT. Biology of sweat glands and their disorders. I. Normal sweat gland function. J Am Acad Dermatol. 1989;20:537–63.
102. Minor V. Ein neues Verfahren zu der klinischen Untersuchung der Schweissabsonderung. Dtsch Z Nervenheilkd. 1927;101:302–8.
103. Glogau RG. Hyperhidrosis and botulinum toxin A: patient selection and techniques. Clin Dermatol. 2004;22:45–52.
104. Sato KT, Richardson A, Timm DE, Sato K. One-step iodine starch method for direct visualization of sweating. Am J Med Sci. 1988;295:528–31.
105. Dulguerov P, Quinodoz D, Cosendai G, Piletta P, Lehmann W. Frey syndrome treatment with botulinum toxin. Otolaryngol Head Neck Surg. 2000;122:821–7.
106. Adie R. Gustatory sweating. Aust N Z J Surg. 1968;38:98–103.
107. Dole VP, Thaysen JH. Variation in the functional power of human sweat glands. J Exp Med. 1953;98:129–44.
108. Adar R, Kurchin A, Zweig A, Mozes M. Palmar hyperhidrosis and its surgical treatment: a report of 100 cases. Ann Surg. 1977;186(1):34–41.
109. Leung AK, Chan PY, Choi MC. Hyperhidrosis. Int J Dermatol. 1999;38(8):561–7.
110. Hornberger J, Grimes K, Naumann M, Glaser DA, Lowe NJ, Naver H, et al. Recognition, diagnosis, and treatment of primary focal hyperhidrosis. J Am Acad Dermatol. 2004;51(2):274–86.
111. Lakraj AA, Moghimi N, Jabbari B. Hyperhidrosis: anatomy, pathophysiology and treatment with emphasis on the role of botulinum toxins. Toxins (Basel). 2013;5(4):821–40.
112. Montoya FJ, Riddell CE, Caesar R, Hague S. Treatment of gustatory hyperlacrimation (crocodile tears) with injection of botulinum toxin into the lacrimal gland. Eye (Lond). 2002;16(6):705–9.
113. de Oliveira D, Gomes-Ferreira PH, Carrasco LC, de Deus CB, Garcia-Júnior IR, Faverani LP. The importance of correct diagnosis of crocodile Tears syndrome. J Craniofac Surg. 2016;27(7):e661–2.
114. Boddie AW, Guillamondegui OM, Byers RM. Gustatory rhinorrhea developing after radical parotidectomy—a new syndrome? Arch Otolaryngol. 1976;102(4):248–50.
115. Gunter AE, Llewellyn CM, Perez PB, Hohman MH, Roofe SB. First Bite syndrome following rhytidectomy: a case report. Ann Otol Rhinol Laryngol. 2021;130(1):92–7.
116. Linkov G, Morris LG, Shah JP, Kraus DH. First bite syndrome: incidence, risk factors, treatment, and outcomes. Laryngoscope. 2012;122(8):1773–8.
117. Charles-Harris H, Rodriguez B. First Bite syndrome: presentation of a patient status-post right carotid endarterectomy. Vasc Endovasc Surg. 2021;55(1):64–8.
118. Durgut O, Basut O, Demir UL, Ozmen OA, Kasapoglu F, Coskun H. Association between skin flap thickness and Frey's syndrome in parotid surgery. Head Neck. 2013;35(12):1781–6.
119. Taylor SM, Yoo J, Matthews TW, Lampe HB, Trites JR. Frey's syndrome and parotidectomy flaps: a retrospective cohort study. Otolaryngol Head Neck Surg. 2000;122(2):201–3.

120. Zeng XT, Tang XJ, Wang XJ, Li MZ, Guo Y, Huang W, Niu YM, Leng WD. AlloDerm implants for prevention of Frey syndrome after parotidectomy: a systematic review and meta-analysis. Mol Med Rep. 2012;5(4):974–80.
121. Govindaraj S, Cohen M, Genden EM, Costantino PD, Urken ML. The use of acellular dermis in the prevention of Frey's syndrome. Laryngoscope. 2001;111(11 Pt 1):1993–8.
122. Fiacchini G, Cerchiai N, Tricò D, Sellari-Franceschini S, Casani AP, Dallan I, Seccia V. Frey syndrome, First Bite syndrome, great auricular nerve morbidity, and quality of life following parotidectomy. Eur Arch Otorhinolaryngol. 2018;275(7):1893–902.
123. Bonanno PC, Palaia D, Rosenberg M, Casson P. Prophylaxis against Frey's syndrome in parotid surgery. Ann Plast Surg. 2000;44(5):498–501.
124. Wille-Bischofberger A, Rajan GP, Linder TE, Schmid S. Impact of the SMAS on Frey's syndrome after parotid surgery: a prospective, long-term study. Plast Reconstr Surg. 2007;120(6):1519–23.
125. Yu LT, Hamilton R. Frey's syndrome: prevention with conservative parotidectomy and superficial musculoaponeurotic system preservation. Ann Plast Surg. 1992;29(3):217–22.
126. Allison GR, Rappaport I. Prevention of Frey's syndrome with superficial musculoaponeurotic system interposition. Am J Surg. 1993;166(4):407–10.
127. Barberá R, Castillo F, D'Oleo C, Benítez S, Cobeta I. Superficial musculoaponeurotic system flap in partial parotidectomy and clinical and subclinical Frey's syndrome. Cosmesis and quality of life. Head Neck. 2014;36(1):130–6.
128. Sultan MR, Wider TM, Hugo NE. Frey's syndrome: prevention with temporoparietal fascial flap interposition. Ann Plast Surg. 1995;34(3):292–6.
129. Kierner AC, Aigner M, Zelenka I, Riedl G, Burian M. The blood supply of the sternocleidomastoid muscle and its clinical implications. Arch Surg. 1999;134(2):144–7.
130. Filho WQ, Dedivitis RA, Rapoport A, Guimarães AV. Sternocleidomastoid muscle flap preventing Frey syndrome following parotidectomy. World J Surg. 2004;28(4):361–4.
131. Curry JM, King N, Reiter D, Fisher K, Heffelfinger RN, Pribitkin EA. Meta-analysis of surgical techniques for preventing parotidectomy sequelae. Arch Facial Plast Surg. 2009;11(5):327–31.
132. Kornblut AD. Sternocleidomastoid muscle transfer in the prevention of Frey's syndrome. Laryngoscope. 1991;101(5):571–2.
133. Sanabria A, Kowalski LP, Bradley PJ, Hartl DM, Bradford CR, de Bree R, Rinaldo A, Ferlito A. Sternocleidomastoid muscle flap in preventing Frey's syndrome after parotidectomy: a systematic review. Head Neck. 2012;34(4):589–98.
134. Needles W. The auriculotemporal syndrome. With a suggestion regarding therapy. Arch Neurol Psychiatr. 1936;35:357–60.
135. Dawson AK, Orr JA. Long-term results of local excision and radiotherapy in pleomorphic adenoma of the parotid. Int J Radiat Oncol Biol Phys. 1985;11:451–5.
136. Drobik C, Laskawi R. Frey's syndrome: treatment with botulinum toxin. Acta Otolaryngol. 1995;115(3):459–61.
137. Clayman MA, Clayman SM, Seagle MB. A review of the surgical and medical treatment of Frey syndrome. Ann Plast Surg. 2006;57(5):581–4.
138. Hays LL. The Frey syndrome: a review and double blind evaluation of the topical use of a new anticholinergic agent. Laryngoscope. 1978;88(11):1796–824.
139. Hemenway WG. Gustatory sweating and flushing. The auriculo-temporal syndrome—Frey's syndrome. Laryngoscope. 1960;70:84–90.
140. Shelley WB, Horvath PN. Comparative study on the effect of anticholinergic compounds on sweating. J Invet Dermatol. 1951;16:267–74.
141. Hays LL, Novack AJ, Worsham JC. The Frey syndrome: a simple, effective treatment. Otolaryngol Head Neck Surg. 1982;90:419–25.
142. May JS, McGuirt WF. Frey's syndrome: treatment with topical glycopyrrolate. Head Neck. 1989;11:85–9.
143. Black MJ, Gunn A. The management of Frey's syndrome with aluminium chloride hexahydrate antiperspirant. Ann R Coll Surg Engl. 1990;72:49–52.

144. Huttenbrink KB. Die Therapie des gustatorischen Schwitzens nach Parotidektomie. Freysches syndrom. Laryngol Rhinol Otol (Stuttg). 1986;65:135–7.
145. Schmelzer A, Rosin V, Steinbach E. Zur Therapie des Freyschen Syndroms durch ein Anhidrotisches gel. Laryngorhinootologie. 1992;71:59–63.
146. Laccourreye O, Bonan B, Brasnu D, et al. Treatment of Frey's syndrome with topical 2% diphemanil methylsulfate (Prantal): a double-blind evaluation of 15 patients. Laryngoscope. 1990;100:651–3.
147. Drobik C, Laskawi R. Frey's syndrome: treatment with botulinum toxin. Acta Otolaryngol. 1995;115:459–61.
148. Arad-Cohen A, Blitzer A. Botulinum toxin treatment for symptomatic Frey's syndrome. Otolaryngol Head Neck Surg. 2000;122:237–40.
149. Beerens AJ, Snow GB. Botulinum toxin A in the treatment of patients with Frey syndrome. Br J Surg. 2002;89:116–9.
150. Bjerkhoel A, Trobbe O. Frey's syndrome: treatment with botulinum toxin. J Laryngol Otol. 1977;111:839–44.
151. Guntinas-Lichius O. Increased botulinum toxin type A dosage is more effective in patients with Frey's syndrome. Laryngoscope. 2002;112:746–9.
152. Kuttner C, Troger M, Dempf R, Eckardt A. Effektivitat von Botulinum-toxin A in der Behandlung des gustatorischen Schwitzens. Nervenarzt. 2001;72:787–90.
153. Laccourreye O, Akl E, Gutierrez-Fonseca R, Garcia D, Brasnu D, Bonan B. Recurrent gustatory sweating (Frey syndrome) after intracutaneous injection of botulinum toxin type A: incidence, management, and outcome. Arch Otolaryngol Head Neck Surg. 1999;125:283–6.
154. Laccourreye O, Muscatelo L, Naude C, et al. Botulinum toxin type A for Frey's syndrome: a preliminary prospective study. Ann Otol Rhinol Laryngol. 1998;107:52–5.
155. Naumann M, Zellner M, Toyka KV, Reiners K. Treatment of gustatory sweating with botulinum toxin. Ann Neurol. 1997;42:973–5.
156. Quinodoz D, Dulguerov P, Cosenday G, Arechulde A, Piletta P. Traitement du syndrome de Frey avec la toxine botulinique. Med Hyg. 1997;55:2070–3.
157. Cantarella G, Berlusconi A, Mele V, Cogiamanian F, Barbieri S. Treatment of Frey's syndrome with botulinum toxin type B. Otolaryngol Head Neck Surg. 2010;143(2):214–8.
158. Jankovic J, Hallet M. Therapy with botulinum toxin. New York, NY: Marcel Dekker Inc.; 1994.
159. Kreyden OP, Scheidegger EP. Anatomy of the sweat glands, pharmacology of botulinum toxin, and distinctive syndromes associated with hyperhidrosis. Clin Dermatol. 2004;22:40–4.
160. Montecucco C, Schiavo G, Tugnoli V, de Grandis D. Botulinum neurotoxins: mechanism of action and therapeutic applications. Mol Med Today. 1996;2:418–24.
161. Blasi J, Chapman ER, Link E, Binz T, Yamasaki S, De Camilli P, et al. Botulinum neurotoxin A selectively cleaves the synaptic protein SNAP-25. Nature. 1993;365:160–3.
162. Coffield JA, Considine RV, Simpson LL. The site and mechanism of action of botulinum neurotoxin. In: Jankovic J, Hallett M, editors. The site and mechanism of action of botulinum neurotoxin. New York, NY: Marcel Drekker Inc.; 1994.
163. Gualberto GV, Sampaio FMS, Madureira NAB. Use of botulinum toxin type A in Frey's syndrome. An Bras Dermatol. 2017;92(6):891–2.
164. Dressler D, Hallett M. Immunological aspects of Botox, Dysport and Myobloc/NeuroBloc. Eur J Neurol. 2006;13(Suppl. 1):11–5.
165. Jankovic J, Vuong KD, Ahsan J. Comparison of efficacy and immunogenicity of original versus current Botulinum toxin in cervical dystonia. Neurology. 2003;60:1186–8.
166. Nigam PK, Nigam A. Botulinum toxin. Indian J Dermatol. 2010;55(1):8–14.
167. Smith RO, Hemenway WG, Stevens KM, Ratzer ER. Jacobson's neurectomy for Frey's syndrome. Am J Surg. 1970;120(4):478–81.
168. Leriche R. Behandlung der permanenten parotis Fisteln durch die Entnervung der Speicheldruse Ausreissen des N. auriculotemporalis. Zentralblatt Chir. 1914;41:754–5.
169. Debets JM, Munting JD. Parotidectomy for parotid tumours: 19-year experience from The Netherlands. Br J Surg. 1922;79:1159–61.

170. Coldwater KB. Surgical treatment of the auriculotemporal syndrome. AMA Arch Surg. 1954;69:54–7.
171. Harrison K, Donaldson I. Frey's syndrome. J R Soc Med. 1979;72:503–8.
172. Blumenfeld RJ, Friedman JE. Intratympanic surgical treatment of Frey's syndrome. Arch Otolaryngol. 1967;86(1):2–7.
173. Gardner WJ, McCubbin JW. Auriculotemporal syndrome; gustatory sweating due to misdirection of regenerated nerve fibers. J Am Med Assoc. 1956;160:272–7.
174. Golding-Wood PH. Tympanic neurectomy. J Laryngol Otol. 1962;76:683–93.
175. Parisier SC, Binder WJ, Blitzer A, Friedman WH, Marovitz WF. Evaluation of tympanic neurectomy and chorda tympanectomy for gustatory sweating and benign salivary gland disease. Ear Nose Throat J. 1978;57:213–23.
176. Sessions RB, Roark DT, Alford BR. Frey's syndrome—a technical remedy. Ann Otol. 1976;85:734–9.
177. Wallis KA, Gibson T. Gustatory sweating following parotidectomy: correction by a fascia lata graft. Br J Plast Surg. 1978;31:68–71.
178. Rubinstein RY, Rosen A, Leeman D. Frey syndrome: treatment with temporoparietal fascia flap interposition. Arch Otolaryngol Head Neck Surg. 1999;125:808–11.
179. Torretta S, Pignataro L, Capaccio P, Brevi A, Mazzola R. Fat injections for the management of post-parotidectomy Frey syndrome: a technical note. J Craniomaxillofac Surg. 2012;40(2):173–6.
180. Lee CC, Chan RC, Chan JY. Predictors for Frey syndrome development after parotidectomy. Ann Plast Surg. 2017;79(1):39–41.
181. Laccourreye O, Akl E, Gutierrez-Fonseca R, Garcia D, Brasnu D, Bonan B. Recurrent gustatory sweating (Frey syndrome) after intracutaneous injection of botulinum toxin type A: incidence, management, and outcome. Arch Otolaryngol Head Neck Surg. 1999;125(3):283–6.
182. Dai XM, Liu H, He J, Tu MS, Yu LF, Liu L. Treatment of postparotidectomy Frey syndrome with the interposition of temporalis fascia and sternocleidomastoid flaps. Oral Surg Oral Med Oral Pathol Oral Radiol. 2015;119(5):514–21.
183. Baek CH, Chung MK, Jeong HS, Son YI, Jung SC, Jeon HK, Ryu NG, Cho HJ, Cho JK, Jang JY. Questionnaire evaluation of sequelae over 5 years after parotidectomy for benign diseases. J Plast Reconstr Aesthet Surg. 2009;62(5):633–8.
184. Gunsoy B, Vuralkan E, Sonbay ND, Simsek G, Tokgoz SA, Akin I. Quality of life following surgical treatment of benign parotid disease. Indian J Otolaryngol Head Neck Surg. 2013;65(Suppl. 1):105–11.

Extra-temporal Facial Nerve Reconstruction

20

20.1 Introduction

The facial nerve is the "connecting cable" between the central nervous system (CNS) and the facial muscles. The vital conditions of this threefold system have to be taken into account, especially in cases of delayed reconstruction. Any severe facial nerve damage leads to "axon degeneration" with the following consequences: (1) centrally, retrograde changes to the motor neurons and their cellular environment [1–9]; and (2) peripherally, the degeneration of muscle fibers [10, 11]. Reversibility or irreversibility of these degenerative processes depends on the time that has elapsed between nerve injury and reinnervation of the musculature.

Facial nerve denervation and paralysis imposes significant psychological and functional impairment negatively affecting quality of life (QOL). Facial paralysis can inhibit and mar facial expression, communication, symmetrical smile, eye protection, and oral competence. While the inability to close the eye, breathe easily through the nose, or maintain oral competence can be very problematic, losing the ability to smile or even to appear symmetric at rest can be even more significant for many patients, especially young women, and may lead to depression in addition to decreased QOL [12, 13].

When the facial nerve is transected, "immediate" surgical repair with primary neurorrhaphy is generally the preferred treatment option [14, 15]. If coaptation without tension is impossible, a cable graft interposition using the greater auricular or sural nerves may be necessary. The success rate of nerve repair, defined as a return to House–Brackmann grade-III function or better, varies in the literature from 5% to 86% [16, 17]. When the proximal facial nerve is unavailable to reconnect to the distal stump, a nerve transfer may be the best method of restoring facial function [17].

Any technique employed other than direct coaptation of the severed facial nerve stumps at the time of injury will have associated risks. "Delayed" primary repair often requires a facial nerve exploration, which risks injury to other facial structures. Interposition grafting and nerve transfer introduce the potential for donor site morbidity, a critical factor when planning for and counseling patients before surgery.

© The Author(s), under exclusive license to Springer Nature Switzerland AG 2024
M. Sakr, *Surgery of the Salivary Glands*,
https://doi.org/10.1007/978-3-031-82069-4_20

The physician must accurately evaluate and examine the patient and determine the etiology, duration, and the scale of the paralysis. Regardless of the technique employed, the return of function after a facial nerve transection injury is a slow process, affecting many aspects of facial function and aesthetics. For this reason, an interprofessional team consisting of not only a peripheral nerve surgeon such as a plastic surgeon or otolaryngologist but also an ophthalmologist and physical and speech therapists is the most effective means of providing holistic care for patients with facial nerve paralysis.

20.2 Surgical Anatomy

20.2.1 Intra-temporal Course

The facial nerve, or seventh cranial nerve (CN-VII), originates in the lower pons and crosses the cerebellopontine angle (CPA) to enter the internal auditory meatus alongside the cochlear nerve and the superior and inferior vestibular nerves [18]. The facial nerve is located in the anterosuperior quadrant within the internal auditory canal (IAC). At the distal aspect of the IAC, the facial nerve turns anteriorly into the labyrinthine segment. This segment is approximately 4 mm long and ends at the geniculate ganglion. Here the nerve takes a 180° turn and gives off the greater superficial petrosal nerve. The canal housing the facial nerve as it travels through the temporal bone is the "Fallopian canal," the narrowest portion of which is the labyrinthine segment. At only 0.7 mm in diameter, the labyrinthine segment is where the facial nerve is particularly susceptible to impingement from bony fractures or intraneural edema [19, 20]. As the nerve leaves the Fallopian canal, it courses posteriorly for 9–10 mm through the middle ear.

As the nerve passes into the mastoid cavity, it turns 90° inferiorly; this is the "mastoid" or "vertical" segment, which is 11–12 mm long. Within the mastoid, the approximate 6000 facial nerve axons begin to organize somatotopically as the fascicles prepare to separate within the parotid gland at the pes anserinus. Leaving the pes anserinus, branches of the facial nerve will control the mimetic muscles in the upper face, midface, lower face, and superficial neck [21]. The chorda tympani branch of the facial nerve splits off the main trunk within the mastoid and travels superiorly to exit the temporal bone through the petrotympanic fissure of Huguier and travel to the oral cavity to carry gustatory sensation from the anterior two-thirds of the tongue [22]. The intra-temporal course of the facial nerve ends when the main trunk passes through the stylomastoid foramen to enter the infratemporal fossa.

20.2.2 Extra-temporal Course

Extra-temporally, the facial nerve travels for approximately 14 mm before dividing into what is classically described as five main branches: frontal, zygomatic, buccal, marginal mandibular, and cervical. The anatomy is variable, with six branching patterns characterized by Davis et al. in 1956 [23] as summarized in Table 20.1.

Table 20.1 Branching patterns of the extra-temporal facial nerve

Pattern	Frequency	Description
Type I	13%	The main trunk branches into upper (temporofacial) and lower (cervicofacial) divisions, with the buccal branch leaving the upper division proximally while the frontal (temporal) and zygomatic branches separate slightly more distally; the marginal mandibular and cervical branches leave form the lower division
Type II	20%	The main trunk branches into upper and lower divisions, with the frontal and zygomatic branches, as well as an upper buccal branch, forming a common upper facial trunk. The upper buccal branch anastomoses distally with the zygomatic branch, but there is also a separate lower buccal branch. The marginal mandibular and cervical branches leave form the lower division
Type III	28%	The main trunk branches into upper and lower divisions, with the frontal and zygomatic branches running together in the upper division until the zygomatic branch separates distally and anastomoses with the buccal branch, which runs with but leaves the lower division proximally. The marginal mandibular and cervical branches leave form the remainder of the lower division
Type IV	24%	The main trunk branches simultaneously into frontal and zygomatic branches and a lower division. The zygomatic branch splits into upper and lower branches proximally, with the frontal and upper zygomatic branches anastomosing proximally. The buccal branch leaves the lower division proximally and anastomoses with the lower zygomatic branch distally. The marginal mandibular and cervical branches leave form the lower division
Type V	9%	The main trunk branches into upper and lower divisions, with the frontal and upper and lower zygomatic branches constituting the upper division. The upper and lower buccal branches and the marginal mandibular and cervical branches comprise the lower division. The upper buccal branch anastomoses proximally with the lower zygomatic branch and the lower buccal branch anastomoses distally with the upper zygomatic branch and the combined lower-zygomatic–upper-buccal complex
Type VI	6%	The main trunk branches into upper and lower divisions, with significant early ramification and anastomosis between frontal and zygomatic branches within the upper division. Within the lower division, an upper buccal branch leaves proximally and anastomoses proximally with the lower aspect of the fronto-zygomatic complex. The cervical branch separates proximally from a common trunk, giving off a lower buccal branch and the marginal mandibular branch more distally—the lower buccal branch then anastomoses with the zygomatic–upper buccal complex distally

20.2.3 Surgical Significance

Despite this substantial anatomical variability among individuals, several surface landmarks facilitate reliable identification of the main extra-temporal facial nerve branches. The "line of Pitanguy," which runs from a point 5 mm inferior to the tragus to a point 15 mm superior to the lateral brow, approximates the course of the frontal branch [24]. The "point of Zuker," halfway between the root of the helix and the oral commissure, consistently overlies the buccal branch that innervates the zygomaticus major muscle, which is particularly useful for masseteric nerve transfer-based smile reanimation [25]. The marginal mandibular nerve (MMN), which is the most commonly injured individual facial nerve branch, is reliably located superior to the inferior margin of the mandible anterior to the point where it crosses the facial artery, just anterior to the mandibular angle; posterior to that, it lies inferior to the margin of the mandible in only 20% of patients [26–28]. The cervical branch can be found 10 mm inferior to the midpoint between the mentum and the tip of the mastoid process [29].

The extra-temporal branches course through the parotid gland, separating its superficial and deep lobes. They exit the gland at its anterior border and run deep to the superficial musculoaponeurotic system (SMAS) of the face, ultimately innervating the mimetic muscles from their deep surfaces, except for the levator anguli oris, buccinator, and mentalis muscles, which are innervated superficially due to their deep location within the face. The SMAS is a fibrofatty layer superficial to the parotid gland that extends superiorly to the zygomatic arch, beyond which it is contiguous with the temporoparietal fascia [30]. Inferiorly, the SMAS is contiguous with the platysma muscle, and anteriorly, it joins the mimetic muscles.

The frontal branch of the facial nerve innervates the muscles of the forehead and upper eyelid: frontalis, corrugator supercilii, procerus muscles, and superior aspect of the orbicularis oculi. The zygomatic branch also controls the orbicularis oculi and some of the upper midface muscles, while the buccal branch innervates the remaining midface muscles and orbicularis oris. The MMN primarily controls the depressor anguli oris and mentalis muscles, while the cervical branch controls the largest mimetic muscle, the platysma, and the mentalis.

20.3 Applied Physiology

The extent of flaccid paralysis in the acute post-traumatic period and the occurrence and degree of synkinesis are dependent upon the severity and location of injury. The severity of motor nerve injury is commonly described using two similar scales, described by Sunderland [31] (Table 20.2) and Seddon [32] (Table 20.3), relating the degree of dysfunction to the microanatomy of the injury. Each motor axon is surrounded by myelin produced by Schwann cells, and around the myelin is a connective tissue membrane called the endoneurium. Axons, wrapped in myelin and endoneurium, are grouped into fascicles, each surrounded by perineurium. Multiple fascicles, surrounded by epineurium, constitute the nerve itself.

The Sunderland and Seddon classification systems illustrate the relationship between injury severity and the development of synkinesis. While all traumatic facial nerve injuries present with weakness, only the most severe injuries characterized by anatomical discontinuity of the nerve result in permanent flaccid paralysis; this emphasizes the importance of nerve repair for improving outcomes.

Table 20.2 Sunderland classification of severity of motor nerve injury

Severity	Description of injury	Prognosis
Class I	Temporary conduction block due to focal demyelination with axonal integrity	Complete recovery
Class II	Axonal disruption with intact endoneurium	Complete recovery
Class III	Axonal disruption with endoneurial violation; the perineurium remains intact	Mild to moderate synkinesis
Class IV	Axonal disruption with endoneurial and perineural violation; only the epineurium remains intact	Severe synkinesis
Class V	Disruption of all nerve components, including the epineurium; a transection injury	Persistent flaccid paralysis

Table 20.3 Seddon classification of severity of motor nerve injury

Severity	Description of injury	Prognosis
Neuropraxia	Equivalent to Sunderland Class I injury	Complete recovery
Axonotomesis	Axonal injury without nerve transection, equivalent to Sunderland Classes II through IV injuries	Variable degree of synkinesis
Neuronotomesis	Nerve transection, equivalent to Sunderland Class V injury	Persistent flaccid paralysis

An axonal disruption that leaves some amount of internal neural architecture intact may result in synkinesis; the degree of which is dictated by which membranes are violated. Endoneurial disruption with intact perineurium portends a better prognosis than an injury to both layers. Axonal disruption also results in Wallerian degeneration, the disintegration of the injured axon between the node of Ranvier just proximal to the site of injury and the neuromuscular junction, following which the immune system clears the debris. Wallerian degeneration occurs approximately 72 h after a neural transection injury, but may persist for days or weeks after a neural crush injury [19, 33]. This timeline of Wallerian degeneration is clinically significant; facial nerve exploration and repair conducted within 72 h of injury can be performed with the aid of a nerve stimulator, and later-attempted repairs may not.

Similarly, the electrophysiological consequences of Wallerian degeneration, reduced compound muscle action potential (CMAP) amplitude, may be of prognostic significance. Electroneuronography (ENoG) is a form of evoked electromyography (EMG) in which a transcutaneous electrical stimulator is placed at the mastoid tip, and surface electrodes are placed over the facial muscles to record the CMAP, allowing for comparison between the injured and unaffected sides. If there is a significant decrease in CMAP amplitude on the injured side, Wallerian degeneration has occurred; the injury is at least a Sunderland Class II, and synkinesis may occur. If it is entirely absent, the injury is very likely a Sunderland Class V, which may be confirmed with an ENoG. A lack of voluntary motor unit potentials indicates nerve transection and corroborates the need for nerve repair [34].

ENoG testing should not be performed before 72 h post-injury; if Wallerian degeneration has not had time to occur, the test will not accurately indicate the extent of axonal injury. Ultimately, facial nerve repair aims to convert a Sunderland

Class V injury to a Class IV injury or a completely transected nerve to one with intact epineurium to improve the prognosis from persistent flaccidity to synkinesis.

20.4 Etiology of Facial Paralysis

Etiology of facial paralysis is the most important factor in determining the timing and choice of reconstructive technique. A retrospective study of almost 2000 patients by Hohman and Hadlock (2014) reported Bell's palsy to be the most common cause of facial paralysis (38%), followed by acoustic neuroma resection (10%), cancer (7%), iatrogenic trauma (7%), varicella zoster (7%), benign lesions (5%), congenital palsy (5%), Lyme disease (4%), and other etiologies (17%). In general, trauma is the second most common cause of facial paralysis [35].

20.4.1 Bell's Palsy

Bell's palsy is idiopathic. About 80% of patients begin to recover nerve function spontaneously within 3 weeks; 15% do not have any movement for 3–6 months. Peitersen found 94% of patients with partial paralysis completely recovered in 1 year without medical or surgical intervention; of those with complete paralysis, 71% completely recovered [36]. Thus, irreversible reconstructive methods are not the best in these patients.

20.4.2 Malignancy

Malignancy of the posterior fossa, temporal bone, skull base, or parotid region can present with facial paralysis. If paralysis is caused by a malignancy or its resection, the risk of recurrence and prognosis may influence the choice of reconstruction.

20.4.3 Denervation

The etiology of the denervation dictates the timing of surgical treatment, if anything is to be done. In a patient with a paralyzed face secondary to traumatic surgical disruption, the surgeon should initiate reconstruction as soon as possible, generally within the first month. On the other hand, a patient with an intact nerve can be monitored for recovery for up to 12 months. The duration of the facial paralysis is essential.

20.4.4 Operative Injury (Extra-temporal)

Extra-temporal facial nerve injury may occur during surgery of the parotid or submandibular gland, temporomandibular joint (TMJ) or face-lift procedures, or from traumatic face lacerations. Paralysis of the facial nerve following uncomplicated parotid procedures is reported at a 20% rate of temporary palsy, with a 10% rate of permanent paresis of temporal or mandibular branches.

Children and patients undergoing total parotidectomy are at a higher risk of facial nerve injury during surgery. If the nerve is resected because of a parotid cancer, histopathological confirmation of clear margins is required prior to repair by end-to-end anastomosis (EEA) or graft. Inadvertent transection during face-lift or parotid surgery warrants immediate primary repair. Postoperative paralysis with known facial nerve integrity usually recovers within 6 months. Traumatic transections and division of segmental branches proximal to the lateral canthus should be explored and repaired.

Facial nerve injury following submandibular gland surgery, which usually involves the MMN, is not uncommon. Sacrifice of this branch may be unavoidable because of involvement by the disease process, most commonly chronic infection or tumor.

Procedures of the TMJ may injure the temporal branch or, less commonly, the main trunk of the facial nerve. Facial nerve injury during rhytidectomy is rare, usually temporary, and most often involves segmental branches.

20.5 Diagnosis of Facial Paralysis

20.5.1 Clinical Evaluation

20.5.1.1 Patient History

A thorough history includes onset, initial degree of paralysis, duration, and associated symptoms. The reconstructive options for paralysis of <18–24 months duration and paralysis for >18–24 months differ significantly.

Facial nerve injuries caused by Bell's palsy, trauma, and malignant neoplasm need to be identified, with the reconstructive efforts based on the etiology. For example, a slowly progressive paralysis suggests malignancy, while a sudden onset of complete paralysis suggests Bell's palsy. In addition, the surgical team must investigate previous surgical procedures for reanimation, since these may limit reconstructive options. The patient's overall health, psychological stability, and life expectancy are significant considerations.

20.5.1.2 Physical Examination

The patient with facial palsy should be scrutinized with the face at rest and during voluntary and reflex emotional movement. The physician must determine the involvement of unilateral or bilateral facial nerves, facial asymmetries, and synkinesis. The degree of brow ptosis, ectropion, lid laxity, and oral competence must also be noted. Moreover, the surgical team cannot neglect other cranial nerve or neurological deficits and soft tissue defects in conjunction with the paralysis, in addition to the general condition of the patient.

Assessment of facial nerve function aims to identify abnormalities in any of the main extra-temporal branches of the nerve. The preferred assessment method begins in the upper face and examines the function of each branch in a descending fashion. The initial examination should be performed with the patient "at rest" to identify any gross or subtle asymmetries in muscle tone; these are frequently manifested as brow ptosis, lower eyelid laxity, nasolabial fold effacement, deviation of the upper lip philtrum, or inferior malposition of the oral commissure. Older patients may also demonstrate effacement of platysmal banding on the affected side.

After static assessment, a "dynamic" physical examination should be performed. Raising the eyebrows, closing the eyes gently and again with full effort, smiling, puckering the lips, and depressing the lower lip successively test the functions of the frontal, zygomatic, buccal, marginal mandibular, and cervical branches of the facial nerve. Determining the level of baseline asymmetry and the amount of effort required to close the affected eye, whenever possible, permits grading the severity of the facial paralysis on the House–Brackmann scale, a simple and universally accepted method of assessing facial nerve function [37] (Table 20.4).

The House–Brackmann scale quantifies overall hemifacial paralysis. However, it is not designed to provide a detailed description of severe synkinesis or segmental facial paralysis. Synkinesis is the involuntary movement of some muscles accompanying the voluntary movement of others, such as eye closure with smiling or cheek and neck twitching with eye closure or brow elevation. Synkinesis is often characterized by an increased resting tone in the affected side of the face, which may manifest as a deepened nasolabial fold or face and progressive neck cramping.

To characterize a broader range of facial paralysis presentations, which includes segmental and synkinetic paralysis, other detailed facial function grading systems have emerged such as the Sunnybrook scale developed by Ross et al. in Toronto in 1994 [38] and the eFACE scale developed by Banks et al. at Harvard in 2015 [39].

Table 20.4 House–Brackmann scale for grading the severity of the facial paralysis

Grade	Description
I	Symmetrical at rest and with movement, with no abnormalities
II	Mild weakness, symmetric at rest, minimal asymmetry with movement, complete eye closure with gentle effort, possible mild synkinesis
III	Moderate weakness, symmetric at rest, moderate asymmetry with movement, complete eye closure only with full effort, possible moderate synkinesis
IV	Moderate-to-severe weakness, symmetric at rest, moderate asymmetry with movement, incomplete eye closure
V	Severe weakness, grossly asymmetric at rest, significant asymmetry with movement, incomplete eye closure
VI	No visible movement, grossly asymmetric at rest ("facial droop")

20.5.2 Investigations

20.5.2.1 Audiometry

Audiometric testing, including acoustic reflexes and tympanometry, may be useful in identifying the etiology of facial palsy secondary to retro-cochlear pathology or mass lesions of the middle ear.

20.5.2.2 Imaging Studies

High-resolution computed tomography (CT) scan and magnetic resonance imaging (MRI) are essential in traumatic facial nerve palsy to delineate features of the temporal bone. Scans are also used to evaluate patients with possible parotid, skull base, temporal bone, intracranial, or extra-temporal tumors.

20.5.2.3 Electrodiagnostic Tests

Electrodiagnostic tests of facial nerve function include nerve excitability tests (NET), electroneuronography (ENoG), and electromyography (EMG).

20.5.2.4 Nerve Excitability Testing (NET)

Nerve excitability testing involves percutaneous stimulation of the facial nerve until muscle contraction is observed. The "minimal" NET determines the threshold stimulation required for muscle contraction compared with the unaffected side. The "maximum stimulation test" (MST) is a supramaximal stimulus compared with the unaffected side, and the stimulus is increased until the patient encounters discomfort. The "subjective" nature of the measurements and lack of recorded data limit both methods, and they do not reflect denervation at the moment it is occurring.

20.5.2.5 Electroneurography (ENoG)

Electroneurography (ENoG) is an objective measure of facial nerve function that measures the amplitude of evoked compound muscle action potentials (CMAPs) with electrodes over the skin of the nasolabial fold. The compound action potential is compared between the two sides of the face, and the response of the affected side is expressed as a percentage of the response of the unaffected side. A percentage of nerve fiber degeneration is calculated. A 95% decrease in CMAP compared with the contralateral side signifies a 50% chance that the patient will have unsatisfactory recovery of facial nerve function. Surgery is indicated if a 90% decrease in CMAP is reached within the initial 2 weeks of the onset of paralysis. ENoG is "objective" and is the most accurate reproducible test, but it is expensive and time-consuming.

20.5.2.6 Electromyography (EMG)

Electromyography (EMG) is a measure of volitional muscle response. Needle electrodes are used to monitor activity of facial muscles. Normal muscle exhibits activity upon needle insertion, electrical silence at rest, and diphasic or triphasic action potentials during voluntary contraction. Fibrillation potentials are observed in the denervated muscle, as well as polyphasic potentials in muscle undergoing reinnervation. Complete electrical silence is observed in denervated muscle with significant fibrosis.

Electromyography is useful in evaluating patients with acute or traumatic nerve injury prior to reinnervation procedures. However, it does not show any signs until 3 weeks after paralysis and should not be utilized until 3 weeks after paralysis without signs of recovery.

20.5.2.7 Objective Measures of Facial Motion

Objective measures of facial motion include digital photography and video-recording of the patient at rest and during motion. The "maximum static response assay" quantifies facial motion pre- and serially postoperatively. The patient's face is marked and he/she is asked to perform specific movements (brow lift, eye closure, smiling, frowning, and whistling). Images of the face in repose and the maximum response movements are recorded and processed for computer display. Images are calibrated and normalized, and vectors of movement are determined and measured using a grid and an internal facial coordinate system. Slight improvements in facial movement are detected over the long recovery periods that often accompany facial reanimation procedures.

20.5.2.8 Differential Diagnosis

The differential diagnosis for facial paralysis is extensive. It includes Bell's palsy, Ramsay–Hunt syndrome (also known as herpes zoster oticus—may cause painful shingles rash, facial paralysis, and hearing loss in the affected ear), Lyme disease, cerebellopontine angle (CPA) tumors, temporal bone fractures, parotid malignancies, autoimmune disorders, iatrogenic and traumatic injuries, and many others [16, 35].

20.6 Indications and Contraindications of Facial Nerve Repair

20.6.1 Indications

20.6.1.1 Intraoperative Injury

The primary indication for facial nerve repair is a Sunderland Class V injury to the main trunk or an extra-temporal branch of the facial nerve. When the injury occurs intraoperatively, the severity may be self-evident and the preferred approach is primary repair at the time of injury. However, some facial nerve injuries are not apparent until upon awakening from general anesthesia or in a delayed fashion. When paralysis is delayed, the nerve is intact; repair or transfer is unnecessary. If, on the other hand, paralysis is complete and immediately apparent upon awakening, but was not identified intraoperatively, it may be prudent to evaluate the severity of the axonal injury 3–5 days later via ENoG and proceed with repair or transfer only if testing reveals >90% reduction in CMAP compared to the uninjured side. There must be viable distal and proximal segments of the nerve if either primary coaptation or interposition grafting is to be attempted.

Kannan et al. (2020) reported improved functional outcomes in patients who underwent immediate facial nerve repair as compared to repair delayed by 3 weeks–18 months [14]. When nerve repair or transfer is scheduled 6 or more months after injury, EMG should be performed to verify muscle viability; insertional activity or fibrillation potentials should be present. If EMG demonstrates polyphasic potentials, reinnervation procedures should be delayed to determine the effectiveness of the ongoing axonal recovery. Axons regenerate at approximately 1 mm/day, although many factors may affect this rate, including age, nutritional status, and general health. Therefore, a rough estimate of the time it will take for axons to travel from the repair site to the target muscles can be obtained by measuring the distance from the point of repair or transfer in millimeters [40].

20.6.1.2 Facial Trauma

In case of facial trauma, particularly lacerations, a similar process may be followed to determine candidacy for surgical intervention. Nerve injuries occurring medial to the lateral canthus do not need to be explored or repaired; the nerve branches in that region are small enough that coaptation is very challenging.

20.6.1.3 Proximal Nerve Injury

Facial paralysis due to a very proximal nerve injury, such as at the CPA, or CNS pathology, such as a cavernous brain stem hemangioma, is better addressed with nerve transfer techniques. When considering nerve repair or transfer, there must be a target muscle expected to remain viable long enough to accept axonal ingrowth weeks to months after the procedure. While muscle typically undergoes atrophy and fibrosis after 12–18 months of denervation, this is not consistently the case. There are anecdotal reports of successful reinnervation years after a facial nerve injury. Generally, the muscle will be viable if the repair or nerve transfer is performed within 6 months of injury; nerve transfer is likely more successful than repair in such cases [17].

20.6.1.4 Contraindications

Contraindications to facial nerve repair include incomplete and delayed facial paralysis as the nerve is intact in both situations and should be allowed to recover spontaneously. Additionally, if the facial nerve injury is medial to the lateral canthus, not only would repair be technically difficult but also the redundancy of innervation close to the target muscles is usually sufficient that spontaneous functional recovery is highly likely [41].

The absence of electrical activity, specifically the lack of insertion or fibrillation potentials, on preoperative EMG of the target muscles indicates atrophy of the neuromuscular junction with possible fibrosis of the muscles and an inability to accept reinnervation [42]. Patients whose facial muscles are absent due to extensive facial resection, trauma, or congenital facial palsy may not have target muscles for reinnervation. Thus, facial nerve repair is contraindicated in these circumstances.

Patients with advanced-stage malignancies or other chronic diseases likely to shorten life expectancy may not live long enough to justify the surgical risk of facial reinnervation. In cases of malignancy, facial reinnervation should be delayed until tumor resection is completed. Additionally, patients in a persistent vegetative state or those with severe dementia will be unable to participate in facial retraining, reducing the benefits of facial reinnervation procedures.

Although preexisting dysphagia is not a contraindication to facial reinnervation in general, it is a contraindication for hypoglossal nerve transfer as the procedure may exacerbate the problem, particularly in older patients [43].

20.7 Equipment and Personnel

20.7.1 Equipment

The following equipment is recommended to perform a facial nerve repair:

- Operating microscope
- Microsurgical instruments (jeweler's forceps, straight and curved microscissors, non-locking microneedle holder)
- 10-0 nylon sutures on cutting spatula-tip needles, such as TG 160-4
- Weck cell spears
- Suction tip
- Bipolar jeweler's forceps
- Collagen wrap or other nerve sheaths, such as a vein graft
- Straight Iris or tenotomy scissors
- Retractors (Senn, Ragnell, Cummings, or Lone Star)
- Fibrin glue
- Nerve stimulator
- Other instruments may be required for exploration of the facial nerve and any other nerve to be grafted or transferred such as Metzenbaum, Gorney-Freeman, or Reynolds tenotomy scissors. In addition, petit point Crile clamps, fine right-angle clamps, McCabe dissectors, and DeBakey or Gerald forceps will serve well for nerve dissection.

20.7.2 Personnel

The nerve coaptation is usually performed by a facial plastic surgeon, neurosurgeon, head and neck surgeon, or plastic surgeon. This may be the primary surgeon whose procedure resulted in the facial nerve injury or a consultant whose expertise is required for nerve repair. For cases that require proximal exposure of the facial nerve within the mastoid process of the temporal bone, an otolaryngologist or otologist should perform the mastoidectomy.

In addition to the surgeon, a circulating nurse and a surgical technologist should be present. In some cases, a surgical first assistant may be necessary. An anesthesia provider is also required. The anesthetist should be capable of maintaining a general anesthetic plane deep enough to prevent patient movement without requiring long-acting paralytics, as these preclude the use of intraoperative nerve stimulation.

20.8 Goals and Limitations of Nerve Reconstruction

Dynamic and static reconstruction procedures are employed for facial reanimation in patients suffering from facial nerve paralysis [44]. However, dynamic strategies tend to be more successful and fruitful and should be offered to patients considering reconstruction, unless health risk contraindications exist. The most common approaches for reconstruction are direct facial nerve repair with or without grafting, nerve transfer, cross-facial nerve grafting, and muscle transfer (regional or free) [45–48]. Understanding facial nerve anatomy with precise assessment of the patient's paralysis and health status dictate the potential for recovery and the appropriate reconstructive scheme.

20.8.1 Goals of Reconstruction

The goals of the reconstruction in facial paralysis include the following:

Facial symmetry at rest
Symmetrical smile
Voluntary, coordinated, and spontaneous facial movements
Oral competence and eyelid closure with corneal protection
Absence or limitation of synkinesis and mass movement

20.8.2 Limitations of Surgery

The facial nerve innervates a total of 23 paired muscles and the orbicular oris, but only 18 of these muscles, working in a delicate balance, produce facial animation and expression. No current reconstructive stratagem can reproduce every facial expression and movement. As part of patient counselling, surgeons need to establish realistic patient expectations and determine whether the patient is willing to expend the time and financial resources required for a successful result.

20.9 Time Schedule for Facial Nerve Repair

Recommendations for the time schedule for facial nerve repair are summarized in Table 20.5.

Table 20.5 Time schedule for facial nerve repair

Duration of paralysis (years)	Functional recovery of facial musculature
0–1	Absolutely certain
1–2	Expected, therefore recommendable
2–3	Probable, with delay and decrease in function
3–5	Increasingly questionable, patient must be notified
5+	Improbable, therefore not to be recommended

20.9.1 Immediate Surgical Reconstruction

For recovery of facial expression following partial or subtotal resection of the facial nerve and/or the peripheral nerve plexus, an immediate surgical reconstruction should be performed when at all possible for the following reasons:

- Facial expression plays an extremely important role in patient psychology and social life.
- Reconstruction should be performed as a one-stage operation together with tumor resection or, if a histological analysis is necessary, within 10–14 days at most, otherwise rapid development of scar tissue may jeopardize the success of this delicate surgery.
- The patient's general health is to be considered, since with a reduced tolerance to anesthesia, more complex and longer procedures must be replaced with simpler methods.
- The patient's age plays a role in the choice of procedure. With advancing age, nerve regeneration diminishes and preference is for procedures that make a safe and fast reinnervation of the paralyzed musculature possible (end-to-end anastomoses).
- Psychologically unstable patients may find it more difficult to live with a failed procedure than more stable or indifferent individuals.

The length of the interposition graft has a substantial influence on the final functional result after reconstruction. The longer the graft, the worse the final outcome will be, particularly if longer than 4–5 cm. The main reason for this is that the axons need more time to penetrate the endoneurial tubes, while at the same time, degeneration of the Schwann cells and fibrosis occurs. Penetration of the distal anastomosis will particularly be handicapped through meanwhile development of scar tissue.

20.9.2 Delayed Nerve Reconstruction: Main Questions Prior to Surgery

The following questions regarding the peripheral nervous system, central nervous system, and musculature should be addressed before planning surgery for delayed nerve reconstruction.

20.9.2.1 Peripheral Nervous System (Facial Nerve and Plexus)

To what extent has the nerve plexus been resected? i.e., is there still enough nerve tissue of the main branches in situ to perform successful anastomoses?

How realistic are the chances of identifying and isolating the branches within the scar tissue from the injury or the previous operation?

Is there enough suitable nerve material available for free nerve transplantation?

If the hypoglossal nerve (CN-XII) is to be used for anastomosis, are both CN-XII and CN-V (trigeminal) intact in their extra-cranial course?

In cases of tumor resection, is the remaining facial nerve tissue free from tumor infiltration?

20.9.2.2 Central Nervous System

What is the general condition of the brain? i.e., what is the patient intellectual or emotional status?

Are cranial nerves V and XII functioning normally? It is important to note that the function of both motor nerves (VII and XII) depends on the common afferent input from CN V [49, 50].

20.9.2.3 Musculature

Is it still vital enough to regain its contractibility?

Is it free from tumor infiltration?

Is it free from infection?

20.10 Principles of Nerve Repair

20.10.1 Selection of Repair Technique

An algorithm is provided to guide the selection of evaluation and management techniques for patients with facial nerve trauma.

If the proximal and distal nerve stumps can be approximated without tension, direct end-to-end coaptation is indicated [16].

If the proximal and distal nerve stumps can be approximated within 6 mm of each other without tension, coaptation using a nerve connector is indicated [51, 52].

If both stumps are accessible, but cannot be approximated without tension, an interposition nerve graft is indicated, most commonly utilizing the greater auricular or sural nerve. Ideally, it should only be performed when duration of paralysis is <1 year.

If >50% of the diameter of the nerve has been disrupted, as in a drill injury during mastoidectomy, the injured segment should be resected and primary neurorrhaphy performed when possible; an interposition graft may be used if necessary.

20.10.2 Early Identification and Repair of Nerve Injuries

The most critical factor in achieving good postoperative facial function is early identification and repair of nerve disruption. Several authors reported that earlier repair of the facial nerve produces superior results. Some authors report function in patients who were grafted 18–36 months after injury, but superior results are found with repairs performed within 1 year. Repair within 30 days is preferred based on clinical results and neurobiological investigations that revealed that the regenerative process begins immediately after injury.

Traumatic nerve injuries must be repaired expediently. In the instance of a grossly contaminated wound (e.g., shotgun injury), the nerve ends can be tagged and repaired later. Accidental transection during surgery (e.g., parotidectomy or face-lift) should be dealt with an end-to-end anastomosis (EEA). If the facial nerve is resected because of tumor involvement, frozen sections of both ends can be sent for histopathological examination to exclude microscopic invasion before attempting repair. When margins are clear, either EEA or graft repair can be performed immediately.

20.10.3 Evaluation of Nerve Condition

The condition of the nerve depends on the type of injury or trauma. A patient with preoperative facial palsy secondary to tumor involvement of the facial nerve is unlikely to experience a good result following resection and repair. The amount of functioning nerve fibers existing at the time of surgery does not increase after repair; improved postoperative facial function over preoperative status is not expected.

A sharp facial nerve laceration from glass or a knife should be suitable for EEA. Gunshot wounds, however, either crush or avulse the nerve, which propagates further nerve degeneration/denervation. These injuries should not be repaired in the immediate setting until the extent of the nerve damage has declared itself. In a delayed intervention, scar tissue and neuromas must be removed, and unhealthy nerve ends must be excised. Identifying healthy nerve stumps may necessitate histologic or microscopic confirmation.

20.10.4 Matching of Endoneurial Surfaces

Matching of the endoneurial surfaces is essential in promoting neural regeneration and is more important than a match of the total nerve diameter. The endoneurium is examined more easily by removing the overlying perineurium at the ends of the nerve. Occasionally, a significant mismatch between proximal and distal nerve ends requires a double cable graft (e.g., when grafting from the main facial nerve trunk to segmental branches).

20.10.5 Epineural Versus Perineural Suturing

Various neurorrhaphy techniques and adjunctive measures have been investigated in attempts to improve neural regeneration, including epineural versus perineural sutures, tissue adhesives, laser neurorrhaphy, tubulization, and trophic factors. However, the most efficacious method of re-approximation remains unproven, and no specific adjunctive measure has been found to be beneficial. The use of a minimal number (2 or 4) of epineural or perineural sutures, employing a fine monofilament suture under magnification (microscope or loupe), remains the time-tested criterion for nerve repair.

20.10.6 Tension-Free Anastomosis and Nerve Grafts

Any tension on the nerve ends after repair results in the formation of scar tissue and poor neural regeneration. If tensionless nerve repair is not feasible, then a nerve graft (usually the sural nerve) will be interposed between the proximal trunk and distal branches. Mobilization of the nerve may add up to 2 cm of relative length, but also may result in devascularization and further neural injury. Any defect >2 cm should be tackled with a nerve graft of adequate length, without any tension and with a small amount of slack.

"Cable grafts" function as conduits in which sprouting axons from the proximal nerve stump travel to the motor end-plates. The graft provides cellular and humoral promoters for neural growth, such as Schwann cells, extracellular matrix, and neurotrophic growth factor.

20.10.7 Donor Nerves for Facial Nerve Grafting

The great auricular nerve (GAN) and sural nerve are the most commonly selected nerves for facial nerve grafting [53]. Disadvantages include a sensory deficit of the ear lobe when using the GAN, or of the lateral foot when using the sural nerve. The GAN is harvested easily, since it is located near the surgical field, it tends to be a good match in size, and its extensive arborization allows the anastomosis of the proximal facial nerve stump to several segmental branches. However, only 7–10 cm of the GAN can be harvested safely, which limits its use in extensive repairs. On the other hand, the sural nerve is larger, with a greater axonal volume, and up to 35 cm is harvested easily from the posterior lower leg. It is especially useful in cross-facial grafting.

The patient should not expect return of facial function following nerve grafting for 4–6 months, as regenerating axons travel a distance of 1 mm/day. Improvement in function can be expected for up to 2 years. In general, results after nerve grafting are not as good as those observed with primary repair. Spector et al. found incomplete reinnervation of facial divisions, decreased voluntary contractions, and more severe synkinesis when comparing cable grafts to direct end-to-end anastomoses

[54]. However, 92–95% of patients who undergo facial nerve grafting experience some return of facial function, and 72–79% have good functional results.

20.10.8 Rehabilitation

After surgery, rehabilitation of patients with facial paralysis necessitates EMG protocols, behavioral modification, and patient exercises. The patient needs to obtain voluntary control of facial regions. Another adjuvant therapy is the use of percutaneous electrical stimulation to stimulate motor function.

20.11 Techniques of Nerve Reconstruction

The following methods (techniques) of extra-temporal facial nerve plexus reconstruction are recommended [55]:

End-to-end anastomosis (EEA)
Free nerve transplantation (interposition graft)
Hypoglossal-facial anastomosis (HFA) as EEA
Hypoglossal-facialis jump anastomosis (HFJA) as EEA.
Combined approach (facio-facial anastomosis combined with HFA)
Cross-facial nerve graft

In comparison to the overall excellent functional outcome of the above-mentioned techniques, the "cross-face anastomosis" has several disadvantages leading to suboptimal results: (1) the need to harvest the sural nerve is time-consuming and leads to decreased sensation at its innervation area; (2) implantation of two or three transplants across the face are also time-consuming and bothersome to patients; (3) the anastomosis with facial nerve branches of the opposite side destroys healthy structures; (4) the long transplants need much more time for reinnervation; and (5) long transplants always result in a worse outcome compared to short grafts and especially to EEA.

20.11.1 End-to-End Anastomosis (EEA)/Direct End-to-End Coaptation

Direct end-to-end coaptation is the treatment of choice for facial nerve injury whenever feasible. Functional outcomes are improved when the nerve is repaired immediately after injury; this situation is only likely to occur during iatrogenic trauma [14, 42]. If repair under the same anesthetic as the injury is impossible, facial nerve exploration and repair should ideally be performed within 72 h of injury before completion of Wallerian degeneration; this permits using an intraoperative stimulator to facilitate identification of the distal nerve stump.

Once the nerve stumps have been identified, they should be trimmed back to healthy tissue, as evidenced by pinpoint bleeding within the nerve. When the injury is "fresh," debridement is usually minimal. However, in case of "old" injury with scar tissue formation, more aggressive trimming of the nerve will be required with internal neurolysis, removing the section containing scar tissue, or external neurolysis, dissecting scar tissue away from the outside of the nerve to improve exposure. Intraneural scar tissue prevents proper axonal regeneration across the neurorrhaphy and must be removed completely, even if the removal precludes a tension-free neurorrhaphy and necessitates a nerve sheath or interposition graft. Similarly, if ≥50% of the diameter of the nerve has been injured, the injured segment should be resected and the nerve repaired to reduce the amount of intraneural scar tissue that forms.

The neurorrhaphy itself is typically performed under an operating microscope. The sutures should be placed as interrupted stitches in the epineurium, avoiding overtightening of the knots and pushing the nerve ends together with excessive force, likely distorting the fascicles contained therein. Individual fascicular repair placing sutures in the perineurium rather than the epineurium is rarely performed; there is no reliable way to determine the correlates between proximal and distal stump fascicles. Outcomes are equivalent between perineural and epineural repair; the latter procedure is far less technically challenging [56, 57].

Trimming of the nerve causes shortening of the nerve endings. Lack of tension in the anastomosis is an important prerequisite for a good, functioning result, and a tension-free suture can only be achieved after mobilization of the central and peripheral nerve stumps. The possibilities for such a mobilization are limited, and the following procedure is therefore recommended to relieve tension from the anastomosis. Before performing the nerve suture, an 8/0 suture is inserted through the epineurium of one or both of the nerve stumps a few millimeters from the anastomosis to the right and left, and these sutures are gently pulled toward the anastomosis, securing it in the underlying base of the incision. Such a procedure is naturally only possible when the nerve branches are of sufficient size.

The first stitch is generally placed in the center of the superficial aspect of the epineurium, where it is easiest to sew; once the first suture is placed, two or three more interrupted stitches may be added to approximate the epineurium gently in a circumferential fashion. Alternatively, fibrin glue may be used to coapt the nerve stumps, which appears to produce comparable functional outcomes to suture neurorrhaphy. However, using sutures provides a more stable repair more capable of resisting the tension that may be applied by patient movement [16, 17, 58]. The most common place to employ fibrin glue during facial nerve repair is intracranially in the CPA or internal auditory canal [17].

Regarding the suture technique for EEA, there are two false statements that are frequently found in the literature, supported by unrealistic diagrams [59]. First, according to these opinions, the epineurium should be trimmed back at the ends of the fascicles. Although the epineural sheath is moveable to a certain extent, suture of the epineurium of both nerve endings leads to an additional shortening of this surrounding structure. This can easily lead to an intrafascicular rejection of the fascicle endings, which in turn prevents correct adaptation of the fascicles. The resultant "bulging" of the fascicles within the anastomosis can often be felt against the bordering nerve section through soft palpation with micro-instruments alone. Conversely, suturing the epineuria that overlap the ends of the fascicles leads to an intraneural separation, creating an "empty space." Thus, it is recommended that the nerve endings be "cleaned up" by one sharp section through the entire nerve. Second, claims that a fascicular suture can be performed for facial nerve surgery are particularly unrealistic. This is impossible for three reasons: (1) in contrast to peripheral nerves, which consist of individual fascicles well separated from each other by the perineurium (poly-fascicular form), cranial nerves do not show any clear individual fascicles (mono-fascicular form); (2) consistency of the alleged fascicles is so soft that they would tear while trying the knot on even the most gentle of sutures; (3) the suture material used for such a technique would shift inward, where it would be perceived as a foreign body and interfere with the healing process by inducing granulation tissue.

If tension-free neurorrhaphy between the proximal and distal nerve stumps is impossible, three other commonly employed options exist. The first option is to coapt the nerve ends via a nerve sheath and leave a small gap between them. The second option is to interpose a cable graft from a donor nerve, and the third option is to perform a nerve transfer. Gaps between proximal and distal nerve stumps of $\leq$6 mm can be bridged by regenerating axons during the healing process, providing a sheath, typically made of collagen, connects the nerve ends and encloses the gap; outcomes are comparable to those achieved with primary neurorrhaphy [51, 52]. Gaps >7 mm should be bridged with interposition grafts. However, interposition grafts should be avoided whenever possible; the number of neurorrhaphies required for the repair is doubled and each neurorrhaphy may potentially lose as many as 50% of the axons regenerating across the repair [60]. Despite this, excessive dissection to mobilize the nerve stumps should also be avoided; epineural dissection and stretching of the nerve stumps compromise the vasa nervorum and adversely affects healing.

20.11.2 Free Nerve Transplantation (Interposition or Cable Graft)

20.11.2.1 Indications

If the gap between the proximal and distal nerve stumps is too long to allow primary neurorrhaphy in case of resection of malignant parotid tumors, an "interposition" graft, or "cable" graft, may be employed to span the distance. Placing a cable graft necessarily requires two neurorrhaphies instead of the one in a primary repair; this significantly increases the risk of axonal loss. This risk may be mitigated by reversing the anatomical direction of the grafted nerve; the distal end of the graft is sutured to the proximal nerve stump and vice versa. This practice theoretically allows every fascicle present at the distal end of the graft, now placed proximally, to have a continuous tract all the way to the proximal end of the graft, now located distally.

20.11.2.2 Difficulties

As a consequence of resection of malignant parotid tumors, nerve defects arise in the region of the facial nerve plexus (pes anserinus). This has a unique tree-like branching. There are two problems encountered when trying to overcome severe material defects in the central region of the nerve plexus: (1) a "numerical" discrepancy due the presence of a few (or one) central nerve stump(s) compared with numerous peripheral endings, which result from the tree-like branching out of the facial nerve; and (2) a "size" discrepancy because the central nerve stumps have a larger diameter than the very thin peripheral nerve endings. The extraction of a single graft that imitates this division satisfactorily is only possible in exceptional cases, and one must therefore almost always opt for several individual grafts. Usually, nerve transplants cannot imitate the tree-like branching out of the facial fan.

Excellent functional results have been reported in many cases using the following techniques to overcome the discrepancy in number and size by using interposition grafts [61, 62]:

20.11.2.3 Interventions at the Peripheral Nerve Branches

The ends of the nerve in the region of the peripheral resection are mobilized sufficiently that each of the two neighboring nerve branches can be positioned with their proximal ends about 5 mm alongside each other. If possible, the epineuria at the contact edges are dissected and, finally, the edges are bound together with a 10/0 suture. In this way, a new nerve branch is created from two peripheral nerve branches, now consisting of two fascicles. This allows the number of peripheral branches to be halved, while at the same time doubling their size, resulting in the defect being more easily repairable with a graft (Fig. 20.1). This technique can be taken further when required, using, for example, three or four neighboring nerve branches to make a new large nerve branch.

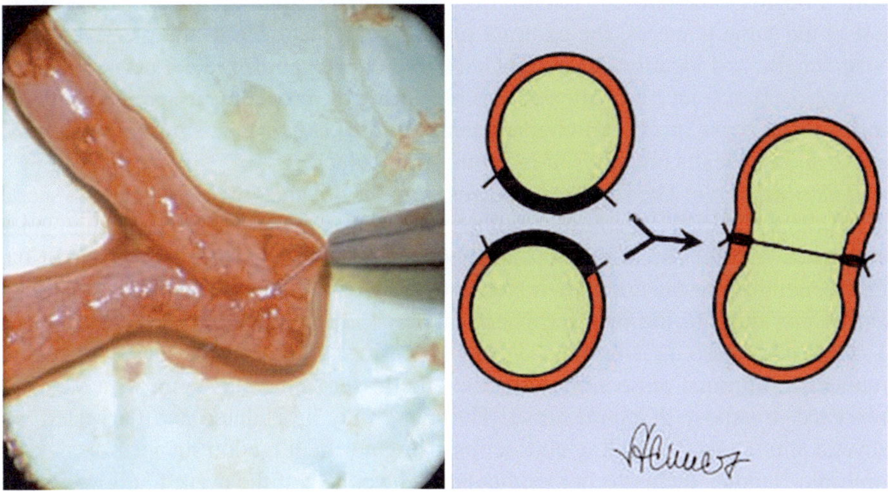

Fig. 20.1 Technique for reduction in number and increase in size. After mobilization and adaptation of amputated nerve endings, epineurium at the site of contact is resected, edges are bound together with a 10/0 suture and thereby the numbers of peripheral branches are halved, while at the same time doubled in their size

20.11.2.4 Interventions with the Graft

When a suitable graft is chosen, its peripheral ends can also be split into individual fascicles, which has a branching effect in addition to the interventions taken at the peripheral nerve endings (so-called diversification). The combination of both methods results in the most suitable synergistic double-effect: the reduction of number and increase in size of the peripheral nerve structures and the increase in number and reduction of size of the central nerve structures.

20.11.3 Nerves Used for Interposition

Typically, sensory nerves are used for graft material: most commonly, the greater auricular or sural nerves and occasionally the medial or lateral antebrachial cutaneous nerves [42]. In rare cases, motor nerves may be used as grafts, generally when they are already being sacrificed as part of a larger graft harvest. Cadaveric nerve allografts also are available, although reported procedural outcomes are inferior to nerve autografts [62–64].

The great auricular nerve (GAN): The GAN arises from the 2nd and 3rd cervical nerve roots (C2, 3), providing sensation to the inferior aspect of the auricle, ear lobule, and part of the skin overlying the mastoid process and parotid gland. It can provide about 7 cm of length, and its diameter is approximately 1.5 mm, making it a suitable size match for the facial nerve [65]. The GAN wraps around the posterior border of the SCM muscle at roughly one-third of the way down the muscle from its insertion on the mastoid tip, a point from which the lesser occipital, transverse cervical, and supraclavicular nerves also emanate. From there, it travels superiorly until it begins to branch 2–3 cm inferior to the lobule, running 1–2 cm posterior to, but in the same plane as, the external jugular vein, just deep to the platysma [65]. Size, length, and location make the GAN very convenient for facial nerve repair; it is easy to extract since it is often accessible during the procedure associated with the initial facial nerve injury. Another advantage of the GAN is that, similar to the facial nerve and its plexus branches, it is "mono-fascicular."

The sural nerve: The sural nerve arises from the 4th and 5th lumbar and 1st sacral nerve roots (L4, 5S1), resulting from the confluence of the medial and lateral sural cutaneous nerves [66]. It rises into a subcutaneous plane between the heads of the gastrocnemius muscle and then travels inferiorly toward the lateral malleolus of the ankle, just deep to the lesser saphenous vein [53]. It is easily approached via a 1–2 cm transverse incision placed 1 cm posterior and 1 cm superior to the lateral malleolus; minimal dissection will reveal the lesser saphenous vein, which can be retracted to expose the sural nerve. The nerve may be isolated and harvested via several approaches, including endoscopy, using a vein or tendon stripper, or making multiple "ladder" incisions perpendicular to the course of the nerve to allow dissection under direct visualization. The sural nerve provides up to 30 cm of length and a diameter of roughly 3.5 mm, slightly more than the facial nerve, but sufficient to transmit an ample number of axons [67]. In addition, donor site morbidity is minimal, typically limited to numbness of the lateral foot and ankle. However, the sural nerve has two considerable disadvantages: its extraction is costly and bifurcations of its nerve branches are very far apart. The sural nerve is particularly well suited to use in cross-face grafting applications.

20.11.4 Direct Hypoglossal-Facial Nerve Anastomosis (HFA) with End-to-End Anastomosis

The hypoglossal nerve (CN-XII) is located superficial to the carotid arteries and deep to the central tendon of the digastric muscle and is typically approached via a high, transverse neck incision. It provides motor innervation to the anterior two-thirds of the tongue and contains approximately 9000 axons, 50% more than the 6000 found in the facial nerve [68]. Because of the relatively high resting tone of the tongue, hypoglossal nerve transfer to the main trunk of the facial nerve is often used to restore resting facial tone. The technique may also be employed specifically for smile rehabilitation; this requires the patient to push their tongue into their cheek to smile. While the high axon count of the hypoglossal nerve makes it a very effective donor for facial reinnervation, the significant morbidity associated with denervating half of the oral tongue has led to the development of multiple variations of the procedure that are designed to limit the functional lingual deficit [43, 69].

The classic HFA procedure involves transecting both the hypoglossal and facial nerves and suturing the proximal hypoglossal stump into the distal facial nerve stump; this procedure is so morbid that it is rarely performed in current practice. Another common procedural variation involves transecting the facial nerve in the mastoid, reflecting the distal facial nerve inferiorly, and performing an end-to-side neurorrhaphy into the hypoglossal nerve. Alternatively, the epineurium of the hypoglossal nerve may be incised, and one-third to one-half of the fascicles may be reflected superiorly to be sewn end-to-side or end-to-end into the main trunk of the facial nerve. However, if some return of facial nerve function is expected, but additional muscle tone is required, hypoglossal-facial nerve transfer without division of the main trunk of the facial nerve is preferable. Lastly, epineural windows may be made, and one-third of the fascicles in the hypoglossal and facial nerves divided so that an interposition or "jump" graft may be sutured end-to-side into both nerves to carry axons from the transected fascicles in the hypoglossal nerve to the transected fascicles in the facial nerve.

HFA is technically easy to perform; success is assured; and it leads to a rapid reinnervation of the paralytic musculature because of its peripheral localization. A review of several large series of patients found that 42–65% of patients experienced good to excellent results, which were described as the presence of tone and symmetry, with fair to good movement and moderate to mild synkinesis [55, 70–73]. Complications following HFA include variable degrees of hemi-tongue atrophy and functional disability, including difficulty with chewing, swallowing, and speaking. In general, these impairments improve over time, and many patients report fewer problems chewing postoperatively than preoperatively. This likely is due to improvement of buccal tone. Regardless of the technique selected, however, the donor site morbidity and facial movement outcomes are inversely proportional; as more axons are transferred to the face, more axons are taken from the tongue.

20.11.5 Hypoglossal-Facial Nerve Anastomosis with "Jump" Anastomosis (HFJA)

This is a very valuable alternative to the classic HFA that was popularized by May et al. [74] (Fig. 20.2). The hypoglossal nerve (CN-XII) is exposed in the retromandibular fossa and a diagonal incision made into its ventral circumference, half-way through the axons and through the epineurium, leaving an open V-shaped wound. A graft (usually from the GAN) is then sutured into this V-shaped incision so that its ends anastomose with the proximal stumps of the dissected axons of the hypoglossal nerve. Finally, the peripheral end of the graft can be sutured with the facial nerve stem as well as with each branch of its plexus. In the plexus region, for overcoming discrepancy in number and size, the same techniques can be used as those described above.

In comparison to direct anastomosis between the two nerve trunks, this technique is more time-consuming and delicate to perform because of the additional need of harvesting and interposing a free nerve graft. However, in the hands of a well-trained microsurgeon, this technique is also a safe method, leading to excellent functional results [75, 76].

Since the functional deficits of the tongue are negligible, the method is especially indicated for all patients with speech occupation and for rehabilitation of irreversible facial palsy after the removal of an acoustic neurinoma, which might be the first manifestation of a Morbus Recklinghausen (type II) disease and then may later also develop

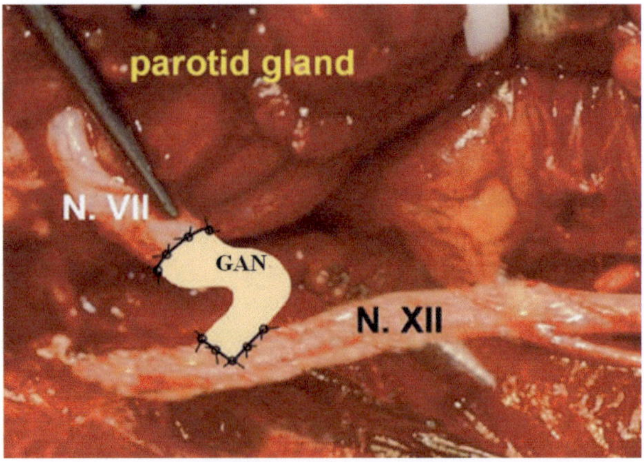

Fig. 20.2 "Hypoglossal-facial jump anastomosis" using the great auricular nerve. The hypoglossal nerve is exposed in the retromandibular fossa and a diagonal incision is made into half of its ventral circumference. The distal end of the interposed nerve transplant is directed toward the proximal stumps of the dissected axons of the hypoglossal nerve. *N.VII* facial nerve, *GAN* great auricular nerve, *N.XII* hypoglossal nerve

on the contralateral side. Good facial movement and expression were noted in 41% of jump graft patients, and the patients experienced less synkinesis than did the nerve transfer patients [48]. Facial motor function generally is not as strong following a jump graft, and recovery of facial function has been found to take longer in jump grafts.

20.11.6 Masseteric Nerve Transfer

While the hypoglossal nerve is relatively conveniently located in the upper neck, not far from the facial nerve, the masseteric nerve lies directly deep to the facial nerve and is easily accessed via the same incision used for facial nerve exposure. The nerve to the masseter muscle is a branch of the mandibular division of the trigeminal nerve. The masseteric nerve exits the skull base via the foramen ovale and traverses the infratemporal fossa before entering the deep surface of the masseter muscle via the sigmoid notch of the mandible. The masseteric nerve contains approximately 1500 axons; this may account for the lower resting tone of the masseter muscle compared to that of the tongue [21]. For this reason, masseteric nerve transfer is not as effective in restoring resting facial tone as hypoglossal nerve transfer. However, the anatomical location of the masseteric nerve makes it ideal for smile rehabilitation.

To locate the masseter nerve, a point is marked 3 cm anterior to the anterior surface of the tragal cartilage and 1 cm inferior to the inferior border of the zygomatic arch. At this point, dissection approximately 1.5 cm deep to the SMAS should reveal the masseteric nerve beneath a tendinous layer within the muscle [77]. The masseteric nerve is dissected distally and transected just before branching, then reflected out of the muscle for coaptation. End-to-end or end-to-side neurorrhaphy into the main trunk of the facial nerve may be performed, or the masseteric nerve may be sutured end-to-end into the buccal branch located at the point of Zuker to rehabilitate a paralytic or synkinetic smile [78–83].

Another advantage of the masseteric nerve transfer over hypoglossal nerve transfer is its comparative lack of donor site morbidity; loss of masseteric function is well tolerated; and not all patients suffer a noticeable loss of facial volume from muscle atrophy. However, as with the hypoglossal nerve transfer, using the masseteric nerve to provide facial movement requires the patient to initiate a conscious movement, such as when biting down or clenching the jaw (see video). Over time, many patients can smile without needing to bite down hard, but achieving a spontaneous smile with either a masseteric or hypoglossal nerve transfer is comparatively uncommon, especially in adult patients [84].

20.11.7 Facio-Facial Anastomosis Combined with HFA (Diversification Technique)

This method is also considered for patients with total loss of facial expression, but only when the resection defect is restricted to the central portion of the facial plexus, i.e., nerve trunk, bifurcation, temporofacial and cervicofacial main branch and immediately adjacent sections of branches extending from this region. The method pays particular attention to the functional anatomy of the facial musculature, which consists of an ocular and oral sphincter system [85, 86].

Experience with the HFA has shown that good functional rehabilitation of the musculature of the "oral sphincter system" can be achieved using the hypoglossal nerve. For this reason, nerve branches that innervate the perioral musculature are supplied either directly or with a jump anastomosis by the hypoglossal nerve.

To innervate musculature of the "ocular sphincter system," a facio-facial anastomosis between the nerve trunk and the cranial nerve branches is made using a free nerve transplant. In this way, the motor neurons (reflex fibers) that are responsible for the blink reflex will have a chance for a more targeted reinnervation of the orbicularis oculi muscle. Here also, the method described for overcoming discrepancy in number and size can be applied for peripheral anastomoses. Using both cranial nerves at the same time leads to a physiologically "diversified" innervation of both independently operating sphincter systems: thus, reducing synkineses, especially in the so-called "mass movements" [86].

20.11.8 Cross-Facial Nerve Graft

From a technical standpoint, cross-face nerve grafting is equivalent to placing a long interposition graft; functionally, it is a nerve transfer, as axons from a different nerve are being redirected into the distal stump of the facial nerve. For this reason, the technique may be indicated in cases where the proximal stump of the ipsilateral facial nerve is unavailable for coaptation, but the distal stumps are available. More frequently, however, the cross-face graft is used to reinnervate a specific muscle group, such as the orbicularis oculi or zygomaticus major and minor muscles, or to control a transferred muscle for facial reanimation, such as the gracilis or sterno-omohyoid muscles [87, 88]. Outcome depends on timing and technique and can provide the best facial reanimation scheme if performed on the right patient.

The surgeon must select appropriate segmental branches of the contralateral facial nerve as donors, with the sural nerve serving as a cable graft. The axon count in the sural nerve is approximately 1100, enough to permit the transit of the approximately 900 axons required for effective reinnervation [89, 90]. Many techniques have been described, such as a single segmental-to-main trunk anastomosis, and multiple anastomoses from segmental branches to segmental branches. The grafts are tunneled above the supraorbital ridge for the orbicularis oculi, the upper lip for the zygomatic and buccal branches, and below the lower lip for the marginal mandibular branch. Facial muscle movement will not emerge until 9–12 months after the procedure (i.e., the allotted time for axonal growth to cross the graft).

Cross-face nerve grafts are notoriously unreliable, particularly when performed in older individuals, patients with long-standing facial paralysis, and patients at increased risk for losing facial function on the donor side, such as those with neurofibromatosis type 2, who are at risk of developing bilateral vestibular schwannomas: such patients are not ideal candidates for the procedure. As with any other nerve transfer procedure, donor site morbidity and axon availability should be considered preoperatively. Because a facial nerve exploration is required on the donor side for cross-face nerve grafting, patients should be aware of the potential for a scar. Additionally, sacrificing a facial nerve branch large enough to provide sufficient axons for effective reinnervation runs the risk of causing weakness. In practice, the weakness is seldom clinically apparent and may help to improve symmetry [89, 90].

20.12 Muscle Transposition

When facial nerve dysfunction has exceeded 18 months, dynamic slings and free muscle transfers can be executed to restore facial and oral motor function. Severe neuro-fibrosis and myo-fibrosis in the distal neuromuscular unit preclude successful reinnervation. Patients with congenital facial paralyses cannot be reinnervated, since the neuromuscular units never developed in these individuals. Regional muscle transposition and free-muscle transfer are the two modalities to reanimate the face in this subset of patients.

20.12.1 Regional Muscle Transfer

Regional muscle transfer can reanimate the lower third of the paralyzed face. This new neuromuscular unit is composed of the transferred muscle with its original nerve and vascular supply. It often produces results slightly better than static strategies, but is limited by anatomical constraints of size and vectors. Regional muscle procedures are appropriate in patients who are in poor health or who will not survive beyond the 12–24-month period of neurotization of a free muscle transfer. Such procedures provide immediate reanimation and are technically less demanding than cross-facial nerve grafting with free muscle transfer.

20.12.2 Temporalis Muscle

The temporalis muscle may improve the symmetry of the commissure of the mouth and reestablish a voluntary smile. The vector of the temporalis muscle resembles that of the zygomaticus major and, thus, results in a lateral smile. Transposition will not produce spontaneous mimetic function. Each movement necessitates a specific volitional action, in which the patient must consciously contract the transposed muscle in conjunction with the smiling. Temporalis muscle transposition can also reanimate the eyelids, but may produce eyelid distortion. To avoid a contour defect, the muscle anterior to the hairline should not be used.

The temporalis muscle is harvested through a vertical incision in front of the ear that extends to the scalp. The middle section of the muscle and fascia is elevated and detached superiorly from the skull while the inferior attachments are preserved. Two tongues are created by bisecting the muscle, and the muscle is tunneled through a subcutaneous pocket from the zygomatic arch to the vermillion border. The ends of the temporalis are secured to the orbicularis and the corner of the mouth. The ends should be secured with enough tension to create some level of overcorrection [91].

The patient initiates a smile by consciously tensing the temporalis muscle. Patients will require therapy to master this technique. In his study, May reported improvement in 95% of patients with temporalis transfer for lower-face reanimation and good to excellent results in 78% of patients. The complication rate was 18%; the most common complications were infection and implant-related complications. Other potential complications include failure of attachment, pulling away of the temporalis muscle from the commissure, and overcorrection of the upper lip. The transfer may also generate excess muscle bulk and a facial deformity, particularly over the zygoma [91].

20.12.3 Masseter Muscle

The masseter muscle is another muscle used for reanimation of the commissure of the mouth, either alone or in conjunction with the temporalis. Unlike the temporalis, the vector of smile of the masseter muscle is in the buccinator-risorius direction, which produces a less natural smile. This muscle is elevated by detaching the anterior portion from its mandibular insertion. It is similarly bisected and secured to the modiolus. The muscle is quite bulky and can create facial irregularity or surface deformity, such as a bulge at the commissure. Postoperatively, patients must train the masseter with aggressive physical therapy to learn how to use the transposed masseter to produce a smile [92].

20.12.4 Digastric Muscle

Conley et al. (1982) developed the modern method of transposing the tendon of the digastric muscle to the orbicularis of the lower lip. The blood supply and nerve to the anterior belly remains intact, and dynamic depression of the lower lip border is achieved. Of 36 patients treated in this manner by Conley, 33 were reported to have satisfactory results. This method is ideal for isolated palsy of the marginal mandibular nerve only, since it can create oral incompetence in patients with more extensive palsy of the lower face [93].

Depressor muscle function is important to dentured smile, as well as to expressions of sadness, anger, and sorrow. The lower lip is animated by interactions of the orbicularis oris, depressor labii inferioris, depressor anguli oris, mentalis, and platysma. Terzis described a technique to improve this type of smile by transfer either of the anterior belly of the digastric tenor or of the platysma [94]. Other authors argue that this symmetrical smile could be achieved with less invasive approaches, including Botox injections or myectomy of the depressor labii inferioris.

20.12.5 Free-Muscle Transfer

20.12.5.1 Principles of Free-Muscle Transfer

The advent of microsurgical technique and free-muscle transfer introduced a new era for facial reconstruction in patients with chronic facial palsy. Free-muscle transfer supplies a new neuromuscular unit to the face via a free-muscle flap and a grafted donor cranial nerve, usually a cross-facial nerve graft. This modality establishes more precise vectors in addition to spontaneous mimetic facial expression.

Cross-facial nerve grafting with micro-neurovascular muscle transfer is the best strategy for facial reanimation when a patient has long-established facial paralysis (>24 months). Other approaches leave residual asymmetry, an unnatural appearance, and unwanted facial movements while eating.

Most commonly, the surgeon executes a two-stage technique of cross-facial nerve graft followed by a delayed free-muscle transfer. The rationale for the delay is to prevent atrophy of the muscle graft while waiting for axons to travel the length of the nerve graft.

20.12.6 Two-Stage Technique

20.12.6.1 Cross-facial Nerve Graft

Occasionally, the proximal segment of the ipsilateral facial nerve is available for grafting to innervate a free-muscle transfer. This situation most commonly occurs in the event of a failed interposition nerve graft, resulting in facial musculature that no longer can be reinnervated.

The contralateral facial nerve is chosen as the donor nerve, and a redundant zygomaticus branch is selected for grafting. The hypoglossal nerve also can act as a donor, either by a direct or jump graft alone or in conjunction with a cross-facial graft. The sural nerve is anastomosed to the contralateral facial nerve or substituted cranial nerve and tunneled subcutaneously from the donor nerve to the planned site of free-muscle transfer, and the distal segment of the graft is tagged. The ideal time for the muscle transfer occurs when a Tinel sign is detected in the distal nerve end, indicating completion of axonal growth.

20.12.6.2 Muscles Suitable for Transfer

Free-muscle transfer is usually performed 9–12 months after nerve graft. A plethora of muscles have been assiduously investigated for free transfer to the paralyzed face, including the gracilis, serratus, pectoralis minor, latissimus dorsi, platysma, rectus abdominis, rectus femoris, and extensor digitorum brevis.

The original report by Harii in 1976 of free-muscle transfer for facial paralysis described the use of the gracilis muscle [95]. It remains the muscle of choice because of its relative ease of dissection, adequate neurovascular pedicle, and muscle fiber length, which corresponds to the action of the zygomaticus major muscle. The vascular pedicle is derived from the medial femoral circumflex artery and provides up to 8 cm of length. Innervation of the gracilis is provided by the anterior branch of the obturator nerve, which can be dissected to a length of 10–12 cm.

During the second-stage procedure, the surgeon must identify the distal end of the nerve graft and send a frozen section for confirmation of viable axons. The muscle flap is harvested and transferred to the face. The flap is secured to the periosteum of the zygomatic arch and the modiolus in a vector that corresponds to the smile on the contralateral face. Subsequently, the micro-anastomosis between the flap and recipient vessels is executed, followed by the nerve anastomosis as close to the muscle as possible. Movement can be expected in 6–9 months, with improvement over the following 2–3 years.

Based on their anatomical findings, Lifchez et al. (2005) endorse the serratus anterior for free-muscle transfer [96]. Each serratus slip, divided along fascial planes, can generate a distinct force vector for facial reanimation, with a total of 5 slips and 10 subslips. This serratus anterior can, therefore, be used as a single donor muscle with multiple vectors of action and multiple functions (e.g., restoration of a symmetrical smile with simultaneous, but independent, eyelid closure).

Terzis and Noah (1997) found no significant effect associated with age, gender, or ischemia time on outcome in their series of 100 free-muscle transfers [97]. They reported moderate or better results in 80% of patients undergoing free-muscle transfer, based on a five-step scale of judgment. O'Brien et al. (1990) reported good-to-excellent results in 51% of 47 patients treated by microvascular free-muscle transfer; the surgeons most commonly used cross-facial nerve grafts and gracilis muscle transfers in their technique [98].

20.12.7 One-Stage Free-Muscle Transfer

In their study of 25 patients, Kumar and Hassan (2002) compared single-stage free-tissue transfer with dual-stage free-tissue transfer for facial reconstruction [99]. The gracilis obturator nerve branch can yield a length of 12 cm, which allows primary anastomosis of this nerve to the contralateral facial nerve. However, this technique produces an additional scar on the cheek. The single-stage transfer has fewer complications and a reduced recovery time with decreased rehabilitation, but the dual-stage approach achieves better overall symmetry.

In their investigation of 166 free gracilis transfers, Manktelow et al. (2006) explored muscle transfer with cross-facial nerve graft versus single-stage transfer to the masseter nerve. The excursion of the free gracilis innervated by the masseter nerves is greater than that of the cross-facial nerve graft. This is probably attributable to the different motor nerve used to reinnervate the muscle. The cross-face nerve graft provides improved spontaneity in terms of movement, which is vital to a normal smile in children. This is a more important characteristic than degree of excursion.

Although the use of the masseter nerve with free-tissue transfer was previously explored and considered only in the setting of "Möbius syndrome," bilateral facial paralysis, and facial paralysis not suitable for cross-facial nerve grafting, the masseter nerve's applicability and role has been recently extended to patients with unilateral facial palsy. This one-stage strategy, incorporating the masseter nerve with free tissue transfer, has become a reasonable alternative (and may become the criterion standard) to the dual-stage approach with cross-facial nerve grafting.

The main advantage of the masseter nerve free-tissue transfer technique is that, unlike the cross-facial nerve, the masseter nerve donor produces a movement and muscle excursion (in relation to smile and commissure excursion) in normal range with consistent movement. Also, this technique obviates the need for a second operation.

A study by Liu et al. (2012) concluded that one-stage reconstruction with free abductor hallucis muscle transfer can effectively restore dynamic facial animation in long-standing, unilateral facial paralysis. The study involved 41 patients who underwent the procedure and were followed up for a mean of 54.6 months. The surgery produced satisfactory results in 37 patients with regard to facial symmetry at rest and voluntary contraction of the transferred muscles; significant increases were achieved in mean values for the Toronto Facial Grading System and the Facial Nerve Function Index, at 2-year follow-up, with even greater increases attained at longer-term follow-up. The remaining four patients experienced complications, including infection, hypertrophic scar, hematoma, and muscle loss [100].

20.12.8 Revisions

Takushima and Harii (2005) determined that predicting muscle bulkiness to obtain symmetry of facial contour is difficult during the initial free-muscle transfer. In their study of a patient population of 486 patients and 183 revisions, Takushima and Harii analyzed excessive muscle bulk and dislocation of the transferred free muscle [101]. Their report illustrated the wide gamut of revisions, including muscle debulking of cheek, adjustment of tension and attachments of transferred free muscle, and lipo-injection to the cheek for better volume symmetry.

20.12.9 Möbius Syndrome

Möbius syndrome involves bilateral facial nerve paralysis and can often attack cranial nerves VI, III, and XII. The syndrome generates psychological disability due to lack of facial animation and lack of emotional expression (immobile face).

The surgical goals for patients with Möbius syndrome are far more modest than for patients who have unilateral developmental facial paralysis. Restoring a true smile in these mask-like faces is impossible. Movement can be restored along only one vector. A detailed neurological evaluation can identify possible motor donors or residual function, which can be used for additional dynamic restorations. Most frequently, the reconstructive surgeon performs free-tissue transfers with bilateral gracilis muscles anastomosed to the masseter nerves on both sides to achieve smile restoration.

20.13 Prognosis

20.13.1 Outcome

Facial paralysis can cause significant reduction in quality of life (QOL) due to social and functional impacts. Facial nerve repair and transfer provide the potential for restoration of mimetic facial function with a good risk-to-benefit ratio, as only minor complications are typically reported. The best results are usually seen in young, healthy patients with distal facial nerve injuries that are repaired immediately, as in facial lacerations or iatrogenic injuries. Worse outcomes are expected when the injury is proximal, the patient is older or in poor health, and the paralysis is chronic, as in advanced parotid malignancies and recurrent cholesteatomas. Patients with slow-growing benign tumors or trauma fare best, while those with malignant and inflammatory pathologies fare worse. The first clinical signs of facial reinnervation can be expected to appear anywhere from 2 to 12 months postoperatively [16].

20.13.2 Complications

20.13.2.1 Procedure Failure

The biggest risk of nerve repair or transfer is no return of function is achieved. Risk factors for procedural failure include prolonged paralysis of >6–12 months before intervention, advanced age, poor health status, and performing multiple neurorrhaphies, as are required for interposition grafting. Each neurorrhaphy introduces additional opportunities for axonal loss. Postoperative radiotherapy (RT) does not appear to affect functional outcomes, although chemotherapy is known to cause facial paralysis [102, 103].

20.13.3 Suboptimal Outcome

20.13.3.1 Synkinesis

When the facial nerve is repaired proximal to the pes anserinus or a nerve transfer to the main trunk is performed, the expected outcome is synkinetic movement, which is not a complication per se but represents a suboptimal outcome. Synkinesis may impair voluntary movements, particularly smiling, resulting in marked facial asymmetry and lower QOL despite restoration of tone and movement. While numerous theories regarding the etiology of synkinesis have been proposed, it is currently thought that a major contributing factor to synkinesis is the misdirection of axons to different neuromuscular junctions from the ones they innervated before the injury [104, 105]. When possible, synkinesis may be avoided or reduced by preferentially reinnervating facial nerve branches rather than the main trunk itself.

20.13.3.2 Discoordinated Movements

Additionally, axons that terminate in multiple rather than single neuromuscular junctions will cause discoordinated movement and increase the basal firing rate of the innervated muscle and its resting tone. Botulinum toxin injections and facial physical therapy are the mainstay treatment options for this problem, but selective neurectomy and myomectomy have also been successfully employed [106–110].

20.13.3.3 Wrong (Suboptimal) Branch Selection

One risk of performing nerve transfers, particularly in the case of the masseteric nerve to buccal branch transfer undertaken >72 h after injury, is the possibility of reinnervating the wrong nerve branch. Without the ability to stimulate the recipient nerve, it is possible to select a suboptimal branch that may not produce the desired precise effect. While suboptimal branch selection is unlikely to result in movements completely different from those intended as long as the recipient branch is in roughly the correct location, it may be that the resulting smile vector, for example, is not entirely symmetric with the uninjured side. Most facial reanimation surgeons prefer to reinnervate native facial muscles whenever possible, but in cases of suboptimal outcomes of nerve transfer, intractable synkinesis, or long-standing paralysis of >12–18 months, free muscle transfer may be employed instead of nerve repair or transfer [111].

20.13.4 Donor Site Morbidity

20.13.4.1 Sensory Nerve Sacrifice

When an uninjured nerve is sacrificed in grafting or transfer, there is always a risk of donor site morbidity. Sensory nerve sacrifice (GAN auricular and sural nerve) commonly causes harvest site hypersthesia; it is predictable, and usually results in nothing more than auricular lobule numbness and lateral ankle and foot numbness, respectively. While uncommon, the potential for developing painful neuromas at these sites does exist. These neuromas can be treated with excision and burying the cut nerve end into muscle.

20.13.4.2 Motor Nerve Sacrifice

Motor nerve sacrifice, on the other hand, may carry a greater risk of morbidity. Masseteric nerve sacrifice is generally well tolerated, with little more than the loss of some facial volume due to muscle atrophy; most patients do not complain of decreased bite force. Cross-face nerve grafting also tends to be well-tolerated, despite requiring sural nerve harvest, and there tends to be minimal morbidity other than a scar from the contralateral dissection required to access the uninjured facial nerve. While sacrificing an uninjured facial nerve branch to supply axons to the cross-face graft may risk weakening the normal side smile, this is rarely seen in practice. The highest risk for donor site morbidity among these procedures occurs with the hypoglossal-facial nerve transfer because of the potential for dysphagia and dysarthria accompanying tongue weakness. When the entire hypoglossal nerve is transferred, facial outcomes are good because of the high axon count in the hypoglossal nerve, but the morbidity is severe [68]. The sacrifice of only part of the hypoglossal nerve via end-to-side coaptation or interfascicular dissection and transfer decreases morbidity dramatically, but also compromises results by reducing the number of axons redirected into the facial nerve [43].

References

1. Blinzinger K, Kreutzberg G. Displacement of synaptic terminals from regenerating motoneurons by microglial cells. Z Zellforsch Mikrosk Anat. 1968;85:145–57.
2. Graeber MB, Kreutzberg GW. Astrocytes increase in glial fibrillary acidic protein during retrograde changes of facial motor neurons. J Neurocytol. 1986;15:363–73.
3. Graeber MB. The role of astrocytes in facial nerve regeneration. Eur Arch Otorhinolaryngol. 1994:S75–7.
4. Guntinas-Lichius O, Gunkel A, Stennert E, Neiss WF. Astroglial response in facial and hypoglossal-facial anastomoses in the rat. Eur Arch Otorhinolaryngol. 1994;S557
5. Guntinas-Lichius O, Gunkel A, Stennert E, Neiss WF. Synaptic stripping in facial and hypoglossal nucleus after hypoglossal-facial anastomoses in the rat. Eur Arch Otorhinolaryngol. 1994;S558
6. Guntinas-Lichius O, Irintchev A, Streppel M, Lenzen M, Grosheva M, Wewetzer K, Neiss WF, Angelov DN. Factors limiting motor recovery after facial nerve transection in the rat: combined structural and functional analyses. Eur J Neurosci. 2005;21:391–402.
7. Kreutzberg GW. Acute neural reaction to injury. In: Nicholls JG, editor. Repair and regeneration of the nervous system. Berlin Heidelberg New York, NY: Springer; 1982. p. 57–69.
8. Streit WJ. The role of microglia in regeneration. Eur Arch Otorhinolaryngol. 1994:S69–70.
9. Tetzlaff W, Graeber MB, Kreutzberg GW. Reactions of motoneurons and their microenvironment to axotomy. Exp Brain Res. 1986;13:3–8.
10. Goebel HH, Schneider I, Tews DS, Gunkel A, Stennert E, Neiss WF. Morphologic studies on human and rodent facial muscles. Eur Arch Otorhinolaryngol. 1994:S24–7.
11. Irintchev A, Wernig A. Denervation and reinnervation of muscle: physiological effects. Eur Arch Otorhinolaryngol. 1994:28–30.
12. Kleiss IJ, Hohman MH, Susarla SM, Marres HA, Hadlock TA. Health-related quality of life in 794 patients with a peripheral facial palsy using the FaCE Scale: a retrospective cohort study. Clin Otolaryngol. 2015;40(6):651–6.
13. Nellis JC, Ishii M, Byrne PJ, Boahene KDO, Dey JK, Ishii LE. Association among facial paralysis, depression, and quality of life in facial plastic surgery patients. JAMA Facial Plast Surg. 2017;19(3):190–6.
14. Kannan RY, Hills A, Shelley MJ, Bisase B, Kapoor K, Norris P, Nduka C. Immediate compared with late repair of extracranial branches of the facial nerve: a comparative study. Br J Oral Maxillofac Surg. 2020;58(2):163–9.
15. Gardetto A, Kovacs P, Piegger J, Rainer C, Meirer R, Piza-Katzer H. Direct coaptation of extensive facial nerve defects after removal of the superficial part of the parotid gland: an anatomic study. Head Neck. 2002;24(12):1047–53.
16. Sánchez-Ocando M, Gavilán J, Penarrocha J, González-Otero T, Moraleda S, Roda JM, Lassaletta L. Facial nerve repair: the impact of technical variations on the final outcome. Eur Arch Otorhinolaryngol. 2019;276(12):3301–8.
17. Prasad SC, Balasubramanian K, Piccirillo E, Taibah A, Russo A, He J, Sanna M. Surgical technique and results of cable graft interpositioning of the facial nerve in lateral skull base surgeries: experience with 213 consecutive cases. J Neurosurg. 2018;128(2):631–8.

18. Seneviratne SO, Patel BC. Facial nerve anatomy and clinical applications. In: StatPearls. Treasure Island, FL: StatPearls Publishing; 2023.
19. Remenschneider AK, Michalak S, Kozin ED, Barber S, De Venecia RK, Hadlock TA, Jung DH. Is serial electroneuronography indicated following temporal bone trauma? Otol Neurotol. 2017;38(4):572–6.
20. Darrouzet V, Duclos JY, Liguoro D, Truilhe Y, De Bonfils C, Bebear JP. Management of facial paralysis resulting from temporal bone fractures: our experience in 115 cases. Otolaryngol Head Neck Surg. 2001;125(1):77–84.
21. Engelmann S, Ruewe M, Geis S, Taeger CD, Kehrer M, Tamm ER, Bleys RLAW, Zeman F, Prantl L, Kehrer A. Rapid and precise semi-automatic axon quantification in human peripheral nerves. Sci Rep. 2020;10(1):1935.
22. Kalaiarasi R, Kiran AS, Vijayakumar C, Venkataramanan R, Manusrut M, Prabhu R. Anatomical features of intratemporal course of facial nerve and its variations. Cureus. 2018;10(8):e3085.
23. Davis RA, Anson BJ, Budinger JM, Kurth LR. Surgical anatomy of the facial nerve and parotid gland based upon a study of 350 cervicofacial halves. Surg Gynecol Obstet. 1956;102(4):385–412.
24. Pitanguy I, Ramos AS. The frontal branch of the facial nerve: the importance of its variations in face lifting. Plast Reconstr Surg. 1966 Oct;38(4):352–6.
25. Dorafshar AH, Borsuk DE, Bojovic B, Brown EN, Manktelow RT, Zuker RM, Rodriguez ED, Redett RJ. Surface anatomy of the middle division of the facial nerve: Zuker's point. Plast Reconstr Surg. 2013;131(2):253–7.
26. Hohman MH, Bhama PK, Hadlock TA. Epidemiology of iatrogenic facial nerve injury: a decade of experience. Laryngoscope. 2014;124(1):260–5.
27. Hazani R, Chowdhry S, Mowlavi A, Wilhelmi BJ. Bony anatomic landmarks to avoid injury to the marginal mandibular nerve. Aesthet Surg J. 2011;31(3):286–9.
28. Batra AP, Mahajan A, Gupta K. Marginal mandibular branch of the facial nerve: an anatomical study. Indian J Plast Surg. 2010;43(1):60–4.
29. Chowdhry S, Yoder EM, Cooperman RD, Yoder VR, Wilhelmi BJ. Locating the cervical motor branch of the facial nerve: anatomy and clinical application. Plast Reconstr Surg. 2010;126(3):875–9.
30. Mitz V, Peyronie M. The superficial musculo-aponeurotic system (SMAS) in the parotid and cheek area. Plast Reconstr Surg. 1976;58(1):80–8.
31. Sunderland S. The anatomy and physiology of nerve injury. Muscle Nerve. 1990;13(9):771–84.
32. Seddon HJ. A classification of nerve injuries. Br Med J. 1942;2(4260):237–9.
33. Lee DH. Clinical efficacy of electroneurography in acute facial paralysis. J Audiol Otol. 2016;20(1):8–12.
34. Andresen NS, Zhu V, Lee A, Sebetka W, Kimura J, Hansen MR, et al. Electrodiagnostic testing in acute facial palsy: outcomes and comparison of methods. Laryngoscope Investig Otolaryngol. 2020;5(5):928–35.
35. Hohman MH, Hadlock TA. Etiology, diagnosis, and management of facial palsy: 2000 patients at a facial nerve center. Laryngoscope. 2014;124(7):E283–93.
36. Peitersen E. The natural history of Bell's palsy. Am J Otol. 1982;4(2):107–11.
37. House JW, Brackmann DE. Facial nerve grading system. Otolaryngol Head Neck Surg. 1985;93(2):146–7.
38. Ross BR, Fradet G, Nedzelski JM. Development of a sensitive clinical facial grading system. Eur Arch Otorhinolaryngol. 1994;S1:80–1.
39. Banks CA, Jowett N, Azizzadeh B, Beurskens C, Bhama P, Borschel G, et al. Worldwide testing of the eFACE facial nerve clinician-graded scale. Plast Reconstr Surg. 2017;139(2):491e–8e.
40. Sulaiman W, Gordon T. Neurobiology of peripheral nerve injury, regeneration, and functional recovery: from bench top research to bedside application. Ochsner J. 2013;13(1):100–8.
41. Danner CJ. Facial nerve paralysis. Otolaryngol Clin North Am. 2008;41(3):619–32.
42. Jandali D, Revenaugh PC. Facial reanimation: an update on nerve transfers in facial paralysis. Curr Opin Otolaryngol Head Neck Surg. 2019;27(4):231–6.

43. Kochhar A, Albathi M, Sharon JD, Ishii LE, Byrne P, Boahene KD. Transposition of the intratemporal facial to hypoglossal nerve for reanimation of the paralyzed face: the VII to XII transposition technique. JAMA Facial Plast Surg. 2016;18(5):370–8.
44. Gordin E, Lee TS, Ducic Y, Arnaoutakis D. Facial nerve trauma: evaluation and considerations in management. Craniomaxillofac Trauma Reconstr. 2015;8(1):1–13.
45. Gousheh J, Arasteh E. Treatment of facial paralysis: dynamic reanimation of spontaneous facial expression-apropos of 655 patients. Plast Reconstr Surg. 2011;128(6):693e–703e.
46. Chan JY, Byrne PJ. Management of facial paralysis in the 21st century. Facial Plast Surg. 2011;27(4):346–57.
47. Robey AB, Snyder MC. Reconstruction of the paralyzed face. Ear Nose Throat J. 2011;90(6):267–75.
48. Meltzer NE, Alam DS. Facial paralysis rehabilitation: state of the art. Curr Opin Otolaryngol Head Neck Surg. 2010;18(4):232–7.
49. Kivelitz R, Loew F, Hubner H. Perspectives on the indications and contraindications of various nerve transplant techniques in cases of facial nerve paralysis after pontine angle tumor operations. Chir Plast (Berl). 1974;2:161–7.
50. Stennert E, Limberg CH. Central connections between fifth, seventh and twelfth cranial nerves and their clinical significance. In: Graham MD, House WF, editors. Disorders of the facial nerve. New York, NY: Raven; 1982. p. 57–65.
51. Liu D, Mi D, Zhang T, Zhang Y, Yan J, Wang Y, et al. Tubulation repair mitigates misdirection of regenerating motor axons across a sciatic nerve gap in rats. Sci Rep. 2018;8(1):3443.
52. Boeckstyns ME, Sørensen AI, Viñeta JF, Rosén B, Navarro X, Archibald SJ, et al. Collagen conduit versus microsurgical neurorrhaphy: 2-year follow-up of a prospective, blinded clinical and electrophysiological multicenter randomized, controlled trial. J Hand Surg Am. 2013;38(12):2405–11.
53. Piedra Buena IT, Fichman M. Sural nerve graft. In: StatPearls. Treasure Island (FL): StatPearls Publishing; 2023.
54. Spector JG, Lee P, Peterein J, Roufa D. Facial nerve regeneration through autologous nerve grafts: a clinical and experimental study. Laryngoscope. 1991;101(5):537–54.
55. Streppel M, Popratiloff A, Angelov DN, Guntinas-Lichius O, Hilgers RD, Stennert E, Neiss WF. Significance of trigeminal sensory input on regrowth of hypoglossal and facial motoneurons after hypoglossal facial anastomosis in rats. Acta Otolaryngol. 1998;118:790–6.
56. Orgel MG. Epineurial versus perineurial repair of peripheral nerves. Clin Plast Surg. 1984;11(1):101–4.
57. Cabaud HE, Rodkey WG, McCarroll HR, Mutz SB, Niebauer JJ. Epineurial and perineurial fascicular nerve repairs: a critical comparison. J Hand Surg Am. 1976;1(2):131–7.
58. Knox CJ, Hohman MH, Kleiss IJ, Weinberg JS, Heaton JT, Hadlock TA. Facial nerve repair: fibrin adhesive coaptation versus epineurial suture repair in a rodent model. Laryngoscope. 2013;123(7):1618–21.
59. Burgess LPA, Goode RL. Reanimation of the paralyzed face. Stuttgart, Germany: Thieme; 1994. p. 16.
60. Van Nest DS, Kahan DM, Ilyas AM. Polyethylene glycol fusion of nerve injuries: review of the technique and clinical applicability. J Hand Microsurg. 2021;13(2):49–54.
61. Stennert E. Prinzipien der Nervenrekonstruktion. In: Naumann HH, Helms J, Herberhold C, Kastenbauer E, editors. Oto-rhino-laryngologie in klinik und praxis. Stuttgart, Germany: Thieme; 1992. p. 744–7.
62. Stennert E, Jungehulsing M. Chirurgie der Glandula parotis einschlieslich rekonstuktiver Fazialis-Chirurgie: Standard und Qualitatssicherung. Laryngorhinootologie. 2001;80(Suppl. 1):156–97.
63. Peters BR, Wood MD, Hunter DA, Mackinnon SE. Acellular nerve allografts in major peripheral nerve repairs: an analysis of cases presenting with limited recovery. Hand (NY). 2023;18(2):236–43.
64. Jowett N, Pineda IR. Acellular nerve allografts in corneal neurotisation: an inappropriate choice. Br J Ophthalmol. 2020;104(2):149–50.

65. Altafulla J, Iwanaga J, Lachkar S, Prickett J, Dupont G, Yilmaz E, et al. The great auricular nerve: anatomical study with application to nerve grafting procedures. World Neurosurg. 2019;125:e403–7.
66. Rinker B, Fink BF, Barry NG, Fife JA, Milan ME, Stoker AR, et al. The effect of cigarette smoking on functional recovery following peripheral nerve ischemia/reperfusion injury. Microsurgery. 2011;31(1):59–65.
67. Mahakkanukrauh P, Chomsung R. Anatomical variations of the sural nerve. Clin Anat. 2002;15(4):263–6.
68. Mackinnon SE, Dellon AL. Fascicular patterns of the hypoglossal nerve. J Reconstr Microsurg. 1995;11(3):195–8.
69. Elkatatny AAAM, Abdallah HAA, Ghoraba D, Amer TA, Hamdy T. Hypoglossal facial nerve anastomosis for post-operative and post-traumatic complete facial nerve paralysis. Open Access Maced J Med Sci. 2019;7(23):3984–96.
70. Neiss WF, Schulte E, Guntinas-Lichius O, Gunkel A, Stennert E. Response of Nissl substance in the facial and hypoglossal nucleus after hypoglossal-facial anastomoses in the rat. Eur Arch Otorhinolaryngol. 1994;S559
71. Streppel M, Popratiloff A, Gruart A, et al. Morphological connections between the hypoglossal and facial nerve in the brain stem of the rat. In: Morphologische Verbindungen zwischen N. hypoglossus und N. facialis im Hirnstamm der Ratte, vol. 48. HNO; 2000. p. 911–6.
72. Stennert E. Hypoglossal facial anastomosis: its significance for modern facial surgery. II. Combined approach in extratemporal facial nerve reconstruction. Clin Plast Surg. 1979;6:471–86.
73. Stennert E. Neurophysiologische und neuroanatomische Untersuchung zur Hypoglossus-Facialis-Anastomose und ihre klinische Bedeutung. Jahrbuch 1996 der Deutschen Akademie der Naturforscher Leopoldina, Halle/Saale. Leopoldina (R. 3). 1997;42:363–85.
74. May M, Sobol SM, Mester SJ. Hypoglossal-facial nerve interpositional-jump graft for facial reanimation without tongue atrophy. Otolaryngol Head Neck Surg. 1991;104:818–25.
75. Manni JJ, Beurskens CHG, Velde van de C, Stokroos RJ. Reanimation of the paralyzed face by indirect hypoglossal-facial nerve anastomosis. Am J Surg. 2001;182:268–73.
76. Manni JJ. Reanimation of the hemiparalysed face with the hypoglossal-facial nerve interpositional graft anastomosis. In: Beurskens CHG, van Gelder RS, Heymans PG, Manni JJ, Nicolai J-PA, editors. The facial palsies. Utrecht: Lemma; 2005. p. 177–85.
77. Borschel GH, Kawamura DH, Kasukurthi R, Hunter DA, Zuker RM, Woo AS. The motor nerve to the masseter muscle: an anatomic and histomorphometric study to facilitate its use in facial reanimation. J Plast Reconstr Aesthet Surg. 2012;65(3):363–6.
78. Klebuc MJA. Facial reanimation using the masseter-to-facial nerve transfer. Plast Reconstr Surg. 2011;127(5):1909–15.
79. Vincent AG, Bevans SE, Robitschek JM, Wind GG, Hohman MH. Masseteric-to-facial nerve transfer and selective neurectomy for rehabilitation of the synkinetic smile. JAMA Facial Plast Surg. 2019;21(6):504–10.
80. Salmerón-González E, Simón-Sanz E, García-Vilariño E, Ruiz-Cases A. Masseter-to-facial nerve transfer: technique and outcomes utilizing a fibrin sealant for coaptation. J Plast Reconstr Aesthet Surg. 2018;71(8):1216–30.
81. Cassoni A, Catalano C, Di Giorgio D, Raponi I, Di Brino M, Perotti S, et al. Masseter-facial neurorrhaphy for facial palsy reanimation: what happens after masseter denervation? Histomorphometric and stomatognathic functional analysis. J Craniomaxillofac Surg. 2020;48(7):680–4.
82. Sakthivel P, Singh CA, Thakar A, Thirumeni G, Raveendran S, Sharma SC. Masseteric-facial nerve anastomosis: surgical techniques and outcomes-a pilot indian study. Indian J Otolaryngol Head Neck Surg. 2020;72(1):92–7.
83. Murphey AW, Clinkscales WB, Oyer SL. Masseteric nerve transfer for facial nerve paralysis: a systematic review and meta-analysis. JAMA Facial Plast Surg. 2018;20(2):104–10.
84. Hontanilla B, Cabello A. Spontaneity of smile after facial paralysis rehabilitation when using a non-facial donor nerve. J Craniomaxillofac Surg. 2016;44(9):1305–9.

85. Stennert E. Das Autoparalytische Syndrom—ein Leitsymptom der postparetischen Fazialisfunktion. Arch Otorhinolarygol. 1982;236:97–114.
86. Stennert E. Synkineses and the autoparalytic syndrome. In: Beurskens CHG, van Gelder RS, Heymans PG, Manni JJ, Nicolai J-PA, editors. The facial palsies. Utrecht: Lemma; 2005. p. 117–33.
87. Bhama PK, Weinberg JS, Lindsay RW, Hohman MH, Cheney ML, Hadlock TA. Objective outcomes analysis following microvascular gracilis transfer for facial reanimation: a review of 10 years' experience. JAMA Facial Plast Surg. 2014;16(2):85–92.
88. Vincent AG, Bevans SE, Robitschek JM, Groom KL, Herr MW, Hohman MH. Sterno-omohyoid free flap for dual-vector dynamic facial reanimation. Ann Otol Rhinol Laryngol. 2020;129(2):195–200.
89. Frey M, Happak W, Girsch W, Bittner RE, Gruber H. Histomorphometric studies in patients with facial palsy treated by functional muscle transplantation: new aspects for the surgical concept. Ann Plast Surg. 1991;26(4):370–9.
90. Terzis JK, Wang W, Zhao Y. Effect of axonal load on the functional and aesthetic outcomes of the cross-facial nerve graft procedure for facial reanimation. Plast Reconstr Surg. 2009;124(5):1499–512.
91. Choi JY, Kim HJ, Moon SY. Management of the paralyzed face using temporalis tendon transfer via intraoral and transcutaneous approach: temporalis tendon transfer. Maxillofac Plast Reconstr Surg. 2018;40(1):24.
92. Hontanilla B, Rodriguez-Losada G. Bilateral reconstruction of smile through muscular transplants neurotized to masseter nerves. J Craniofac Surg. 2011;22(3):1099–100.
93. Conley J, Baker DC, Selfe RW. Paralysis of the mandibular branch of the facial nerve. Plast Reconstr Surg. 1982;70(5):569–77.
94. Terzis JK, Kalantarian B. Microsurgical strategies in 74 patients for restoration of dynamic depressor muscle mechanism: a neglected target in facial reanimation. Plast Reconstr Surg. 2000;105(6):1917–31.
95. Harii K, Ohmori K, Torii S. Free gracilis muscle transplantation, with microneurovascular anastomoses for the treatment of facial paralysis. A preliminary report. Plast Reconstr Surg. 1976;57(2):133–43.
96. Lifchez SD, Gasparri MG, Sanger JR, LoGiudice JA, Godat DM, Tisol WB, et al. Serratus anterior in vivo contractile force study. Plast Reconstr Surg. 2005;116(3):839–45.
97. Terzis JK, Noah ME. Analysis of 100 cases of free-muscle transplantation for facial paralysis. Plast Reconstr Surg. 1997;99(7):1905–21.
98. O'Brien BM, Pederson WC, Khazanchi RK, et al. Results of management of facial palsy with microvascular free-muscle transfer. Plast Reconstr Surg. 1990;86(1):12–22.
99. Kumar PA, Hassan KM. Cross-face nerve graft with free-muscle transfer for reanimation of the paralyzed face: a comparative study of the single-stage and two-stage procedures. Plast Reconstr Surg. 2002;109(2):451–62.
100. Liu AT, Lin Q, Jiang H, Sun MQ, Zhang JL, Zhang YF, et al. Facial reanimation by one-stage microneurovascular free abductor hallucis muscle transplantation: personal experience and long-term outcomes. Plast Reconstr Surg. 2012;130(2):325–35.
101. Takushima A, Harii K, Asato H, Momosawa A. Revisional operations improve results of neurovascular free muscle transfer for treatment of facial paralysis. Plast Reconstr Surg. 2005;116(2):371–80.
102. Gidley PW, Herrera SJ, Hanasono MM, Yu P, Skoracki R, Roberts DB, Weber RS. The impact of radiotherapy on facial nerve repair. Laryngoscope. 2010;120(10):1985–9.
103. Lee RT, Oster MW, Balmaceda C, Hesdorffer CS, Vahdat LT, Papadopoulos KP. Bilateral facial nerve palsy secondary to the administration of high-dose paclitaxel. Ann Oncol. 1999;10(10):1245–7.
104. Pourmomeny AA, Asadi S. Management of synkinesis and asymmetry in facial nerve palsy: a review article. Iran J Otorhinolaryngol. 2014;26(77):251–6.
105. Brown J, Hohman MH, Shermetaro C. Facial nerve intratemporal trauma. In: StatPearls. Treasure Island (FL): StatPearls Publishing; 2023.

106. Jacobson J, Rihani J, Lin K, Miller PJ, Roland JT. Outcomes of direct facial-to-hypoglossal neurorrhaphy with parotid release. Skull Base. 2011;21(1):7–12.
107. Moraleda S, Hachoue Z, Abdel-Muti E, Ruiz G, Díez Sebastián J, Lassaletta L. Satisfaction survey of patients with sequels of peripheral facial palsy treated with botulinum toxin A. Rehabilitacion (Madr). 2020;54(4):254–9.
108. van Veen MM, Quatela O, Tavares-Brito J, Robinson M, Baiungo JH, Werker PMN, et al. Patient-perceived severity of synkinesis reduces quality of life in facial palsy: a cross-sectional analysis in 92 patients. Clin Otolaryngol. 2019;44(3):483–6.
109. Hohman MH, Lee LN, Hadlock TA. Two-step highly selective neurectomy for refractory periocular synkinesis. Laryngoscope. 2013;123(6):1385–8.
110. Henstrom DK, Malo JS, Cheney ML, Hadlock TA. Platysmectomy: an effective intervention for facial synkinesis and hypertonicity. Arch Facial Plast Surg. 2011;13(4):239–43.
111. Mistry RK, Hohman MH, Al-Sayed AA. Facial nerve trauma. In: StatPearls. Treasure Island (FL): StatPearls Publishing; 2023.

Evaluation of the Submandibular Gland 21

21.1 Clinical Evaluation

Despite the availability of modern technology in the diagnosis of salivary gland disorders, great care should be taken during history-taking and physical examination.

21.1.1 History Taking

Patients with submandibular gland disorders usually complain of swelling and pain during meals followed by a reduction in symptoms after meals, which may indicate partial stenosis of Wharton's duct.

The medical profile of the patient may provide helpful clues to diagnosis. Gland dysfunction is often associated with certain systemic disorders such as diabetes mellitus (DM), atherosclerosis, hormonal imbalances, and neurological disorders [1, 2]. A careful dietary and nutrition history should not be neglected, for patients who suffer from chronic dehydration due to bulimia or anorexia or during chemotherapy are at risk for sialadenitis.

The drug history of the patient should also be considered, for salivary function is often affected by certain drugs such as diuretics and other antihypertensive drugs, which may cause xerostomia [1, 2]. Since xerostomia is also a debilitating consequence of radiation therapy to the head and neck, a history of prior irradiation should be sought.

For evaluation of a submandibular mass, it is important to take a history of the submandibular mass duration, rate of growth and presence of pain, marginal mandibular nerve (MMN—branch of the facial nerve) paralysis, cervical lymphadenopathy, eye and joint symptoms, and irradiation exposure.

© The Author(s), under exclusive license to Springer Nature Switzerland AG 2024
M. Sakr, *Surgery of the Salivary Glands*,
https://doi.org/10.1007/978-3-031-82069-4_21

21.1.2 Physical Examination

Extraoral, intraoral, and bimanual examinations (extraoral with one hand and intraoral with the palmar aspects of the fingertips of the other) should be performed to properly evaluate the submandibular glands clinically.

21.1.3 Extraoral Examination

21.1.3.1 Extraoral Inspection

With the patient facing in front of the examiner, 3–4 ft away, the examiner should inspect symmetry, color, pulsations, and discharging sinuses on both sides of the patient. Enlargement of the submandibular gland may be unilateral or bilateral. A submandibular swelling presents just medial and inferior to the angle of the mandible. It is often confused with enlargement of LNs, but a submandibular gland swelling is single and generally larger and smoother. Palpation and bimanual examination are necessary to differentiate between both conditions. Significant neurological deficits should be examined as well. Paralysis of the MMN with a deviation of the angle of the mouth to the sound opposite side should alert the examiner to a malignant submandibular neoplasm.

21.1.3.2 Extraoral Palpation

Owing to the superficial anatomical location of the submandibular gland, the size, tenderness, consistency, mobility, and surface of the gland and associated masses can be easily assessed (Fig. 21.1). If the swelling can be rolled over the lower border of the mandible, it is an enlarged lymph node (LN) (Fig. 21.2) and not a submandibular gland swelling since the latter's mobility is restricted by its fascial covering and attachment to the mylohyoid line of mandible.

21.1.4 Intraoral Examination

21.1.4.1 Extraoral Inspection

Using a torch or headlight, the orifices of the submandibular ducts are inspected and compared using a light source. They lie on either side of the frenulum of the tongue. A "stone" (sialolithiasis) may be seen exuding from the orifice with edema and redness. Saliva may be seen pouring from the non-affected side only. A "swelling" may be seen in the floor of the mouth, and its characteristics are recorded. For example, a ranula is bluish and transparent, whereas a dermoid cyst is yellow and opaque. Dental hygiene and the presence of periodontal disease should also be noted during intraoral inspection.

21.1.4.2 Intraoral Palpation

The gloved index finger of the examiner is inserted into the mouth of the patient, and palpation is started from behind at the end of the alveolus anteriorly. The gland and duct are palpated. A stone may be felt.

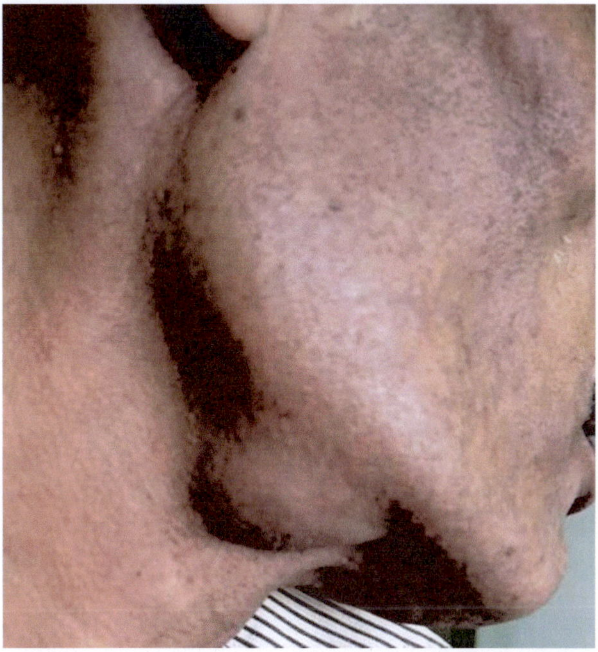

Fig. 21.1 A 41-year-old gentleman with an enlarged right submandibular gland (could not be rolled over the mandible contrary to a submandibular lymph node)

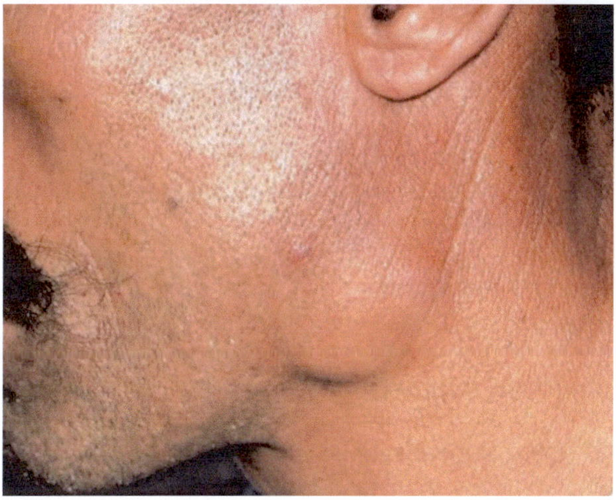

Fig. 21.2 A 43-year-old gentleman with an enlarged left submandibular LN (could be rolled over the mandible contrary to a submandibular gland swelling)

21.1.5 Bimanual Examination

With one or two gloved fingers palpating the floor of the mouth and the fingers of the other hand palpating beneath the jaw, a submandibular gland swelling is felt to have two components: buccal and cervical. It becomes fixed when the patient contracts the mylohyoid muscle. This is done by asking the patient to open the mouth against resistance by the examiner.

If a submandibular gland swelling is felt bimanually, its consistency must be noted. A hard swelling may be a stone or a malignant tumor (carcinoma), while a firm mass may be due to a mixed salivary tumor or chronic sialadenitis. On the other hand, increased salivation from the duct orifice due to external pressure applied to the gland may indicate inflammation.

21.2 Laboratory Studies

21.2.1 Changes in Saliva in Disease

21.2.1.1 Salivary Flow

Most causes of xerostomia (dry mouth) are systemic in nature, but a significant percentage is idiopathic. Dehydration, hospital admission, mental stress, psychopathic emotional states (e.g., depression), fatigue, infection, raised ambient temperature, tranquilizers, ganglionic blockers, and light deprivation decrease salivary flow. In addition, pernicious and iron-deficiency anemia and loss of salivary tissue (due to irradiation, infection, or Sjögren's syndrome) cause decreased flow. After a full course of radiation therapy, flow rates are reduced by 95% or more, and this reduction persists indefinitely [3]. Histopathological studies have shown that the parotid acini and serous cells from the submandibular gland are severely injured, but there is little discernible change in the mucous cells.

On the other hand, cigarette smoking, acute stomatitis, heavy metal poisoning, acrodynia, rabies, ingestion of highly seasoned foods, and schizophrenia increase the flow of saliva. Chewing on one side of the mouth also increases the flow on that side.

21.2.1.2 Salivary Composition

The constituents (composition) of saliva are affected by pregnancy and many pathological conditions as follows:

21.2.1.3 Pregnancy

In pregnancy, the submandibular calcium (Ca^{++}) concentration is reduced, whereas the Na^+ concentration is reduced and the K^+ concentration is increased in both parotid and submandibular saliva [4].

21.2.1.4 Suprarenal Gland Diseases

Primary aldosteronism causes decreased sodium (Na^+) levels with normal potassium (K^+) content. A Na^+-K^+ ratio of 0.3 or less is diagnostic, below 0.5 is suggestive, and above 1.0 rules out aldosteronism (normal, 1.3) [5]. Low Na^+-K^+ ratios are also found in Cushing's disease with a mean ratio of 0.5.24. High ratios occur in Addison's disease with a mean ratio of 5.0 [6].

21.2.1.5 Cystic Fibrosis

The salivary glands, like the other exocrine glands, are affected by "cystic fibrosis" [7]. Total protein, amylase, lysozyme, and glycoprotein concentrations are increased in submandibular but not in parotid saliva [8]. There is no change in the flow rate in the major glands [9], but there is a significant reduction in the minor glands [10].

21.2.1.6 Thyroid and Parathyroid Disease

Thyroid diseases and their treatment may affect the saliva. The salivary glands concentrate iodine to 40 times the plasma level, regardless of the thyroid-stimulating hormone (TSH) level or the state of thyroid function [11]. Hyperparathyroidism (HPT) causes an increased amount of Ca++ and phosphorus (P + 3) in saliva, with the levels paralleling the parathormone levels [12].

21.2.1.7 Essential (Primary) Hypertension

In cases of essential or primary hypertension, both Na + concentration and flow rate are decreased [13].

21.2.1.8 Sarcoidosis

In sarcoidosis, amylase and kallikrein levels are decreased, whereas albumin and lysozyme concentrations are increased [14, 15].

21.2.1.9 Alcoholic Cirrhosis

Alcoholic cirrhosis may cause an increased flow rate with increased concentrations of K+ and amylase [16].

21.2.1.10 Inflammatory Conditions

Inflammatory lesions may also cause changes in saliva composition. Acute pancreatitis may cause an increase in the amount of amylase. In acute infections, the Na + and K+ levels approach those of serum [17]. There is also a pronounced decrease in phosphate concentration. Other elements that are increased in amount include glucose, immunoglobulins (IgA, IgG, IgM), albumin, and transferrin, which leak from plasma, and myeloperoxidase, lactoferrin, and lysozyme, which are produced by the inflammatory infiltrate. IgG dominates the immunoglobulins, reflecting the normal serum pattern rather than the normal salivary pattern, in which IgA dominates.

21.2.1.11 Irradiation

"Irradiation" causes also alteration in the composition of saliva with increased amounts of Ca++, Na+, chloride (Cl-), and protein and a decrease in bicarbonate. These changes lead to a significant rise in the number of dental caries.

21.2.2 Medications/Drugs

Numerous systemically administered drugs can be detected in saliva, including iodide, heavy metals, thiocyanate, morphine, clindamycin, and rifampin [18]. Digitalis toxicity causes greatly elevated levels of K+ and Ca++, and this study can be used to distinguish between toxic and therapeutic doses [19].

21.3 Imaging Studies

For patients with no specific symptoms (swelling and pain) and unclear physical signs, imaging studies can play an important role in clarifying the etiology of the gland and duct disorder and assist in treatment selection and planning. These include conventional radiology (plain X-ray), conventional and digital sialography, ultrasound (US), computed tomography (CT) scan and CT sialography, magnetic resonance imaging (MRI), and MR sialography (MR-Si) [20–22].

21.3.1 Conventional Radiography (Plain X-Ray)

This is the simplest, oldest, and cheapest method of studying the salivary glands. Since the majority (70–80%) of submandibular gland stones (sialolithiasis) is radiopaque, plain radiography using the anteroposterior, lateral, and oblique lateral occlusal views will be valuable in evaluating the presence of such calculi (Fig. 21.3). Plain radiography is also useful in detecting calcifications (as in hemangioma and LNs) and adjacent osseous lesions such as infiltration of the mandible by a malignant neoplasm. A plain chest X-ray may also be helpful in cases of suspected pulmonary metastases.

21.3.2 Sialography

21.3.2.1 Conventional Sialography

The beginnings of the conventional sialographic studies are dated 1902 [20]. Sialography visualizes the ducts (Fig. 21.4) and the parenchyma of the salivary gland, after contrast administration into the main salivary duct. For decades, it has been the main diagnostic method in the salivary glands [23].

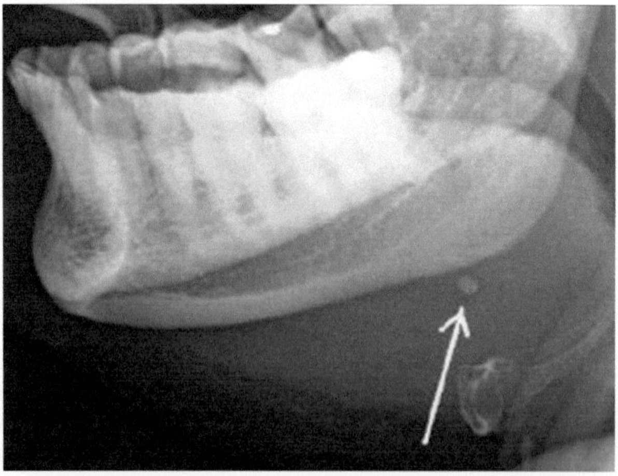

Fig. 21.3 Conventional plain X-ray of the submandibular region in lateral oblique projection showing soft tissue swelling associated with a small calculus (arrow)

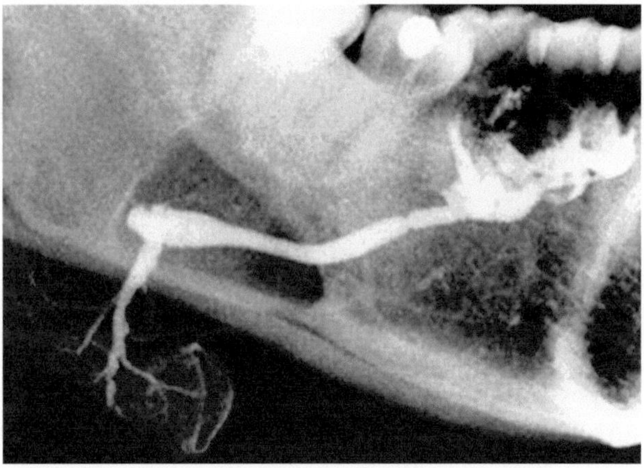

Fig. 21.4 Conventional sialography of submandibular glands showing the ductal system

21.3.2.2 Technique

An initial series of plain films is taken to identify radiopaque calculi. A sialogogue (lemon juice or citric acid) is given to dilate the duct orifice. The duct is intubated by means of a blunt-tipped slightly angulated, metal cannula or fine thin-walled polyethylene catheter with a tapered end. Approximately 0.5–1.5 mL of contrast medium (radiopaque such as Lipiodol Ultrafluid) or a water-soluble medium, e.g., Hypaque (sodium diatrizoate) is slowly injected by hand until the duct system is filled. To complete the examination, a few drops of lemon juice are given to stimulate salivation. After an interval of 10 min, a further plain film is taken, which normally shows most of the contrast medium cleared from the ducts. Any filling defect (e.g., stone), retained sections (e.g., chronic sialadenitis), stricture (e.g., inflammation), extravasation (e.g., Sjögren's syndrome), or irregular borders (e.g., tumor) are noted. Fistulae and abscess cavities can also be displayed with this technique.

21.3.2.3 Indications

The main indication of sialography is chronic sialadenitis unrelated to sialolithiasis. Other indications include sialolithiasis (filling defect) or other obstructive disorders (stricture), chronic sialadenitis (retained secretions), tumors (irregular borders of the submandibular gland and ductal obstruction without the presence of calculus), and duct lesions [21, 24–28]. It is advised to wait approximately 6 weeks from the moment of inflammatory symptom relief until sialography [23]. Sialography is also excellent in revealing and localizing calcifications close to salivary ducts [29]. It also allows for a high-certainty discrimination of stone location; in the salivary duct or in parenchyma, which is crucial for the choice of the appropriate therapeutic method [24]. Fistulae and abscess cavities can also be displayed with this technique.

However, sialography is not a method of choice in salivary gland tumor diagnosis [25, 30–32]. Nowadays, sialography and its modified version, CT sialography, are largely replaced with CT and MRI in salivary gland tumor diagnostics. In suspicion of a malignant tumor, the recommended diagnostic tool is contrast-enhanced MRI [21].

The diagnostic reliability of sialography was improved after the introduction of digital subtraction sialography (DSS) [33]. The use of post-processing enables the subtraction of a bony background and contrast enhancement of the salivary ducts [34].

21.3.2.4 Contraindications

Acute salivary infection (acute sialadenitis) is an absolute contraindication to conventional sialography as it can exacerbate the condition. Sialography should also not be performed in patients with known allergy to iodinated contrast media, as fatal anaphylactic reactions have been reported in the literature. In patients scheduled for thyroid function studies, sialography should be postponed until the thyroid work-up is completed [35, 36].

21.3.2.5 Disadvantages

The disadvantages of conventional sialography include patient's exposure to ionizing radiation and iodine contrast media, pain during contrast medium injection into the salivary ducts, the possibility of calculi dislocation toward the inside of the gland, quality of examination results is operator-dependent, and movement artifacts [21, 37, 38]. Failure to cannulate the ductal orifice may occur if there is calculus at the ductal orifice, with related edema of the surrounding buccal mucosa, or in the absence of any ductal abnormalities. The primary limitation of conventional sialography is that stricture cannot be overcome at most times in cases with duct obstruction; therefore, an examination cannot be carried out, and even if the examination is performed, the proximal segment of the stricture of the submandibular duct cannot be evaluated. In addition, smaller calculi and subtle ductal abnormalities near the ductal orifice may be obscured by the injection of contrast, and overfilling may result in a false-positive diagnosis of sialectasis. When interpreting sialography, it should be remembered that air bubbles, injected together with the contrast medium, may simulate the presence of the calculi leading to false-positive assessments for lithiasis [21, 37, 38].

21.3.2.6 Potential Complications

Potential complications of conventional sialography include damage to the orifice, overfilling and rupture (perforation) of the ductal system, exacerbation of infection, adverse reactions to iodine contrast media, and bleeding.

21.3.2.7 Advantages

Sialography requires a lower X-ray radiation dose as compared to a CT scan and is more accessible than MRI [39]. Moreover, sialography, owing to its possibilities of a detailed visualization of anatomical and pathological structures of the salivary ducts, plays an important role in the qualification of patients for sialendoscopic procedures and in choosing the strategy of the procedure [40].

21.3.2.8 Computed Tomography (CT) Sialography

Several reports have suggested that the sialographic technique can be improved by combining sialography with computed tomography (CT) [41–43]. These authors have reported increased sensitivity and a more precise definition of lesions with this combined technique. However, the technique is invasive, and the presence of metallic dentures or metallic fillings can cause artifacts [44].

21.3.2.9 Magnetic Resonance Sialography (MR-Si)

Despite the advantages of conventional sialography, being an invasive investigation, it has largely been replaced in recent years by the "non-invasive" magnetic resonance sialography (MR-Si) examinations in which the patient's own salivary secretion is used as a natural contrast agent and which can be conducted quickly and without any complications [38, 45–47]. This method is based on the basic principle of using a T2-weighted sequence for monitoring liquids [38, 48]. Its superior properties also include its capability of displaying the duct diameter in its actual value due to the nonuse of the contrast agent (administration of contrast agent increases lumen pressure and makes the diameter look wider than it actually is), as well as displaying the ducts of Rivinus.

The limitations of MR-Si examination include the fact that it cannot be applied in individuals with pacemakers as well as in claustrophobic individuals and that the image is affected by patient mobility and the loss in saliva amount [20, 36, 45].

21.3.2.10 Ultrasonography (US)

Ultrasonography (US) is a quick, noninvasive, and relatively inexpensive method that involves no radiation exposure for assessing submandibular gland pathology. Submandibular (and parotid) glands are examined with US using a 7.5 MHz or higher frequency linear array transducer with the patients' chin turned away from the side being examined. Both glands have homogenous echo patterns with scattered echogenic steaks produced by branch ducts converging into the main duct. The external carotid artery (ECA) and retromandibular vein can both be seen. Cervical lymph nodes (LNs) can also be seen.

Ultrasound remains the initial noninvasive investigation of choice due to its high resolution, easy availability, and ability to guide needle biopsy. It is currently used to evaluate calculi (Fig. 21.5), inflammatory diseases, congenital lesions, and space-occupying lesions of major salivary glands [49]. In combination with fine-needle aspiration cytology (FNAC), it is a powerful tool for characterizing salivary gland tumors and deciding whether a mass lesion is solid or cystic. Ultrasound color Doppler can add to the value of US by depicting the blood flow within the lesion.

However, US is operator-dependent and does not allow complete cross-sectional imaging of the salivary glands. The deepest portion of the submandibular gland may be difficult to visualize. In addition, ultrasound does not allow assessment of the skull base or mandible in infiltrative lesions.

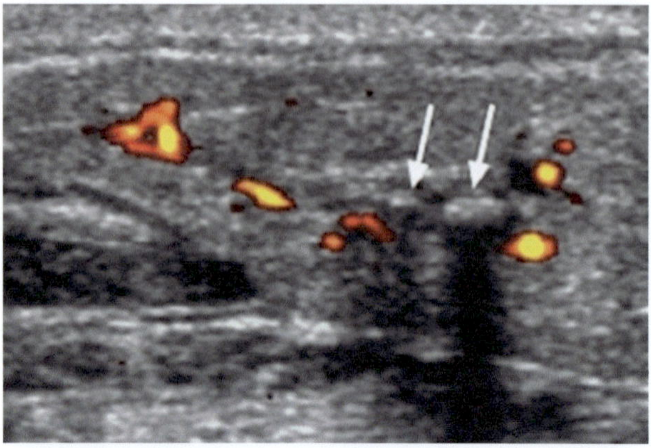

Fig. 21.5 Sialolithiasis and sialadenitis, as seen on color Doppler ultrasound of the submandibular gland. Two small calculi (arrows) are seen as hyper-echoic structures with posterior shadowing. The increased vascularization of the slightly enlarged gland is also noted

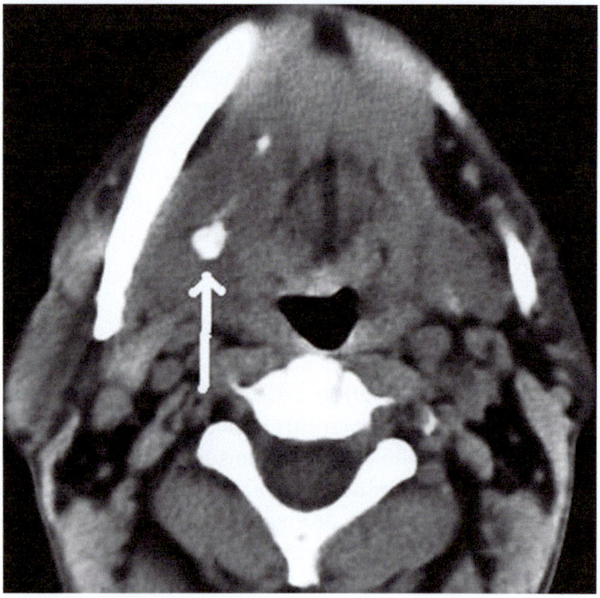

Fig. 21.6 Axial non-contrast-enhanced CT image showing submandibular sialolithiasis on the right side (white arrow) and normal gland on the left side

21.3.2.11 Computed Tomography (CT)

The gland has low attenuation due to its high fat content and is therefore easily discernible by CT scanning. Computed tomography scanning involves radiation exposure without contrast (Fig. 21.6) and with contrast (IV injection of iodinated) enhancement (Fig. 21.7), which increases the conspicuity of masses and affords some prediction of their nature. It is useful in situations where magnetic resonance imaging (MRI) is not readily available.

The advantage of CT imaging is the two-dimensional view of the salivary gland, which can elucidate relationships to adjacent vital structures, differentiate intrinsic from extrinsic disease, and assess the draining cervical lymph nodes (LNs). Differences between intrinsic and extrinsic gland masses, however, are often

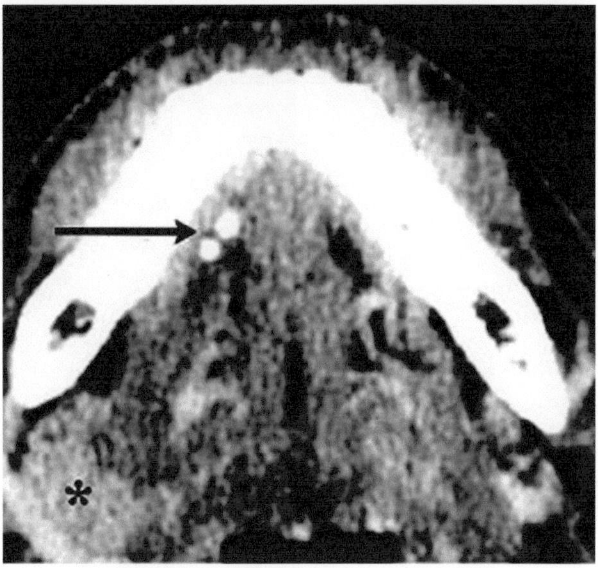

Fig. 21.7 Axial contrast-enhanced CT image at the level of the submandibular gland demonstrates two well-circumscribed stones in the distal right submandibular duct (arrow). There is enlargement and enhancement of the right submandibular gland (*) compared to the normal left submandibular gland

difficult to assess [50]. CT scan is also extremely valuable in defining abscess formation versus phlegmon. In addition, several aspects such as the detection of calculus and the involvement of the mandible are better seen in CT [45]. Although stones can be identified with CT scanning, submandibular sialadenitis is not generally an indication of CT.

In general, a CT scan is limited in evaluating the ductal system unless combined with simultaneous sialography, i.e., CT sialography, which is an alternative method of increasing conspicuity of glandular masses, but the technique is invasive and is not widely practiced as MRI is more beneficial. The presence of metallic dentures/metallic fillings can cause artifacts on CT scanning [44].

21.3.2.12 Magnetic Resonance Imaging (MRI)

Magnetic resonance imaging has been proven useful in the diagnosis of several diseases of the salivary glands, including benign and malignant tumors, Sjögren's syndrome, stones (Fig. 21.8), and infections [51–54]. Magnetic resonance imaging (MRI) gives excellent soft tissue contrast of major salivary gland lesions against a fatty background. T1-weighted images with fat suppression and contrast enhancement show the tumor margins and spread accurately, while T2-weighted images give an insight into the internal architecture of the tumor.

Compared with CT, MRI provides better contrast resolution, exposes the patient to less harmful radiation, reduces artifacts from dental amalgam, and yields detailed images on several different planes without patient repositioning (multi-planar imaging). However, MRI is inferior to CT scanning for the detection of early bone erosion and calcification, the presence of which is important in the diagnosis of pleomorphic adenoma and sialolithiasis. Chronic inflammation of the salivary glands and calculi are not indications of MRI.

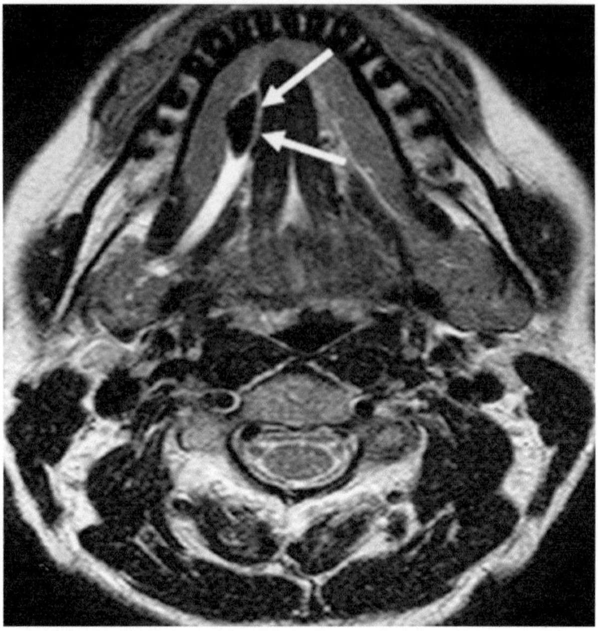

Fig. 21.8 Axial T2-weighted magnetic resonance image showing a stone located in the distal part of the main duct of the right submandibular gland (arrows)

Magnetic resonance sialography (MR-Si) has recently been described using heavy T2W1, which contrasts ductal fluid against stroma. It helps in the diagnosis of sialectasis up to some extent.

21.4 Endoscopy (Sialoendoscopy)

21.4.1 Introduction

Sialendoscopy is a minimally invasive technique that inspects the salivary glands using narrow-diameter, rigid fiberoptic endoscopes, introduced under direct vision through the ductal orifice after its dilatation with a lacrimal probe [55]. It is well tolerated, with minimal complications, and has thus opened up a new frontier for the evaluation and treatment of salivary gland disorders [56].

Direct inspection of the glandular duct and hilum is performed during lavage of the duct. Thus, in one setting, at the time of diagnosis, treatment of benign lesions can be performed [57, 58]. Through a CO2-laser papillotomy, sialolithectomy can be easily performed. Pharmacotherapy and laser ablation can also be performed. This relatively new technique is an efficient yet simple mode of treatment in the diagnosis and treatment of major salivary gland obstructions, strictures, and sialoliths (salivary stones). Depending on the obstruction, sialendoscopy can be conducted under local anesthesia in an outpatient office or in the operating room under general anesthesia.

21.4.2 Indications

Salivary gland stones are one of the major causes of salivary gland infections (sialadenitis). These types of stones can be found in 1.2% of the general population [59]. The second leading cause of salivary obstruction is strictures and adhesions, which may result from prior salivary gland infections. Most strictures could be seen in the parotid duct and mostly in the disease process of chronic recurrent sialadenitis.

21.4.3 Technique

Generally, the salivary duct opening needs to be either dilated or incised prior to the intraoral introduction of the endoscope into the gland through its natural orifice in the oral cavity or by making a small incision in the duct opening. Once the sialendoscope is in place, saline is utilized to dilate the salivary duct and its branching. Once the endoscopes are introduced into the gland, the internal anatomy is explored either for diagnosis or for treatment of a specific disease entity.

21.4.4 Instrumentation

The ability to perform this technique is the result of the development of miniaturized endoscopic imaging tools. Most sialendoscopes, currently in use, are semirigid, which allows for visualization, manipulation, and navigation of the internal salivary anatomy.

Multiple types of micro-instrumentation are available from many companies, including grasping forceps, biopsy forceps, drills, needles, laser fibers, and lithotripters. Different practitioners utilize different systems according to the experience and clinical training of the surgeon.

21.5 Cytology/Biopsy

21.5.1 Fine-Needle Aspiration Cytology (FNAC)

Fine-needle aspiration cytology (FNAC) guided by ultrasound (US) imaging is a widely used diagnostic tool to evaluate both inflammatory and neoplastic lesions of the salivary glands [26–28]. FNAC became popular approximately 40 years ago [60]. It is a minimally invasive procedure that does not require anesthesia [61] and is well tolerated, simple, safe, and cost-effective [62, 63]. Moreover, it can be easily repeated in case of nondiagnostic results, thus improving diagnostic precision [64]. Furthermore, FNAC allows for improved patient selection for surgery since it can identify disorders such as reactive lymph nodes that might mimic parotid tumors clinically.

Nevertheless, the role of FNAC in the preoperative evaluation is not universally established. At present, the debate focuses on the reliability of FNAC as a diagnostic tool and its usefulness in treatment planning. Although in some hospitals, FNAC is performed in every case of major salivary gland mass, some authors support the role of cytology only in a selected group of patients with suspected malignancy, metastatic carcinoma, or lymphoma [65]. However, Butsakis et al. stated that pre-surgical FNAC does not impact the surgical handling of these lesions [66].

At present, there is no consensus regarding the effective role of FNAC in the diagnostic work-up of salivary gland masses [65, 67]. In the recent literature, sensitivity ranges from 57% to 98%, specificity from 56% to 100%, and accuracy from 78 to 98% [60, 64, 65, 68–76]. Different causes could account for this variability including the different methods adopted by different authors to classify and diagnose [77].

Ultrasound guidance increases the diagnostic accuracy of FNAC by enabling avoidance of necrotic or cystic regions and by targeting higher yield areas of the lesion for tissue extraction [78–80]. Ultrasound guidance also allows the operator to confirm that the needle tip is inserted within the lesion.

21.5.2 Ultrasound Core Biopsy (USCB)

The perceived and real diagnostic limitations associated with FNAC have led operators to explore alternative biopsy techniques. USCB is a safe and successful technique for the diagnosis of parotid lesions where FNAC is nondiagnostic [81] and is developing into an established technique. The technique [81, 82] requires an operator, usually a radiologist trained in head and neck US and biopsy techniques. The procedure requires local anesthetic infiltration, a small skin incision, and the use of an automated spring-loaded biopsy device. The throw is deployed under US guidance.

The core of tissue is then processed by paraffin section histology. Sections from the core can be used for grading, staging, and immunohistochemical (IHC) analysis, allowing planning of appropriate operative or nonoperative management. Immunofluorescence analysis is particularly useful for hematological malignancies [81, 82].

This technique is already well-established in other areas of image-guided biopsy including the breast and abdomen [83] and is now widely accepted by histopathologists and oncologists as a sufficient technique to allow tumor grading and typing [84].

A recent meta-analysis incorporates 12 studies and provides substantial evidence supporting the potentially superior diagnostic yield of USCB over FNAC as it showed a higher sensitivity (96%) and specificity (100%) compared to FNAC, a low complication rate (1.6% hematoma rate), and no variation in accuracy between locations [85]. The low complication rate is attributed to the ability of US to visualize the vessels and allow the operator to infer the position of facial nerve branches.

A systematic observational clinicopathological study demonstrated USCB of salivary gland lesions to have a sensitivity of 94%, a specificity of 100%, an accuracy of 96%, a positive predictive value of 100%, and a negative predictive value of 90% [86]. A study by Eom et al. (2012) [87] also showed that trainees had a significantly lower accuracy with FNAC than USCB when diagnosing malignant tumors when compared to USCB with lymphomas being diagnosed much more accurately using USCB as reported by Huang et al. (2015) [88].

Despite generally favorable outcomes and diagnostic advantages, USCB is not yet considered the reference standard in parotid lesion biopsy, and the optimum technique remains controversial. The potential problems with USCB include possible false-negative results, complications of a slightly more invasive technique, and tumor seeding. Haldar et al. [89] described two cases which were malignant clinically, on imaging and in the resected specimen, but benign on USCB (false negative). Also, some cases of well-differentiated malignancy require direct histological assessment of the whole excised lesion capsule to demonstrate invasiveness; USCB will miss this. This emphasizes that USCB should not be used alone in parotid lesion assessment.

21.5.3 Intraoperative Frozen Section (IOFS)

Another salivary gland biopsy technique is intraoperative frozen section (IOFS), which is used in a small number of specialist centers as an alternative to FNAC or where FNAC is not performing well. Results can be telephoned to the surgeon within 20–30 min. This is useful where no preoperative diagnosis is available, for example, in deep parotid lesions not amenable to percutaneous biopsy or for lesions that are suspicious on clinical/imaging assessment but benign or considered nonrepresentative on FNAC/USCB. Intraoperative frozen section can be employed to guide further surgical management while the patient is still on the operating table [90].

Intraoperative frozen section (IOFS) cannot be recommended as a first-line diagnostic technique, which cannot be widely supported outside dedicated histopathology units. Most pathologists are reluctant to diagnose complex parotid lesions on the table in the absence of further techniques including immunofluorescence. The pitfalls and failures outlined above for USCB also apply to IOFS. In general, IOFS can be used as an adjunct to the less invasive options described where diagnostic suspicion and uncertainty remain [90].

References

1. Graamans K, von der Akker HP. History and physical examination. In: Graamans AK, editor. Diagnosis of salivary gland disorders. Dordrecht, Germany: Kluwer Academic Publishers; 1991. p. 1–3.
2. Mason D, Chisholm D. Salivary glands in health and disease. London, UK: WB Saunders; 1975.
3. Dreizen S, Daley TE, Drane JB, Brown LR. Oral complications of cancer radiotherapy. Postgrad Med. 1977;61:85–92.
4. Marder MX, Wotman S, Mandel ID. Salivary electrolyte changes during pregnancy-I. Normal pregnancy. Am J Obstet Gynecol. 1972;112:233–6.

5. Lawler DP, Hickler RB, Thorn GW. The salivary sodium-potassium ratio. N Engl J Med. 1962;267:1136–7.
6. Frawley TF, Thurn FW. The relation of the sodium-potassium ratio to adrenal cortical activity. In: Mote JR, editor. Proceedings of second annual ACTH conference. London, UK: Churchill Livingstone; 1951.
7. Di Sant' Agnese PA, Davis PB. Research in cystic fibrosis. N Engl J Med. 1976;295(1 of 3 pt):481–5.
8. Mandel ID, Kutscher AH, Denning CR, Thompson RH, Zegarelli EV. Salivary studies in cystic fibrosis. Am J Dis Child. 1967;113:431–8.
9. Bloomfield J, Rush AR, Allars H, Brown JM. Parotid gland function in children with cystic fibrosis and child control subjects. Pediatr Res. 1976;10:574–8.
10. Kurscher AH, Denning CR, Zegarelli EV, Kessler W, Eriv A, Mandel ID, et al. Capillary tube test for minor salivary gland secretion in cystic fibrosis of pancreas. NY State J Med. 1968;68:2812–3.
11. Mason DK, Harden RMG, Alexander WB. The salivary and thyroid glands. Br Dent J. 1967;122:485–9.
12. Weinberger A, Sperling O, De Vries A. Calcium and inorganic phosphate in saliva of patients with primary hyperparathyroidism. Clin Chim Acta. 1974;50:5–7.
13. Niedermeier W, Dreizen S, Stone RE, Spies TD. Sodium and potassium concentrations in the saliva of normotensive and hypertensive subjects. Oral Surg. 1956;9:426–31.
14. Bhoola KD, McNichol NW, Oliver S, Foran J. Changes in salivary enzymes in patients with sarcoidosis. N Engl J Med. 1969;281:877–9.
15. Beeley JA, Chisholm DM. Sarcoidosis with salivary gland involvement: biochemical studies on parotid saliva. J Lab Clin Med. 1976;88:276–81.
16. Abelson DC, Mandel ID, Karmiol M. Salivary studies in alcoholic cirrhosis. Oral Surg. 1976;41:188–92.
17. Masson PL, Heremans JF, Prignot JJ, Wauters G. Immunohistochemical localization and bacteriostatic properties of an iron-binding protein from bronchial mucus. Thorax. 1966;21:538–44.
18. Mandel ID. Sialochemistry in diseases and clinical situations affecting salivary glands. CRC Crit Rev Clin Lab Sci. 1980;12:321–66.
19. Wotman S, Bigger TJ, Mandel ID, Bartelstone HJ. Salivary electrolytes in the detection of digitalis toxicity. N Engl J Med. 1971;285:871–6.
20. Jager L, Menauer F, Holzknecht N, Scholz V, Grevers G, Reiser M. Sialolithiasis: MR sialography of the submandibular duct—an alternative to conventional sialography and US? Radiology. 2000;216(3):665–71.
21. Kalinowski M, Heverhagen JT, Rehberg E, Klose KJ, Wagner HJ. Comparative study of MR sialography and digital subtraction sialography for benign salivary gland disorders. AJNR Am J Neuroradiol. 2002;23(9):1485–92.
22. White SC, Pharoah MJ, Wydawnictwo C, Wyd I. Radiologia stomatologiczna. 2002; pp. 621–628.
23. Forman WH. Subtraction sialography. Radiology. 1977;122(2):533.
24. Białek EJ, Jakubowski W, Zajkowski P, Szopinski KT, Osmolski A. US of the major salivary glands: anatomy and spatial relationships, pathologic conditions, and pitfalls. Radiographics. 2006;26(3):745–63.
25. Yu C, Zheng L, Yang C, Shen N. Causes of chronic obstructive parotitis and management by sialoendoscopy. Oral Surg Oral Med Oral Pathol Oral Radiol Endod. 2008;105(3):365–70.
26. Forman WH. Subtraction sialography. Radiology. 1977;122(2):536–339.
27. Kalk WW, Vissink A, Fred KL, Möller JM, Roodenburg JL. Morbidity from parotid sialography. Oral Surg Oral Med Oral Pathol Oral Radiol Endod. 2001;92(5):572–5.
28. Szolar DH, Groell R, Braun H, Preidler K, Stiskal M, Kern R, et al. Ultrafast computed tomography and three-dimensional image processing of CT sialography in patients with parotid masses poorly defined by magnetic resonance imaging. Acta Otolaryngol. 1996;116(1):112–8.
29. Obaid H, Sinha R, Robinson L. Submandibular sialogram performed through a Wharton's duct fistula: technical adaptation of conventional technique. Eur J Radiol. 2006;60(1):56–7.

30. Eyjólfsson O, Nordshus T, Dahl T. Sialography and CT-sialography in the diagnosis of parotid masses. Acta Radiol Diagn (Stockh). 1984;25(5):361–4.
31. Bryan RN, Miller RH, Ferreyro RI, Sessions RB. Computed tomography of the major salivary glands. AJR Am J Roentgenol. 1982;139(3):547–54.
32. Nixon PP, Lancer J, Bradley MJ. Case report: percutaneous Sialography. Clin Radiol. 1998;53(5):381–3.
33. Kalk WW, Vissink A, Spijkervet FK, Bootsma H, Kallenberg CG, Roodenburg JL. Parotid sialography for diagnosing Sjögren syndrome. Oral Surg Oral Med Oral Pathol Oral Radiol Endod. 2002;94(1):131–7.
34. Buckenham TM, George CD, McVicar D, Moody AR, Coles GS. Digital sialography: imaging and intervention. Br J Radiol. 1994;67(798):524–9.
35. Sakamoto M, Sasano T, Higano S, et al. Evaluation of pulse sequences used for magnetic resonance sialography. Dentomaxillofac Radiol. 2001;30(5):276–84.
36. Murakami R, Baba Y, Nishimura R, Baba T, Matsumoto N, Yamashita Y, et al. MR sialography using half-fourier acquisition single-shot turbo spin-echo (HASTE) sequences. AJNR Am J Neuroradiol. 1998;19(5):959–61.
37. Jäger L, Menauer F, Holzknecht N, Scholz V, Grevers G, Reiser M. Sialolithiasis: MR sialography of the submandibular duct—an alternative to conventional sialography and US? Radiology. 2000;216(3):665–71.
38. Becker M, Marchal F, Becker CD, Dulguerov P, Georgakopoulos G, Lehmann W, et al. Sialolithiasis and salivary ductal stenosis: diagnostic accuracy of MR sialography with a three-dimensional extended-phase conjugate-symmetry rapid spin-echo sequence. Radiology. 2000;217(2):347–58.
39. Drage NA, Brown JE, Wilson RF. Pain and swelling after sialography: is it a significant problem? Oral Surg Oral Med Oral Pathol Oral Radiol Endod. 2000;90(3):385–8.
40. Hasson O. Sialoendoscopy and sialography: strategies for assessment and treatment of salivary gland obstructions. J Oral Maxillofac Surg. 2007;65(2):300–4.
41. Carter BL, Karmody CS. Computed tomography of the face and neck. Semin Roentgenol. 1978;13:257–66.
42. Mancuso A, Rice D, Hanafee W. Computed tomography of the parotid gland during contrast sialography. Radiology. 1979;132:211–3.
43. Som PM, Biller HF. The combined CT-sialogram. Radiology. 1980;13:387–90. (Stuttg) 1 977; 56: 740–748.
44. Quinn HJ Jr. Symposium: management of tumors of the parotid gland. II. Diagnosis of parotid gland swelling. Laryngoscope. 1976;86(1):22–4.
45. Yousem DM, Kraut MA, Chalian AA. Major salivary gland imaging. Radiology. 2000;216(1):19–29.
46. Haring JI. Diagnosing salivary stones. J Am Dental Ass. 1991;122(6):75–6.
47. Jungehulsing M, Fischbach R, Schroder U, Kugel H, Damm M, Eckel HE. Magnetic resonance sialography. Otolaryngol Head Neck Surg. 1999;121(4):488–94.
48. Varghese JC, Thornton F, Lucey BC, Walsh M, Farrell MA, Lee MJ. A prospective comparative study of MR sialography and conventional sialography of salivary duct disease. Am J Roentgenol. 1999;173(6):1497–503.
49. Gritzmann N, Rettenbacher T, Hollerweger A, Macheiner P, Hubner E. Sonography of the salivary glands. Eur Radiol. 2003;13(5):964–75.
50. Som PM, Biller HF. The combined computerized tomography-sialogram. A technique to differentiate deep lobe parotid tumors from extraparotid pharyngomaxillary space tumors. Ann Otol Rhinol Laryngol. 1979;88(5 Pt 1):590–5.
51. Teresi LM, Lufkin RB, Wortham DG, Abemayor E, Hanafee WN. Parotid masses: MR imaging. Radiology. 1987;163:405–9.
52. Mandelblatt SM, Braun IF, Davis PC, Fry SM, Jacobs LH, Hoffman JC Jr. Parotid masses: MR imaging. Radiology. 1987;153:411–4.
53. Izumi M, Eguchi K, Ohki M, Uetani M, Hayashi K, Kita M, et al. MR imaging of the parotid gland in Sjögren's syndrome: a proposal for a new diagnostic criteria. AJR Am J Roentgenol. 1996;166:1483–7.

54. Izumi M, Eguchi K, Nakamura H, Nagataki S, Nakamura T. Premature fat deposition in the salivary glands associated with Sjögren's syndrome: MR and CT evidence. AJNR Am J Neuroradiol. 1997;18:951–8.
55. Nahlieli O, Baruchin AM. Sialoendoscopy: three years' experience as a diagnostic and treatment modality. J Oral Maxillofac Surg. 1997;55(9):912–8.
56. Ziegler CM, Hedemark A, Brevik B, Idris M, Isaksen R. Endoscopy as minimal invasive routine treatment for sialolithiasis. Acta Odontol Scand. 2003;61(3):137–40.
57. Nahlieli O, Baruchin AM. Long-term experience with endoscopic diagnosis and treatment of salivary gland inflammatory diseases. Laryngoscope. 2000;110(6):988–93.
58. Rauch SGR. Diseases of the salivary glands. 6th ed. St.Louis, MO: Mosby; 1970. p. 997.
59. Katz P. Endoscopy of the salivary glands. Ann Radiol (Paris). 1991;34:110–3.
60. Frable MA, Frable WJ. Fine needle aspiration biopsy of salivary glands. Laryngoscope. 1991;101:245–9.
61. David OD, Blaney S, Hearp M. Parotid gland fine-needle aspiration cytology: an approach to differential diagnosis. Diagn Cytopathol. 2007;35:47–56.
62. Alphs HH, Eisele DW, Westra WH. The role of fine needle aspiration in the evaluation of parotid masses. Curr Opin Otolaryngol Head Neck Surg. 2006;14:62–6.
63. O'Donnell ME, Salem A, Badger SA, Sharif MA, Kamalapurkar D, Lieo T, et al. Fine needle aspiration at a regional head and neck clinic: a clinically beneficial and cost-effective service. Cytopathology. 2009;20:81–6.
64. Stewart CJ, MacKenzie K, McGarry GW, Mowat A. Fine-needle aspiration cytology of salivary gland: a review of 341 cases. Diagn Cytopathol. 2000;22:139–46.
65. Cohen EG, Patel SG, Lin O, Boyle JO, Kraus DH, Singh B, et al. Fine-needle aspiration biopsy of salivary gland lesions in a selected patient population. Arch Otolaryngol Head Neck Surg. 2004;130:773–8.
66. Batsakis JG, Sueige N, El-Naggar AK. Fine-needle aspiration of salivary gland: its utility and tissue effects. Ann Otol Rhinol Laryngol. 1992;101:185–8.
67. Wong DS, Li GK. The role of fine-needle aspiration cytology in the management of parotid tumors: a critical clinical appraisal. Head Neck. 2000;22:469–73.
68. Zurrida S, Alasio L, Tradati N, Bartoli C, Chiesa F, Pilotti S. Fine needle aspiration of parotid masses. Cancer. 1993;72:2306–11.
69. Jayaram G, Verma AK, Sood N, Khurana N. Fine needle aspiration cytology of salivary gland lesions. J Oral Pathol Med. 1994;23:256–61.
70. Atula T, Greénman R, Laippala P, Klemi PJ. Fine-needle aspiration biopsy in the diagnosis of parotid gland lesions: evaluation of 438 biopsies. Diagn Cytopathol. 1996;153:185–90.
71. Cristallini EG, Ascani S, Farabi R, Liberati F, Macciò T, Peciarolo A, et al. Fine needle aspiration biopsy of salivary gland, 1985-1995. Acta Cytol. 1997;41:1421–5.
72. Cajulis RS, Gokaslan ST, Yu GH, Frias-Hidvegi D. Fine needle aspiration biopsy of the salivary glands. A five-year experience with emphasis on diagnostic pitfalls. Acta Cytol. 1997;41:1412–20.
73. Al-Khafaji BM, Nestok BR, Katz RL. Fine needle aspiration of 154 parotid masses with histologic correlation: ten-year experience at the University of Texas, MD Anderson Cancer Center. Cancer. 1998;84:153–9.
74. Que-Hee CG, Perry CF. Fine-needle aspiration cytology of parotid tumours: is it useful? ANZ J Surg. 2001;71:345–8.
75. Bajaj Y, Singh S, Cozens N, Sharp J. Critical clinical appraisal of the role of ultrasound guided fine needle aspiration cytology in the management of parotid tumours. J Laryngol Otol. 2005;119:289–92.
76. Carrillo JF, Ramirez R, Flores L, Ramirez-Ortega MC, Arrecillas MD, Ibarra M, et al. Diagnostic accuracy of fine needle aspiration biopsy in preoperative diagnosis of patients with parotid gland mass. J Surg Oncol. 2009;100:133–8.
77. McIvor NP, Freeman JL, Salem S, Elden L, Noyek AM, Bedard YC. Ultrasonography and ultrasound-guided fine-needle aspiration biopsy of head and neck lesions: a surgical perspective. Laryngoscope. 1994;104:669–74.

78. Robinson IA, Cozens NJ. Does a joint ultrasound guided cytology clinic optimize the cytological evaluation of head and neck masses? Clin Radiol. 1999;54:312–6.
79. Sharma G, Jung AS, Maceri DR, Rice DH, Martin SE, Grant EG. US-guided fine-needle aspiration of major salivary gland masses and adjacent lymph nodes: accuracy and impact on clinical decision making. Radiology. 2011;259:471–8.
80. Buckland JR, Manjaly G, Violaris N, Howlett DC. Ultrasound-guided cutting-needle biopsy of the parotid gland. J Laryngol Otol. 1999;113:988–92.
81. Kesse KW, Manjaly G, Violaris N, Howlett DC. Ultrasound-guided biopsy in the evaluation of focal lesions and diffuse swelling of the parotid gland. Br J Oral Maxillofac Surg. 2002;40:384–8.
82. Zinzani PL, Colecchia A, Festi D, Magagnoli M, Larocca A, Ascani S, et al. Ultrasound-guided core-needle biopsy is effective in the initial diagnosis of lymphoma patients. Haematologica. 1998;83:989–92.
83. Burke C, Thomas R, Inglis C, Baldwin A, Ramesar K, Grace R, Howlett DC. Ultrasound-guided core biopsy in the diagnosis of lymphoma of the head and neck. A 9-year experience. Br J Radiol. 2011;84:727–32.
84. Witt BL, Schmidt RL. Ultrasound-guided core-needle biopsy of salivary gland lesions: a systematic review and meta-analysis. Laryngoscope. 2014;124:695–700.
85. Pfeiffer J, Ridder GJ. Diagnostic value of ultrasound-guided core needle biopsy in patients with salivary gland masses. Int J Oral Maxillofac Surg. 2012;41:437–43.
86. Eom HJ, Lee JH, Ko MS, Choi YJ, Yoon RG, Cho KJ, et al. Comparison of fine-needle aspiration and core needle biopsy under ultrasonographic guidance for detecting malignancy and for the tissue-specific diagnosis of salivary gland tumors. AJNR Am J Neuroradiol. 2015;36:1188–93.
87. Huang YC, Wu CT, Lin G, Chuang WY, Yeow KM, Wan YL. Comparison of ultrasonographically guided fine-needle aspiration and core needle biopsy in the diagnosis of parotid masses. J Clin Ultrasound. 2012;40:189–94.
88. Halder S, Mandalia U, Skelton E, Chow V, Turner SS, Ramesar K, et al. Diagnostic investigation of parotid neoplasms: a 16-year experience of freehand fine needle aspiration cytology and ultrasound-guided core needle biopsy. Int J Oral Maxillofac Surg. 2015;44:151–7.
89. Schmidt RL, Hunt JP, Hall BJ, Wilson AR, Layfield LJ. A systematic review and meta-analysis of the diagnostic accuracy of frozen section for parotid gland lesions. Am J Clin Pathol. 2011;136:729–38.
90. Halder S, Sinnott JD, Tekeli KM, Turner SS, Howlett DC. Biopsy of parotid masses: review of current techniques. World J Radiol. 2016;8(5):501–5.

Sialolithiasis: Calculi of the Submandibular Gland

22

22.1 Overview

The term "sialolithiasis" is derived from the Greek words "sialon" (saliva) and "lithos" (stone), and the Greek "iasis" means "process" or "morbid condition." A calculus is a hard, stone-like concretion that forms within an organ or duct inside the body. Sialolithiasis (salivary calculi or stones) is a benign condition where a calcified mass or sialolith forms within a salivary gland, usually in the duct of the submandibular gland (Wharton's duct), less commonly in the parotid gland, or rarely in the sublingual gland or a minor salivary gland [1].

Sialolithiasis is the most frequent cause of salivary gland swelling, accounting for about 50% of all diseases occurring in the major salivary glands and causing symptoms in about 0.45% of the general population. Individuals aged 30–60 years and males are more likely to develop sialolithiasis [2].

The usual symptoms of submandibular calculi are pain and swelling of the affected gland, both of which get worse when salivary flow is stimulated as with the sight, thought, smell, or taste of food or with hunger or chewing (peri-prandial). This is often termed "meal-time syndrome" [2]. Inflammation or infection of the gland (sialadenitis), or in rare cases, abscess formation, may develop as a result of duct obstruction. Sialolithiasis may also develop because of the presence of existing chronic infection of the glands, dehydration (e.g., use of phenothiazines), Sjögren's syndrome, and/or increased local levels of calcium (Ca), but in many instances, the cause is unknown, i.e., idiopathic. Modern diagnostic techniques involve point-of-care ultrasound (US), computed tomography (CT), magnetic resonance imaging (MRI), and direct visualization with sialoendoscopy [3, 4]. A variety of treatment options exist for sialolithiasis, including sialogogues, direct massage of distal stones out of the duct, and other procedures including interventional sialography, lithotripsy, sialoendoscopy, and surgery [4, 5].

© The Author(s), under exclusive license to Springer Nature Switzerland AG 2024
M. Sakr, *Surgery of the Salivary Glands*,
https://doi.org/10.1007/978-3-031-82069-4_22

22.2 Incidence/Epidemiology

The incidence of sialolithiasis is estimated at one in 10,000–30,000 individuals. The prevalence of salivary stones in the general population is about 1.2% according to postmortem studies, but the prevalence of symptomatic salivary stones is about 0.45% in the general population [2]. Sialolithiasis is the most common disorder of major salivary glands [6] accounting for about 50% of all diseases occurring in major salivary glands and for about 66% of all obstructive salivary gland diseases. The majority of salivary calculi (80–95%) occur in the submandibular gland making it the most common location for sialolithiasis, whereas approximately 5–20% of stones are found in the parotid gland [6–13]. The difference in incidence is attributed to a number of factors such as the difference in the composition of the saliva produced by each gland (the submandibular gland produces predominately mucinous saliva) and the dependence of the submandibular (Wharton's) duct, which hinders easy drainage of its viscid secretions. The submandibular gland also produces more alkaline saliva, which predisposes to the precipitation of inorganic salts (i.e., calcium and phosphate), further leading to salivary stone formation. Sialothiasis rarely affects the sublingual gland and the minor salivary glands (1–2%) [14, 15].

Approximately 75% of stones are single, and 25% are multiple [6, 8, 9, 12]. The mean number of stones per patient is 1.67 (range 1–5) [2]. Salivary gland stones are twice as common in males as in females. The most symptomatic sialolithiasis can be observed in patients between 30 and 60 years old [7]. Sialolithiasis is uncommon in children [2].

22.3 Classification

22.3.1 Anatomical Classification

Salivary stones may be divided according to which gland they form in. About 80–95% of stones occur in the submandibular gland [16] and 5–20% in the parotid gland [2]. In about 0–2% of cases, the sublingual gland or a minor salivary gland is affected [2]. When minor glands are involved, calculi are more likely in the minor glands of the buccal mucosa and the maxillary labial mucosa [17]. Submandibular stones are further classified as anterior or posterior in relation to an imaginary transverse line drawn between the mandibular first molar teeth.

22.3.2 Radiological Classification

Stones or calculi may be "radio-opaque" showing up on conventional radiographs or "radio-lucent" not visible.

22.3.3 Clinical Classification

Stones or calculi may also be "symptomatic" or "asymptomatic," according to whether they cause any problems or not.

22.4 Histopathology/Composition

Salivary stones are composed of "organic" substances such as glycoproteins, cellular debris, bacteria, and mucopolysaccharides [4, 18] and "inorganic" substances, mainly phosphates and calcium carbonates [19]. The organic substances are mainly found at the core of the stone, while the inorganic substances are in its periphery arranged in a lamellae (layers) fashion. Inorganic materials include hydroxyapatite, whitlockite, and octacalcium phosphate, with hydroxyapatite (calcium phosphate) being the most prevalent component present throughout the calculus. The exact ratios of inorganic material found within a sialolith depend on the chemical environment in which it forms.

Studies utilizing scanning electron microscopy (SEM) and polymerase chain reaction (PCR) have demonstrated bacteria within sialoliths, predominantly the *Streptococcus* genus [20, 21]. Bacteria are not present in all sialoliths suggesting they are not necessary for their formation.

The annual growth rate of an established stone is about 1 mm per year, and the average size is about 3.4 mm (range 1.5–9 mm) [7]. Calculi within a major duct tend to be smooth and rounded, whereas those within the gland tend to be irregular in shape.

22.5 Etiology

A series of stages that lead to the formation of a calculus (lithogenesis) is believed to exist. Initially, factors such as abnormalities in calcium (Ca) metabolism [16], dehydration due to decreased fluid intake, and pharmacological side effects resulting in decreased salivary production (e.g., diuretics) [2], reduced salivary flow rate [2], altered acidity (pH) of saliva caused by oropharyngeal infections [2], and altered solubility of crystalloids [2], leading to precipitation of mineral salts, are involved. Other authors stated that no systemic abnormality of Ca or phosphate metabolism is responsible [22]. The next stage involves the formation of a "nidus," which is successively layered with organic and inorganic material, eventually forming a calcified mass [2, 16]. In about 15–20% of cases, the sialolith will not be sufficiently calcified to appear radio-opaque on a radiograph [16] and therefore be difficult to detect.

Other authors suggest a retrograde theory of lithogenesis, where food debris, bacteria, or foreign bodies from the mouth enter the ducts of a salivary gland and are trapped by abnormalities in the sphincter mechanism of the duct opening (papilla), which are reported in 90% of cases. Fragments of bacteria from salivary calculi were reported to be Streptococci species, which are part of the normal oral microbiota and are present in dental plaque [2]. Accordingly, the formation of the salivary gland calculi results from a deposition of Ca salts around a "core" made of desquamated epithelial cells, foreign bodies, bacteria, or mucus. Salivary gland calculi are of a "laminal" structure.

In recent years, tobacco smoking has been discussed as a potential risk factor for the formation of salivary stones. Tobacco may induce inflammation within the salivary ducts and decrease the production of salivary amylase [4, 22].

Stone formation occurs most commonly in the submandibular gland for several reasons: (1) saliva produced by the submandibular gland contains a relatively high concentration of hydroxyapatites and phosphates; (2) the concentration of Ca in saliva produced by the submandibular gland is twice that of the saliva produced by the parotid gland [2, 16]; (3) the submandibular gland saliva is also relatively alkaline and mucous [6, 9]; (4) the submandibular duct (Wharton's duct) is long, meaning that saliva secretions must travel further before being discharged into the mouth [7, 16]; (5) the duct possesses two bends, the first at the posterior border of the mylohyoid muscle and the second near the duct orifice [16]; (6) the flow of saliva from the submandibular gland is against gravity due to variations in the location of the duct orifice [16]; (7) the orifice itself is smaller than that of the parotid [16] and is narrower than the diameter of the whole duct; and (8) the orifice of the duct being in the floor of the mouth renders it more liable to be obstructed by a stone, inflammation, and foreign bodies such as a small piece of a tooth brush or food particles. All of these factors promote slowing and stasis of saliva in the submandibular duct, making the formation of an obstruction with subsequent calcification more likely [9, 12, 19, 23].

Salivary calculi sometimes are associated with other salivary diseases, e.g., sialoliths occur in two-thirds of cases of chronic sialadenitis [17], although obstructive sialadenitis is often due to sialolithiasis. Gout may also cause salivary stones, although in this case, they are composed of uric acid crystals rather than the normal composition of salivary stones [17].

22.6 Pathogenesis

The exact pathogenesis of sialolithiasis is not well understood, but factors that are believed to affect salivary stone formation are divided into two major groups: anatomical, affecting saliva formation or flow (e.g., duct stenosis or inflammation), and compositional (e.g., increased Ca content or altered enzyme function). It can thus be concluded that salivary gland stone formation appears to be mainly related to the following conditions: (1) salivary stagnation (stasis), (2) duct obstruction, (3) epithelial injury along the duct causing nidus formation, and (4) precipitation of Ca salts, mainly calcium phosphate and calcium carbonate, in association with other salts (magnesium phosphate) and organic material such as glycoproteins, desquamated cellular residue, and mucopolysaccharides [2, 16].

22.7 Clinical Presentation

Clinical diagnosis of sialolithiasis can be challenging as patients may not be symptomatic unless the stone obstructs the salivary ducts. Signs and symptoms of submandibular lithiasis (stones) are variable and depend largely upon whether the obstruction of the duct is complete or partial and how much resultant pressure is created within the gland [22]. The development of infection in the gland also influences the signs and symptoms.

The clinical presentations (signs and symptoms) of patients with submandibular calculi can be summarized as follows:

Pain, which is intermittent, may suddenly get worse before meal times, and then slowly get better due to the slow flow of saliva into the oral cavity. This denotes "partial obstruction" [5, 16] and helps to differentiate it from pain of dental origin.

Swelling of the gland, which simulates a tumor (Fig. 22.1), but is also usually intermittent, often suddenly appearing or increasing before meal times, and then slowly going down (also denoting partial obstruction) [5, 16].

Intake of lemon juice (lemon juice test) causes aggravation of pain and an increase in the size of the swelling.

Tenderness on palpation of the involved gland [16].

Palpable hard lump: With bimanual examination, a stone may be felt within the duct or within the gland [1, 16]. If the stone is near the submandibular duct orifice, the lump may be felt under the tongue, and its tip may be visible (Fig. 22.2). Salivary stones typically demonstrate an oval or round shape and a white or yellow color on inspection [24–26].

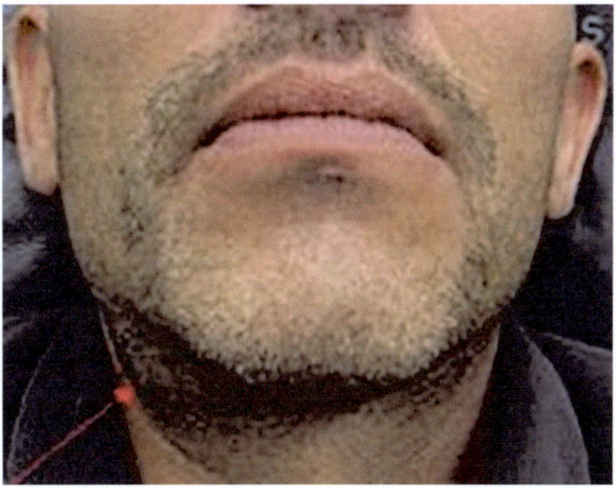

Fig. 22.1 Swelling of the right submandibular gland as seen from the outside (red arrow)

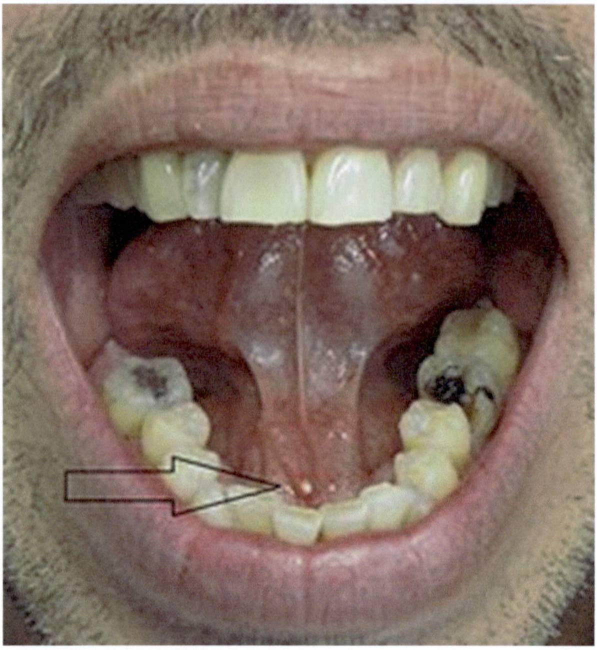

Fig. 22.2 A stone seen at the orifice of the right submandibular duct in the floor of the mouth (arrow) of the same patient in Fig. 22.1

Salivary stones' size and weight vary. Sialoliths' diameter ranges between 2.1 and 10 mm, and only 7.6% exceeds 15 mm in diameter [14]. Submandibular stones are usually larger than parotid ones [28]. Sialoliths weigh 300 mg on average, ranging between 1 mg and 5 g [27].

Lack of saliva coming from the duct (total obstruction) [16]; oral examination of the duct orifice reveals saliva pouring on the unaffected side, with little or no secretion seen ejecting from the swollen (affected) side.

Erythema (redness) and swelling of the papilla and floor of the mouth (infection) [16] (Fig. 22.3).

Pus discharging from the duct (infection) [16].

Cervical lymphadenitis (infection) [16].

Foul breathe [16].

Complications of sialolithiasis may be encountered and include acute suppurative sialadenitis, ductal ulceration, and stricture [6, 29].

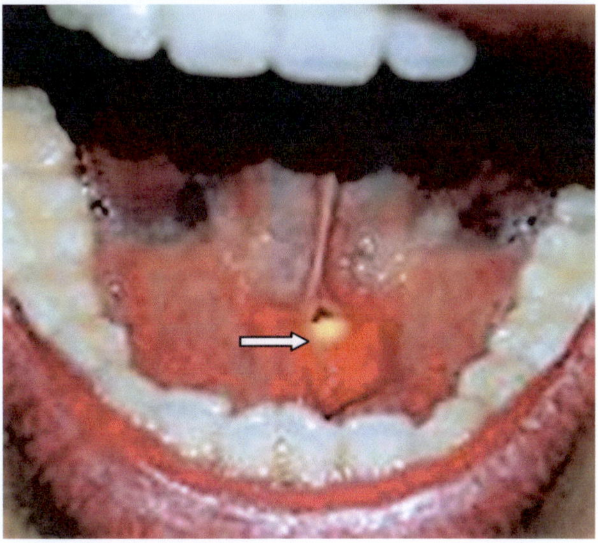

Fig. 22.3 Erythema (redness) and swelling of the papilla in the floor of the mouth. Note the visible tip of the stone (arrow)

22.8 Investigations

Calculi must be differentiated from stenosis of the duct caused by repeated trauma and fibrosis. The basic imaging methods of sialolithiasis are plain X-ray images, X-ray sialography, ultrasonography (US), computed tomography (CT) scan, and magnetic resonance imaging (MRI). Sialoendoscopy, which is also a therapeutic method, is becoming increasingly common.

In the USA, a major role in sialolithiasis diagnostics is played by unenhanced CT, while in Europe, this is US and digital subtraction sialography (DSS) [3]. Recently, MR sialography (MR-Si) is also gaining popularity.

22.8.1 Plain X-Rays

Conventional radiographs using occlusal views were the initial diagnostic choice in the past. These can detect large radio-opaque ductal stones relatively well (Fig. 22.4), but they miss smaller and parenchymal stones. It is reported that stones of the submandibular gland produce opacity in up to 80–90% of cases, while radio-opaque stones of the parotid gland are seen in only 60% of cases [1, 6, 8]. Radiolucent calculi are undetectable by plain radiography.

While conventional radiography can still be useful in the initial work-up of salivary stones, modern imaging techniques using US or CT scans can accurately diagnose the sialoliths and provide their exact location [4].

A single plain X-ray is normally performed before contrast administration for sialography.

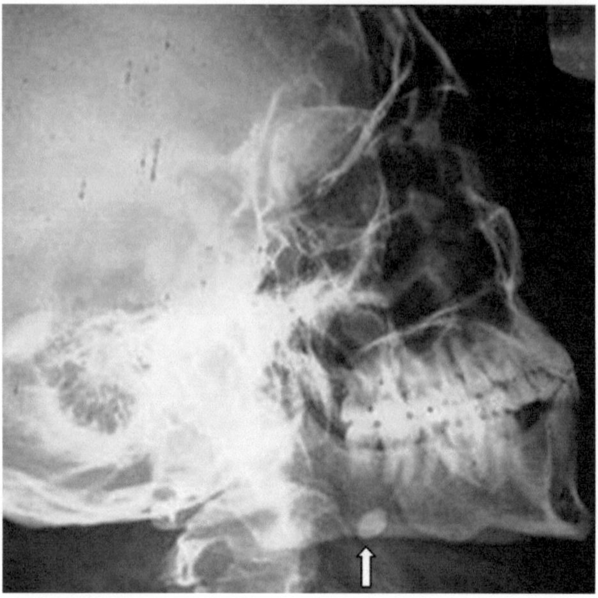

Fig. 22.4 Plain X-ray showing an oval radio-opaque shadow (arrow) (right submandibular calculus)

22.8.2 Conventional Sialography

Sialography has traditionally been regarded as the "gold standard" for diagnosing sialolithiasis as it allows excellent visualization of the salivary ducts and underlying ductal pathology. In this technique, contrast is injected via a small needle, enabling radiographic visualization, acting as a sialogogue, and allowing passage of smaller stones. Disadvantages include radiation exposure and risk of contrast reaction [4, 30].

Submandibular stones are seen on sialography as a filling defect if they were radiolucent (Fig. 22.5). The sensitivity of conventional sialography in calculi detection ranges between 64 and 100%, while its specificity is between 88 and 100%. Digitalization of that examination, with the use of subtraction (digital subtraction sialography (DSS)), increased its sensitivity of stone detection up to 96–100% and its specificity to 88–91% [10].

22.8.3 Ultrasonography (US)

Ultrasonography (US) can be used to differentiate between solid and cystic lesions of the submandibular gland. It can be used to differentiate intrinsic from extrinsic disease and is helpful in the identification of abscess formation. It is regarded by some authors as a noninvasive method of choice in salivary stone diagnostics. In calculi detection, it has a sensitivity of 94%, a specificity of 100%, and an accuracy of 96% [6, 9, 23]. Ultrasonography has also been reported to allow for "non-opaque" calculi detection with a sensitivity of 80–96% [11, 12]. Reported sensitivities are

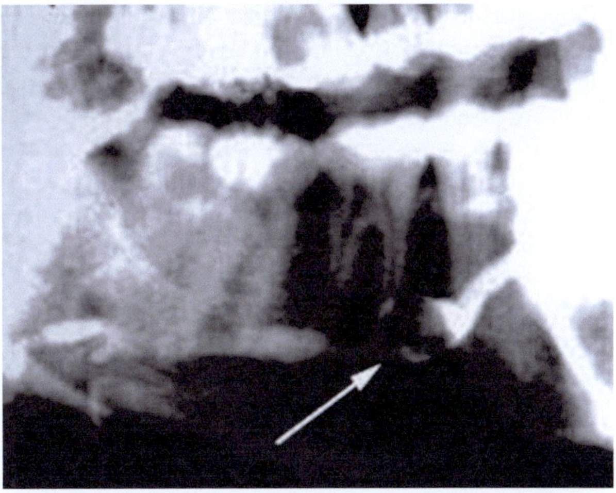

Fig. 22.5 Sialography showing a filling defect in the right submandibular gland indicative of a radiolucent calculus

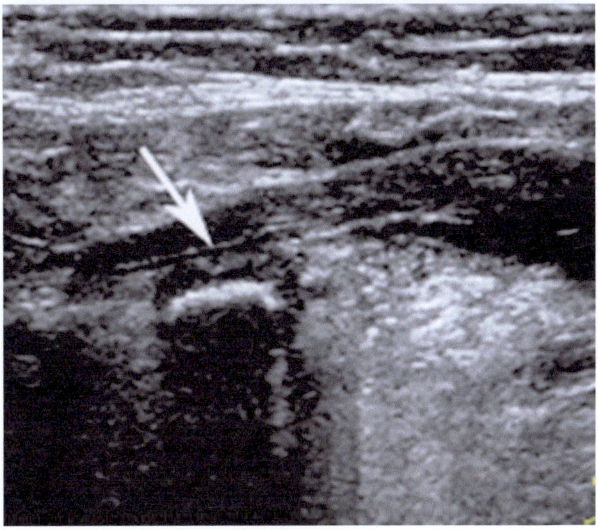

Fig. 22.6 Ultrasound showing a stone (white arrow) with an acoustic shadow behind the calculus

best for stones greater than 2–3 mm in size. Recent research has demonstrated sensitivity and specificity for stones greater than 3 mm in size comparable to conventional NCCT and sialendoscopy [31].

A typical US image of a stone involves an echogenic, round, or oval structure, producing an acoustic shadow (Fig. 22.6) [6, 11, 30].

Stones in salivary ducts may lead to the distension of the duct above the obstacle, which may be shown on US [12]. Stones smaller than 2 mm may not produce any acoustic shadow [6, 10, 12]. The detection of fine stones may be helped by sialogogue injection, which causes salivary duct dilatation and thus facilitates calculi visualization [6, 11]. In about 50% of the sialolithiasis cases, US images show features of inflammation.

Benefits of US include no radiation exposure, real-time image interpretation, and widespread availability. Ultrasound is often available at the point of care and can provide rapid diagnostic information. However, US is highly operator-dependent, and despite the many advantages of US, it turns out to be less precise in differentiating a cluster of stones from a single, large stone [9]. Diagnostic mistakes may concern very small stones in intraparenchymal ducts, with no duct distension [6, 11]. Moreover, hyper-echogenic air bubbles, mixed with saliva and simulating stones, may also be misleading [13].

22.8.4 Computed Tomography (CT) Scanning

Computed tomography (CT) scan is useful in differentiating intrinsic from extrinsic glandular disease. It can be also used in defining abscess formation versus phlegmon. According to some authors, non-contrast computed tomography (NCCT) is a widely used modality for the evaluation of sialolithiasis. It is a valid tool for diagnosing sialolithiasis when it is big enough or when the radiographic slices are done every millimeter [4]. It has also been considered by several authors to be the best method in the detection of sialolithiasis in case of painful salivary glands and suspicion of a few, very tiny calculi [6, 9]. Advantages of NCCT include excellent sensitivity and specificity for calcified stones, fast acquisition time, and widespread availability. Disadvantages, however, include radiation exposure, relatively high cost, and limited evaluation of the ductal system or underlying pathology (i.e., obstructing masses) [7].

The administration of intravenous contrast has been used only as an adjunct to NCCT due to concerns that small vessels may simulate calcifications resulting in false-positive results. A recent study by Purcell et al. in 2017 comparing contrast-enhanced CT (CECT) and NCCT demonstrated excellent sensitivity and specificity with no false-positive results. Benefits of initial contrast-enhanced CT include better evaluation of the ductal system, improved soft tissue contrast in assessing salivary masses, and decreased radiation dose (compared to dual-phase NCCT with CECT) [32].

22.8.5 Cone Beam Computed Tomography (CBCT)

Recently, some authors reported encouraging results on the use of volumetric tomography (alternatively called cone beam computed tomography (CBCT)) in sialolithiasis diagnostics [33]. This method produces high-resolution, 3D images of bony structures of the head and neck, with the use of up to 15 times lower ionizing radiation dose and being much cheaper [34, 35].

22.8.6 Computed Tomography (CT) Sialography

CT sialography requires cannulation of the duct opening. Moreover, it exposes patients to a higher dose of radiation, as compared to conventional sialography. This method allows for simultaneous visualization of the glandular tissue and the salivary ducts. The salivary glands may be shown in 3D reconstruction. However, CT sialography cannot visualize the secondary and tertiary branches of the duct [10].

22.8.7 Magnetic Resonance Imaging (MRI)

Magnetic resonance imaging (MRI) does not allow evaluation of the ductal system, and it is not helpful in defining calcifications. It is an excellent tool, however, for soft tissue definition (invaluable in suspected neoplasia) [36].

22.8.8 Magnetic Resonance Sialography (MR-Si)

Being a noninvasive method, magnetic resonance sialography (MR-Si) does not require cannulation of the salivary duct opening and does not expose patients to ionizing radiation or iodine contrast administration. It allows for a precise morphological evaluation of the salivary ducts, enabling the visualization of their tertiary branches [37]. Moreover, the examination may be carried out in acute inflammation of the salivary gland. It is considered an alternative to digital subtraction sialography (DDS), especially in cases of acute sialadenitis or failure of salivary opening cannulation [37–40].

Capaccio et al. (2008) compared the results of MR-Si versus US. Examinations were performed before and after stimulation with lemon juice. MR-Si showed secondary branches of the salivary ducts within the submandibular salivary glands and tertiary branches within the parotid glands. Thus, MR-Si allowed visualization of very tiny stones that could not be found with US [36].

According to Becker et al. (2000) [40], MR-Si is a better method for salivary gland evaluation than conventional sialography or US, as it allows visualization of distal salivary ducts. Moreover, by adding extra MRI sequences for parenchymal imaging, it is possible to detect some lesions located outside the system of the salivary ducts [8].

Becker et al. (2000) [40] compared MR-Si precision in the detection of calculi as compared to conventional sialography, US, and sialoendoscopy. MR-Si showed a sensitivity of 91%, a specificity of 94–97%, a positive predictive value of 93–97%, and a negative predictive value of 91%. False-negative results were obtained in calculi measuring 2–3 mm, located in undilated salivary ducts. MR-Si did not distinguish a stone from a dense mucosal plug. Moreover, amalgam fillings veiled tiny calculi and stenoses of the salivary ducts. Results also revealed that the peripheral salivary ducts could be better visualized with the conventional sialography than with MR-Si. The limitation of MR-Si is also connected with its lower spatial resolution enabling the differentiation between partial and complete occlusions of the salivary ducts [38]. Disadvantages include cost, image acquisition time, and limited availability compared to NCCT and US [4, 15].

22.8.9 Sialendoscopy

Sialendoscopy enabled the surgeons to examine the salivary ducts from the inside, thus providing excellent sensitivity and specificity. The causes of salivary duct stenosis remain unknown by imaging modalities in 5–10% of cases. The diagnostic gap is filled by sialendoscopy that allows direct visualization of the salivary duct lumen, i.e., visualization of calculi, mucosal plugs, foreign bodies, and polyps. Some authors recommend dilatation of the ductal openings before performing sialoendoscopy. Others recommend papillotomy [29]. During sialendoscopy, the operators use very small tools and a camcorder, to reach the proximal parts of the salivary ducts. At the end of the sialendoscopic procedure, a stent, 2–3 cm long, is left in the salivary duct for 7–10 days to facilitate healing and drainage.

In addition to aiding in the diagnosis of sialolithiasis, clinicians increasingly use sialendoscopy for therapy and stone removal with the use of the Dormia basket, given the advancements in endoscopic technology [3]. Research has shown sialendoscopy to be a safe and effective alternative to conventional open surgical techniques with a more favorable complication profile [41], as in dilatation of the stenosed salivary ducts with the use of balloons [42]. Additionally, sialendoscopy is performed in the outpatient setting utilizing local anesthesia.

22.8.10 Conclusions

Conventional X-ray sialography (especially DSS) combined with US is the method of choice in the visualization of salivary gland calculi. Sialography precisely shows the location and number of stones. Interventional sialography is less invasive than surgical treatment. Moreover, sialography and US are inevitable in a patient's qualification for diagnostic and therapeutic sialendoscopy, thus avoiding sialadenectomy. An alternative, noninvasive diagnostic method of salivary gland calculi and salivary duct stenosis detection is MRI or MR-Si. These methods neither require cannulation of the salivary duct openings nor the administration of the contrast medium or exposure to ionizing radiation. In addition, MR-Si may also be carried out in acute sialoadenitis. As the last resort in search for very fine and multiple calculi, it is possible to apply the NCCT scan of the salivary glands.

22.9 Differential Diagnosis

The differential diagnosis of submandibular salivary gland swelling includes sialolithiasis, sialadenitis (inflammatory or infectious), and neoplasm. However, the clinical presentation can vary, and the differential diagnosis of the pathology of the oral cavity and face can be extensive and relies heavily on physical examination findings and clinical history. Conditions that can have a similar presentation include cellulitis, poor dentition and dental abscess formation, infection of the buccal or masticator space, herpes zoster, and neoplasm. The different imaging techniques in addition to sialoendoscopy can settle the diagnosis of sialolithiasis.

22.10 Treatment

Treatment options of submandibular calculi include (1) noninvasive treatment, (2) minimally invasive therapy, and (3) surgical methods (intraoral/cervical) as summarized in Table 22.1.

22.10.1 Noninvasive Treatment

22.10.1.1 Medical Treatment

For small stones, hydration, moist heat therapy, nonsteroidal anti-inflammatory drugs (NSAIDs), and having the patient take any food or beverage that is bitter and/or sour such as sucking on citrus fruits (lemon or orange) may increase salivation and promote spontaneous expulsion of the stone (e.g., size 2–10 mm) [43]. To prevent infection while the stone is lodged in the duct, antibiotics are sometimes used. Signs of infection, including cervical lymphadenopathy, purulent discharge from the salivary ducts, or erythema surrounding the salivary ducts, indicate the need for antibiotic therapy [5, 24].

22.10.1.2 Massage

Some small stones in the submandibular duct may be massaged out of the oral cavity by a specialist.

22.10.1.3 External Lithotripsy

New therapeutic modalities use extracorporeal or intracorporeal crushing of the salivary gland calculi. The crushed stones can be flushed out with saliva, through natural salivary duct openings [7]. The advent of external lithotripsy in the early 1990s paved the way for conservative treatment of all calculi, with a success rate of only 40% in the submandibular gland and 75% in the parotid gland.

Table 22.1 Treatment options of submandibular calculi

Method	Options
Conservative (noninvasive) methods	Medical treatment Massage Extracorporeal shock wave lithotripsy (ESWL)
Minimally invasive methods	Interventional sialendoscopy
Surgical methods	Trans-oral approach Transcervical approach

Unfortunately, the results are considered discouraging, specifically in patients with large calculi (larger than 7–10 mm) [44–47]. In general, ultrasonic lithotripsy for submandibular gland calculi is rarely effective. Still, however, extracorporeal shock wave lithotripsy (ESWL) may be indicated for smaller stones that are not palpable clinically and not visualized endoscopically [24, 48–50].

22.10.2 Minimally Invasive Treatment

22.10.2.1 Interventional Sialendoscopy

Interventional sialendoscopy, first described in the 1990s, offered much less invasive therapeutic options than submandibular sialadenectomy and became popular with technological improvements after 2000 [4, 51–55]. Interventional sialendoscopy can be used to retrieve stones from the ducts (Fig. 22.7) and to dilate ductal strictures. When the diameter of the stone is 5 mm or less, it can be removed purely by an endoscopic technique, particularly when the stone is located above the muscles that comprise the floor of the mouth.

The four common techniques used to remove the salivary gland stones are (1) the grasping technique, (2) using a small wire basket retrieval system, (3) mechanical fragmentation, and (4) laser fragmentation [56]. Nevertheless, success rates of interventional sialendoscopy with intraductal laser fragmentation and basket extraction of calculi remained possible in only 80% of patients [4]. Unsuccessful treatment was attributed to large-sized calculi (6 mm and larger) and to associated ductal stenosis [57]. In such cases, the only solution is to remove the gland, with its associated potential morbidity [44–46].

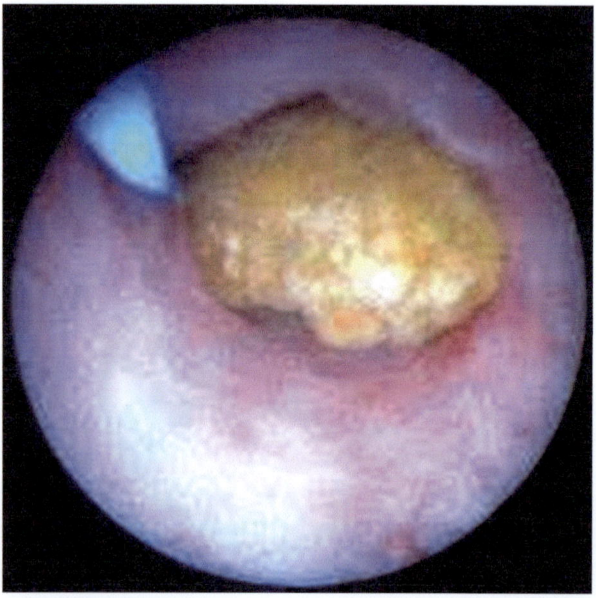

Fig. 22.7 Sialendoscopy showing interior stone in Wharton's duct (intraductal stone)

When the diameter is larger than 5 mm, a twofold (endoscopic-assisted) approach can also be utilized. The endoscope is introduced, and the stone is localized, then dissected, and removed through an intraoral approach. After a sialolith is removed from an affected gland, a silastic stent is inserted into the duct for 2–4 weeks for the duration of the healing process of the oral region and until normal function of the gland is restored. This prevents scar formation, which can develop over the ductal opening into the mouth.

In the presence of strictures or adhesions, the diagnosis and exact location of obstruction are established using a sialogram. The surgeon can use the endoscopic method. The first step is anesthetizing and lavaging the duct with 2% lidocaine and saline solution. If there is no improvement, the surgeon then can insert a dilation balloon, which can be inflated up to 3 mm. The pressure created by inflation is sufficient to dilate most strictures. Another technique for dilating strictures is to expand the stricture region with grasping forceps used as a dilator.

22.10.3 Surgical Treatment

22.10.3.1 Transcervical Approach

Surgical excision of the submandibular gland is considered by several authors to be a last resort for the management of submandibular calculi. However, patients with deep intraparenchymal, multiple, or recurrent stones should be treated with submandibular sialadenectomy on an elective basis [24, 48–50].

22.10.3.2 Trans-oral Approach

Calculi in the proximity of Wharton's duct (close to the duct orifice) are removed by ductal cannulation, dilation, and massage or by longitudinal slitting of the duct and releasing the stone via a trans-oral approach.

For ductal calculi in the floor of the mouth, a stitch is passed under the duct proximal to the stone to stop the stone from slipping backward. An incision is made in the mucosa over the duct, which is then mobilized and a stay suture is passed under the duct to bring it up into the top of the wound and to control it while the wall is incised to release the stone (Fig. 22.8).

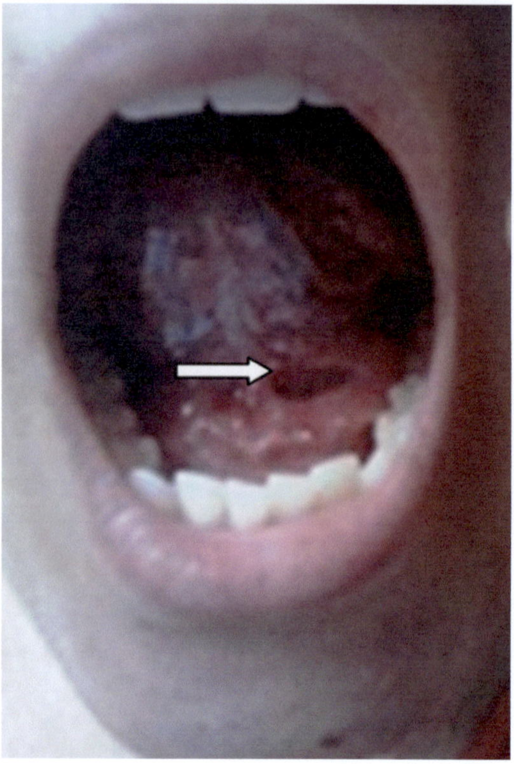

Fig. 22.8 Trans-oral approach: submandibular gland stone extracted and the hole left behind in the floor of the mouth from the operation (arrow)

22.11 Prognosis

22.11.1 Outcome

Sialolithiasis has an excellent prognosis, and the majority of patients can be managed conservatively with sialogogues and NSAIDs. Minimally invasive procedures have excellent success rates with minimal morbidity compared to traditional surgical techniques. Sialadenectomy for the treatment of sialolithiasis is rarely necessary with modern treatment techniques [49].

In cases in which only the calculus is removed, the recurrence rate may be as high as 18% because the underlying cause, which is unknown, has not been corrected.

22.11.2 Complications

The primary complications of sialolithiasis are the development of sialadenitis, acute or chronic, and atrophy of the affected salivary gland. Obstruction of the salivary glands by a sialolith blocks the flow of saliva resulting in swelling and pain. Additionally, this blockage of flow prevents the removal of bacteria and debris from the salivary duct, resulting in bacterial infection. If obstruction is chronic, the blocked flow of saliva will damage the salivary glands' acinar cells, resulting in local inflammation. Without proper treatment, it can result in permanent fibrosis and atrophy of the gland [18].

References

1. Neville BW, Damm DD, Allen CA, Bouquot JE. Oral and maxillofacial pathology. 2nd ed. Philadelphia, PA: WB Saunders; 2002. p. 393–5.
2. Capaccio P, Torretta S, Ottavian F, Sambataro G, Pignataro L. Modern management of obstructive salivary diseases. Acta Otorhinolaryngol Ital. 2007;27(4):161–72.
3. Rzymska-Grala I, Stopa Z, Grala B, Gołębiowski M, Wanyura H, Zuchowska A, Sawicka M, Zmorzyński M. Salivary gland calculi—contemporary methods of imaging. Pol J Radiol. 2010;75(3):25–37.
4. Marchal F, Dulguerov P. Sialolithiasis management: the state of the art. Arch Otolaryngol Head Neck Surg. 2003;129(9):951–6.
5. Diebold S, Overbeck M. Soft tissue disorders of the mouth. Emerg Med Clin North Am. 2019;37(1):55–68.
6. Madani G, Beale T. Inflammatory conditions of the salivary glands. Semin Ultrasound CT MRI. 2006;27(6):440–51.
7. Drage NA, Brown JE, Escudler MP, McGurk M. Interventional radiology in the removal of salivary calcluli. Radiology. 2000;214(1):139–42.
8. Rabinov JD. Imaging of salivary gland pathology. Radiol Clin North Am. 2000;38(5):1047–57.
9. Yousem DM, Kraut MA, Chalian AA. Major salivary gland imaging. Radiology. 2000;216(1):19–29.
10. Jäger L, Menauer F, Holzknecht N, et al. Sialolithiasis: MR sialography of the submandibular duct—an alternative to conventional sialography and US? Radiology. 2000;216(3):665–71.
11. Koischwitz D, Gritzmann N. Ultrasound of the neck. Radiol Clin North Am. 2000;38(5):1029–45.
12. Alyas F, Lewis K, Williams M, Moody AB, Wong KT, Ahuja AT, et al. Diseases of the submandibular gland as demonstrating using high resolution ultrasound. Br J Radiol. 2005;78(928):362–9.
13. Białek EJ, Jakubowski W, Zajkowski P, Szopinski KT, Osmolski A. US of the major salivary glands: anatomy and spatial relationships, pathologic conditions, and pitfalls. Radiographics. 2006;26(3):745–63.
14. Rabinov K, Weber AL. Radiology of the salivary glands. Boston, MA: G.K. Hall Medical Publishers; 1985.
15. Andretta M, Tregnaghi A, Prosenikliev V, Staffieri A. Current opinions in sialolithiasis diagnosis and treatment. Acta Otorhinolaryngol Ital. 2005;25(3):145–9.
16. Hupp JR, Ellis E, Tucker MR. Contemporary oral and maxillofacial surgery. 5th ed. St. Louis, MO: Mosby Elsevier; 2008. p. 398, 407–409.
17. Rice DH. Advances in diagnosis and management of salivary gland diseases. West J Med. 1984;140(2):238–49.
18. Harrison JD. Causes, natural history, and incidence of salivary stones and obstructions. Otolaryngol Clin N Am. 2009;42(6):927–47.
19. Langlais RP. Diagnostic imaging of the jaws. Philadelphia, PA: Williams and Wilkins; 1995. p. 623–7.
20. Teymoortash A, Wollstein AC, Lippert BM, Peldszus R, Werner JA. Bacteria and pathogenesis of human salivary calculus. Acta Otolaryngol. 2002;122(2):210–4.
21. Brady JM, McKinney L, Stanback JS. Scanning electron microscopy of submandibular sialoliths: a preliminary report. Dentomaxillofac Radiol. 1989;18(1):42–4.
22. Huoh KC, Eisele DW. Etiologic factors in sialolithiasis. Otolaryngol Head Neck Surg. 2011;145(6):935–9.

23. Wong KT, Ahuja AT, Yuen HY, King AD. Ultrasound of salivary glands. ASUM Ultrasound Bulletin. 2003;6(3):18–22.
24. Koch M, Zenk J, Iro H. Algorithms for treatment of salivary gland obstructions. Otolaryngol Clin N Am. 2009;42(6):1173–92.
25. Arifa SP, Christopher PJ, Kumar S, Kengasubbiah S, Shenoy V. Sialolithiasis of the submandibular gland: report of cases. Cureus. 2019;11(3):e4180.
26. Pachisia S, Mandal G, Sahu S, Ghosh S. Submandibular sialolithiasis: a series of three case reports with review of literature. Clin Pract. 2019;9(1):1119.
27. Avishai G, Ben-Zvi Y, Ghanaiem O, Chaushu G, Gilat H. Sialolithiasis-do early diagnosis and removal minimize post-operative morbidity? Medicina (Kaunas). 2020;56(7):332.
28. Escudier MP, McGurk M. Symptomatic sialoadenitis and sialolithiasis in the English population, an estimate of the cost of hospital treatment. Br Dent J. 1999;186(9):463–6.
29. Yu C, Zheng L, Yang C, King AD. Causes of chronic obstructive parotitis and management by sialoendoscopy. Oral Surg Oral Med Oral Pathol Oral Radiol Endod. 2008;105(3):365–70.
30. Terraz S, Poletti PA, Dulguerov P, Dfouni N, Becker CD, Marchal F, et al. How reliable is sonography in the assessment of sialolithiasis? AJR Am J Roentgenol. 2013;201(1):W104–9.
31. Goncalves M, Schapher M, Iro H, Wuest W, Mantsopoulos K, Koch M. Value of sonography in the diagnosis of sialolithiasis: comparison with the reference standard of direct stone identification. J Ultrasound Med. 2017;36(11):2227–35.
32. Purcell YM, Kavanagh RG, Cahalane AM, Carroll AG, Khoo SG, Killeen RP. The diagnostic accuracy of contrast-enhanced CT of the neck for the investigation of sialolithiasis. AJNR Am J Neuroradiol. 2017;38(11):2161–6.
33. Drage NA, Brown JE. Cone beam computed sialography of sialoliths. Dentomaxillofac Radiol. 2009;38(5):301–5.
34. Ludlow JB, Ivanovic M. Comparative dosimetry of dental CBCT devices and 64-slice CT for oral and maxillofacial radiology. Oral Surg Oral Med Oral Pathol Oral Radiol Endod. 2008;106(1):106–14.
35. Scarfe WC, Farman AG, Sukovic P. Clinical applications of cone-beam computed tomography in dental practice. J Can Dent Assoc. 2006;72(1):75–80.
36. Capaccio P, Cuccarini V, Ottaviani F, Minorati D, Sambataro G, Cornalba P, et al. Comparative ultrasonographic, magnetic resonance sialographic, and videoendoscopic assessment of salivary duct disorders. Ann Otol Rhinol Laryngol. 2008;117(4):245–52.
37. Obaid H, Sinha R, Robinson L. Submandibular sialogram performed through a Wharton's duct fistula: technical adaptation of conventional technique. Eur J Radiol. 2006;60(1):56–7.
38. Kalinowski M, Heverhagen JT, Rehberg E, Klose KJ, Wagner HJL. Comparative study of MR sialography and digital subtraction sialography for benign salivary gland disorders. AJNR Am J Neuroradiol. 2002;23(9):1485–92.
39. McGahan JP, Walter JP, Bernstein L. Evaluation of the parotid gland. Comparison of sialography, non-contrast computed tomography and CT sialography. Radiology. 1984;152(2):453–8.
40. Becker M, Marchal F, Becker CD, Dulguerov P, Georgakopoulos G, Lehmann W, et al. Sialolithiasis and salivary ductal stenosis: diagnostic accuracy of MR sialography with a three-dimensional extended-phase conjugate-symmetry rapid spin-ECHO sequence. Radiology. 2000;217(2):347–58.
41. Strychowsky JE, Sommer DD, Gupta MK, Cohen N, Nahlieli O. Sialendoscopy for the management of obstructive salivary gland disease: a systematic review and meta-analysis. Arch Otolaryngol Head Neck Surg. 2012;138(6):541–7.
42. Nahlieli O, Shacham R, Yoffe B, Eliav E. Diagnosis and treatment of strictures and kinks in salivary gland ducts. J Oral Maxillofac Surg. 2001;59:484–90.
43. Bhansali S, Sarrami N. Oral surgery: self-milking the sialolith. Br Dental J. 2016;220:154.
44. Aidan P, De Kerviler E, LeDuc A, Monteil JP. Treatment of salivary stones by extracorporeal lithotripsy. Am J Otolaryngol. 1996;17(4):246–50.
45. Capaccio P, Ottaviani F, Manzo R, Schindler A, Cesana B. Extracorporeal lithotripsy for salivary calculi: a long-term clinical experience. Laryngoscope. 2004;114(6):1069–73.

46. Iro H, Zenk J, Waldfahrer F, Benzel W, Schneider T, Ell C. Extracorporeal shock wave lithotripsy of parotid stones. Results of a prospective clinical trial. Ann Otol Rhinol Laryngol. 1998;107(10 Pt 1):860–4.
47. Gutmann R, Ziegler G, Leunig A, Jacob K, Feyh J. Endoscopic and extracorporeal shock wave lithotripsy of salivary calculi. Laryngorhinootologie. 1995;74(4):249–53.
48. Park HS, Pae SY, Kim KY, Chung SM, Kim HS. Intraoral removal of stones in the proximal submandibular duct: usefulness of a surgical landmark for the hilum. Laryngoscope. 2013;123(4):934–7.
49. Capaccio P, Torretta S, Pignataro L. The role of adenectomy for salivary gland obstructions in the era of sialendoscopy and lithotripsy. Otolaryngol Clin N Am. 2009;42(6):1161–71.
50. Capaccio P, Torretta S, Pignataro L. Extracorporeal lithotripsy techniques for salivary stones. Otolaryngol Clin N Am. 2009;42(6):1139–59.
51. Marchal F, Becker M, Dulguerov P, Lehmann W. Interventional sialendoscopy. Laryngoscope. 2000;110(2 Pt 1):318–20.
52. Marchal F, Dulguerov P, Lehmann W. Interventional sialendoscopy. N Engl J Med. 1999;341(16):1242–3.
53. Marchal F, Dulguerov P, Becker M, Barki G, Disant F, Lehmann W. Specificity of parotid sialendoscopy. Laryngoscope. 2001;111(2):264–71.
54. Marchal F, Dulguerov P, Becker M, Barki G, Disant F, Lehmann W. Submandibular diagnostic and interventional sialendoscopy: new procedure for ductal disorders. Ann Otol Rhinol Laryngol. 2002;111(1):27–35.
55. Nahlieli O, Baruchin AM. Endoscopic technique for the diagnosis and treatment of obstructive salivary gland diseases. J Oral Maxillofac Surg. 1999;57(12):1394–401.
56. Nahlieli O, Nakar LH, Nazarian Y, Turner MD. Sialoendoscopy: a new approach to salivary gland obstructive pathology. J Am Dent Assoc. 2006;137:1394–400.
57. Marchal F. A combined endoscopic and external approach for extraction of large stones with preservation of parotid and submandibular glands. Laryngoscope. 2007;117(2):373–7.

Inflammatory Disorders of the Submandibular Gland

23

23.1 Epidemiology

The exact prevalence of submandibular sialadenitis is unclear. The submandibular gland is suggested to account for approximately 10% of all cases of sialadenitis of the major salivary glands. It accounts for about 0.001–0.002% of all hospital admissions. Sialadenosis is the most common cause of salivary gland swelling in the USA. There is no racial, gender, or age predilection for submandibular sialadenitis; however, in general, it tends to occur in older, debilitated, or dehydrated patients [1].

23.2 Etiology/Classification

Submandibular sialadenitis can be classified according to etiology into the following forms:

23.2.1 Acute Sialadenitis

Chronic non-autoimmune sialadenitis: non-calcular or calcular (sialolithiasis)

23.2.2 Autoimmune Sialadenitis

Individual causes of submandibular sialadenitis could be infectious (bacterial [often polymicrobial], viral, others), inflammatory, obstructive, drug-induced, or granulomatous as listed in Table 23.1.

© The Author(s), under exclusive license to Springer Nature Switzerland AG 2024
M. Sakr, *Surgery of the Salivary Glands*,
https://doi.org/10.1007/978-3-031-82069-4_23

Table 23.1 Causes of submandibular sialadenitis

Causes	Examples
Infectious bacterial	*Staphylococcus aureus*: the most common organism *Haemophilus influenzae* Gram-negative aerobes (e.g., Enterobacteriaceae) Anaerobes: *Prevotella, Fusobacterium, Peptostreptococcus*
Viral	Mumps Human immunodeficiency virus (HIV) Parainfluenza Epstein-Barr virus (EBV)
Others	Actinomycosis Tuberculosis (TB)
Inflammatory	Postradiation sialadenitis Contrast-induced sialadenitis [2] Radioiodine treatment (131I)
Obstructive	Sialolithiasis Ductal stricture Ductal foreign body, e.g., fish bone, hair, and grass blade External compression of duct, e.g., denture flanges Postoperative acute sialadenitis (after intubation)
Drug-induced	Clozapine L-asparaginase Phenylbutazone
Autoimmune	Sjögren's syndrome IgG4-related disease [3]
Granulomatous	Sarcoidosis Xantho-granulomatous sialadenitis

23.3 Pathophysiology

The main risk factors for the development of submandibular sialadenitis include reduced salivary secretion and duct obstruction. Hyposecretion of saliva can occur in dehydrated people, postoperative patients, and immuno-compromised and undernourished subjects. Medications that decrease salivary flow such as antihistamines, anticholinergic agents, diuretics, and beta-blockers can predispose to sialadenitis. Decreased salivary production can also occur in patients with a history of radiation to the head and neck region and long-standing xerostomia (e.g., Sjögren's syndrome) and those with chronic illness. Salivary duct obstruction is usually due to sialolithiasis, ductal stricture, ductal foreign body, and external compression of the duct by a tumor.

Other risk factors include old age, poor oral hygiene, and intubation [4]. Stasis of salivary flow through the ducts and parenchyma promotes acute suppurative infection. Retrograde contamination of salivary ducts and parenchymal tissues by bacteria inhabiting the oral cavity is common. Usually, submandibular sialadenitis is polymicrobial. *Staphylococcus aureus* is the most frequently isolated organism. Viral sialadenitis can result from mumps, parainfluenza, EBV, and HIV.

23.4 Histopathology

In acute suppurative submandibular sialadenitis, interstitial neutrophilic infiltration and necrosis with acinar destruction are often present. However, vacuolar changes in the acini cells and lymphocytic infiltration are more common in viral sialadenitis. On the other hand, dilated ducts with calculi, chronic inflammation, and fibrosis are evident in chronic sialadenitis mostly due to sialolith. In sialadenosis, there may be atrophy of parenchymal tissue and a compensatory increase in the amount of adipose tissue, but inflammatory infiltrates are absent.

23.5 Clinical Presentation

23.5.1 History-Taking

The diagnostic work-up of any submandibular enlargement begins with a thorough history-taking. This should include the number of glands involved, onset, duration of symptoms (acute versus chronic), recurrence, recent operative history, recent dental work, thorough drug history, immunization history (specifically measles, mumps, rubella [MMR] vaccine), medical comorbidities (e.g., alcohol use, diabetes mellites, bulimia, liver disease, autoimmune disease), past surgical history, and history of radiation therapy.

Symptoms to be inquired about include the presence of a mass, discomfort associated with swelling, aggravating factors (association with meals or salivary stimulants), bilaterality or unilaterality, skin changes, lymphadenopathy, dental pain, foul taste in the mouth, and skin discharge, in addition to constitutional symptoms such as associated fever or chills, viral prodrome, and weight loss and systemic symptoms such as joint pain, dry eyes/keratitis, shortness of breath, and oral discharge.

23.5.2 Physical Examination

23.5.2.1 Local Examination

Physical examination should begin with the gland itself. It includes "inspection" to observe the number of glands involved, erythema of overlying skin, and look for lingual papillary atrophy and loss of enamel from the tooth surface. "Palpation" of the gland is essential to note gland size, texture (consistency), tenderness, and the presence of calculi, and the ductal opening should be examined for purulence (massage of the gland may reveal purulent saliva at the ductal orifice). On examination, the gland is swollen, indurated, and tender. Cervical lymphadenitis may be present in cases of infections.

Acute unifocal salivary gland swelling due to obstructive sialadenitis is usually the result of salivary gland stones and/or strictures and is characterized by intermittent gland swelling occurring with the stimulation of meals. Mechanical obstruction of salivary flow within the duct causes swelling of the gland. Chronic or recurrent sialadenitis causes repeated episodes of pain and swelling, often with meals and recurrent infections.

Palpation should extend into the floor of the mouth as well as the soft tissue of the tongue, cheek, and neck. All of the major salivary glands should be examined for masses, symmetry, and the presence of discharge. An examination of cervical lymph nodes (LNs) is also required to detect the presence of lymphadenopathy.

23.5.2.2 Systemic Examination

Fever may be present. Viral sialadenitis (e.g., mumps) presents with acute multifocal salivary gland swelling accompanied by constitutional symptoms, including fever, headache, malaise, and myalgia. The eyes should be examined for any presence of interstitial keratitis. A focused cranial nerve examination should be conducted with particular attention to the facial nerve (CN-VII) especially the marginal mandibular nerve (MMN), trigeminal nerve (CN-V), and hypoglossal nerve (CN-XII). The lungs should be examined and a chest radiograph ordered if suspected pulmonary involvement exists.

23.6 Investigations

23.6.1 Laboratory Tests

Laboratory investigations should begin with the culture and sensitivity of exudate from the duct of the offending gland. This should be conducted before the initiation of empiric antibiotic therapy; the appropriate antibiotic is tailored according to sensitivity thereafter. As a rule, needle aspiration of a suspected abscess is not indicated. Blood cultures should be obtained if the patient is exhibiting bacteremia or sepsis.

Serum electrolytes and a complete blood count (CBC) with differential should be obtained to assess for any evidence of dehydration or systemic infection. If a diagnosis of autoimmunity is entertained, serum analysis for antinuclear antibody (ANA), SSA/anti-Ro, SSB/anti-La, and erythrocyte sedimentation rate (ESR) should be conducted.

23.6.2 Imaging Studies [5]

Numerous imaging techniques are available in submandibular imaging. Deciding which study to obtain first is often difficult.

23.6.3 Plain Radiography

Of all the radiological examinations available, one of the simplest examinations is conventional plain radiography [6]. Anteroposterior (AP), lateral, and oblique intraoral occlusal views are used. This technique is particularly valuable in evaluating the presence of calculi, which are radio-opaque in approximately 70–80% of cases. However, these radiographs do not provide any information about the ductal system or soft tissues.

23.6.4 Sialography

Sialography can be used to evaluate sialolithiasis or other obstructive entities, as well as inflammatory and neoplastic disease. In this technique, a water-soluble medium such as meglumine diatrizoate is injected into Wharton's duct, and lateral, oblique, and AP plain radiographs are obtained in order to assess the ductal arborization. Contraindications for this test are iodine allergy and acute sialadenitis.

Any filling defects (e.g., calculi), retained secretions (e.g., chronic sialadenitis), stricture formation (e.g., inflammation), extravasation (e.g., Sjögren's disease), or irregularly contoured borders (e.g., neoplasm) are noted.

23.6.5 Ultrasonography (US)

Ultrasonography (US) can be used to differentiate between solid versus cystic lesions of the gland. It can demonstrate sialolith (>1 mm), can also be used to differentiate intrinsic from extrinsic disease, and can be helpful in the identification of abscess formation. A 2009 study by Bozzato et al. determined that the application of ascorbic acid (vitamin C) as a contrast agent can aid in the US assessment of obstructive sialadenitis of the parotid and submandibular glands [7].

23.6.6 Computed Tomography (CT) Scan

Computed tomography (CT) scanning is indicated if conventional plain films are negative or when the clinical presentation is severe. Computed tomography (CT) scanning is an excellent modality in differentiating intrinsic versus extrinsic glandular disease. In chronic sclerosing sialadenitis, the salivary gland may be enlarged or atrophic. It is also extremely valuable in defining abscess formation versus phlegmon. It can demonstrate sialolith, but in general, it is limited in evaluating the ductal system unless combined with simultaneous sialography (CT sialography).

23.6.7 Magnetic Resonance Imaging (MRI)

Magnetic resonance imaging (MRI) is of little utility in sialadenitis or sialadenosis. It does not allow evaluation of the ductal system and is not helpful in defining calcifications. However, it is an excellent tool for soft tissue definition and is invaluable in instances of suspected neoplasia.

23.6.8 Biopsy Procedures

Biopsy procedures in cases of submandibular sialadenitis include fine-needle aspiration cytology (FNAC) and biopsy if suspicion of a solid neoplasm masquerading as sialadenitis is significant. Chronic sclerosing sialadenitis can present similarly to a tumor; FNA is useful to exclude the presence of a neoplasm [8]. An open biopsy of the lip should be considered when the diagnosis of Sjögren's disease is contemplated.

23.7 Differential Diagnosis

Differentials of submandibular sialadenitis include the following:

Infectious causes: bacterial (e.g., *Staphylococcus aureus*) or viral (e.g., mumps)
Granulomatous causes: tuberculosis (TB), sarcoidosis, cat scratch disease, actinomycosis
Autoimmune causes: Sjögren's disease, systemic lupus erythematosus (SLE)
Tumors: pleomorphic adenoma (PA), oncocytoma, ductal papilloma, adenoid cystic carcinoma (AdCC), squamous cell carcinoma (SCC), mucoepidermoid carcinoma (MEC)
Endocrine and metabolic causes: hypothyroidism, diabetes mellitus, bulimia, cirrhosis, vitamin deficiency, malabsorption
Drug-related disorder: e.g., thiourea

23.8 Treatment

Most patients with "acute sialadenitis" receive conservative medical management; this includes hydration, warm compresses, massage, pain relief with analgesics, and sialogogues. Empiric antibiotic therapy starts with amoxicillin/clavulanate or clindamycin. The selection of antibiotics should be according to culture and sensitivity reports. Intravenous antibiotics may be necessary in severe cases. If soft tissue swelling is significant and there is no contraindication, corticosteroid therapy is an option. Rarely, acute suppurative sialadenitis can lead to abscess formation; in such cases, surgical incision and drainage are indicated.

Medical management of "chronic sialadenitis" is with hydration, oral hygiene, pain relief, and sialogogues. In case of infection, broad-spectrum antibiotics are added. In the presence of sialolithiasis, salivary gland stone removal should take place, using interventional sialendoscopy or direct surgical removal [9, 10]. Extracorporeal shock wave lithotripsy (EWSL) under ultrasonic guidance is used for intraglandular duct stone removal. For recurrent sialadenitis (>3 episodes/year) or in chronic sclerosing sialadenitis, excision of the salivary gland itself (submandibular sialadenectomy) is recommended.

23.9 Prognosis

23.9.1 Outcome

Acute sialadenitis has an excellent prognosis. Complete resolution is usually the expectation following conservative outpatient management. Most of the acute symptoms resolve in a week; however, edema takes a longer time to disappear. Chronic sialadenitis can have multiple relapses and remissions.

The outcome of treatment is dependent on the etiology. If sialoliths require surgery, the prognosis is good. Symptoms of autoimmune sialadenitis often improve following medical management of the underlying condition (such as Sjögren's syndrome). With the treatment of the underlying cause, sialadenosis has an excellent prognosis.

23.9.2 Complications

The main complications of submandibular sialadenitis include the following:

23.9.3 Recurrence

Abscess formation: Infection may spread along the fascial planes of the neck, causing a potentially serious complication. Incision and drainage are required.

Dental decay: Hypofunction of the salivary gland with reduced saliva production causes decreased protection from acid erosion, promoting dental decay.

23.10 Acute Submandibular Sialadenitis

23.10.1 Etiology

Acute submandibular sialadenitis is an acute inflammation of the submandibular salivary gland. Causes may be bacterial or viral. Acute sialadenitis is usually secondary to obstruction of Wharton's duct and is often recurrent. The most common organism is *Staphylococcus aureus*. Other bacterial organisms include *Streptococcus viridans*, *Haemophilus influenzae*, *Streptococcus pyogenes*, and *Escherichia coli*. Infection is often the result of dehydration with overgrowth of the oral flora. The most common causes are postoperative dehydration, radiation therapy, and immunosuppression. Though rare in the neonate and prepubescent child, infection of the submandibular gland can result from other pathogens such as *Pseudomonas aeruginosa* and group B streptococci.

Though less common than bacteria, several viruses have been implicated in acute submandibular sialadenitis including mumps virus (typically affects the parotid gland), HIV, Coxsackievirus, parainfluenza types I and II, influenza, and herpes.

Acute postoperative sialadenitis can be caused by duct obstruction or submandibular gland injury [4]. Uchino et al. (2015) reported two cases of postoperative acute submandibular sialadenitis after neurosurgery. On postoperative day 1, the patients developed severe left neck swelling. Computed tomography (CT) scan revealed a profoundly edematous left submandibular gland. They suggested that patients who develop postoperative acute sialadenitis may experience severe upper airway swelling and obstruction, thus necessitating intubation [11].

23.10.2 Pathology

23.10.2.1 Gross Appearance

Grossly, for both acute bacterial and viral sialadenitis, the lobular architecture of the salivary gland is maintained, though the lobules may be expanded and friable with the color ranging from red to yellow. Areas of liquefaction indicative of abscess formation may be present. Cytomegalovirus (CMV) sialadenitis may show no gross abnormalities.

23.10.2.2 Microscopic Picture

Microscopically, acute bacterial sialadenitis is characterized by acinar destruction with interstitial infiltrates comprised mainly of neutrophils. Multiple small abscesses with necrosis are common. Occasionally, the bacteria can be seen with special stains such as gram stain and acid-fast stain, particularly in cases where antibiotics have not yet been administered. Acute viral sialadenitis is rarely examined histopathologically but consists of a lymphocytic and monocytic infiltrate in the interstitium with vacuolar change in the acini. CMV sialadenitis shows minimal inflammation but instead may show viral inclusions in both the acini and ducts [12].

23.10.3 Pathogenesis

23.10.3.1 Bacterial Sialadenitis

Bacterial sialadenitis typically occurs as a result of salivary stasis and subsequent retrograde contamination of the salivary ducto-acinar units by oral flora [13, 14].

The parotid is thought to be more prone to bacterial infection since its secretions are predominantly serous and thus lack the protective constituents (IgA, sialic acid, lysozymes) seen in mucinous secretions of the submandibular and sublingual salivary glands [15, 16].

Causes of salivary stasis include postsurgical setting, dehydration, medical illness, advanced age, radiation, medications, neonatal setting [17], sialectasia, and sialolithiasis Bacterial sialadenitis is often polymicrobial. The most common bacterial isolate in acute sialadenitis is *Staphylococcus aureus*. Streptococcal species, most notably the *viridans* streptococcal organisms, are also common, and more recently, the contributing role of anaerobic bacteria such as Bacteroides, peptostreptococcal, and fusobacterial species has been recognized.

Rarely, mycobacterial infection may present as an acute sialadenitis rather than a chronic granulomatous sialadenitis [13, 14, 18–20].

23.10.3.2 Viral Sialadenitis

Viral sialadenitis is typically systemic and can be most commonly attributed to the mumps paramyxovirus. Additional viral isolates include influenza, parainfluenza, Coxsackie A and B, Epstein-Barr (EBV), echovirus, and lymphocytic choriomeningitis virus [13, 20]. In the setting of human immunodeficiency virus (HIV), CMV and adenovirus have also rarely been implicated in acute viral sialadenitis [13].

23.10.3.3 Postoperative Acute Sialadenitis

Although rarely presented, it is thought that during head and neck surgery, the intraoperative head position and endotracheal intubation may lead to compression of the submandibular gland and surrounding tissues, thereby effectively limiting drainage and resulting in acute sialadenitis [11].

23.10.4 Clinical Picture

23.10.4.1 History-Taking

There is no age predilection; however, sialadenitis in general tends to occur in older, debilitated, or dehydrated patients [21]. No race or gender predilection exists.

The patient usually complains of a painful and tender unilateral swelling in the submandibular region and salivary colic, i.e., pain and swelling of the gland with meals. Pain may be referred to teeth or tongue. Infection of the submandibular gland can result in the formation of a submandibular abscess (Fig. 23.1). In such cases, the patient may

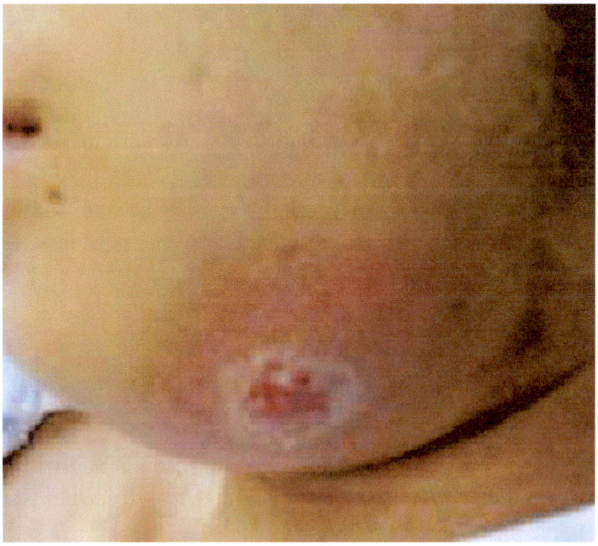

Fig. 23.1 A 33-year-old lady with a left submandibular gland abscess with overlying erythema and edema

appear toxic with features similar to acute sialadenitis and, sometimes, spiking fever. The infection may spread to other deep spaces of the neck. Trismus may be indicative of para-pharyngeal space involvement. Progression to Ludwig angina, a life-threatening infection of the submental and sublingual spaces, although rare, may occur.

Acute viral sialadenitis, in contrast, is preceded by prodromal symptoms including fever, myalgia, and headache and is typically bilateral [13, 20].

23.10.5 Physical Examination

Physical examination should begin with the gland itself. A tender swelling is felt bimanually. A stone in the duct may also be felt. The orifice of the duct will appear congested and edematous. It may pour drops of purulent saliva on squeezing the duct. Palpation should extend to include the floor of the mouth, tongue, cheek, and neck. All of the major salivary glands should be examined for masses, symmetry, and the presence of discharge. Cervical lymphadenopathy should also be noted. Both eyes should be examined for interstitial keratitis, and a cranial nerve examination should be conducted with particular attention to cranial nerves VII and XII.

23.10.6 Investigations (Work-Up)

23.10.6.1 Laboratory Tests

Laboratory investigations should begin with the culture of the gland prior to administration of antibiotics, in addition to blood cultures in the presence of bacteremia or sepsis. Needle aspiration of a suspected abscess is not indicated. Electrolytes and CBC should be obtained to assess for any evidence of dehydration or systemic infection.

23.10.6.2 Imaging Studies

Imaging studies should begin with a conventional plain X-ray, which is particularly valuable in evaluating the presence of calculi. Sialography is contraindicated in acute sialadenitis. Ultrasonography can differentiate between solid versus cystic lesions of the gland and is helpful in the identification of abscess formation. Computed tomography scanning is an excellent modality not only in differentiating intrinsic versus extrinsic glandular disease, but also in defining abscess formation versus phlegmon. Magnetic resonance imaging is of little utility in sialadenitis (or sialadenosis).

23.10.7 Treatment

Management of acute submandibular sialadenitis involves a wide range of approaches, from conservative medical treatment to more aggressive surgical intervention.

23.10.7.1 Medical Treatment

Medical management focuses on eliminating the causative factor, and the goals of pharmacotherapy are to eradicate the infection, reduce morbidity, and prevent complications. Adequate hydration should be ensured and electrolyte imbalances corrected. Sialogogues may temporarily increase salivary flow, but this frequently is short-lived, and better results are obtained by an overall increased fluid intake [22]. Patients are most often treated on an outpatient basis, with the administration of a single dose of parenteral antibiotics in an emergency department, followed by oral antibiotics for a period of 7–10 days. Clindamycin (900 mg IV q8h or 300 mg PO q8h) is an excellent choice and provides good coverage against typical organisms. In patients refractory to antibiotics, viral and atypical bacterial causes should be considered. In addition to antibiotics, patients may be treated with nonsteroidal anti-inflammatory medications, and narcotics may be needed in severe cases.

When possible, patients are instructed to empty the gland by external massage. The submandibular gland is best emptied by a constant compressive motion, starting below the mandible near the angle, with the hand sliding upward toward the chin. A short course of high-dose steroids reduces the peri-ductal inflammation and facilitates massage.

Patients who are septic, severely dehydrated, or exhibiting significant morbidity should be admitted to the hospital, and CT scanning of the affected area should be performed. Small abscesses usually respond to conservative methods; however, if a large abscess is noted, incision and drainage should be considered. Patients with sialolithiasis are initially treated with hydration, warm compresses, and gland massage, as well as antibiotics for the infected gland.

23.10.7.2 Surgical Treatment

Surgical management includes incision and drainage in case of abscess formation and excision of the gland, during a period of quiescence, in patients with recurrent acute sialadenitis. Endoscopic management of sialadenitis frequently obviates the need for gland excision. Results follow a learning curve [7].

23.10.8 Prognosis

The prognosis of acute submandibular sialadenitis is very good. Most cases are easily treated with conservative medical measures, and hospital admission is the exception, not the rule. Generally, prognosis is largely dependent on the patient's underlying disease and its successful treatment.

Acute symptoms of acute submandibular sialadenitis usually resolve within 5–7 days; however, edema in the area may last several weeks. A small number will progress to chronic sialadenitis after resolution of the acute sialadenitis [13]. Patients with sialolithiasis require definitive surgical treatment in the quiescent stage, in most cases, which results in an excellent prognosis and resolution of signs and symptoms.

23.11 Chronic Non-autoimmune Submandibular Sialadenitis

23.11.1 Etiology

Chronic sialadenitis is associated with conditions linked to decreased salivary flow, rather than dehydration. These conditions include salivary stasis, a change in the fluid and electrolyte composition of the gland, and mechanical obstruction of Wharton's duct. Proximal to the site of chronic obstruction, the duct will be dilated with retention of secretions and chronic infection. Causes of obstruction include calculi, strictures, edema or fibrosis of the papilla, pressure on the duct by adjacent masses, or duct invasion by a malignant neoplasm.

23.11.2 Papillary Stenosis

Ulceration of the papilla of the submandibular duct may follow trauma from a denture. The obstruction and recurrent swelling will subside as the ulcer heals. Repeated trauma results in fibrosis which is only relieved by papillotomy with suture of the duct lining to the oral mucosa.

23.11.3 Sialolithiasis

Salivary calculi (sialolithiasis) relate to the formation and deposition of concretions within the ductal system of the gland. Approximately 85% of all salivary calculi occur in the submandibular gland [23] with approximately 70% of these demonstrable as radio-opacities on routine plain radiography. The calculi vary in size and may be single or multiple. The formation of calculi is associated with chronic sialadenitis and, in particular, the recurrent nature of the problem. The exact mechanism of stone formation is unclear, but it appears to be related to the following conditions:

Salivary stagnation (stasis): The secretion of the submandibular gland is more viscid than that of the parotid gland, and Wharton's duct is independent (directed forwards and upwards).

Duct obstruction: The end of the duct opens in the floor of the mouth and is more liable to be obstructed by a stone, inflammation, and foreign bodies such as a small piece of a toothbrush or food particles.

Epithelial injury along the duct: This results in sialolith formation, which acts as a nidus for further stone formation.

Precipitation of calcium salts: The stones themselves are typically composed of calcium phosphate, calcium carbonate, and magnesium phosphate, in association with other salts and organic material such as glycoproteins, desquamated cellular residue, and mucopolysaccharides.

23.11.4 Granulomatous Sialadenitis

Granulomatous sialadenitis can result from tuberculosis, mycosis, sarcoidosis, or duct obstruction from calculi or malignant tumors. In the latter instance, granulomas result from the rupture of ducts and may contain small pools of mucin.

23.11.5 Tuberculosis (TB)

Tuberculosis (TB) is a necrotizing granulomatous disease with a high morbidity and mortality. Extrapulmonary tuberculosis accounts for at least 30% of TB in certain regions of the world such as India [24]. Involvement of the salivary glands is rare and may take place secondary to systemic dissemination from a distant focus, especially the lungs, or, less commonly, as a primary tuberculous sialadenitis. Both, Mycobacterium tuberculosis (TB) and atypical mycobacterium, can affect LNs adjacent to salivary glands or intraglandular LNs. Primary involvement presents with a myriad of clinical features, and therefore, a high index of suspicion is necessary to diagnose this entity.

23.11.6 Sarcoidosis

Sarcoidosis is a systemic disease involving multiple organs. Its etiology remains unclear, but several hypotheses have been made, including auto-antigens and infectious organisms. It resembles TB but with no caseation. Salivary glands are usually affected, specifically the parotid glands. Symptoms include swellings and xerostomia. Sometimes, the disease may present as a mass, and the diagnosis is only made after surgical excision of the presumed tumor—the sarcoid pseudotumor. Laboratory diagnosis is made through amylase, kallikrein, and the ACE test. Radiological and histological evidence of non-caseous epithelial granulomas is confirmatory. Corticosteroids are the best therapeutic option.

Heerfordt's syndrome is a rare form of sarcoidosis that involves parotid swelling, anterior uveitis, facial palsy, and fever (uveoparotid fever). It usually affects young patients in their third decade of life [25].

23.11.7 Pathogenesis

The predilection of sialoliths (calculi) to form in the submandibular gland is thought to be a result of the alkaline pH and high mucin content of its secretions. The nidus for stone formation has been postulated to arise from bacterial or organic debris [13, 20]. However, recent scanning electron microscopy and X-ray crystallography studies refuted this as a major cause, finding only hydroxyapatite crystals rich in calcium phosphates [26].

The mechanisms for radiation sialadenitis are not entirely understood, but recent T-cell subset evaluations suggest a possible immune-mediated component of injury [27, 28].

Two theories can explain the pathogenesis of tuberculous sialadenitis. Most commonly, the involvement of salivary glands is "secondary" to systemic dissemination from a distant focus, especially the lungs, via hematogenous or lymphatic spread. Secondary TB involves the submandibular and sublingual glands more frequently than the parotid glands. Rarely, an infected source of mycobacteria in the oral cavity, such as tonsils or teeth, liberates these bacilli, which then spread to the nearby salivary gland through direct inoculation by sputum, retrograde ascent of bacilli through the salivary duct, or by afferent lymphatics to its associated LNs. This "primary" tuberculous involvement of the salivary glands is rare, and unlike the secondary form, the most common site of involvement in the literature seems to be the parotid gland (70%) [29]. A review by van der Walt and Leake (2001) showed that tuberculous sialadenitis comprised 14% (8/57) of cases of granulomatous sialadenitis [30].

23.11.8 Pathology

23.11.8.1 Gross Appearance

Chronic sialadenitis on gross examination ranges from unremarkable to a firm tan with expansion or atrophy of the lobular architecture depending on the degree of inflammation and chronicity. With sialolithiasis, stones may be grossly evident with associated obstructive changes of sialectasia and periductal fibrosis. Mucus extravasation may be noted as well [12].

Radiation sialadenitis may show a fibrous white cut surface with the involvement of adjacent soft tissue. When the residual lobules are noted, they may be attenuated with interstitial fibrosis.

23.11.8.2 Microscopic Picture

Microscopically, the classic findings of chronic sialadenitis are a chronic inflammatory infiltrate composed of lymphocytes, plasma cells and macrophages, fibrosis, acinar atrophy, and mucous cell metaplasia of the ductal system (Fig. 23.2) [20].

A common regenerative phenomenon is the presence of intercalated duct hyperplasia that may be diffuse or nodular. In sialolithiasis, dark calcific stone fragments are noted within the ducts which may have a concomitant squamous metaplasia. Infectious granulomatous sialadenitis ranges from the caseating granulomatosis seen in tuberculosis to foamy histiocytic aggregates seen in atypical mycobacterial infections. Intra- and peri-parotid lymph node (LN) involvement may be seen in the latter [31]. Acid-fast stains will highlight the mycobacterial organisms.

The presence of granuloma with central necrosis surrounded by epithelioid cells and Langhan's giant cells is the histopathological hallmark for diagnosis of tuberculous sialadenitis.

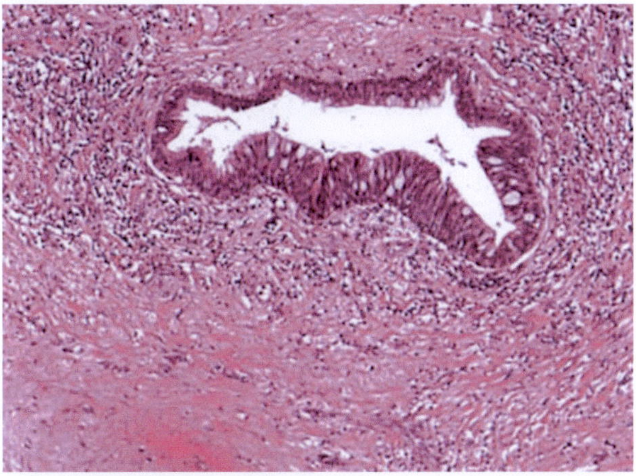

Fig. 23.2 Chronic sialadenitis with periductal fibrosis and a mixed chronic inflammatory infiltrate around a large duct that shows mucinous metaplasia (H&E, ×100)

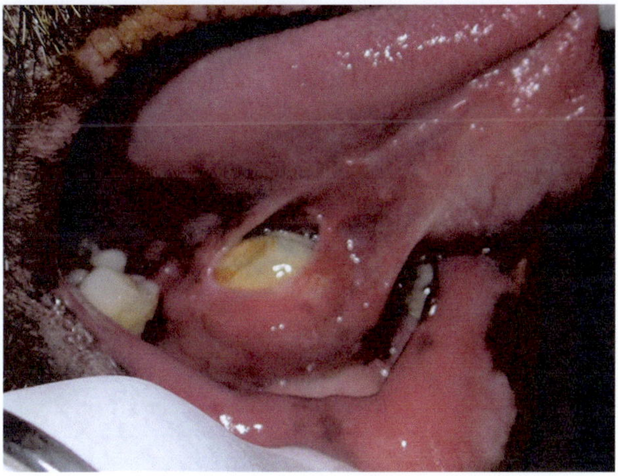

Fig. 23.3 A huge Wharton duct stone causing chronic calcular submandibular sialadenitis (non-autoimmune)

23.11.9 Clinical Picture

Chronic non-autoimmune sialadenitis is often attributable to a specific etiologic factor such as recurrent obstruction (i.e., sialolithiasis; Fig. 23.3), irradiation, granulomatous disease [12, 20], or rarely infectious granulomatous disease [12, 19].

Clinically, chronic non-autoimmune sialadenitis is characterized by a variety of symptoms ranging from a long-standing swelling or mass to xerostomia and superinfection. Chronic sialadenitis, often resulting in xerostomia, is a common and dreaded complication of radiotherapy for head and neck malignant neoplasms [27, 28]. Chronic sialadenitis is typically less painful than acute sialadenitis and is associated with recurrent enlargement of the gland (often following meals) typically without erythema (Fig. 23.4).

The patient usually presents with a firm or hard submandibular swelling, which simulates a tumor and increases in size with meals. Pain is associated with meals,

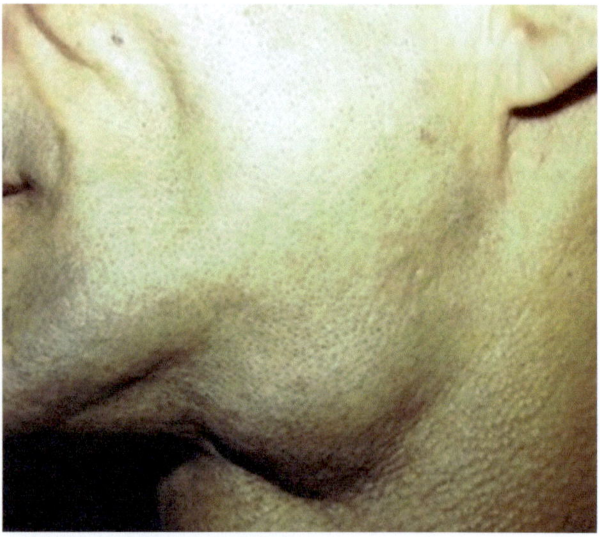

Fig. 23.4 A 56-year-old gentleman with left chronic submandibular sialadenitis. It could not be rolled over the lower edge of the mandible

and this helps to differentiate it from pain of dental origin. Intake of lemon juice (lemon juice test) causes aggravation of pain and an increase in the size of the swelling.

Oral examination of the orifice of the duct reveals saliva pouring on the unaffected side, with little or no secretion seen ejecting from the swollen (affected) side. With bimanual examination, a stone may be felt within the duct or within the gland. The swelling itself may also be felt.

In the case of tuberculous sialadenitis, the patient may suffer from one or more of the systemic manifestations of TB such as low-grade fever, night sweating, and anemia. The enlarged submandibular gland (Fig. 23.5) is firm and nodular but may become cystic with sinuses and little pain.

23.11.10 Investigations

Submandibular calculi are relatively easy to demonstrate by plain radiography. Sialography may show a filling defect, if the stone is translucent. The application of ascorbic acid as a contrast agent can aid in the ultrasound assessment of obstructive sialadenitis of the submandibular (and parotid) glands.

Different diagnostic modalities of tuberculous sialadenitis include FNAC, acid-fast staining, mycobacterial culture, and tuberculosis-polymerase chain reaction (TB-PCR), which is considered the best preoperative laboratory diagnostic tool [32]. However, a definite diagnosis is only confirmed with histopathology after the excision of the involved gland.

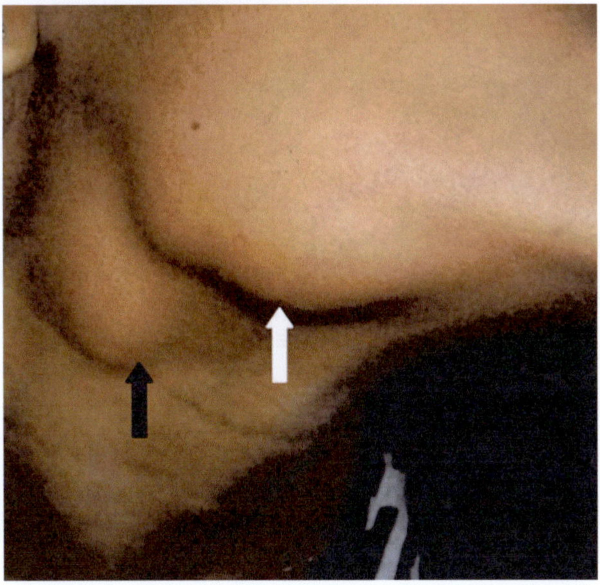

Fig. 23.5 A 33-year-old lady with right tuberculous submandibular sialadenitis (white arrow) and associated cervical lymphadenopathy (black arrow)

23.11.11 Treatment

Chronic non-calcular sialadenitis is usually considered a medical disease, with surgical intervention reserved for intractable symptoms of pain and swelling.

In patients with calculi in the proximity of Wharton's duct opening, the duct can be cannulated and dilated and the stone removed via a trans-oral approach. For ductal calculi in the floor of the mouth, a stitch is passed under the duct proximal to the stone to stop the stone from slipping backward. An incision is made in the mucosa over the duct, which is then mobilized, and a stay suture is passed under the duct to bring it up into the top of the wound and to control it while the wall is incised to release the stone. Patients with deep intraparenchymal, recurrent, or multiple stones should have their glands excised (submandibular sialadenectomy) on an elective basis. Ultrasonic lithotripsy is rarely effective.

For tuberculous sialadenitis, the timely institution of specific treatment is essential for establishing a cure. It includes multidrug therapy for an average of 1 year together with exposure to direct sunlight, good aeration, and well-balanced nutrition to enhance general health and immunity. A four-drug regimen (rifampicin, isoniazid, ethambutol, and pyrazinamide) in the intensive phase followed by two drugs (rifampicin and isoniazid) in the continuation phase is the recommended treatment [33, 34].

23.11.12 Prognosis

The prognosis depends on the etiological factor, if identified, and the severity of the disease. While surgical treatment of chronic sialadenitis leads to the resolution of symptoms of pain and prevention of superinfection with fistula or sinus tract formation [35], xerostomia, often seen in radiation sialadenitis, does not resolve [27, 28].

23.12 Chronic Autoimmune Submandibular Sialadenitis

23.12.1 General Features

23.12.1.1 Etiology (Types)

The majority of autoimmune sialadenitis is in the histopathological spectrum of myoepithelial sialadenitis (MESA) [36], also known as benign lymphoepithelial lesions.

The clinical correlates are varied and include terms such as Mikulicz's disease, sicca complex, Sjögren's syndrome, and chronic punctate sialadenitis [12]. Other systemic autoimmune diseases that can affect the salivary glands, usually the parotid, include Wegener's granulomatosis, sarcoidosis, Kimura's disease [25], and a subset of chronic sclerosing sialadenitis (Küttner's tumor) [37].

23.12.1.2 Pathogenesis

While Sjögren's syndrome often has a characteristic serology, including anti-SS-A, anti-SS-B, and occasionally ANA and rheumatoid factor, the pathogenesis of the disease is not entirely clear and is multifactorial as with most autoimmune diseases [38]. In addition to HLA-DR associations, recent studies suggest that polymorphisms in genes, such as minor histocompatibility antigen HA-1, and TNF may play a role in the disease process. Humoral dysregulation and B-cell hyperactivity are thought to be another pathogenic mechanism for Sjögren's syndrome [38, 39].

Similarly, though the serological manifestations are well known, the pathogenesis of Wegener's granulomatosis, sarcoidosis, Kimura's disease, and chronic sclerosing sialadenitis is not well understood. The classic serological manifestation of Wegener's granulomatosis is a positive C-ANCA. Sarcoidosis often manifests with hypergammaglobulinemia as well as non-serological laboratory abnormalities such as hypercalcemia, elevated alkaline phosphatase, and angiotensin-converting enzyme levels. Kimura's disease is characterized by elevated IgE levels. Sialadenitis with elevated IgG4 levels has been noted recently [25, 37, 40].

23.12.2 Pathology

23.12.2.1 Gross Appearance

The gross manifestations of myoepithelial sialadenitis are similar to chronic nonimmune sialadenitis, ranging from diffuse to multinodular expansion. In some cases, the gross cut surface is a tan pink reminiscent of a lymph node (LN); however, the lobular architecture is maintained distinguishing this from lymphoma. Wegener's granulomatosis may show areas of liquefaction necrosis as a result of vasculitis. Sarcoidosis and Kimura's disease may show preferential enlargement of the intra/periparotid LNs. Chronic sclerosing sialadenitis on gross examination resembles a salivary gland neoplasm and with a well-circumscribed tan-white appearance.

23.12.2.2 Microscopic Picture

The histological hallmark of MESA is the presence of epithelial-myoepithelial islands infiltrated by lymphocytes (Fig. 23.6).

However, the process begins as a collection of lymphocytes centered on an intralobular duct. This lymphoid infiltrate, when a cluster of at least 50 lymphocytes/4 mm^2 defines a lymphoid focus, is the basis for grading labial minor salivary gland biopsies for the diagnosis of Sjögren's syndrome [41, 42]. As these lymphoid infiltrates progress, germinal centers may form, and acinar atrophy ensues. A proliferation of ductal epithelium-myoepithelium arises, obliterating duct lumina and eventually giving rise to classic epithelial-myoepithelial islands. A few studies suggest that these islands may not contain a myoepithelial component but are composed of metaplastic intercalated ducts with an altered immunophenotype [43, 44].

Salivary glands in the setting of secondary Sjögren's syndrome due to progressive systemic sclerosis may show peri-glandular fibrosis without inflammation in addition to MESA [42]. Wegener's granulomatosis manifests as a classic triad of vasculitis, necrosis, and granulomatous inflammation; however, only 16% of cases with parotid involvement have the complete triad [25]. Sarcoid disease is characterized by tight epithelioid granulomas and a lymphoid infiltrate. Biopsies of minor salivary glands present in the lip for the diagnosis of sarcoid show granulomas in 53% of cases [45].

Chronic sclerosing sialadenitis bears a remarkable similarity to lymphoplasmacytic sclerosing pancreatitis [40]. It is characterized by peri-ductal fibrosis with a dense lymphoplasmacytic infiltrate with lymphoid follicles. Eosinophils are variably

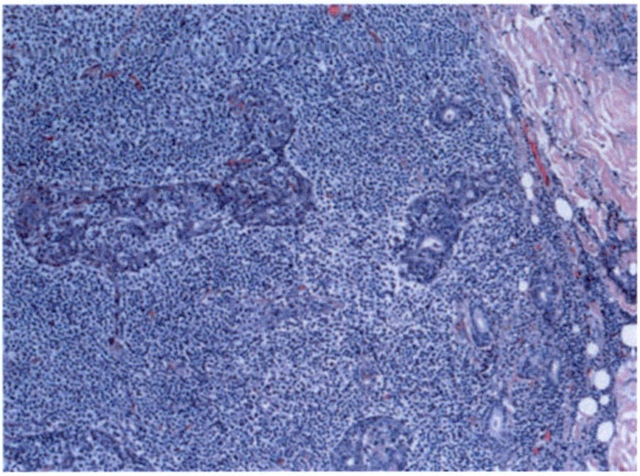

Fig. 23.6 Myoepithelial sialadenitis (MESA) with a florid lymphoid infiltrate and prominent epithelial myoepithelial islands permeated by lymphocytes (H&E, ×100)

present. Kitagawa et al. (2005) demonstrated the presence of obliterative phlebitis in all cases of chronic sclerosing sialadenitis as demonstrated by elastic stain [37].

23.12.3 Clinical Features

23.12.3.1 Myoepithelial Sialadenitis

Myoepithelial sialadenitis may present as unilateral or bilateral enlargement of salivary glands, at any age with or without autoimmune disease, but most commonly manifests in females in their 5th–sixth decade as a reflection of the close association with Sjögren's syndrome [20].

23.12.3.2 Sjögren's Syndrome

Sjögren's syndrome is an autoimmune exocrinopathy characterized by keratoconjunctivitis, xerostomia, and often other extra-salivary manifestations. It can exist as a primary disease or as a secondary disease associated with other systemic autoimmune diseases, typically rheumatoid arthritis and occasionally progressive systemic sclerosis [38].

23.12.3.3 Wegener's Granulomatosis

Involvement of salivary glands in Wegener's granulomatosis is characterized by upper and lower respiratory tract and renal disease and is rare with the parotid being most commonly affected [25]. Fauci et al. (1983) [46] reported an incidence of <1% ($n = 158$) in their experience.

23.12.3.4 Sarcoidosis

Sarcoidosis involvement of the salivary gland is not infrequent, ranging from 4–30%. A rare syndromic variant of sarcoidosis known as Heerfordt syndrome is characterized by uveitis, bilateral parotitis, and facial nerve palsy [25].

23.12.3.5 Kimura's Disease

Kimura's disease occurs typically in young Asian males and is characterized clinically by painless lymphadenopathy of the head and neck region, including periparotid and intra-parotid LNs [44, 46].

23.12.3.6 Chronic Sclerosing Sialadenitis

Chronic sclerosing sialadenitis presents as a firm localized swelling of the salivary gland mimicking a neoplasm, most commonly involving the submandibular glands [20].

23.12.4 Prognosis

As with most sialadenitis, the prognosis of chronic autoimmune sialadenitis is related to the severity and treatment of the underlying disorder [47]. It is noteworthy that patients with Sjögren's syndrome have a 40-fold increased risk for the development of small B-cell lymphomas of mucosa-associated lymphoid tissue (MALT) type [38].

23.12.5 Sjögren's Syndrome (SS)

23.12.5.1 Clinical Presentation

Sjögren's syndrome (SS) is an autoimmune disease involving the parotid glands more frequently than the submandibular glands. Females are affected more than males (10:1). The disease, which is associated with keratoconjunctivitis sicca, xerostomia (due to progressive destruction of both salivary and lacrimal glands), salivary gland enlargement, and lingual papillary atrophy, is confirmed through a biopsy of the minor salivary glands of the lip. The diseased gland is occasionally enlarged and is occasionally painful. Secondary bacterial ascending infection may occur as a result of dry mouth.

23.12.5.2 Diagnosis

Numerous laboratory tests are also used to confirm the diagnosis, such as autoantibodies Sjögren's syndrome A (SS-A) and Sjögren's syndrome B (SS-B), rheumatoid factor, and antinuclear antibodies. Erythrocyte sedimentation rate should also be conducted. Lack of lacrimal secretion can be shown by the Schirmer test and keratitis by Rose Bengal and fluorescein staining.

Computed tomography (CT) scan and MRI show bilateral gland enlargement with heterogeneously enhancing parenchyma. The CT scan may show a honeycomb appearance with low-density foci in a generally enhancing gland.

Histologically, primary SS is characterized by massive progressive lymphocytic infiltration, acinar cell destruction, and ductal epithelial cell proliferation (causing blockage of smaller ducts) affecting all salivary and lacrimal glands. Intense infiltration of the gland with lymphocytes can result in diffuse enlargement or the formation of localized nodules, which must be distinguished from neoplasms. Mucous gland metaplasia of the duct epithelium leads to the formation of gelatinous saliva in some patients.

Secondary Sjögren's syndrome differs from the primary type in that it is associated with a connective tissue disorder, symptoms are less severe, and the incidence of lymphomatous transformation (most commonly monocytoid B-cell lymphoma) is also less common [38].

23.12.6 Treatment

There is no known specific treatment available to stop Sjögren's syndrome, and thus, management is totally symptomatic. Artificial tears and periodic ophthalmological examination are mandatory to avoid corneal ulcerations. Lateral tarsorrhaphy may be indicated in some cases. Artificial salivary substitutes (sprays, rinses, etc.) are available, and their importance increases in the dentate patient where fluoride should be added as well. Usually, the patient consumes a large amount of water daily. Artificial nasal sprays are also available for dryness of the nasal mucosa [48]. Steroids and immunosuppressive agents generally alter the course of the disease but are rarely used in view of their side effects and the increased risk of ascending infection. Gland excision is rarely indicated [48].

23.12.7 Mikulicz's Disease/Syndrome

Mikulicz (Johann von Mikulicz-Radecki, 1850–1905, a Polish surgeon) described this autoimmune disease in 1892, as a triad that includes (1) symmetrical bilateral enlargement of all the salivary glands, (2) narrowing of the palpebral fissures due to enlargement of the lacrimal glands, and (3) parchment-like dryness of the mouth. Mikulicz's disease (MD) is also called a "benign lympho-epithelial lesion" or "myoepithelial sialadenitis" [49].

The disease almost always occurs in association with another underlying disease such as tuberculosis, syphilis, sarcoidosis, leukemia, lymphoma, or systemic lupus erythematosus. In such cases, it is referred to as "Mikulicz's syndrome." Patients may experience recurring fever [22].

Mikulicz's disease affects the parotid glands in 85% of cases and the submandibular in 15%. It occurs more among women (60–80%) with a mean age of 50 years and causes firm, diffuse enlargement of the affected gland. Patients are usually asymptomatic but may complain of mild pain and are at a higher risk of developing lymphomas. It is believed by some authors to be a variant of SS. In Mikulicz's disease, there is lymphocytic infiltration, parenchymal atrophy, myoepithelial islands, and duct changes signifying chronic inflammation. Actually, the main clinical difference between Mikulicz's disease and SS is the preservation of the lacrimation and salivation in Mikulicz's disease due to much less gland cell apoptosis than that found in SS [38].

23.12.8 Benign Lymphoepithelieal Lesion (Myoepithelial Sialadenitis [MESA])

Benign lymphoepithelial lesion (myoepithelial sialadenitis) (MESA) mostly affects females over 50 years of age. Patients present with a diffusely enlarged, firm, and often painful parotid gland, which is bilateral in 20% of cases. Sialography shows sialectasia, which ranges from punctuate to cavitary. Management is usually parotidectomy to establish a final diagnosis.

Histopathological examination of the excised gland carries the very same previously described histopathological features of Sjögren's syndrome, and so the differentiation between both is only done on clinical grounds. Prolonged follow-up of such patients is mandatory as 20% of them will develop lymphoma at a certain time [50].

23.12.9 Other Autoimmune Sialadenitis

23.12.9.1 Wegener's Granulomatosis

Wegener's granulomatosis is an autoimmune disease characterized by upper and lower respiratory and renal disease. The most common salivary gland to be involved is the parotid gland [25]; however, this occurs in less than 1% of the cases [46].

23.12.9.2 Chronic Sclerosing Sialadenitis (Küttner's Tumor)

Immunoglobulin G4-related diseases (IgG4-RD) are a recently emerged entity [3]. They are defined as a systemic fibro-inflammatory disorder of unknown origin which can affect virtually every organ of the body. They have a predilection for the Japanese and Chinese populations [51]. Chronic sclerosing sialadenitis is a part of the IgG4-RD spectrum [52]. It presents as a painless, firm, localized mass lesion in any of the major or minor salivary glands and often mimics malignancy. Küttner's tumor is a fibro-inflammatory disorder which classically affects the submandibular salivary gland [53].

Chronic sclerosing sialadenitis presents as a firm localized swelling of the salivary gland mimicking a neoplasm, most commonly involving the submandibular gland. It may be associated with autoimmune extra-salivary diseases such as primary sclerosing cholangitis and idiopathic retroperitoneal fibrosis [50].

23.13 Special Consideration

23.13.1 Myoepithelial Sialadenitis and Mucosa-Associated Lymphoid Tissue (MALT) Lymphomas

Most salivary gland lymphomas are of the MALT type and arise in the setting of MESA. This association was noted as early as 1971 by Azzopardi and Evans [54]. The transition from MESA to MALT lymphoma is postulated to occur as a result of antigenic stimulation, though, unlike gastric MALT lymphoma, the etiological agent (*H. pylori* in gastric MALT lymphoma) has not been identified [55]. The histological distinction of MESA from early MALT lymphoma is obfuscated by the detection of clonal proliferations in otherwise typical appearing MESA [56, 57].

These MESA clones have a limited VH repertoire even among different patients, suggesting antigenic stimulation from a common epitope [55]. While these clones say eventually give rise to MALT lymphoma, clonality in the setting of typical or even atypical MESA without a significant mass lesion does not indicate lymphoma. The earliest histological changes of MALT lymphoma are the presence of "halos" of monocytoid or centrocyte-like B cells that are slightly paler on low power magnification [58]. These coalesce into sheets and eventually form mass lesions. Involvement of intra- and peri-parotid lymph nodes is often seen. Immunohistochemical and flow cytometric analyses show a population of B cells that are CD19-positive, CD20-positive, CD5-negative, CD10-negative, and

CD23-negative. CD43, typically seen on T cells, may be aberrantly expressed. MALT lymphomas will often but not always show light chain restriction [59].

Mucosa-associated lymphoid tissue lymphomas have several associated characteristic translocations and trisomies, though the frequencies of these vary by site. In the salivary gland, the most common translocation is (q32;q21), which is the fusion of IGH/MALT1 [22, 34], while trisomy 3 was the most common alteration overall. The significance of these alterations is unclear at this point [60].

23.13.2 Myoepithelial Sialadenitis and Carcinoma

In rare instances, MESA can have a malignant transformation of the epithelial component. Carcinomas arising in MESA are typically lymphoepithelial carcinomas resembling undifferentiated non-keratinizing nasopharyngeal carcinoma, though keratinizing squamous cell carcinomas have been described [61–63].

Lymphoepithelial carcinomas of the salivary gland are often associated with Epstein-Barr virus (EBV) infection. Wu et al. demonstrated the presence of EBV small RNA-1 (EBER-1) in MESA with carcinomatous transformation in both the benign and malignant areas, while typical MESA was negative for EBER [64].

23.13.3 Necrotizing Sialometaplasia (NSM)

23.13.3.1 Clinical Features

Necrotizing sialometaplasia (NSM), originally described by Abrams et al. in 1973 [65], is a benign self-healing salivary gland lesion that can mimic malignancy. It typically occurs in the fourth decade (mean age 45.9 years) with a male predilection with a ratio of 2:1 [20, 66–68]. Although the palate is the most frequently involved site, NSM has been described in mucoserous glands throughout the upper and lower respiratory tract [66, 69–71]. The usual presentation is that of a single unilateral ulcer at the junction of the hard and soft palate [20, 66, 67]. Roughly 10% are bilateral, and 15% are asymptomatic [66].

23.13.3.2 Pathology

Grossly, NSM is typically a well-demarcated, raised, erythematous ulcer. The underlying salivary tissue is a soft friable gray tan [12, 20]. In a review of 184 cases, the mean size was 1.9 cm (range 0.7–5.0 cm) [66].

The defining microscopic features are ulceration with pseudo-epitheliomatous hyperplasia of the adjacent mucosa; infarction of the salivary lobule, with mucus extravasation; varying degrees of fibrosis; and squamous metaplasia of the ducto-acinar units. The latter may be prominent and thus misread as mucoepidermoid carcinoma (MEC) or squamous cell carcinoma (SCC). However, the key distinguishing feature of NSM from the malignant lesions that it may mimic is the maintenance of the lobular architecture despite the often extensive squamous metaplasia. On small biopsy specimens, this may be difficult to assess. Though a high index of suspicion of this lesion is the main requirement for its diagnosis in such a situation, a recent study suggests that NSM in contrast to SCC does not show evidence of immunohistochemical (IHC) staining for p53, Ki-67, and bcl-2 and thus may be a useful adjunct for distinguishing between these lesions [72].

23.13.3.3 Pathogenesis

The classic NSM is thought to be the result of spontaneous infarction of mucoserous glands. However, a clinically and histologically identical picture is seen as a result of surgery, radiation, trauma, or vasculitis among other distortive injuries [73, 74]. The self-limiting nature and histologic features suggest a vascular compromise with ischemic injury and subsequent regeneration as the main pathogenic mechanism [20, 66]. The occasional association with repeated emesis seen in bulimia and other disorders raises the possibility of chemical injury as a contributing factor [75, 76].

23.13.3.4 Prognosis

The prognosis of necrotizing sialometaplasia is excellent. It is a self-limiting lesion lasting from a few days to a few months and does not recur [66].

23.13.3.5 Postradiation Sialadenitis

Radiation-induced sialadenitis is frequently seen in patients who receive radiation for the treatment of oropharyngeal cancer. The first clinical sign is reduced saliva flow which has been reported to occur with radiation dose thresholds as low as 15 Gy [77]. The classical imaging findings of radiation-induced sialadenitis include hyper-enhancement of the salivary glands that progresses to atrophy over time. This hyper-enhancement occurs with doses >45 Gy and is thought to represent contrast expanding the extracellular space that was once occupied by acinar cells lost from radiation [78]. Over time, chronic scarring/fibrosis leads to volume loss and magnetic resonance imaging typically demonstrates low-to-intermediate signal intensity on all sequences [79].

References

1. Chandak R, Degwekar S, Chandak M, Rawlani S. Acute submandibular sialadenitis-a case report. Case Rep Dent. 2012;2012:615375.
2. Lucarelli A, Perandini S, Borsato A, Strazimiri E, Montemezzi S. Iodinated contrast-induced sialadenitis: a review of the literature and sonographic findings in a clinical case. J Ultrason. 2018;18(75):359–64.
3. Gurwale SG, Gore CR, Gulati I, Dey I. Immunoglobulin G4-related chronic sclerosing sialadenitis: an emerging entity. J Oral Maxillofac Pathol. 2020;24(Suppl 1):S135–8.
4. Urits I, Orhurhu V, Chesteen G, Yazdi C, Viswanath O. Acute sialadenitis after intubation. Turk J Anaesthesiol Reanim. 2020;48(3):263.
5. Abdel Razek AAK, Mukherji S. Imaging of sialadenitis. Neuroradiol J. 2017;30(3):205–15.
6. Isacsson G, Isberg A, Haverling M, Lundquist PG. Salivary calculi and chronic sialoadenitis of the submandibular gland: a radiographic and histologic study. Oral Surg Oral Med Oral Pathol. 1984;58(5):622–7.

7. Bozzato A, Hertel V, Koch M, Zenk J, Iro H. [Vitamin C as contrast agent in diagnosis of salivary duct obstruction]. Laryngorhinootologie. 2009;88(5):290–2.
8. Zhang YY, Hong X, Wang Z, Li W, Su JZ, Chen Y, et al. Diagnostic utility of submandibular and labial salivary gland biopsy in IgG4-related sialadenitis. Clin Rheumatol. 2020;39(12):3715–21.
9. Klinovskaya AS, Gurgenadze AP, Bazikyan EA, Abrahamyan KD, Chunikhin AA. Sialendoscopy in diagnosis and treatment of salivary gland disorders. Stomatologiia (Mosk). 2020;99(3):83–6.
10. Hammett JT, Walker C. Sialolithiasis. In: StatPearls. Treasure Island, FL: StatPearls Publishing; 2022.
11. Uchino H, Motegi H, Kobayashi H, Kamoshima Y, Kazumata K, Terasaka S, et al. Postoperative acute submandibular sialadenitis after neurosurgery: two case reports and a review of the literature. NMC Case Rep J. 2015;3:1–4.
12. Eversole L. Salivary gland pathology. In: Fu Y, Wenig BM, Abemayor E, Wenig BL, editors. Head and neck pathology: with clinical correlations. Philadelphia, PA: Churchill-Livingstone; 2001. p. 242–91.
13. McQuone SJ. Acute viral and bacterial infections of the salivary glands. Otolaryngol Clin N Am. 1999;32:793–811.
14. Silvers AR, Som PM. Salivary glands. Radiol Clin North Am. 1998;36:941–66.
15. Tabak LA. In defense of the oral cavity: structure, biosynthesis, and function of salivary mucins. Annu Rev Physiol. 1995;57:547–64.
16. Tabak LA, Levine MJ, Mandel ID, Ellison SA. Role of salivary mucins in the protection of the oral cavity. J Oral Pathol. 1982;11:1–17.
17. McAdams RM, Mair EA, Rajnik M. Neonatal suppurative submandibular sialadenitis: case report and literature review. Int J Pediatr Otorhinolaryngol. 2005;69:993–7.
18. Raad II, Sabbagh MF, Caranasos GJ. Acute bacterial sialadenitis: a study of 29 cases and review. Rev Infect Dis. 1990;12:591–601.
19. Brook I. Acute bacterial suppurative parotitis: microbiology and management. J Craniofac Surg. 2003;14:37–40.
20. Peel R. Diseases of the salivary gland. In: Barnes L, editor. Surgical pathology of the head and neck. New York: Marcel-Dekker; 2001. p. 634–90.
21. Gillespie MB, Koch M, Iro H, Zenk J. Endoscopic-assisted gland-preserving therapy for chronic sialadenitis: a German and US comparison. Arch Otolaryngol Head Neck Surg. 2011;137(9):903–8.
22. Blatt IM. Studies in Sialolithiasis. III. Pathogenesis, diagnosis and treatment. South Med J. 1964;57:723–9.
23. Conley J, Myers E, Cole R. Analysis of 115 patients with tumors of the submandibular gland. Ann Otol Rhinol Laryngol. 1972;81(3):323–30.
24. Virmani N, Dabholkar J. Primary tubercular sialadenitis—a diagnostic dilemma. Iran J Otorhinolaryngol. 2019;31(102):45–50.
25. Mandel L, Surattanont F. Bilateral parotid swelling: a review. Oral Surg Oral Med Oral Pathol Oral Radiol Endod. 2002;93(3):221–37.
26. Kasaboglu O, Er N, Tumer C. Micromorphology of sialoliths in submandibular salivary gland: a scanning electron microscope and X-ray diffraction analysis. J Oral Maxillofac Surg. 2004;62:1253–8.
27. Grotz KA, Wustenberg P, Kohnen R, Al-Nawas B, Henneicke-von Zepelin HH, Bockisch A, et al. Prophylaxis of radiogenic sialadenitis and mucositis by coumarin/troxerutine in patients with head and neck cancer—a prospective, randomized, placebo-controlled, double-blind study. Br J Oral Maxillofac Surg. 2001;39:34–9.
28. Teymoortash A, Simolka N, Schrader C, Tiemann M, Werner JA. Lymphocyte subsets in irradiation-induced sialadenitis of the submandibular gland. Histopathology. 2005;47:493–500.
29. Lee IK, Liu JW. Tuberculous parotitis: case report and literature review. Ann Otol Rhinol Laryngol. 2005;114:547–51.

30. van der Walt JD, Leake J. Granulomatous sialadenitis of the major salivary glands. A clinicopathological study of 57 cases. Histopathology. 1987;11:131–44.
31. Jervis PN, Lee JA, Bull PD. Management of nontuberculous mycobacterial peri-sialadenitis in children: the Sheffield otolaryngology experience. Clin Otolaryngol. 2001;26:243–8.
32. Singh KK, Muralidhar M, Kumar A, Chattopadhyaya TK, Kapila K, Singh MK, et al. Comparison of in-house polymerase chain reaction with conventional techniques for the detection of mycobacterium tuberculosis DNA in granulomatous lymphadenopathy. J Clin Pathol. 2000;53(5):355–61.
33. Thakur J, Thakur A, Mohindroo N, Mohindroo S, Sharma D. Bilateral parotid tuberculosis. J Glob Infect Dis. 2011;3(3):296–9.
34. Ozcan C, Apa DD, Aslan G, Gulhan S, Gorur K. Mycobacterium tuberculosis infection within parotid gland Warthin tumor. J Craniofac Surg. 2008;19(6):1561–5.
35. Arriaga MA, Myers EN. The surgical management of chronic parotitis. Laryngoscope. 1990;100:1270–5.
36. Donath K, Seifert G. Ultrastructure and pathogenesis of myoepithelial sialadenitis. Occurrence of myoepithelial cells in the benign lymphoepithelial lesion (Sjogren's syndrome). Virchows Arch Pathol Anat. 1972;356(9482):315–29.
37. Kitagawa S, Zen Y, Harada K, Sasaki M, Sato Y, Minato H, et al. Abundant IgG4-positive plasma cell infiltration characterizes chronic sclerosing sialadenitis (Kuttner's tumor). Am J Surg Pathol. 2005;29:783–91.
38. Fox RI. Sjogren's syndrome. Lancet. 2005;366:321–31.
39. Hansen A, Lipsky PE, Dorner T. Immunopathogenesis of primary Sjogren's syndrome: implications for disease management and therapy. Curr Opin Rheumatol. 2005;17:558–65.
40. Kamisawa T, Nakajima H, Egawa N, Funata N, Tsuruta K, Okamoto A. IgG4-related sclerosing disease incorporating sclerosing pancreatitis, cholangitis, sialadenitis and retroperitoneal fibrosis with lymphadenopathy. Pancreatology. 2005;6:132–7.
41. Daniels TE. Labial salivary gland biopsy in Sjogren's syndrome. Assessment as a diagnostic criterion in 362 suspected cases. Arthritis Rheum. 1984;27:147–56.
42. Osial TA Jr, Whiteside TL, Buckingham RB, Singh G, Barnes EL, Pierce JM, et al. Clinical and serologic study of Sjogren's syndrome in patients with progressive systemic sclerosis. Arthritis Rheum. 1983;26:500–8.
43. Ihrler S, Zietz C, Sendelhofert A, Riederer A, Löhrs U. Lymphoepithelial duct lesions in Sjogren-type sialadenitis. Virchows Arch. 1999;434:315–23.
44. Kjorell U, Ostberg Y. Distribution of intermediate filaments and actin microfilaments in parotid autoimmune sialoadenitis of Sjogren syndrome. Histopathology. 1984;8:991–1011.
45. Nessan VJ, Jacoway JR. Biopsy of minor salivary glands in the diagnosis of sarcoidosis. N Engl J Med. 1979;301:922–4.
46. Fauci AS, Haynes BF, Katz P, Wolff SM. Wegener's granulomatosis: prospective clinical and therapeutic experience with 85 patients for 21 years. Ann Intern Med. 1983;98(1):76–85.
47. Bowman SJ. Collaborative research into outcome measures in Sjogren's syndrome. Update on disease assessment. Scand J Rheumatol Suppl. 2002;116:23–7.
48. Petrone D, Condemi JJ, Fife R, Gluck O, Cohen S, Dalgin P. A double-blind, randomized, placebo-controlled study of cevimeline in Sjogren's syndrome patients with xerostomia and keratoconjunctivitis sicca. Arthritis Rheum. 2002;46(3):748–54.
49. Yamamoto M, Takahashi H, Ohara M, Suzuki C, Naishiro Y, Yamamoto H, et al. A new conceptualization for Mikulicz's disease as an IgG4-related plasmacytic disease. Mod Rheumatol. 2006;16:335–40.
50. Peel R. Diseases of the salivary gland. In: Barnes L, editor. Surgical pathology of the head and neck. New York, NY: Marcel-Dekker; 2001. p. 634–757.
51. Zen Y, Nakanuma Y. Pathogenesis of IgG4-related disease. Curr Opin Rheumatol. 2011;23:114–8.
52. Geyer JT, Ferry JA, Harris NL, Stone JH, Zukerberg LR, Lauwers GY, et al. Chronic sclerosing sialadenitis (Küttner tumor) is an IgG4-associated disease. Am J Surg Pathol. 2010;34:202–10.

53. Küttner H. About inflammatory tumors of the submaxillary gland. Beitr Klin Chir. 1896;15:815–28.
54. Azzopardi JG, Evans DJ. Malignant lymphoma of parotid associated with Mikulicz disease (benign Lymphoepithelial lesion). J Clin Pathol. 1971;24:744–52.
55. Bahler DW, Swerdlow SH. Clonal salivary gland infiltrates associated with myoepithelial sialadenitis (Sjogren's syndrome) begin as nonmalignant antigen-selected expansions. Blood. 1998;91:1864–72.
56. Fishleder A, Tubbs R, Hesse B, et al. Uniform detection of immunoglobulin-gene rearrangement in benign Lymphoepithelial lesions. N Engl J Med. 1987;316:1118–21.
57. Knowles DM, Athan E, Ubriaco A, McNally L, Inghirami G, Wieczorek R, et al. Extranodal noncutaneous lymphoid hyperplasias represent a continuous spectrum of B-cell neoplasia: demonstration by molecular genetic analysis. Blood. 1989;73:1635–45.
58. Hyjek E, Smith WJ, Isaacson PG. Primary B-cell lymphoma of salivary glands and its relationship to myoepithelial sialadenitis. Hum Pathol. 1988;19:766–76.
59. Abbondanzo SL. Extranodal marginal-zone Bcell lymphoma of the salivary gland. Ann Diagn Pathol. 2001;5:246–54.
60. Streubel B, Simonitsch-Klupp I, Mullauer L, Müllauer L, Lamprecht A, Huber D, et al. Variable frequencies of MALT lymphoma-associated genetic aberrations in MALT lymphomas of different sites. Leukemia. 2004;18:1722–6.
61. Batsakis JG, Bernacki EG, Rice DH, Stebler ME. Malignancy and the benign lymphoepithelial lesion. Laryngoscope. 1975;85:389–99.
62. Brauneis J, Laskawi R, Schroder M, Eilts M. Squamous cell carcinoma in the area of the parotid gland. Metastasis or primary tumor? HNO. 1990;38:292–4.
63. Nagao K, Matsuzaki O, Saiga H, Akikusa B, Sugano I, Shigematsu H, et al. A histopathologic study of benign and malignant lymphoepithelial lesions of the parotid gland. Cancer. 1983;52:1044–52.
64. Wu LY, Cheng J, Lu Y, Zhou ZY, Saku T. Epstein-Barr virus infection in benign lymphoepithelial lesions with malignant transformation of salivary glands. Zhonghua Kou Qiang Yi Xue Za Zhi. 2004;39:291–3.
65. Abrams AM, Melrose RJ, Howell FV. Necrotizing sialometaplasia: a disease simulating malignancy. Cancer. 1973;32:130–5.
66. Brannon RB, Fowler CB, Hartman KS, Necrotizing sialometaplasia. A clinicopathologic study of sixty-nine cases and review of the literature. Oral Surg Oral Med Oral Pathol. 1991;72:317–25.
67. Fowler CB, Brannon RB. Subacute necrotizing sialadenitis: report of 7 cases and a review of the literature. Oral Surg Oral Med Oral Pathol Oral Radiol Endod. 2000;89:600–9.
68. Imbery TA, Edwards PA. Necrotizing sialometaplasia: literature review and case reports. J Am Dent Assoc. 1996;127:1087–92.
69. Maisel RH, Johnston WH, Anderson HA, Cantrell RW. Necrotizing sialometaplasia involving the nasal cavity. Laryngoscope. 1977;87:429–34.
70. Romagosa V, Bella MR, Truchero C, Moya J. Necrotizing sialometaplasia (adenometaplasia) of the trachea. Histopathology. 1992;21:280–2.
71. Zschoch H. Mucus gland infarct with squamous epithelial metaplasia in the lung. A rare site of so-called necrotizing sialometaplasia. Pathologe. 1992;13:45–8.
72. Mohammed BS, Liu Z, Tang W. BCL-2, Ki67 and P53 expression in oral necrotizing sialometaplasia and squamous cell carcinoma. Mod Pathol. 2006;19:105A.
73. Aydin O, Yilmaz T, Ozer F, Saraç S, Sökmensüer C. Necrotizing sialometaplasia of parotid gland: a possible vasculitic cause. Int J Pediatr Otorhinolaryngol. 2002;64:171–4.
74. Rye LA, Calhoun NR, Redman RS. Necrotizing sialometaplasia in a patient with Buerger's disease and Raynaud's phenomenon. Oral Surg Oral Med Oral Pathol. 1980;49:233–6.
75. Aframian D, Milhem II, Kirsch G, Markitziu A. Necrotizing sialometaplasia after silastic ring vertical gastroplasty: case report and review of literature. Obes Surg. 1995;5:179–82.
76. Schoning H, Emshoff R, Kreczy A. Necrotizing sialometaplasia in two patients with bulimia and chronic vomiting. Int J Oral Maxillofac Surg. 1998;27:463–5.

77. Cheng SC, Wu VW, Kwong DL, Ying MT. Assessment of post-radiotherapy salivary glands. Br J Radiol. 2011;84:393–402.
78. Bronstein AD, Nyberg DA, Schwartz AN, Shuman WP, Griffin BR. Increased salivary gland density on contrast-enhanced CT after head and neck radiation. Am J Roentgenol. 1987;149:1259–63.
79. Houweling AC, van den Berg CA, Roesink JM, Terhaard CH, Raaijmakers. Magnetic resonance imaging at 3.0T for submandibular gland sparing radiotherapy. Radiother Oncol. 2010;97:239–43.

24 Sialadenosis (Sialosis) of the Submandibular Gland

24.1 Introduction

Sialadenosis is a chronic, diffuse, noninflammatory, nonneoplastic disorder, in association with acinar hypertrophy and ductal atrophy causing diffuse enlargement of salivary glands, usually the parotid glands, and less commonly the submandibular [1–3] and minor salivary glands [4].

24.2 Etiology

Causes of sialadenosis fall into five major categories (nutritional, metabolic, endocrinal, inflammatory/autoimmune, and neurochemical/drugs) as shown in Table 24.1. In general, any disorder that affects the digestion of food over a prolonged period of time can result in sialadenosis, and malnutrition may contribute to sialadenosis in alcoholics.

Among the wide range of drugs that may induce sialadenosis, antihypertensive agents are prominent; others include thiouracil (antithyroid) and phenothiazines (heterocyclic antipsychotic). However, it is worth mentioning that in many cases, no underlying disorder can be detected.

© The Author(s), under exclusive license to Springer Nature Switzerland AG 2024
M. Sakr, *Surgery of the Salivary Glands*,
https://doi.org/10.1007/978-3-031-82069-4_24

Table 24.1 Causes of sialadenosis

Etiology	Examples
Nutritional	Alcoholism, bulimia, anorexia nervosa [5], kwashiorkor disease, and pellagra (deficiency of niacin [vitamin B3])
Metabolic	Obesity, liver cirrhosis, and malabsorption
Endocrinal	Diabetes mellitus, thyroid disorders (e.g., acromegaly and hypothyroidism), pregnancy, gonadal dysfunction, and post-oophorectomy
Inflammatory/ autoimmune	Sjögren's disease, Heerfordt syndrome (a triad of parotid enlargement, uveitis, and facial nerve palsy)
Neurochemical/ drugs	Vegetative state, lead and mercury poisoning, iodine, thiouracil (antithyroid), isoproterenol (sympathomimetic), phenothiazines (antipsychotic), thiourea, and valproic acid (used in various neurological and psychiatric disorders) [6]

24.3 Pathogenesis

The proposed pathogeneses of sialadenosis include prolonged malnutrition with resultant glandular atrophy and fatty replacement. Sialadenosis is also thought to be a neurosecretory disorder. Diabetic neuropathy may be the clue causing acinar cell atrophy in some cases. Ultrastructural and animal studies point to a disturbance in the autonomic innervation of salivary glands (autonomic neuropathy), which is considered to be the initiating factor for sialadenosis [2, 3, 7–9].

Multiple emetic episodes (bulimia) cause autonomic neuropathy. With sympathetic nerve impairment, individual acinar cells enlarge because of zymogen granule engorgement. One explanation is that the sympathetic nerve supply to the secreting acinar cell is concerned with the production and secretion of zymogen, the precursor of amylase. Because of sympathetic nerve dysfunction, there may be an increase in zymogen storage in the cell, owing to increased production and/or decreased secretion of the granules. The ensuing cellular enlargement, which is evidenced by fine-needle aspiration biopsy (FNAB), leads to clinically visible bilateral gland enlargement [2, 3, 7–9].

24.4 Pathology

Grossly, there is only diffuse enlargement of the affected gland. Histologically, the condition is characterized by acinar hypertrophy and fatty infiltration (Fig. 24.1) [10]. Zymogen granules are increased in size and number by light and electron microscopy. No inflammation or fibrosis can be detected, which differentiates sialadenosis from sialadenitis. While amyloidosis may also present with diffuse enlargement of the salivary glands, histologically, there will be interstitial fibrosis as well as the characteristic pale amyloid deposition that can be demonstrated with a Congo red stain [11].

Diabetics with sialosis have smaller acini, greater fatty infiltration in the glandular stroma, and normal-appearing epithelium, while alcoholic sialosis is identified by a reduction in the proportion of fatty tissue of stroma with an enlargement in the

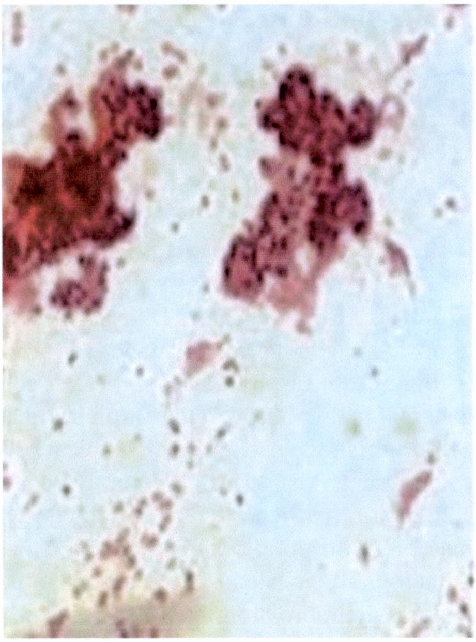

Fig. 24.1 Microscopy showing moderately cellular smears having acinar epithelial cells arranged in clusters, papillae, glandular pattern, and scattered singly. Inflammatory infiltrates are absent

ductal epithelium that contributes to an increased caliber of the striated ducts. Also noted in alcoholic sialosis are accumulation of secretory granules in the acinar cells' cytoplasm and enlarged excretory ducts [12].

24.5 Clinical Picture

Sialadenosis is usually bilateral and has an equal gender distribution. Most of the patients are between 40 and 70 years of age. Usually, there is painless, soft, and diffuse enlargement of both parotid glands giving the patient a striking facial feature, known as the "hamster-like appearance." Less commonly, the submandibular glands are affected presenting with painless bilateral submandibular enlargement and may be associated with mild discomfort. Approximately 50% of cases are associated with recognized risk factors, including diabetes mellitus, metabolic syndrome, alcoholism, bulimia, malnutrition, and liver disease.

24.6 Investigations

24.6.1 Laboratory Tests

Blood tests may reveal hyperglycemia (diabetes mellitus), abnormal liver function tests (cirrhosis, alcoholism), or abnormal thyroid hormone levels (hypothyroidism). Sialo-chemistry may show increased serum potassium and calcium levels.

24.6.2 Imaging Studies

Imaging studies including ultrasonography (US), computed tomography (CT) scan, magnetic resonance imaging (MRI), or sialography help differentiate space-occupying lesions in the major salivary glands.

24.6.3 Biopsy/Cytology

Biopsy is rarely indicated. If performed, the biopsy shows enlarged acinar cells to almost twice the normal diameter and packed cytoplasm with enzyme granules.

Fine-needle aspiration (FNA) yields cellular smears having acinar epithelial cells adherent to thin fibrovascular stroma and large numbers of naked nuclei of epithelial cell origin in the background. Atypical cells or inflammatory cells are characteristically absent. A similar condition that can mimic sialadenosis is a low-grade acinic cell tumor (particularly on cytology), which generally yields abundant cellular material with poorly formed micro-acinar groupings [13]. Naked nuclei that are numerous in sialadenosis are absent in acinic cell tumors, while atypical nuclear features are more prominent in acinic cell tumors as compared to sialadenosis. The distinguishing cellular features of acinic cell carcinoma include large nuclei, grainy eosinophilic cytoplasm, and neoplastic cells arranged singly or in small clusters. In addition, usually, there is an absence of other normal salivary gland structures such as duct epithelium and interstitial adipose tissue.

24.7 Differential Diagnosis

The diagnosis of sialadenosis must exclude inflammatory causes of salivary gland swelling, particularly Sjögren's syndrome, human immunodeficiency virus (HIV) infection, sarcoidosis, and lymphoepithelial diseases by relevant investigations. On histopathology, other conditions of sialadenitis will be excluded by the presence of inflammatory cells in the background.

24.8 Treatment

Usually, no specific treatment is necessary. Treatment in the form of controlling the underlying disorder or withdrawing the incriminated drug helps sialosis to resolve. Unnecessary surgical intervention can be avoided by excluding other pathological conditions. There is usually little morbidity associated with the condition itself, and surgery (submandibular sialadenectomy) is resorted to only in case of significant disfigurement and cosmetic complaints.

In some instances, anorexic or bulimic patients may seek advice about removal of the glands. Anorexia or bulimia would need to be treated first before any such surgery could be contemplated. Mahler and Wallace (1993) [14] and Park et al.

(2009) [15] reported that pilocarpine has proved to be beneficial in the treatment of sialadenosis in bulimic patients.

24.9 Prognosis

The persistence of sialadenosis is dependent on the severity and duration of the underlying disease. However, there is usually little morbidity associated with the condition itself; most surgical treatment is performed for cosmetic purposes.

References

1. Peel R. Diseases of the salivary gland. In: Barnes L, editor. Surgical pathology of the head and neck. New York, NY: Marcel-Dekker; 2001. p. 634–757.
2. Chilla R. Sialadenosis of the salivary glands of the head. Studies on the physiology and pathophysiology of parotid secretion. Adv Otorhinolaryngol. 1981;26:1–38.
3. Donath K. Sialadenosis of the parotid gland. Ultrastructural, clinical and experimental findings in disturbances of secretion (author's transl). Veroff Pathol. 1976;(103):1–122.
4. Mignogna MD, Fedele S, Lo RL. Anorexia/bulimia-related sialadenosis of palatal minor salivary glands. J Oral Pathol Med. 2004;33(7):441–2.
5. Steiger R, Storck C. [CME ORL 5. Bilateral pre-auricular swelling. Sialadenitis of all salivary glands in bulimia]. Praxis (Bern 1994). 2012;101(11):748–9.
6. Mauz PS, Mörike K, Kaiserling E, Brosch S. Valproic acid-associated sialadenosis of the parotid and submandibular glands: diagnostic and therapeutic aspects. Acta Otolaryngol. 2005;125(4):386–91.
7. Chilla R, Witzemann V, Opaitz M, Arglebe C. Possible involvement of parotid beta-adrenergic receptors in the etiology of sialadenosis. Arch Otorhinolaryngol. 1981;230(2):113–20.
8. Donath K, Seifert G. Ultrastructural studies of the parotid glands in sialadenosis. Virchows Arch A Pathol Anat Histol. 1975;365(2):119–35.
9. Donath K, Spillner M, Seifert G. The influence of the autonomic nervous system on the ultrastructure of the parotid acinar cells. Experimental contribution to the neurohormonal sialadenosis. Virchows Arch A Pathol Anat Histol. 1974;364(1):15–33.
10. Gupta S, Sodhani P. Sialadenosis of parotid gland: a cytomorphologic and morphometric study of four cases. Anal Quant Cytol Histol. 1998;20(3):225–8.
11. Eversole L. Salivary gland pathology. In: Fu Y, Wenig BM, Abemayor E, Wenig BL, editors. Head and neck pathology: with clinical correlations. Philadelphia, PA: Churchill-Livingstone; 2001. p. 242–91.
12. Merlo C, Bohl L, Carda C, Gómez de Ferraris ME, Carranza M. Parotid sialosis: morphometrical analysis of the glandular parenchyma and stroma among diabetic and alcoholic patients. J Oral Pathol Med. 2010;39:10–5.
13. Henry-Stanley MJ, Beneke J, Bardales RH, Stanley MW. Fine-needle aspiration of normal tissue from enlarged salivary glands: sialosis or missed target? Diagn Cytopathol. 1995;13:300–3.
14. Mehler PS, Wallace JA. Sialadenosis in bulimia. A new treatment. Arch Otolaryngol Head Neck Surg. 1993;119(7):787–8.
15. Park KK, Tung RC, de Luzuriaga AR. Painful parotid hypertrophy with bulimia: a report of medical management. J Drugs Dermatol. 2009;8(6):577–9.

Tumors of the Submandibular Gland 25

25.1 Benign Tumors (BTs)

25.1.1 Epidemiology

The submandibular gland encompasses 10–15% of all salivary gland tumors with an even distribution of benign and malignant neoplasms. The most common benign submandibular tumor is a pleomorphic adenoma (PA), which consists of 36% of all submandibular tumors [1, 2].

25.1.2 Etiology

The etiology of benign salivary tumors in general is exactly unknown but has been linked to radiation (with 50% of radiation-induced tumors being PAs) [3], smoking (Warthin's tumor) [4, 5], oral trauma (ductal papilloma), human papillomavirus (HPV) (inverted type of ductal papilloma) [6, 7], and genetics (chromosomal translocation involving 8q12 and rearrangement at 12q13–15 activates the PA gene 1 [PLGA1]) [8–10]. Moreover, the increased IgG4-positive plasma cells in lymphadenoma suggest a role for immunomodulation in its development [11].

25.1.3 Pathophysiology

Benign salivary gland tumors are heterogeneous in their morphology and are postulated to develop from the same stem cell differentiation pathways as normal salivary gland tissues. Four main theories have been proposed as follows [12, 13]:

Basal reserve cell theory: Basal cells of both excretory and intercalated ducts develop into functional salivary units and are capable of tumor development [14].

© The Author(s), under exclusive license to Springer Nature Switzerland AG 2024
M. Sakr, *Surgery of the Salivary Glands*,
https://doi.org/10.1007/978-3-031-82069-4_25

Pluripotent unicellular reserve cell theory: Basal cells of the excretory ducts are responsible for developing the functional salivary unit and tumor differentiation [15].

Semi-pluripotent bicellular reserve cell theory: Basal cells of the excretory duct form the progenitor cells of the intercalated ducts, which then form the striated ducts and acinar units. The basal cells of the excretory duct and the progenitor cells of the intercalated ducts are capable of cellular division and tumor development. In contrast, the acinar unit and striated ducts are terminally differentiated and cannot undergo either [15]. This is the most common theory of salivary gland tumor histogenesis [14].

Multicellular theory: All cellular types in normal salivary glands, including those of acinar units and striated ducts, can undergo cellular division and development into salivary tumors. Each tumor develops from a specific cell of origin [16].

25.1.4 Pleomorphic Adenoma (PA)

25.1.4.1 Incidence

The most commonly encountered benign tumor (BT) of the submandibular gland (50–65%) is "pleomorphic adenoma" (PA) that has histological features and biological behavior which are similar to those of the parotid gland, but with an incidence of 1:10, respectively.

Pleomorphic adenoma (PA) is a mixed salivary tumor that represents 75–80% of all benign parotid tumors. It may affect as well the submandibular and minor salivary glands. Its incidence is slightly higher in females and affects most commonly patients between 30 and 50 years of age [17–19]. Though uncommon, it has been reported in the first two decades of life. It is uncommon to be bilateral [20]. It is usually a solitary lesion, although synchronous or metachronous involvement of two or more salivary glands can occur.

25.1.4.2 Pathology

Gross Appearance

Grossly, PA is a well-defined tumor, but with small extensions into the adjacent normal tissue through an incomplete capsule, which explains, at least in part, recurrence after enucleation. It has a pleomorphic matrix, with a non-cystic cut section that may show some islets of cartilage.

Microscopic Picture

Microscopically, it is formed of epithelial cells intermingled with a pleomorphic mesenchymal stroma (Fig. 25.1). The epithelial elements give rise to ducts, whereas the mesenchymal elements give rise to cartilaginous, osseous, hyaline, and myxoid tissues. The mesenchymal component develops from a metaplastic process of the myoepithelial cells. It is categorized into 4 types: (1) principally myxoid, (2) mixed myxoid and cellular components in equal proportions, (3) predominantly cellular, and (4) cellular [21].

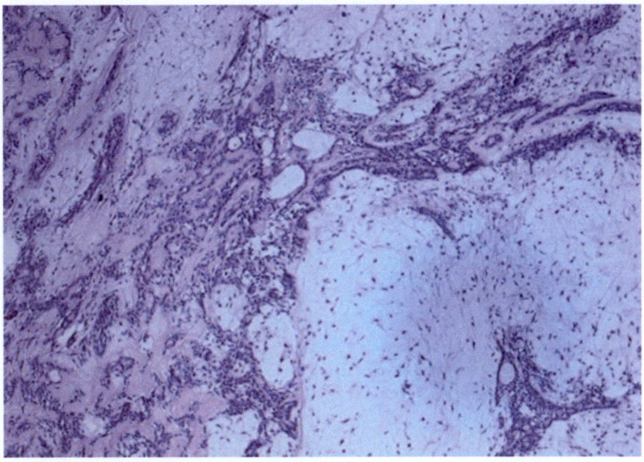

Fig. 25.1 Microscopy of pleomorphic adenoma showing biphasic population of epithelial and mesenchymal cells. Epithelial cells assume tubular profiles, cords, or nests. Stroma is myxoid. (H&E, ×100)

Pleomorphic adenoma of the major salivary glands is "encapsulated," whereas those from minor salivary glands are not [22]. It often has an irregular border with finger-like projections (pseudopodia) that grow into the surrounding tissue making local recurrence a frequent occurrence if these tumors are not completely excised [23].

Pleomorphic adenoma carries a malignant potential of 2–10%. The presence of hyalinized stroma is the most predictive histological parameter of malignant transformation. The tumor may rarely metastasize without having the histological features of malignancy, but this almost always occurs after inadequate surgical excision, possibly due to altered anatomy secondary to surgery, which gave access to vascular and lymphatic channels. In metastasizing pleomorphic adenoma (MPA), the histology resembles the original PA with occasional mitotic figures and pleomorphism but is not overtly histologically malignant [24].

Approximately 70% of PAs have cytogenetic alterations that likely play a major role in tumorigenesis and can be categorized into four groups: (1) tumors with 8q12 rearrangements, (2) those with 12q13–15 rearrangements, (3) those with miscellaneous clonal changes, and (4) those that are karyotypically normal [25, 26].

25.1.4.3 Clinical Presentation

The patient with PA typically presents with a painless, slowly growing, spherical mass (Fig. 25.2) of variable size ranging from pea-sized to a large mass [27–29]. The patient's complaint is usually disfigurement. The mass is of heterogonous consistency and mobile, being neither attached to the skin nor to the deep structures. Bosselation of the tumor is demonstrable if it is bigger than 3 cm. The draining lymph nodes (LNs) are not enlarged. Malignant transformation (2–10%) may occur, particularly in long-standing tumors or in those that have recurred.

25.1.4.4 Investigations

Imaging Studies

As for any submandibular gland mass, ultrasonography (US), computed tomography (CT) scan, and magnetic resonance imaging (MRI) are the best imaging tools.

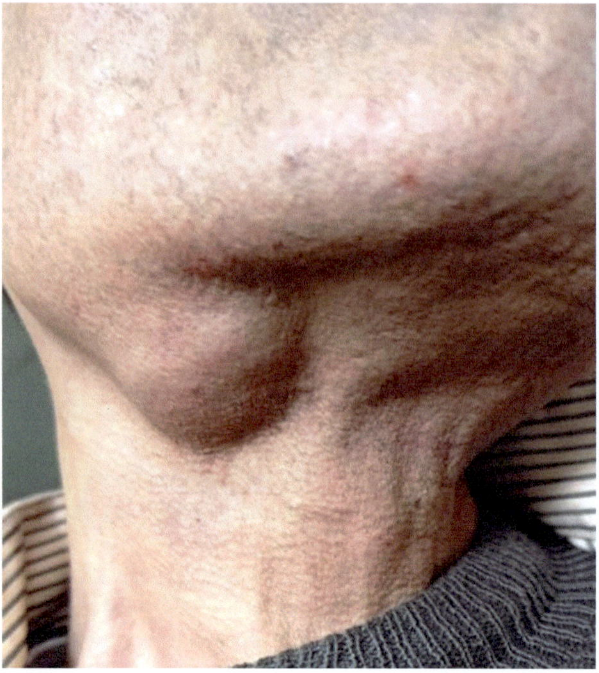

Fig. 25.2 A 47-year-old gentleman with a slowly growing right submandibular mass (proven histologically to be a pleomorphic adenoma)

Ultrasonography (US)

Ultrasonography (US) is the initial noninvasive modality for localizing superficial tumors, distinguishing solid masses from cystic collections, and helping guide fine-needle aspiration biopsy (FNAB) [30, 31].

Computerized Tomography (CT) Scan

Conventional CT scan and MRI have similar sensitivity and specificity in determining tumor location, tumor margin, and tumor infiltration [32]. Although CT scan has a lower resolution than MRI for soft tissue, it provides an advantage in detecting early cortical bony invasion of the mandible [32].

Magnetic Resonance Imaging (MRI)

Magnetic resonance imaging (MRI) provides an accurate location and extent of the tumor for preoperative planning purposes [22]. It can quantify the diffusion properties of water in tumor tissue into the apparent diffusion coefficient (ADC). Diffusion-weighted MRI is useful for PA due to its higher ADC [33].

Positron Emission Tomography (PET)

Compared with a conventional CT scan, PET may be more accurate in demonstrating tumor extension, nodal involvement, local recurrence, and distant metastasis due to the tissues' higher levels of standardized uptake values (SUV) [34, 35]. However, PET is unable to differentiate between benign and malignant tumors due to PA and Warthin's tumor both exhibiting high glucose uptake values [36].

Cytopathology

Imaging alone may not be able to completely distinguish between benign and malignant lesions. Obtaining histological samples is the key to determining treatment options. Fine-needle aspiration cytology (FNAC) is a recognized safe diagnostic tool for obtaining preoperative diagnosis and is advised to be done after imaging for the fear of hemorrhage. It has a high level of accuracy including sensitivity and specificity of 73% and 91%, respectively, in distinguishing benign from malignant tumors [37–39].

Several studies showed that the use of "flow cytometry" as a biological parameter for the prediction of recurrence in PAs should be considered. Tumors of a larger size showed a higher percentage of cells in the S-phase fraction and probably a greater tendency for recurrence [40–43].

Ultrasound-guided core needle biopsy (CNB) is able to obtain larger tissue specimens with histologic architecture, which improves recognition of tumor grading and subtyping. However, the disadvantages of CNB include more pain, the need for local anesthesia, and an increased risk of nerve injury and hematoma [44]. The intraoperative frozen section has a sensitivity and specificity of 90% and 99%, respectively, in distinguishing between benign and malignant lesions [45].

25.1.4.5 Treatment

The mainstay treatment of submandibular PA is complete surgical excision in the form of submandibular sialadenectomy.

25.1.4.6 Prognosis

Recurrence of PA has been reported in 1–5% of cases at 7–10 years after initial treatment, most likely secondary to incomplete excision, capsule rupture, pseudopodia presence, and satellite lesions [46–48]. Metastasizing pleomorphic adenoma (MPA) is a rare condition with PA developing in bone (36.6%), lung (33.8%), and cervical LNs (20.1%), liver, and skin without any metastatic features on histology [49–51]. MPA has been associated with incomplete excision, with 90% of cases also displaying local recurrence [52, 53]. Patients with MPA have a 5-year disease-specific survival rate of 58% [54]. Carcinoma ex-pleomorphic adenoma (CEPA) can develop in 2–15% of cases and is the malignant transformation of PA arising from its epithelial components [22, 55–57].

25.1.5 Other Benign Tumors

Other types of adenomas, such as the basal cell adenoma, are much less common, and other benign tumors, such as Warthin's tumor, oncocytomas, and myoepitheliomas, are very rarely encountered in submandibular (and sublingual) glands. Basal cell adenoma accounts for about 1.8–5% of all salivary gland tumors. Around 75–80% is seen in the parotid glands, followed by 5% in the submandibular glands. It has a predilection for females and patients in the seventh decade of life and in Western countries [57–59].

Hemangiomas affect mainly the parotid gland (90% of cases), but occasionally, the submandibular gland is affected, as a part of massive facial lesions.

25.2 Malignant Tumors (MTs)

25.2.1 Classification

Malignant neoplasms of the submandibular (and sublingual glands) can be classified into three major categories (Table 25.1):

Tumors of epithelial origin
Tumors of non-epithelial origin
Secondary tumors

Among malignant tumors, the most frequent is adenoid cystic carcinoma (AdCC), accounting for 36–63% of cases [60–64] followed by mucoepidermoid carcinoma (MEC) (17–22.2%), squamous cell carcinoma (SCC) (17.3%), and adenocarcinoma (15.4%) [64].

25.2.2 Epidemiology

The majority of salivary gland malignancies occur in the parotid, followed by the submandibular, sublingual, and minor salivary glands [65]. The probability of malignancy in a parotid mass ranges from 15–32%, compared to 41–50% in a submandibular mass, 70–90% in minor salivary gland masses, and almost 100% in sublingual masses [66]. Salivary gland tumors in children are more likely to be malignant [4].

The submandibular gland harbors 10–15% of all salivary gland tumors with nearly equal distribution of benign and malignant neoplasms [67]. The most

Table 25.1 Malignant tumors of the submandibular gland

Origin	Examples
Epithelial tumors	Adenoid cystic carcinoma (AdCC) Mucoepidermoid carcinoma (MEC) Acinic cell carcinoma (ACC) Carcinoma ex-pleomorphic adenoma (CEPA) True malignant mixed tumor (TMMT) Basal cell adenocarcinoma (BCAC) Squamous cell carcinoma (SCC) Salivary duct carcinoma (SDC)
Non-epithelial tumors	Sarcoma Lymphoma: non-Hodgkin's lymphoma (NHL)
Secondary tumors	Metastases most commonly from skin cancer of the head and neck, mainly squamous cell carcinoma (SCC) and malignant melanoma

common malignant neoplasm in the submandibular gland is AdCC followed by MEC and CEPA. Less common tumors include ACC, salivary duct carcinoma, epi-myoepithelial carcinoma, carcinosarcoma, oncocytic carcinoma, and SCC [67]. Malignant submandibular tumors are more common in the sixth decade with a predilection for men [68].

25.2.3 Etiology

The exact etiology of salivary gland cancer is unknown, but various mechanisms have been proposed [69–75], including radiation (MEC [3, 76], PSSC [77, 78]), viruses (EBV and HIV), autoimmune disease (non-Hodgkin's lymphoma [NHL] [79, 80]), ultraviolet light exposure, occupational exposures in rubber or nickel industries, exposure to tobacco and alcohol (MEC [8, 82]), prior diagnosis of medulloblastoma, prior diagnosis of basal cell carcinoma, androgen receptor expression, and genetics.

25.2.4 Adenoid Cystic Carcinoma (AdCC)

Adenoid cystic carcinoma (AdCC) has been given many names since it was first described by Robin and colleagues in 1853. From these names, "cylindroma" was particularly discouraged to avoid confusion with the benign cutaneous appendage tumor carrying the same name. This tumor arises not only from major and minor salivary glands, but also from seromucous glands throughout the body [83, 84]. It is the second most common salivary malignancy and affects patients between 40 and 60 years of age with no difference in gender, although it tends to be more common in the submandibular gland in women [4, 85, 86].

Over 50% of AdCC tumors contain the t(6;9)(q22–23;p23–24) translocation, which fuses the MYB proto-oncogene on chromosome 6q to the NFIB gene on chromosome 9p, resulting in an overexpression of MYB-NFIB fusion oncogene and worse prognosis [87–89].

Adenoid cystic carcinoma usually develops over a short time as a submandibular mass (Fig. 25.3) with rapid growth and is frequently associated with pain and fixation to the mandible. Regional LN metastases may occur in approximately 30% of patients. This tumor has a propensity to invade nerves, thus posing a risk of perineural spread through the mandibular or cervical branches of the facial nerve, and through the lingual and hypoglossal nerves toward the skull base. The risk of distant metastases and the development of late recurrences are similar to those observed in the parotid gland [61].

Histologically, AdCC presents as a nonencapsulated, well-circumscribed mass with biphasic ductal and myoepithelial components and three distinct patterns: tubular, cribriform, and solid [4, 90]. The tubular variant consists of ducts lined by one to two layers of myoepithelial-like cells. The cribriform variant presents with a "Swiss-cheese" appearance containing cylindrical pseudocysts lined with epithelial

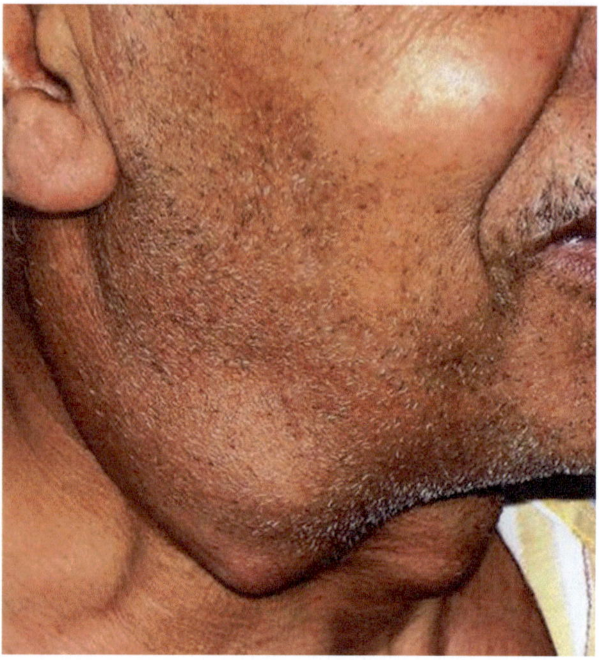

Fig. 25.3 A 62-year-old gentleman with a right submandibular mass of rapid growth, proven by histopathology to be an adenoid cystic carcinoma (AdCC)

cells and filled with hyaline material. The solid variant has solid epithelial islands with central areas of necrosis [91, 92]. The solid variant is the most aggressive of the three and has a tendency for hematogenous metastasis in 40–60% of cases with perineural invasion [92–94].

According to histological grade, low-grade (Fig. 25.4) and high-grade (Fig. 25.5) variants of AdCC are recognized.

The best results of treatment are obtained through radical surgery and postoperative radiotherapy (RT). The tumor is radiosensitive, but not radio-curable. Although controversial, neck dissection may be reserved for patients with clinically positive LNs [95–97].

Some studies showed that age over 45 years, advanced clinical stage, paresthesia, and increased expression of p53 are associated with poor prognosis [84, 95]. The prognostic significance of perineural invasion and DNA ploidy remains controversial. The solid pattern histology has the worst prognosis [4, 98–100].

25.2.5 Mucoepidermoid Carcinoma (MEC)

Mucoepidermoid carcinoma (MEC) is the most common salivary gland malignancy in adults and children [4]. Approximately 8.4% of MECs occur in the submandibular gland [101]. It mostly occurs around the age of 50 years [102, 103]. In some series, MEC is more common in women by a ratio of 3:2, while in others, there is no sex predominance [104].

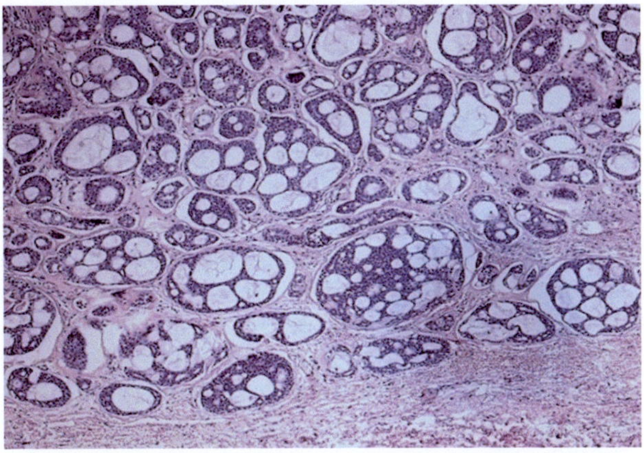

Fig. 25.4 Low-grade adenoid cystic carcinoma (AdCC) with a notable cribriform pattern (H&E, ×100)

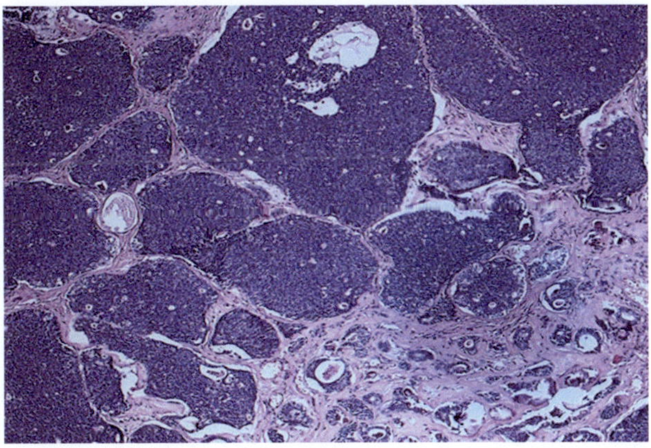

Fig. 25.5 High-grade adenoid cystic carcinoma (AdCC) with a predominant (>70%) solid pattern. The lower right corner still depicts tubular structures (H&E, ×100)

Histologically, MEC can be composed of up to six different types of cells, including maternal, intermediate, epidermoid, clear, columnar, and mucous cells [105, 106]. It may be low, intermediate, or high grade in histological appearance depending on the quantity of aggressive, epidermoid tissue, with eventual outcome dependent upon this grading. Low-grade tumors are usually well circumscribed, resemble benign mixed tumors grossly, and recur after excision in approximately 15% of patients. Histologically, they have well-formed cystic spaces with high glandular composition. Intermediate-grade MEC tends to have more solid nests of epidermoid and intermediate cells with less prominent cystic spaces. High-grade MEC, on the other hand, has limited mucous cells with large amounts of solid, squamous cells that can often be misdiagnosed as squamous cell carcinoma [107, 108]. They are aggressive and invade locally, causing fixation and extension to nerves. When MEC arises in the submandibular gland, it is known to behave aggressively regardless of its histological grading [4].

The most common genetic finding in MEC is the chromosomal translocation t(11;19)(q21:p13), leading to the fusion of MECT1 and MAML2 genes, which is responsible for disrupting the NOTCH signaling pathway. This translocation is found in 50–70% and is more often seen in low-grade tumors associated with a better prognosis [109, 110].

Metastases from MEC occur in LNs, lungs, and bones [111]. On presentation, up to 50% of patients with high-grade tumors have LN metastases [60, 61], and the risk of local failure can be as high as 40% [61].

Treatment is surgical resection with neck dissection being reserved for high-grade variants [111]. Prognosis is influenced by the grade and stage of the tumor and the patient's age (above 45 years is associated with poor prognosis) and gender. Histological grade is considered one of the most important factors in prognosis. The overall 5-year survival rates range from 92–100% for low-grade tumors and 0–43% for high-grade tumors [112]. The overall 10-year survival rate for MEC is about 53% [98].

25.2.6 Carcinoma Ex-pleomorphic Adenoma (CEPA)

Carcinoma ex-pleomorphic adenoma (CEPA) is by definition the malignant transformation of a long-standing PA, which occurs in about 5–25% of such cases over a 15-year period [67, 97, 113, 114]. Epigenetic mutations involving DNA promoter methylation of tumor suppressor genes can lead to transcriptional inactivation and increase the risk of the transformation of PA into CEPA (and SDC) [115, 116].

Carcinoma ex-pleomorphic adenoma (CEPA) occurs in the major salivary glands in 80% of the cases, of which again 80% occur in the parotid gland. The average age at diagnosis is 50–60 years, which is approximately 10 years older than most individuals with PA. It is extremely uncommon in individuals below the age of 20 years [97, 117]. The female-to-male ratio is 1.2–3:1.

Clinical features predictive of malignant transformation are age, tumor size (rapid rate of growth), harder consistency, fixation to the underlying muscles or the overlying skin, and submandibular location. Histologically, the presence of hyalinized stroma is the most predictive parameter for malignant transformation. The carcinoma is usually a high-grade adenocarcinoma or an undifferentiated carcinoma, although numerous other types including SCC, MEC, AdCC, myoepithelial carcinoma, clear cell carcinoma, papillary carcinoma, and terminal duct carcinoma have been reported [118, 119]. Microscopically, CEPA can present with varying extents of invasion, including intracapsular, minor extracapsular (<5 mm beyond the capsule), and wide extracapsular (>5 mm beyond the capsule). The latter presents with a high risk of recurrence and distant metastasis [90, 118, 119].

CEPA metastasizes in up to 70% of the cases to distant sites rather than regionally, with a special affinity to the lungs and vertebral column. Clinical neck metastasis is present in 33% of patients with CEPA and occult neck metastasis in 16% [120]. Treatment of CEPA is surgical resection usually with neck dissection. "In-situ variant" is a tumor that did not invade the capsule of a PA and thence was diagnosed postoperatively. In this case, the performed standard resection is curative.

Depending on the extent of differentiation and invasion, CEPA can display a wide range of recurrence and survival rates. Tumors with wide extracapsular invasion beyond 5 mm of the capsule have a high risk of recurrence and distant metastasis [90, 118, 119]. The 5-year survival rate (SR) of CEPA ranges from 30–96% depending on the histological variant [118, 121]. The overall 10-year survival rate for CEPA is 62% [98]. The presence of regional metastasis in CEPA reduces the 5-year survival rate from 67% to 16% [122].

25.2.7 True Malignant Mixed Tumor (TMMT)

True malignant mixed tumor is a very rare neoplasm that may be regarded as "carcinosarcoma" since both epithelial and stromal components are histologically malignant, and both can metastasize. Such metastases are more commonly via a hematogenous rather than lymphatic route, with the lungs and bones being the most frequent sites [123–125]. There is a wide range of age affection (14–87 years), and there is no sex predilection [125, 126]. Clinical presentation is similar to that of CEPA. Treatment is surgical resection, combined with radiation and chemotherapy. Even with such radical treatment, most patients die within 5 years [117].

25.2.8 Acinic Cell Carcinoma (ACC)

Acinic cell carcinoma (ACC) is a rare tumor, which is indistinguishable clinically from benign neoplasms being of low-grade malignancy [127, 128]. However, it can rarely dedifferentiate into an aggressive high-grade tumor and present with complete loss of acinar differentiation, desmoplasia, tumor necrosis, frequent mitosis, and cervical or distant metastasis [127, 129, 130]. The parotid gland is the most common site (80%) followed by the minor salivary glands (16%) and the submandibular gland (4%). It has a predilection for women and more commonly occurs in the fifth decade [4, 86, 104].

Acinic cell carcinoma (ACC) develops from tumorigenesis of cells responsible for acinar development, namely, the reserve cells of the intercalated ducts and terminal tubule. It has a higher expression of mTOR compared to other salivary malignancies [75]. It presents with several growth patterns, including solid (most common), papillary-cystic, follicular, and microcystic [131]. Microscopically, it appears well circumscribed by a lymphoid stroma or a capsule. Individual cells can be granulated serous-type cells, primitive tubule cells, or undifferentiated polymorphous cells [131, 132]. Although acinic cell carcinoma is usually considered a low-grade malignancy, it can undergo high-grade transformation into high-grade adenocarcinoma or undifferentiated carcinoma.

Patients typically present with a slowly enlarging painless mass that is not fixed to the surrounding soft tissue or skin. Pain occurs in approximately 22% of patients [4]. Treatment is complete surgical resection. Neck dissection is usually not recommended because of the relatively low incidence of metastases to regional LNs [4].

Cervical neck metastasis occurs in only 6–10% and distant metastasis in 12–15% of cases. ACC is usually radio-resistant; however, RT is resorted to when complete resection is not achieved, in case of perineural invasion, and if LNs are affected [133, 134]. The recurrence rate averages 10–35% [4, 135]. Overall survival is influenced by male gender, age >45 years, tumor size >3 cm, and presence of distant metastasis [136]. The overall SR at 5 years is 75–96% and at 20 years is 56% [132, 137–140].

25.2.9 Basal Cell Adenocarcinoma (BCAC)

Basal cell adenocarcinoma (BCAC) is the malignant counterpart of basal cell adenoma (BCA). It is an uncommon low-grade malignancy that accounts for about 1.5% of all salivary gland tumors and 3% of all salivary gland malignancies [141]. There is no sex predilection [142], and most patients are in their sixth or seventh decade, though cases have been reported in patients as young as 2 months and as old as 92 years [141–146]. Most of these tumors arise de novo. Origin in a preexisting BCA is uncommon and usually involves the membranous subtype [142, 143, 146]. Approximately 90% of tumors arise in the major salivary glands, mostly parotid [147]. Patients present with a slowly growing asymptomatic mass; pain and tenderness are uncommon [148]. In 10–15% of cases, it occurs in conjunction with dermal cylindromas and trichoepitheliomas as compared to 40% of BCA [149]. Treatment is complete surgical excision, with neck dissection being reserved for patients with clinically positive LNs [150, 151].

25.2.10 Myoepithelial Carcinoma

Myoepithelial carcinoma (also known as "malignant myo-epithelioma") is the malignant counterpart of myoepithelioma. By definition, it is composed of myoepithelial cells with an infiltrative growth pattern. It is a rare tumor accounting for only 0.2% of all epithelial salivary gland tumors [152] and involving most commonly (75%) the parotid glands followed by the submandibular gland [149, 150, 152]. Approximately 50% of cases arise in a preexisting benign tumor, usually a pleomorphic adenoma or a myoepithelioma. It is most common in the sixth and seventh decades and occurs with no sex predilection [152]. A painless mass is usually the only clinical complaint. Treatment is a complete surgical excision. The clinical behavior of this tumor is unpredictable and unrelated to histological features [151].

25.2.11 Cystadenocarcinoma

Cystadenocarcinomas of the salivary glands are low-grade cystic neoplasms, which are twice as common in the major salivary glands as in the minor salivary glands, and most frequently occur in the parotid [153]. The majority of patients (75%) are over the age of 50 years [153]. Recognizing these tumors as carcinomas is predicated on finding areas of infiltrative growth. Perineural invasion is not a feature of this neoplasm. Complete surgical excision is usually curative as these tumors are of low-grade malignancy [154].

25.2.12 Salivary Duct Carcinoma (SDC)

Salivary duct carcinoma (SDC) is a rare high-grade tumor (7–10% of all salivary gland tumors) thought to arise from large excretory ducts [155]. The peak incidence of this tumor occurs in the sixth and seventh decades [4, 90, 156]. It is more common in men than women (2.5:1). It occurs most commonly in the parotid gland (78%) followed by the submandibular gland (12%) and the minor salivary glands (10%) [154]. Salivary duct carcinoma tends to overexpress erb-B2, which has been associated with a worse prognosis [157, 158]. Histologically, SDC is similar to high-grade duct carcinoma of the breast [159] and can present with cribriform, solid, cystic, or papillary growth patterns [90].

Many patients present with signs and symptoms reflecting the aggressive behavior of this tumor including a rapidly enlarging painful mass and facial nerve paresis or paralysis. In the series by Hosal et al. (2003), approximately two-thirds of patients presented with T3 or T4 tumors [154]. The presence of calcifications has been reported to be seen on CT scans in also one-third of the patients with salivary duct carcinoma [160–166].

The differential diagnosis includes metastatic adenocarcinoma from the prostate and metastatic ductal carcinoma of the breast. Immuno-perioxidase staining for prostate-specific antigens aids in ruling out metastatic prostate carcinoma [167]. Identifying areas of intraductal (in situ) tumor would serve to distinguish SDC from both metastatic prostate and breast carcinoma [154].

Because of its aggressive clinical behavior, SDC is treated by complete surgical excision of the primary combined with neck dissection and adjuvant RT. Cervical LN metastases are present in 60–80% of cases. The incidence of distant metastases ranges from 33–66%. Two-thirds of patients die of their disease usually within 3–4 years of treatment, usually from distant metastases, which occur most commonly to the lungs and bone [107, 156, 168–170]. The 5-year overall survival ranges from 20–50% [4, 107, 171].

25.2.13 Primary Squamous Cell Carcinoma (PSCC)

The presence of SCC in the salivary glands is suspected to arise from several sources including (1) malignant squamous portion of MEC, (2) metastasis from a cutaneous or mucosal head and neck source, (3) metastasis from distant primary carcinoma, or (4) primary squamous cell carcinoma (PSCC) [172].

Primary squamous cell carcinomas of the salivary glands (PSSC) are rare, extremely aggressive neoplasms, the majority of patients presenting with advanced disease [77, 173]. In a review of 2807 salivary gland tumors, PSSC accounted for only 1.9% [77]. About 9% of patients have a history of prior radiation exposure [77]. The parotid gland is involved in over two-thirds of cases, and the remaining involves the submandibular gland [77]. PSSC is twice as common in men as in women [174]. Histologically, SCC presents with intracellular keratinization, intercellular bridging, and keratin-pearl formation without any intracellular mucin [106].

Although PSCC has been reported in all decades of life, it is most common in the seventh decade. It is extremely uncommon in individuals below the age of 20 years [175]. Squamous cell carcinoma (SCC) usually presents as a hard mass, often fixed, with a short history of 1 year or less. It is often asymptomatic but may be painful in 20% of patients, and nodal metastases can occur in nearly 50% of patients.

It is important to ensure that this tumor is a primary tumor of the gland and not a metastatic lesion to the submandibular LNs from other SCCs in the head and neck. Differentiating it from MEC must also be confirmed. In general, differential diagnosis includes squamous metaplasia, necrotizing sialometaplasia, teratocystoma, high-grade MEC, and metastatic SCC. Metastatic SCC in salivary glands is more common than PSSC [176]. The presence of a focus on SCC in situ distinguishes PSSC from metastatic SCC.

Since this is an aggressive tumor, radical resection with neck dissection is usually indicated. Up to 75% of patients have histologically positive cervical LNs. Locoregional recurrence can occur in approximately 50% of cases [61], which has led to the use of postoperative RT in many instances. Distant metastases occur in 20–30% of patients. The overall 5-year SR ranges from 50–80% for early-stage tumors and 15% for advanced-stage tumors [77, 78, 177]. Advanced age, facial nerve palsy, and regional LN metastasis are poor prognostic factors [177, 178].

25.3 Clinical Presentation of Submandibular Tumors

25.3.1 History-Taking

Benign and malignant tumors of the submandibular gland usually present with a painless (72–87%), firm, lobulated, solitary mass in the submandibular region [60, 63]. The presence of pain suggests malignancy, but sialadenitis must be ruled out first. The discharge of purulent saliva from the salivary duct is usually diagnostic of an inflammatory glandular process. Nevertheless, it must be borne in mind that a salivary gland tumor can coexist with obstructive sialopathy leading to sialadenitis.

A detailed history, including pain, the onset of the mass, growth rate, swallowing difficulties, and facial weakness symptoms, should be obtained. Past medical history, surgical history, family history of malignancies, and social risk factors (such as smoking, past radiation exposure, and occupational hazards) should also be elicited.

25.3.2 Physical Examination

Physical examination should include a focused head and neck examination. Both benign and malignant tumors can present as painless, fixed masses [4]. Clinical examination, including bimanual palpation, is important in order to elicit the tumor size and mobility and to evaluate its extension to adjacent structures. Sensory (lingual nerve) and motor (hypoglossal and marginal mandibular branch of the facial nerve) deficits denote malignancy [63, 179]. Occasionally, MTs may fungate by direct extension through the skin or in association with dermal lymphatic permeation.

25.4 Work-Up of Submandibular Tumors

25.4.1 Diagnostic Imaging

The main objectives of imaging major salivary gland lesions in general are (1) to establish whether the mass is intrinsic or extrinsic, (2) to determine its relationship to the nerves, and (3) to evaluate its full extent and possible invasion of surrounding structures. If there is any radiological evidence of malignancy, the study is extended to include the neck.

25.4.2 Plain X-Ray, Sialography, and Nuclear Scan

Plain radiographs, sialography, and nuclear scans add very little to the diagnostic information and are seldom indicated for evaluation of submandibular (and sublingual) gland tumors.

25.4.3 Ultrasonography (US)/Color Doppler Sonography

Ultrasonography (US) is the first noninvasive option for evaluating major salivary gland tumors. It can differentiate between solid and cystic masses and between intra- and extra-glandular nodules and help guide FNAB. It can also provide important information regarding the contents of the mass, its size, and limits. Nevertheless, there are no definitive US criteria to differentiate between benign and malignant tumors [180], although heterogenous echogenicity, local invasion, poorly defined margins, and lymphadenopathy have been reported to be sonographic signs of malignancy [30, 31].

Color Doppler sonography usually shows enhanced vascularization in MTs when compared with the normal parenchyma or with BTs. Low-grade MECs, particularly those <2 cm, however, usually have a homogeneous structure and present with smooth borders and may be erroneously considered benign. High-grade MECs, in contrast, have irregular borders and typical heterogeneous echo patterns. It is noteworthy, however, that patterns of extra-glandular spread, such as perineural invasion and infiltration of the parapharyngeal space, mandible, and base of the skull, are not easily visible at US [180].

25.4.4 Computed Tomography (CT) Scan and Magnetic Resonance Imaging (MRI)

Computed tomography (CT) and magnetic resonance imaging (MRI) permit better visualization of masses within the salivary glands. Both are equally satisfactory in differentiating cystic from solid lesions and allow evaluation of the relationship of the tumor with adjacent structures, including soft tissues and bones [90]. However, CT scans are especially useful in the assessment of bone erosion, while MRI better evaluates soft tissue involvement and may also detect tumor extension along cranial nerves [181]. Heterogenous contrast enhancement, local soft tissue invasion, poorly defined margins, hypointensity on T2-weighted imaging, and lymphadenopathy on MRI are characteristics of malignancy [30, 182].

25.4.5 Positron Emission Tomography (PET)

The role of PET is to detect locoregional and distant metastasis. Compared with conventional CT, PET is more accurate in demonstrating tumor extension, nodal involvement, local recurrence, and distant metastasis due to the tissues' higher levels of standardized uptake values (SUV) [34, 35].

25.4.6 Cytopathological Diagnosis

25.4.6.1 Fine-Needle Aspiration Cytology (FNAC)

Fine-needle aspiration cytology (FNAC) can accurately establish cytological diagnosis in over 90–95% of patients in experienced hands [183]. Diagnosis of PA poses no difficulties in cytopathological specimens. Aspirates are highly cellular containing both myxo-cartilaginous stroma and large sheets or small aggregates of epithelial cells.

Determining the histopathological type of the primary tumor preoperatively can help in deciding the extent of the surgical procedure (with or without neck dissection). High-grade cancers such as adenocarcinomas and SCCs should be considered for neck dissection based on significantly increased rates of occult LN metastases. On the other hand, sarcomas, AdCC, and other histological types, which are unlikely to involve LNs, may not benefit from elective treatment of the neck [184].

25.4.6.2 Tissue Biopsy

An US-guided core needle biopsy can obtain larger tissue specimens with histological architecture, which improves recognition of tumor grade to allow further subtyping [185]. Disadvantages of core biopsy include more pain, increased risk of nerve injury, and hematoma formation [44]. Intraoperative frozen section biopsy has a sensitivity and specificity of 90% and 99%, respectively, in distinguishing between benign and malignant lesions [45].

25.4.7 Patterns of Spread of Malignant Tumors

Malignant tumors of the submandibular gland may extend through the capsule to involve the adjacent mandible, mylohyoid muscle, tongue, and the lingual and hypoglossal nerves. Moderate to severe pain is usually associated with advanced tumors, while nerve deficits involving cranial nerves V, VII, and XII may be found in 14% of patients [186]. Skin invasion, ulceration, and extension to the oral cavity can occur in advanced cases.

The incidence of LN metastases in submandibular carcinomas at the time of initial presentation varies from 8–33%. The risk of occult nodal metastases is higher in anaplastic, high-grade MEC, SCC, adenocarcinoma, and salivary duct carcinoma than in low-grade MEC, AdCC, ACC, and sarcoma [60, 61, 187, 188].

25.5 Differential Diagnosis of Submandibular Tumors

A primary submandibular gland neoplasm should mainly be differentiated from sialadenitis and metastatic SCC to a LN. It should also be differentiated from other causes of cervical lymphadenopathy such as atypical mycobacteria infection, cervicofacial actinomycosis, sarcoidosis, acquired or congenital cysts, benign follicular lymphadenopathy, and cat-scratch disease [186].

Episodic pain and mass are the hallmarks of inflammatory disease (sialadenitis), although one-third of the lesions may be asymptomatic. Obstructive sialadenitis, due to stricture or duct calculus, is a common cause of submandibular gland enlargement. In such cases, pain and swelling are associated with eating, receding after several hours. Erythema may occur over the mass, and a stone may be palpated in the duct which may drain purulent saliva when the gland is compressed [186, 189]. A solitary SCC metastatic to a submandibular LN in the absence of an obvious primary lesion in the oral cavity (occult primary) is rather uncommon.

Differentials of submandibular gland tumors include the following:

Salivary cysts
Sialadenitis
Sialoliths
Lymphadenopathy (from infectious or inflammatory causes)
Tuberculosis (TB)
Infectious Mononucleosis (IMN)
Chronic sclerosing sialadenitis (Küttner's tumor)
Branchial cleft cysts

Lymphoepithelial cysts (especially in immuno-compromised patients such as HIV patients)
Metastases from tumors of other body sites

25.6 Treatment of Submandibular Tumors

25.6.1 Management of Benign Tumors

The mainstay of treatment for benign submandibular tumors is complete surgical excision with negative margins. Through a cervical incision under general anesthesia, a subfascial dissection is usually performed to remove the submandibular gland without a cuff of surrounding normal tissue in cases of benign diseases such as small BTs and sialolithiasis or sialadenitis refractory to conservative management. This technique is rapid and has a low complication rate. Alternatively, Weber et al. (1990) [187] recommended level-I neck dissection (submental [level Ia] and submandibular [level Ib] LNs) during the routine resection of submandibular gland tumors as this would provide adequate margins in the treatment of BTs and also serve to sample LNs adjacent to the gland in the treatment of MTs [187].

Extirpation of the entire submandibular gland for treatment of benign submandibular tumors can lead to decreased resting salivary production. Studies that evaluated grand-preserving "partial sialadenectomy" for benign submandibular tumors showed that patients had higher postoperative resting saliva rates and less facial deformity with no difference in local control [190, 191]. Gland preservation surgery is contraindicated for malignant tumors and central gland lesions that would risk damage to the vascular and ductal integrity of the remaining salivary tissue after partial sialadenectomy [190]. Repeated surgical interventions, in case of recurrent tumors, increase the risk of tumor spillage and nerve injury [192–194].

25.6.2 Management of Malignant Tumors

Comprehensive management of MTs of the submandibular gland includes definitive treatment of the primary tumor and treatment (therapeutic or elective) of the neck; eventually, only neck observation is advised, as many neoplasms have a low propensity for lymphatic spread. Most of the clinical variables required to predict survival can often be obtained before definitive surgery. Based on findings of clinical evaluation, MRI, and FNAC, patients may be counseled as to surgical approach, need for neck dissection, and need for postoperative radiotherapy (RT).

25.6.3 Factors Influencing Selection of Therapy

The size of the primary tumor and histological grade are the most important tumor factors affecting the choice of initial therapy. Clinical (advanced stage and submandibular site) and histological (higher cancer grade, presence of perineural invasion, presence of LN metastases) parameters are considered independent predictors of poorer clinical outcomes in most series of major salivary gland MTs [60, 63, 64, 187, 195]. Vander Poorten et al. (1999) [63] reported that age at diagnosis ($p = 0.0006$), T stage ($p = 0.001$), and clinical skin invasion ($p = 0.005$) were the most significant predictors of poor survival among their patients.

Interestingly, Hocwald et al. (2001) [195] reported that older patients tend to have a higher incidence of more aggressive tumors as compared to younger patients (79% versus 56%, respectively). They also observed that men tended to present with higher T-stage tumors at diagnosis than did women, 53% versus 26% ($p = 00.02$). More recently, Bhattacharyya (2004) [64] identified patients with younger age, decreased tumor grade, and the addition of radiation therapy as factors associated with improved survival ($p < 0.001$, 0.005, and 0.015, respectively) in his series. Factors predicting tumor recurrence in most series include higher TNM stages, perineural growth, and LN metastases [60, 61, 63, 64, 187, 188, 195].

25.6.4 Resectable Tumors

Low-grade, low-stage MTs can be treated by excision of the submandibular gland with nodal dissection of level I. High-grade, high-stage MTs, however, require supra-omohyoid neck dissection (SOND), in conjunction with the excision of the submandibular gland. For advanced (locoregional) tumors, more radical local resection and neck dissection are indicated [61, 186, 187]. Morbidity secondary to sacrifice of the hypoglossal, lingual, and marginal branches of the facial nerve is better tolerated than that after loss of the entire facial nerve.

Reconstruction with regional and sometimes microvascular free flaps may be necessary. Adjuvant postoperative RT may be indicated, in selected cases, in an attempt at improving local and regional control. High-grade malignancies, recurrent tumors, gross or microscopic residual disease, tumors adjacent to the nerves, regional nodal metastases, and invasion of muscle, bone, skin, or nerve are all strong indications for postoperative RT [188, 196].

25.6.5 Advanced Non-resectable Tumors

Advanced non-resectable tumors of the submandibular gland are generally treated by RT with palliative intent. Treatment with neutron beam therapy is of particular value for adenoid cystic carcinomas (AdCCs).

25.6.6 Management of the Neck

Although the role of neck dissection in clinically proven metastases in salivary gland cancer is straightforward, routine elective treatment of the negative neck remains controversial. Some investigators recommend neck dissection only for patients with clinically evident LNs, whereas others also recommend elective neck dissection for tumors based on various prognostic factors [60, 61, 64, 187]. The incidence of LN metastases in submandibular carcinomas at the time of initial presentation varies from 8 to 33% [187, 188, 196], which reduces the 5-year survival rates from 40% to 9% [188, 197–203].

25.6.7 Predictive Factors for Cervical Metastases

Several authors have attempted to determine predictive factors for cervical metastases in salivary gland malignancy. Several studies have shown that the risk of occult nodal metastases is higher in anaplastic, high-grade MEC, SCC, adenocarcinoma, and salivary duct carcinoma than in low-grade MEC, AdCC, acinic cell carcinoma, and sarcoma [60, 61, 187, 199–201]. An increased risk of occult metastases is also associated with advanced-stage primary cancer.

25.6.8 Indications of Elective Neck Dissection

Medina (1998) [204] summarized the indications reported in the literature for elective neck dissection in salivary gland cancers as follows: high-grade tumors, T3–4 tumors, tumors >3 cm, facial nerve (neural) invasion, age >54 years, extra-glandular extension, and perilymphatic invasion [60–62, 187, 188, 196–204].

25.6.9 Treatment of Clinically Positive Node Metastases

The treatment of clinically positive node metastases is surgical. The extent of neck dissection is determined by the grossly involved LNs, and an attempt should be made to preserve vital structures. The most common levels of neck involvement in submandibular (and sublingual) malignant tumors are levels I–III [199, 201]. Since contralateral neck involvement is rare, only the ipsilateral neck is treated.

25.6.10 Treatment of the Clinically Negative Neck

Treatment of the clinically negative neck includes observation, elective neck dissection, and primary radiation. Currently, treatment of the N0 neck is only appropriate when the risk for occult metastases is high.

The general guidelines for the treatment of submandibular gland cancer are summarized in Table 25.2.

Table 25.2 General guidelines for the treatment of submandibular gland cancer

	Low grade (T1/T2 N0)	High grade (T1/T2 N0N1)	High grade (T3/T4 N0N+)
Tumor type	MEC (low grade) ACC (low grade) Adenocarcinoma (low grade)	MEC (high grade) ACC (high grade) Adenocarcinoma (high grade) AdCC CEPA SDC SCC	Any histological type
Treatment	Level I ND	Supraomohyoid ND (N0) Comprehensive ND (N+) Postoperative RT	Supraomohyoid ND (N0) Comprehensive ND (N+) Postoperative RT

MEC mucoepidermoid carcinoma; *ACC* acinic cell carcinoma; *AdCC* adenoid cystic carcinoma; *CEPA* carcinoma ex-pleomorphic adenocarcinoma; *SDC* salivary duct carcinoma; *SCC* squamous cell carcinoma; *ND* neck dissection; *RT* radiotherapy

25.6.11 Chemotherapy

The role of chemotherapy in the treatment of salivary gland MTs has been confined to metastatic disease and locoregional disease not amenable to either salvage surgery or RT. The most studied "single agent" is cisplatin. Licitra et al. (1991) [205] analyzed the results obtained from 25 patients treated for advanced carcinoma in a phase II trial (100 mg/m^2 of cisplatin every 3 weeks). They observed a response rate of 7 and 18% rate in metastatic lesions and locoregional recurrence, respectively. The median response duration was 7 months, and the median survival time was 14 months.

For "combination chemotherapy" with cisplatin, the most common agents used include 5-fluorouracil, cyclophosphamide, and doxorubicin. A regimen using all four drugs was used in 17 patients, and a 50% response rate was observed. The median duration of response was 8 months, and the median survival was 18 months [206].

Several "molecular targets" have been identified in salivary gland cancer such as C-kit proto-oncogene, EGFR, HER2 proto-oncogene, androgen receptors, p53 protein, and VEGF. These may ultimately provide useful information into diagnosis, biological behavior, and management of cancer of the salivary glands [207–214].

25.7 Prognosis of Submandibular Malignant Tumors

25.7.1 Outcome

In general, the prognosis of salivary malignancies is better for children and adolescents than that for adults due to lower frequencies of cervical metastasis, absence of local soft tissue invasion, and more differentiated histologies. The 5-year overall survival for children after surgical treatment is 85% compared with 60% for adults [215, 216].

Regardless of malignant sub-type, negative prognostic factors for survival include advanced age, high-stage disease, high-grade histology, cervical metastasis, male gender, presence of pain, facial nerve involvement, perineural invasion, local soft tissue invasion, positive or close margins, distant metastasis, and comorbidities [216–223]. Smoking and alcohol statuses were controversial, with some studies showing no significant influence on overall survival or disease-free survival [224, 225], whereas others found them to be poor prognostic factors [70, 81].

Overexpression of epidermal growth factor receptor (EGFR) and human epidermal growth factor receptor 2 (HER2) has been identified in several salivary gland malignancies, such as SDC. They tend to predict a higher incidence of cervical metastasis and worse survival [90]. The absence of C-kit expression in AdCC is correlated with poorer prognosis [170].

Distant metastasis, the main cause of mortality [226], most commonly involves the lungs (40–91%) followed by bone (13–40%), liver (4–19%), soft tissue (9%), distant nodal basins (8%), and the brain (4–7%) [227].

25.7.2 Complications

Patients who undergo submandibular gland resection or neck dissection for cervical LN metastasis have a risk of neurological damage to the sympathetic trunk, spinal accessory, phrenic, hypoglossal, lingual, vagus nerves, and the marginal mandibular branch of the facial nerve [228–230].

Complications from RT include skin erythema, mucositis, dysphagia, dysgeusia, xerostomia, soft tissue fibrosis, osteoradionecrosis, and radiation-induced malignancy [65, 226]. Mandibular osteoradionecrosis (<2%) and radiation-induced malignancy (1%) at 10–25 years are rare complications [226, 231, 232].

References

1. Carlson ER, McCoy JM. Margins for benign salivary gland neoplasms of the head and neck. Oral Maxillofac Surg Clin North Am. 2017;29(3):325–40.
2. Ord RA, Carlson ER. Pediatric Salivary gland malignancies. Oral Maxillofac Surg Clin North Am. 2016;28(1):83–9.
3. Rice DH, Batsakis JG, McClatchey KD. Postirradiation malignant salivary gland tumor. Arch Otolaryngol. 1976;102(11):699–701.
4. Bradley PJ. Frequency and histopathology by site, major pathologies, symptoms and signs of Salivary gland neoplasms. Adv Otorhinolaryngol. 2016;78:9–16.
5. Kotwall CA. Smoking as an etiologic factor in the development of Warthin's tumor of the parotid gland. Am J Surg. 1992;164(6):646–7.
6. Haberland-Carrodeguas C, Fornatora ML, Reich RF, Freedman PD. Detection of human papillomavirus DNA in oral inverted ductal papillomas. J Clin Pathol. 2003;56(12):910–3.
7. Sala-Pérez S, España-Tost A, Vidal-Bel A, Gay-Escoda C. Inverted ductal papilloma of the oral cavity secondary to lower lip trauma. A case report and literature review. J Clin Exp Dent. 2013;5(2):e112–6.

8. Martins C, Fonseca I, Roque L, Pereira T, Ribeiro C, Bullerdiek J, Soares J. PLAG1 gene alterations in salivary gland pleomorphic adenoma and carcinoma ex-pleomorphic adenoma: a combined study using chromosome banding, in situ hybridization and immunocytochemistry. Mod Pathol. 2005;18(8):1048–55.
9. Mito JK, Jo VY, Chiosea SI, Dal Cin P, Krane JF. HMGA2 is a specific immunohistochemical marker for pleomorphic adenoma and carcinoma ex-pleomorphic adenoma. Histopathology. 2017;71(4):511–21.
10. Andreasen S, von Holstein SL, Homøe P, Heegaard S. Recurrent rearrangements of the PLAG1 and HMGA2 genes in lacrimal gland pleomorphic adenoma and carcinoma ex pleomorphic adenoma. Acta Ophthalmol. 2018;96(7):e768–71.
11. Kim J, Song JS, Roh JL, Choi SH, Nam SY, Kim SY, Cho KJ. Increased immunoglobulin g4-positive plasma cells in lymphadenoma of the salivary gland: an immunohistochemical comparison among lymphoepithelial lesions. Appl Immunohistochem Mol Morphol. 2018;26(6):420–4.
12. Cheuk W, Chan JK. Advances in salivary gland pathology. Histopathology. 2007;51(1):1–20.
13. Dwivedi N, Agarwal A, Raj V, Chandra S. Histogenesis of salivary gland neoplasms. Indian J Cancer. 2013;50(4):361–6.
14. Sreeja C, Shahela T, Aesha S, Satish MK. Taxonomy of salivary gland neoplasm. J Clin Diagn Res. 2014;8(3):291–3.
15. Regezi JA, Batsakis JG. Histogenesis of salivary gland neoplasms. Otolaryngol Clin N Am. 1977;10(2):297–307.
16. Dardick I, Jeans MT, Sinnott NM, Wittkuhn JF, Kahn HJ, Baumal R. Salivary gland components involved in the formation of squamous metaplasia. Am J Pathol. 1985;119(1):33–43.
17. Buenting JE, Smith TL, Holmes DK. Giant pleomorphic adenoma of the parotid gland: case report and review of the literature. Ear Nose Throat J. 1998;77(8):634–40.
18. Honda T, Yamamoto Y, Isago T, Nakazawa H, Nozaki M, Hirayama T. Giant pleomorphic adenoma of the parotid gland with malignant transformation. Ann Plast Surg. 2005;5(5):524–7.
19. Kici S, Peytral C. Giant pleomorphic adenoma of the parotid gland: a case report and review of the literature. Ann Otolaryngol Chir Cervicofac. 2001;118(5):330–2.
20. Eveson JW, Kusafuka K, Stenman G. Pleomorphic adenoma. In: Barnes EL, Eveson JW, Reichart P, Sidransky D, editors. Pathology and classification of head and neck Tumours. Lyon: IARC; 2005.
21. Chaplin AJ, Darke P, Patel S. Tyrosine-rich crystals in pleomorphic adenomas of parotid glands. J Oral Pathol. 1983;12(5):342–6.
22. Lingam RK, Daghir AA, Nigar E, Abbas SA, Kumar M. Pleomorphic adenoma (benign mixed tumour) of the salivary glands: its diverse clinical, radiological, and histopathological presentation. Br J Oral Maxillofac Surg. 2011;49(1):14–20.
23. Henriksson G, Westrin KM, Carlsöö B, Silfverswärd C. Recurrent primary pleomorphic adenomas of salivary gland origin: intrasurgical rupture, histopathologic features, and pseudopodia. Cancer. 1998;82(4):617–20.
24. Soteldo J, Aranaga N. Metastasizing pleomorphic adenoma of the parotid gland. Ecancermedicalscience. 2017;11:758.
25. Kas K, Voz ML, Roijer E, Astrom AK, Meyen E, Stenman G, et al. Promoter swapping between the genes for a novel zinc finger protein and beta-catenin in pleiomorphic adenomas with t(3;8)(p21;q12) translocations. Nat Genet. 1997;15(2):170–4.
26. Voz ML, Astrom AK, Kas K, Mark J, Stenman G, Van de Ven WJ. The recurrent translocation t(5;8)(p13;q12) in pleomorphic adenomas results in upregulation of PLAG1 gene expression under control of the LIFR promoter. Oncogene. 1998;16(11):1409–16.
27. Lee KC, Chan JK, Chong YW. Ossifying pleomorphic adenoma of the maxillary antrum. J Laryngol Otol. 1992;106(1):50–2.
28. Seifert G, Donath K, Schafer R. Lipomatous pleomorphic adenoma of the parotid gland. Classification of lipomatous tissue in salivary glands. Pathol Res Pract. 1999;195(4):247–52.
29. Skalova A, Starek I, Simpson RH, Kucerova V, Dvorackova J, Curik R, et al. Spindle cell myoepithelial tumours of the parotid gland with extensive lipomatous metaplasia. A report

of four cases with immunohistochemical and ultrastructural findings. Virchows Arch. 2001;439(6):762–7.
30. Lee YY, Wong KT, King AD, Ahuja AT. Imaging of salivary gland tumours. Eur J Radiol. 2008;66(3):419–36.
31. Kovacević DO, Fabijanić I. Sonographic diagnosis of parotid gland lesions: correlation with the results of sonographically guided fine-needle aspiration biopsy. J Clin Ultrasound. 2010;38(6):294–8.
32. Koyuncu M, Seşen T, Akan H, Ismailoglu AA, Tanyeri Y, Tekat A, Unal R, Incesu L. Comparison of computed tomography and magnetic resonance imaging in the diagnosis of parotid tumors. Otolaryngol Head Neck Surg. 2003;129(6):726–32.
33. Yerli H, Agildere AM, Aydin E, Geyik E, Haberal N, Kaskati T, Oguz D, Ozluoglu LN. Value of apparent diffusion coefficient calculation in the differential diagnosis of parotid gland tumors. Acta Radiol. 2007;48(9):980–7.
34. Roh JL, Kim HS, Park CI. Randomized clinical trial comparing partial parotidectomy versus superficial or total parotidectomy. Br J Surg. 2007;94(9):1081–7.
35. Jeong HS, Chung MK, Son YI, Choi JY, Kim HJ, Ko YH, Baek CH. Role of 18F-FDG PET/CT in management of high-grade salivary gland malignancies. J Nucl Med. 2007;48(8):1237–44.
36. Keyes JW, Harkness BA, Greven KM, Williams DW, Watson NE, McGuirt WF. Salivary gland tumors: pretherapy evaluation with PET. Radiology. 1994;192(1):99–102.
37. Hughes JH, Volk EE, Wilbur DC. Cytopathology Resource Committee, College of American Pathologists. Pitfalls in salivary gland fine-needle aspiration cytology: lessons from the College of American Pathologists Interlaboratory Comparison Program in Nongynecologic Cytology. Arch Pathol Lab Med. 2005;129(1):26–31.
38. Bajaj Y, Singh S, Cozens N, Sharp J. Critical clinical appraisal of the role of ultrasound guided fine needle aspiration cytology in the management of parotid tumours. J Laryngol Otol. 2005;119(4):289–92.
39. Das DK, Anim JT. Pleomorphic adenoma of salivary gland: to what extent does fine needle aspiration cytology reflect histopathological features? Cytopathology. 2005;16(2):65–70.
40. Seifert G, Donath K. Multiple tumours of the salivary glands—terminology and nomenclature. Eur J Cancer B Oral Oncol. 1996;32 B(1):3–7.
41. Yu GY, Ma DQ, Zhang Y, Peng X, Cai ZG, Gao Y, et al. Multiple primary tumours of the parotid gland. Int J Oral Maxillofac Surg. 2004;33(6):531–4.
42. Eveson JW, Cawson RA. Salivary gland tumours. A review of 2410 cases with particular reference to histological types, site, age and sex distribution. J Pathol. 1985;146(1):51–8.
43. Junquera L, Alonso D, Sampedro A, Fresno F, Albertos JM, Lopez-Arranz JS. Pleomorphic adenoma of the salivary glands: prospective clinicopathologic and flow cytometric study. Head Neck. 1999;21(7):652–6.
44. Schmidt RL, Hall BJ, Layfield LJ. A systematic review and meta-analysis of the diagnostic accuracy of ultrasound-guided core needle biopsy for salivary gland lesions. Am J Clin Pathol. 2011;136(4):516–26.
45. Schmidt RL, Hunt JP, Hall BJ, Wilson AR, Layfield LJ. A systematic review and meta-analysis of the diagnostic accuracy of frozen section for parotid gland lesions. Am J Clin Pathol. 2011;136(5):729–38.
46. Ellis GL. Salivary gland neoplasms. Ear Nose Throat J. 1984;63(8):358–69.
47. Laskawi R, Schott T, Schröder M. Recurrent pleomorphic adenomas of the parotid gland: clinical evaluation and long-term follow-up. Br J Oral Maxillofac Surg. 1998;36(1):48–51.
48. Witt RL. The significance of the margin in parotid surgery for pleomorphic adenoma. Laryngoscope. 2002;112(12):2141–54.
49. Ethunandan M, Pratt CA, Morrison A, Anand R, Macpherson DW, Wilson AW. Multiple synchronous and metachronous neoplasms of the parotid gland: the Chichester experience. Br J Oral Maxillofac Surg. 2006;44(5):397–401.
50. Chen I, Hy T. Pleomorphic adenoma of the parotid gland metastasizing to the cervical lymph node. Otolaryngol Head Neck Surg. 2000;122(3):455–7.

51. Marioni G, Marino F, Stramare R, Marchese-Ragona R, Staffieri A. Benign metastasizing pleomorphic adenoma of the parotid gland: a clinicopathologic puzzle. Head Neck. 2003;25(12):1071–6.
52. Nouraei SA, Ferguson MS, Clarke PM, Sandison A, Sandhu GS, Michaels L, Rhys-Evans P. Metastasizing pleomorphic salivary adenoma. Arch Otolaryngol Head Neck Surg. 2006;132(7):788–93.
53. Raja V, China C, Masaki KH, Nakano G. Unusual presentations of uncommon tumors: case 1. Benign metastasizing pleomorphic adenoma. J Clin Oncol. 2002;20(9):2400–3.
54. Snyderman C, Johnson JT, Barnes EL. Extraparotid Warthin's tumor. Otolaryngol Head Neck Surg. 1986;94(2):169–75.
55. Andreasen S, Therkildsen MH, Bjørndal K, Homøe P. Pleomorphic adenoma of the parotid gland 1985-2010: a Danish nationwide study of incidence, recurrence rate, and malignant transformation. Head Neck. 2016;38(Suppl 1):E1364–9.
56. Gnepp DR. Sebaceous neoplasms of salivary gland origin: a review. Pathol Annu. 1983;18(Pt 1):71–102.
57. Hellquist H, Paiva-Correia A, Vander Poorten V, Quer M, Hernandez-Prera JC, Andreasen S, Zbären P, Skalova A, Rinaldo A, Ferlito A. Analysis of the clinical relevance of histological classification of benign epithelial Salivary gland Tumours. Adv Ther. 2019;36(8):1950–74.
58. Tian Z, Li L, Wang L, Hu Y, Li J. Salivary gland neoplasms in oral and maxillofacial regions: a 23-year retrospective study of 6982 cases in an eastern Chinese population. Int J Oral Maxillofac Surg. 2010;39(3):235–42.
59. Wilson TC, Robinson RA. Basal cell adenocarcinoma and basal cell adenoma of the salivary glands: a clinicopathological review of seventy tumors with comparison of morphologic features and growth control indices. Head Neck Pathol. 2015;9(2):205–13.
60. Spiro RH. Salivary neoplasms: overview of a 35-year experience with 2,807 patients. Head Neck Surg. 1986;8:177–84.
61. Shah JP, Ihde JK. Salivary gland tumors. Curr Probl Surg. 1990:803–11.
62. Sykes AJ, Slevin NJ, Birzgalis AR, Gupta NK. Submandibular gland carcinoma; an audit of local control and survival following adjuvant radiotherapy. Oral Oncol. 1999;35:187–90.
63. Vander Poorten VLM, Balm AJM, Hilgers FJM, et al. Prognostic factors for long term results of the treatment of patients with malignant submandibular gland tumors. Cancer. 1999;85:2255–64.
64. Bhattacharyya N. Survival and prognosis for cancer of the submandibular gland. J Oral Maxillofac Surg. 2004;62:427–30.
65. Thomson DJ, Slevin NJ, Mendenhall WM. Indications for salivary gland radiotherapy. Adv Otorhinolaryngol. 2016;78:141–7.
66. Spiro RH. Management of malignant tumors of the salivary glands. Oncology (Williston Park). 1998;12(5):671–80.
67. Ord RA, Ghazali N. Margin analysis: malignant Salivary gland neoplasms of the head and neck. Oral Maxillofac Surg Clin North Am. 2017;29(3):315–24.
68. Camilleri IG, Malata CM, McLean NR, Kelly CG. Malignant tumours of the submandibular salivary gland: a 15-year review. Br J Plast Surg. 1998;51(3):181–5.
69. Goldstein AM, Yuen J, Tucker MA. Second cancers after medulloblastoma: population-based results from the United States and Sweden. Cancer Causes Control. 1997;8(6):865–71.
70. Horn-Ross PL, Ljung BM, Morrow M. Environmental factors and the risk of salivary gland cancer. Epidemiology. 1997;8(4):414–9.
71. Milán T, Pukkala E, Verkasalo PK, Kaprio J, Jansén CT, Koskenvuo M, Teppo L. Subsequent primary cancers after basal-cell carcinoma: a nationwide study in Finland from 1953 to 1995. Int J Cancer. 2000;87(2):283–8.
72. Fan CY, Wang J, Barnes EL. Expression of androgen receptor and prostatic specific markers in salivary duct carcinoma: an immunohistochemical analysis of 13 cases and review of the literature. Am J Surg Pathol. 2000;24(4):579–86.

73. Nasser SM, Faquin WC, Dayal Y. Expression of androgen, estrogen, and progesterone receptors in salivary gland tumors. Frequent expression of androgen receptor in a subset of malignant salivary gland tumors. Am J Clin Pathol. 2003;119(6):801–6.
74. Schwarz-Furlan S, Brase C, Stockmann P, Furlan I, Hartmann A. Hereditary head and neck tumors. Pathologe. 2010;31(6):477–84.
75. Ettl T, Schwarz-Furlan S, Haubner F, Müller S, Zenk J, Gosau M, Reichert TE, Zeitler K. The PI3K/AKT/mTOR signalling pathway is active in salivary gland cancer and implies different functions and prognoses depending on cell localisation. Oral Oncol. 2012;48(9):822–30.
76. Boukheris H, Ron E, Dores GM, Stovall M, Smith SA, Curtis RE. Risk of radiation-related salivary gland carcinomas among survivors of Hodgkin lymphoma: a population-based analysis. Cancer. 2008;113(11):3153–9.
77. Shemen LJ, Huvos AG, Spiro RH. Squamous cell carcinoma of salivary gland origin. Head Neck Surg. 1987;9(4):235–40.
78. Spitz MR, Batsakis JG. Major salivary gland carcinoma. Descriptive epidemiology and survival of 498 patients. Arch Otolaryngol. 1984;110(1):45–9.
79. Voulgarelis M, Dafni UG, Isenberg DA, Moutsopoulos HM. Malignant lymphoma in primary Sjögren's syndrome: a multicenter, retrospective, clinical study by the European concerted action on Sjögren's syndrome. Arthritis Rheum. 1999;42(8):1765–72.
80. Turner MD. Salivary gland disease in Sjögren's syndrome: sialoadenitis to lymphoma. Oral Maxillofac Surg Clin North Am. 2014;26(1):75–81.
81. Hayes RB, Bravo-Otero E, Kleinman DV, Brown LM, Fraumeni JF, Harty LC, Winn DM. Tobacco and alcohol use and oral cancer in Puerto Rico. Cancer Causes Control. 1999;10(1):27–33.
82. Sadetzki S, Oberman B, Mandelzweig L, Chetrit A, Ben-Tal T, Jarus-Hakak A, Duvdevani S, Cardis E, Wolf M. Smoking and risk of parotid gland tumors: a nationwide case-control study. Cancer. 2008;112(9):1974–82.
83. Lee DJ, Smith RR, Spaziani JT, Rostock R, Holliday M, Moses H. Adenoid cystic carcinoma of the nasopharynx. Case reports and literature review. Ann Otol Rhinol Laryngol. 1985;94(3):269–72.
84. Bradley PJ. Adenoid cystic carcinoma of the head and neck: a review. Curr Opin Otolaryngol Head Neck Surg. 2004;12(2):127–32.
85. Martínez-Rodríguez N, Leco-Berrocal I, Rubio-Alonso L, Arias-Irimia O, Martínez-González JM. Epidemiology and treatment of adenoid cystic carcinoma of the minor salivary glands: a meta-analytic study. Med Oral Patol Oral Cir Bucal. 2011;6(7):e884–9.
86. Bishop JA, Yonescu R, Batista D, Eisele DW, Westra WH. Most nonparotid "acinic cell carcinomas" represents mammary analog secretory carcinomas. Am J Surg Pathol. 2013;37(7):1053–7.
87. Mitani Y, Li J, Rao PH, Zhao YJ, Bell D, Lippman SM, et al. Comprehensive analysis of the MYB-NFIB gene fusion in salivary adenoid cystic carcinoma: incidence, variability, and clinicopathologic significance. Clin Cancer Res. 2010;16(19):4722–31.
88. Brill LB, Kanner WA, Fehr A, Andrén Y, Moskaluk CA, Löning T, et al. Analysis of MYB expression and MYB-NFIB gene fusions in adenoid cystic carcinoma and other salivary neoplasms. Mod Pathol. 2011;24(9):1169–76.
89. Brayer KJ, Frerich CA, Kang H, Ness SA. Recurrent fusions in MYB and MYBL1 define a common, transcription factor-driven oncogenic pathway in Salivary gland adenoid cystic carcinoma. Cancer Discov. 2016;6(2):176–87.
90. Ettl T, Schwarz-Furlan S, Gosau M, Reichert TE. Salivary gland carcinomas. Oral Maxillofac Surg. 2012;16(3):267–83.
91. Batsakis JG, Regezi JA. The pathology of head and neck tumors: salivary glands, part 1. Head Neck Surg. 1978;1(1):59–68.
92. Yaga US, Gollamudi N, Mengji AK, Besta R, Panta P, Prakash B, Rajashekar E. Adenoid cystic carcinoma of the palate: case report and review of literature. Pan Afr Med J. 2016;24:106.
93. DeAngelis AF, Tsui A, Wiesenfeld D, Chandu A. Outcomes of patients with adenoid cystic carcinoma of the minor salivary glands. Int J Oral Maxillofac Surg. 2011;40(7):710–4.

94. Shimamoto H, Chindasombatjaroen J, Kakimoto N, Kishino M, Murakami S, Furukawa S. Perineural spread of adenoid cystic carcinoma in the oral and maxillofacial regions: evaluation with contrast-enhanced CT and MRI. Dentomaxillofac Radiol. 2012;41(2):143–51.
95. Gurney TA, Eisele DW, Weinberg V, Shin E, Lee N. Adenoid cystic carcinoma of the major salivary glands treated with surgery and radiation. Laryngoscope. 2005;115(7):1278–82.
96. Rapidis AD, Givalos N, Gakiopoulou H, Faratzis G, Stavrianos SD, Vilos GA, et al. Adenoid cystic carcinoma of the head and neck. Clinicopathological analysis of 23 patients and review of the literature. Oral Oncol. 2005;41(3):328–35.
97. Gerughty RM, Scofield HH, Brown FM, Hennigar GR. Malignant mixed tumors of salivary gland origin. Cancer. 1969;24(3):471–86.
98. Rinaldo A, Ferlito A, Pellitteri PK, Robbins KT, Shaha AR, Bradley PJ, Kowalski LP, Wei WI. Management of malignant submandibular gland tumors. Acta Otolaryngol. 2003;123(8):896–904.
99. Hamper K, Lazar F, Dietel M, Caselitz J, Berger J, Arps H, Falkmer U, Auer G, Seifert G. Prognostic factors for adenoid cystic carcinoma of the head and neck: a retrospective evaluation of 96 cases. J Oral Pathol Med. 1990;19(3):101–7.
100. Perzin KH, Gullane P, Clairmont AC. Adenoid cystic carcinomas arising in salivary glands: a correlation of histologic features and clinical course. Cancer. 1978;42(1):265–82.
101. Eversole LR. Mucoepidermoid carcinoma: review of 815 reported cases. J Oral Surg. 1970;28(7):490–4.
102. Waldron CA, Koh ML. Central mucoepidermoid carcinoma of the jaws: report of four cases with analysis of the literature and discussion of the relationship to mucoepidermoid, sialodontogenic, and glandular odontogenic cysts. J Oral Maxillofac Surg. 1990;48(8):871–7.
103. Browand BC, Waldron CA. Central mucoepidermoid tumors of the jaws. Report of nine cases and review of the literature. Oral Surg Oral Med Oral Pathol. 1975;40(5):631–43.
104. Krolls SO, Trodahl JN, Boyers RC. Salivary gland lesions in children. A survey of 430 cases. Cancer. 1972;30(2):459–69.
105. Jakobsson PA, Blanck C, Eneroth CM. Mucoepidermoid carcinoma of the parotid gland. Cancer. 1968;22(1):111–24.
106. Batsakis JG, Chinn E, Regezi JA, Repola DA. The pathology of head and neck tumors: salivary glands, part 2. Head Neck Surg. 1978;1(2):167–80.
107. Foote FW, Frazell EL. Tumors of the major salivary glands. Cancer. 1953;6(6):1065–133.
108. Healey WV, Perzin KH, Smith L. Mucoepidermoid carcinoma of salivary gland origin. Classification, clinical-pathologic correlation, and results of treatment. Cancer. 1970;26(2):368–88.
109. O'Neill ID. t(11;19) translocation and CRTC1-MAML2 fusion oncogene in mucoepidermoid carcinoma. Oral Oncol. 2009;45(1):2–9.
110. Tonon G, Modi S, Wu L, Kubo A, Coxon AB, Komiya T, et al. t(11;19)(q21;p13) translocation in mucoepidermoid carcinoma creates a novel fusion product that disrupts a Notch signaling pathway. Nat Genet. 2003;33(2):208–13.
111. Boahene DK, Olsen KD, Lewis JE, Pinheiro AD, Pankratz VS, Bagniewski SM. Mucoepidermoid carcinoma of the parotid gland: the Mayo clinic experience. Arch Otolaryngol Head Neck Surg. 2004;130(7):849–56.
112. Smith A, Winkler B, Perzin KH, Wazen J, Blitzer A. Mucoepidermoid carcinoma arising in an intraparotid lymph node. Cancer. 1985;55(2):400–3.
113. LiVolsi VA, Perzin KH. Malignant mixed tumors arising in salivary glands. I. Carcinomas arising in benign mixed tumors: a clinicopathologic study. Cancer. 1977;39(5):2209–30.
114. Milford CA, Mugliston TA, O'Flynn P, McCarthy K. Carcinoma arising in a pleomorphic adenoma of the epiglottis. J Laryngol Otol. 1989;103(3):324–7.
115. Conley J, Arena S. Parotid gland as a focus of metastasis. Arch Surg. 1963;87:757–64.
116. Gottenberg JE, Cagnard N, Lucchesi C, Letourneur F, Mistou S, Lazure T, et al. Activation of IFN pathways and plasmacytoid dendritic cell recruitment in target organs of primary Sjögren's syndrome. Proc Natl Acad Sci USA. 2006;103(8):2770–5.

117. Gnepp DR. Malignant mixed tumors of the salivary glands: a review. Pathol Annu. 1993;28(1):279–328.
118. Lewis JE, Olsen KD, Sebo TJ. Carcinoma ex pleomorphic adenoma: pathologic analysis of 73 cases. Hum Pathol. 2001;32(6):596–604.
119. Weiler C, Zengel P, van der Wal JE, Guntinas-Lichius O, Schwarz S, Harrison JD, et al. Carcinoma ex pleomorphic adenoma with special reference to the prognostic significance of histological progression: a clinicopathological investigation of 41 cases. Histopathology. 2011;59(4):741–50.
120. Olsen KD, Lewis JE. Carcinoma ex pleomorphic adenoma: a clinicopathologic review. Head Neck. 2001;23(9):705–12.
121. Tortoledo ME, Luna MA, Batsakis JG. Carcinomas ex pleomorphic adenoma and malignant mixed tumors. Histomorphologic indexes. Arch Otolaryngol. 1984;110(3):172–6.
122. Chen AM, Garcia J, Bucci MK, Quivey JM, Eisele DW. The role of postoperative radiation therapy in carcinoma ex pleomorphic adenoma of the parotid gland. Int J Radiat Oncol Biol Phys. 2007;67(1):138–43.
123. Eneroth CM, Zetterberg A. Malignancy in pleomorphic adenoma. A clinical and microspectrophotometric study. Acta Otolaryngol. 1974;77(6):426–32.
124. Barnes L, Appel BN, Perez H, El-Attar AM. Myoepithelioma of the head and neck: case report and review. J Surg Oncol. 1985;28(1):21–8.
125. Kwon MY, Gu M. True malignant mixed tumor (carcinosarcoma) of parotid gland with unusual mesenchymal component: a case report and review of the literature. Arch Pathol Lab Med. 2001;125(6):812–5.
126. Fowler MH, Fowler J, Ducatman B, Barnes L, Hunt JL. Malignant mixed tumors of the salivary gland: a study of loss of heterozygosity in tumor suppressor genes. Mod Pathol. 2006;19(3):350–5.
127. Lewis JE, Olsen KD, Weiland LH. Acinic cell carcinoma. Clinicopathologic review. Cancer. 1991;67(1):172–9.
128. Mehta RP, Faquin WC, Deschler DG. Pathology quiz case 1. Acinic cell carcinoma of the parotid gland with ductal extension. Arch Otolaryngol Head Neck Surg. 2004;130(6):790–3.
129. Gomez DR, Katabi N, Zhung J, Wolden SL, Zelefsky MJ, Kraus DH, et al. Clinical and pathologic prognostic features in acinic cell carcinoma of the parotid gland. Cancer. 2009;115(10):2128–37.
130. Skálová A, Sima R, Vanecek T, Muller S, Korabecna M, Nemcova J, et al. Acinic cell carcinoma with high-grade transformation: a report of 9 cases with immunohistochemical study and analysis of TP53 and HER-2/neu genes. Am J Surg Pathol. 2009;33(8):1137–45.
131. Abrams AM, Cornyn J, Scofield HH, Hansen LS. Acinic cell adenocarcinoma of the major salivary glands. A clinicopathologic study of 77 cases. Cancer. 1965;18:1145–62.
132. Eneroth CM, Jakobsson PA, Blanck C. Acinic cell carcinoma of the parotid gland. Cancer. 1966;19(12):1761–72.
133. Chong GC, Beahrs OH, Woolner LB. Surgical management of acinic cell carcinoma of the parotid gland. Surg Gynecol Obstet. 1974;138(1):65–8.
134. Neto AG, Pineda-Daboin K, Spencer ML, Luna MA. Sinonasal acinic cell carcinoma: a clinicopathologic study of four cases. Head Neck. 2005;27(7):603–7.
135. Miki H, Masuda E, Ohata S, Komaki K, Hirokawa M, Uehara H, et al. Late recurrence of acinic cell carcinoma of the parotid gland. J Med Investig. 1999;46(3–4):213–6.
136. Neskey DM, Klein JD, Hicks S, Garden AS, Bell DM, El-Naggar AK, et al. Prognostic factors associated with decreased survival in patients with acinic cell carcinoma. JAMA Otolaryngol Head Neck Surg. 2013;139(11):1195–202.
137. El-Naggar AK, Batsakis JG, Luna MA, McLemore D, Byers RM. DNA flow cytometry of acinic cell carcinomas of major salivary glands. J Laryngol Otol. 1990;104(5):410–6.
138. Skalova A, Leivo I, Von Boguslawsky K, Saksela E. Cell proliferation correlates with prognosis in acinic cell carcinomas of salivary gland origin. Immunohistochemical study of 30 cases using the MIB 1 antibody in formalin-fixed paraffin sections. J Pathol. 1994;173(1):13–21.

139. Spiro RH, Huvos AG, Strong EW. Cancer of the parotid gland. A clinicopathologic study of 288 primary cases. Am J Surg. 1975;130(4):452–9.
140. Hickman RE, Cawson RA, Duffy SW. The prognosis of specific types of salivary gland tumors. Cancer. 1984;54(8):1620–4.
141. Muller S, Barnes L. Basal cell adenocarcinoma of the salivary glands. Report of seven cases and review of the literature. Cancer. 1996;78(12):2471–7.
142. Gross M, Maly B, Goldfarb A, Eliashar R. Basal cell adenocarcinoma in a buccal minor salivary gland. Acta Otolaryngol. 2004;124(2):213–6.
143. Jayakrishnan A, Elmalah I, Hussain K, Odell EW. Basal cell adenocarcinoma in minor salivary glands. Histopathology. 2003;42(6):610–4.
144. Nagao T, Sugano I, Ishida Y, Hasegawa M, Matsuzaki O, Konno A, et al. Basal cell adenocarcinoma of the salivary glands: comparison with basal cell adenoma through assessment of cell proliferation, apoptosis, and expression of p53 and bcl-2. Cancer. 1998;82(3):439–47.
145. Warrick PD, Irish JC, Mancer K, Dardick I, Pynn BR, Gullane P. Basal cell adenocarcinoma: a rare malignancy of the salivary glands. J Otolaryngol. 2000;29(2):102–9.
146. de Sousa SO, Schwarzschild M, de Araujo NS, de Araujo VC. Basal cell adenocarcinoma of the palate with squamous metaplasia. J Clin Pathol. 2000;53(2):153–6.
147. Ellis GL, Wiscovitch JG. Basal cell adenocarcinomas of the major salivary glands. Oral Surg Oral Med Oral Pathol. 1990;69(4):461–9.
148. Seifert G. Classification and differential diagnosis of clear and basal cell tumors of the salivary glands. Semin Diagn Pathol. 1996;13(2):95–103.
149. Chhieng DC, Paulino AF. Cytology of myoepithelial carcinoma of the salivary gland. Cancer. 2002;96(1):32–6.
150. Said S, Campana J. Myoepithelial carcinoma ex pleomorphic adenoma of salivary glands: a problematic diagnosis. Oral Surg Oral Med Oral Pathol Oral Radiol Endod. 2005;99(2):196–201.
151. Foss RD, Ellis GL, Auclair PL. Salivary gland cystadenocarcinomas. A clinicopathologic study of 57 cases. Am J Surg Pathol. 1996;20(12):1440–7.
152. Savera AT, Sloman A, Huvos AG, Klimstra DS. Myoepithelial carcinoma of the salivary glands: a clinicopathologic study of 25 patients. Am J Surg Pathol. 2000;24(6):761–74.
153. Kleinsasser O, Klein HJ, Hubner G. Salivary duct carcinoma. A group of salivary gland tumors analogous to mammary duct carcinoma. Arch Klin Exp Ohren Nasen Kehlkopfheilkd. 1968;192(1):100–5.
154. Hosal AS, Fan C, Barnes L, Myers EN. Salivary duct carcinoma. Otolaryngol Head Neck Surg. 2003;129(6):720–5.
155. Jaehne M, Roeser K, Jaekel T, et al. Clinical and immunohistologic typing of salivary duct carcinoma: a report of 50 cases. Cancer. 2005;103:2526–33.
156. Gilbert MR, Sharma A, Schmitt NC, Johnson JT, Ferris RL, Duvvuri U, Kim S. A 20-year review of 75 cases of salivary duct carcinoma. JAMA Otolaryngol Head Neck Surg. 2016;142(5):489–95.
157. Sugano S, Mukai K, Tsuda H, Hirohashi S, Furuya S, Shimosato Y, Ebihara S, Takeyama I. Immunohistochemical study of c-erbB-2 oncoprotein overexpression in human major salivary gland carcinoma: an indicator of aggressiveness. Laryngoscope. 1992;102(8):923–7.
158. Wang BY, Lawson W, Robinson RA, Perez-Ordonez B, Brandwein M. Malignant melanomas of the parotid: comparison of survival for patients with metastases from known vs unknown primary tumor sites. Arch Otolaryngol Head Neck Surg. 1999;125(6):635–9.
159. Huan AT, Tang C, Bell D, Yener M, Izquierdo L, Frank SJ, El-Naggar AK, Hanna EY, Weber RS, Kupferman ME. Prognostic factors in adenocarcinoma of the salivary glands. Oral Oncol. 2015;51(6):610–5.
160. Brandwein MS, Jagirdar J, Patil J, et al. Salivary duct carcinoma (cribriform salivary carcinoma of excretory ducts). A clinicopathologic and immunohistochemical study of 12 cases. Cancer. 1990;65:2307–14.
161. Delgado R, Vuitch F, Albores-Saavedra J. High grade salivary duct carcinoma. Mod Pathol. 1992;5:71A.

162. Haines K, Murad T. Infiltrating salivary duct carcinoma of the parotid. Lab Investig. 1989;60:36A.
163. Lewis JE, McKinney BC, Weiland LH, Ferreiro JA, Olsen KD. Salivary duct carcinoma. Clinicopathologic and immunohistochemical review of 26 cases. Cancer. 1996;77:223–30.
164. Murrah VA, Batsakis JG. Salivary duct carcinoma. Ann Otol Rhinol Laryngol. 1994;103:244–7.
165. Ockner DM, Mills SE, Swanson PE. Salivary duct carcinoma: an immunohistologic comparison with invasive ductal carcinoma of the breast. Lab Investig. 1994;70:100A.
166. Smith JA, Warhol MJ, Brodsky GL. An immunohistochemical study of a carcinoma of the parotid gland exhibiting both ductal and acinic cell differentiation. Oral Surg Oral Med Oral Pathol. 1983;55:267–73.
167. Barnes L, Rao U, Krause J, Contis L, Schwartz A, Scalamogna P. Salivary duct carcinoma. Part I. A clinicopathologic evaluation and DNA image analysis of 13 cases with review of the literature. Oral Surg Oral Med Oral Pathol. 1994;78:64–73.
168. Brandwein-Gensler M, Hille J, Wang BY, Urken M, Gordon R, Wang LJ, et al. Lowgrade salivary duct carcinoma: description of 16 cases. Am J Surg Pathol. 2004;28:1040–4.
169. Delgado R, Klimstra D, Albores-Saavedra J. Low grade salivary duct carcinoma. A distinctive variant with a low-grade histology and a predominant intraductal growth pattern. Cancer. 1996;78:958–67.
170. Ettl T, Schwarz S, Kleinsasser N, Hartmann A, Reichert TE, Driemel O. Overexpression of EGFR and absence of C-KIT expression correlate with poor prognosis in salivary gland carcinomas. Histopathology. 2008;53(5):567–77.
171. Guzzo M, Di Palma S, Grandi C, Molinari R. Salivary duct carcinoma: clinical characteristics and treatment strategies. Head Neck. 1997;19(2):126–33.
172. Taxy JB. Squamous carcinoma in a major salivary gland: a review of the diagnostic considerations. Arch Pathol Lab Med. 2001;125(6):740–5.
173. Marciani RD, Trodahl JN, Dauchess VG, Canlas MS. Squamous cell carcinoma of the submandibular gland. J Oral Surg. 1976;34:646–50.
174. Li S, Baloch ZW, Tomaszewski JE, LiVolsi VA. Worrisome histologic alterations following fine-needle aspiration of benign parotid lesions. Arch Pathol Lab Med. 2000;124:87–91.
175. Nagao T, Serizawa H, Iwaya K, Shimizu T, Sugano I, Ishida Y, et al. Keratocystoma of the parotid gland: a report of two cases of an unusual pathologic entity. Mod Pathol. 2002;15(9):1005–10.
176. Lewis JE, Olsen KD. Tumors of salivary glands. In: Barnes EL, Eveson J, Reichart P, Sidransky D, editors. Pathology and genetics head and neck tumors. Lyon: IARC; 2005. p. 245–6.
177. Gaughan RK, Olsen KD, Lewis JE. Primary squamous cell carcinoma of the parotid gland. Arch Otolaryngol Head Neck Surg. 1992;118(8):798–801.
178. Lee S, Kim GE, Park CS, Choi EC, Yang WI, Lee CG, et al. Primary squamous cell carcinoma of the parotid gland. Am J Otolaryngol. 2001;22(6):400–6.
179. Weber RS, Byers RM, Petit B, Wolf P, Ang K, Luna M. Submandibular gland tumors. Adverse histologic factors and therapeutic implications. Arch Otolaryngol Head Neck Surg. 1990;116(9):1055–60.
180. Gritzmann N, Rettenbacher T, Hollerweger A, Macheiner P, Hübner E. Sonography of the salivary glands. Eur Radiol. 2003;13:964–75.
181. Hanna E, Vural E, Prokopakis E, Carrau R, Snyderman C, Weissman J. The sensitivity and specificity of high-resolution imaging in evaluating perineural spread of adenoid cystic carcinoma to the skull base. Arch Otolaryngol Head Neck Surg. 2007;133(6):541–5.
182. Burke CJ, Thomas RH, Howlett D. Imaging the major salivary glands. Br J Oral Maxillofac Surg. 2011;49(4):261–9.
183. Stewart CJ, MacKenzie K, McGarry GW, Mowat A. Fine needle aspiration cytology of salivary gland: a review of 341 cases. Diagn Cytopathol. 2000;22:139–46.

184. Luna MA, Tortoledo ME, Ordonez NG, Frankenthaler RA, Batsakis JG. Primary sarcomas of the major salivary glands. Arch Otolaryngol Head Neck Surg. 1991;117:302–6.
185. Routsias JG, Goules JD, Charalampakis G, Tzima S, Papageorgiou A, Voulgarelis M. Malignant lymphoma in primary Sjögren's syndrome: an update on the pathogenesis and treatment. Semin Arthritis Rheum. 2013;43(2):178–86.
186. Rice DH. Salivary gland disorders: neoplastic and nonneoplastic. Med Clin North Am. 1999;83:197–218.
187. Weber RS, Byers RM, Petit B, Wolf P, Ang K, Luna M. Submandibular gland tumors: adverse histologic factors and therapeutic implications. Arch Otolaryngol Head Neck Surg. 1990;116:1055–60.
188. Armstrong JG, Harrison LB, Thaler HT, Friedlander-Klar H, Fass DE, Zelefsky MJ, et al. The indications for elective treatment of the neck in cancer of the major salivary glands. Cancer. 1992;69:615–9.
189. Gallia TD, Johnson JT. The incidence of neoplastic versus inflammatory disease in major salivary gland masses diagnosed by surgery. Laryngoscope. 1981;91:512–5.
190. Ge N, Peng X, Zhang L, Cai ZG, Guo CB, Yu GY. Partial sialadenectomy for the treatment of benign tumours in the submandibular gland. Int J Oral Maxillofac Surg. 2016;45(6):750–5.
191. Springborg LK, Møller MN. Submandibular gland excision: long-term clinical outcome in 139 patients operated in a single institution. Eur Arch Otorrinolaringol. 2013;270(4):1441–6.
192. Buchman C, Stringer SP, Mendenhall WM, Parsons JT, Jordan JR, Cassisi NJ. Pleomorphic adenoma: effect of tumor spill and inadequate resection on tumor recurrence. Laryngoscope. 1994;104(10):1231–4.
193. Robertson BF, Robertson GA, Shoaib T, Soutar DS, Morley S, Robertson AG. Pleomorphic adenomas: post-operative radiotherapy is unnecessary following primary incomplete excision: a retrospective review. J Plast Reconstr Aesthet Surg. 2014;67(12):e297–302.
194. Mendenhall WM, Mendenhall CM, Werning JW, Malyapa RS, Mendenhall NP. Salivary gland pleomorphic adenoma. Am J Clin Oncol. 2008;31(1):95–9.
195. Hocwald E, Korkmaz H, Yoo GH, Adsay V, Shibuya TY, Abrams J, et al. Prognostic factors in major salivary gland cancer. Laryngoscope. 2001;111:1434–9.
196. Shah JP. Management of regional metastasis in salivary and thyroid cancer. In: Larson DL, Ballantyne AJ, Guillamondegui M, editors. Cancer of the neck: evaluation and treatment. New York, NY: Macmillan; 1986. p. 253–6.
197. Spiro RH, Hadju SL, Strong EW. Tumors of the submandibular gland. Am J Surg. 1976;132:463–8.
198. Castro EB, Huvos AG, Strong EW, Foote FW Jr. Tumors of the major salivary glands in children. Cancer. 1972;29:312–7.
199. Gold DR, Annino DJ. Management of the neck in salivary gland carcinoma. Otolaryngol Clin N Am. 2005;38:99–105.
200. Bhattacharyya N, Fied MP. Nodal metastasis in major salivary gland cancer: predictive factors and effects on survival. Arch Otolaryngol Head Neck Surg. 2002;128:904–8.
201. Shah JP. Cervical lymph nodes. In: Shah JP, Patel SG, editors. Head and neck surgery & oncology. 3rd ed. Edinburgh, UK: Mosby; 2003. p. 353–94.
202. Stennert E, Kisner D, Jungehuelsing M, Guntinas-Lichius O, Schröder U, Eckel HE, et al. High incidence of lymph node metastasis in major salivary gland cancer. Arch Otolaryngol. 2003;129:720–3.
203. Lima RA, Tavares MR, Dias FL, Kligerman J, Nascimento MF, Barbosa MM, et al. Clinical prognostic factors in malignant parotid gland tumors. Otolaryngol Head Neck Surg. 2005;133(5):702–8.
204. Medina JE. Neck dissection in the treatment of cancer of major salivary glands. Otolaryngol Clin N Am. 1998;31:815–22.
205. Licitra L, Marchini S, Spinazze S, Rossi A, Rocca A, Grandi C, et al. Cisplatin in advanced salivary gland carcinoma. A phase II study of 25 patients. Cancer. 1991;1:1874–7.

206. Dimery IW, Legha SS, Shirinian M, Hong WK. Fluorouracil; doxorubicin. Cyclophosphamide and cisplatin combination chemotherapy in advanced or recurrent salivary gland carcinoma. J Clin Oncol. 1990;8:1056–62.
207. Dodd RL, Slevin NJ. Salivary gland adenoid cystic carcinoma: a review of chemotherapy and molecular therapies. Oral Oncol. 2006;42:759–69.
208. Harari PM, Huang SM. Modulation of molecular targets to enhance radiation. Clin Cancer Res. 2000;6:323–5.
209. Vered M, Braunstein E, Buchner A. Immunohistochemical study of epidermal growth factor receptor in adenoid cystic carcinoma of salivary gland origin. Head Neck. 2002;24:632–6.
210. Sugano S, Mukai K, Tsuda H, Hirohashi S, Furuya S, Shimosato Y, et al. Immunohistochemical study of c-erbB-2 oncoprotein overexpression in human major salivary gland carcinoma: an indicator of aggressiveness. Laryngoscope. 1992;102:923–7.
211. Nagler RM, Kerner H, Ben-Eliezer S, Minkov I, Ben-Itzhak O. Prognostic role of apoptotic, Bcl-2, erbB-2, and p53 tumor markers in salivary gland malignancies. Oncology. 2003;64:389–98.
212. Nasser SM, Faquin WC, Dayal Y. Expression of androgen, estrogen, and progesterone receptors in salivary gland tumors. Frequent expression of androgen receptor of malignant salivary gland tumors. Am J Clin Pathol. 2003;119:801–6.
213. Nemunaitis J, Khouri F, Ganly I, Arseneau J, Posner M, Vokes E, et al. Phase II trial of intratumoral administration of ONYX-015, a replication-selective adenovirus, in patients with refractory head and neck cancer. J Clin Oncol. 2001;19:289–98.
214. Kaban K, Herbst RS. Angiogenesis as a target for cancer therapy. Hematol Oncol Clin North Am. 2002;16:1125–71.
215. Sultan I, Rodriguez-Galindo C, Al-Sharabati S, Guzzo M, Casanova M, Ferrari A. Salivary gland carcinomas in children and adolescents: a population-based study, with comparison to adult cases. Head Neck. 2011;33(10):1476–81.
216. Kupferman ME, de la Garza GO, Santillan AA, Williams MD, Varghese BT, Huh W, et al. Outcomes of pediatric patients with malignancies of the major salivary glands. Ann Surg Oncol. 2010;17(12):3301–7.
217. Renehan AG, Gleave EN, Slevin NJ, McGurk M. Clinico-pathological and treatment-related factors influencing survival in parotid cancer. Br J Cancer. 1999;80(8):1296–300.
218. Therkildsen MH, Christensen M, Andersen LJ, Schiødt T, Hansen HS. Salivary gland carcinomas—prognostic factors. Acta Oncol. 1998;37(7–8):701–13.
219. Schwarz S, Stiegler C, Müller M, Ettl T, Brockhoff G, Zenk J, Agaimy A. Salivary gland mucoepidermoid carcinoma is a clinically, morphologically and genetically heterogeneous entity: a clinicopathological study of 40 cases with emphasis on grading, histological variants and presence of the t(11;19) translocation. Histopathology. 2011;58(4):557–70.
220. Bhattacharyya N, Fried MP. Determinants of survival in parotid gland carcinoma: a population-based study. Am J Otolaryngol. 2005;26(1):39–44.
221. Speight PM, Barrett AW. Prognostic factors in malignant tumours of the salivary glands. Br J Oral Maxillofac Surg. 2009;47(8):587–93.
222. Hocwald E, Korkmaz H, Yoo GH, Adsay V, Shibuya TY, Abrams J, Jacobs JR. Prognostic factors in major salivary gland cancer. Laryngoscope. 2001;111(8):1434–9.
223. Kelley DJ, Spiro RH. Management of the neck in parotid carcinoma. Am J Surg. 1996;172(6):695–7.
224. Oliveira LR, Soave DF, Oliveira-Costa JP, Zorgetto VA, Ribeiro-Silva A. Prognostic factors in patients with malignant salivary gland neoplasms in a Brazilian population. Asian Pac J Cancer Prev. 2011;12(2):363–8.
225. Becker C, Dahlem KKK, Pfeiffer J. Prognostic value of comorbidities in patients with carcinoma of the major salivary glands. Eur Arch Otorrinolaringol. 2017;274(3):1651–7.
226. Guzzo M, Locati LD, Prott FJ, Gatta G, McGurk M, Licitra L. Major and minor salivary gland tumors. Crit Rev Oncol Hematol. 2010;74(2):134–48.
227. Glazer TA, Shuman AG. Distant metastases and palliative care. Adv Otorhinolaryngol. 2016;78:182–8.

228. Kolokythas A. Long-term surgical complications in the oral cancer patient: a comprehensive review. Part I. J Oral Maxillofac Res. 2010;1(3):e1.
229. Kim DD, Ord RA. Complications in the treatment of head and neck cancer. Oral Maxillofac Surg Clin North Am. 2003;15(2):213–27.
230. Schauber MD, Fontenelle LJ, Solomon JW, Hanson TL. Cranial/cervical nerve dysfunction after carotid endarterectomy. J Vasc Surg. 1997;25(3):481–7.
231. Dawson AK, Orr JA. Long-term results of local excision and radiotherapy in pleomorphic adenoma of the parotid. Int J Radiat Oncol Biol Phys. 1985;11(3):451–5.
232. Barton J, Slevin NJ, Gleave EN. Radiotherapy for pleomorphic adenoma of the parotid gland. Int J Radiat Oncol Biol Phys. 1992;22(5):925–8.

Submandibular Sialadenectomy 26

26.1 Introduction

Submandibular gland (SMG) excision (submandibular sialadenectomy) is traditionally performed via a trans-cervical approach [1, 2]. Although this approach provides a wide operative field, it sometimes results in an unsatisfactorily conspicuous scar and does not prevent injury to the marginal mandibular nerve (MMN) (branch of the facial nerve), lingual nerve, or hypoglossal nerve nor does it prevent postoperative infection or bleeding [3].

Surgical incisions that provide access to head-neck lesions have rapidly evolved from the traditional incisions along natural skin creases to more cosmetically acceptable incisions in the local region or from remote locations that permit comprehensive surgery. These access incisions are often smaller and complemented by endoscopy, robotic instrumentation, and laparoscopic techniques that allow the surgeon to achieve and maintain excellent operative exposure and view. The impetus to move to more minimally invasive techniques has been that these procedures are associated with better cosmesis, less scarring, diminished blood loss, shorter hospital stays, and lower morbidity. Recently, there have been several articles discussing novel approaches to excise the SMG.

26.2 Relevant Surgical Anatomy

26.2.1 Submandibular Triangle

The submandibular triangle is bound superiorly by the inferior border of the mandible, inferiorly by the posterior belly of the digastric muscle, anteriorly by the anterior belly of the digastric muscle, and posteriorly by the posterior border of the submandibular gland. Anteriorly, the floor of the triangle is the mylohyoid muscle;

© The Author(s), under exclusive license to Springer Nature Switzerland AG 2024
M. Sakr, *Surgery of the Salivary Glands*,
https://doi.org/10.1007/978-3-031-82069-4_26

posteriorly, it is the hyoglossus muscle [4]. The SMG occupies most of this triangle, below the mylohyoid muscle [5]. A part of the gland extends around the free edge of the mylohyoid muscle that divides the gland into a smaller anterior and larger posterior part. The mylohyoid muscle must be retracted in order to gain access to both parts of the gland [6].

26.2.2 Submandibular Duct (Wharton's Duct)

The submandibular duct (Wharton's duct) is approximately 5 cm in length and arises from the anterior portion of the gland. It traverses the floor of the mouth between the mylohyoid and genioglossus muscles alongside the tongue. Its opening is found at the base of the frenulum of the tongue just posterior to the inferior incisors on the submandibular carbuncle via one to three orifices [4, 5].

26.2.3 Sublingual Space

The sublingual space lies between the tongue and the mandibular ramus containing the deep portion of the sublingual gland, the anterior portion of Wharton's duct, and the lingual nerve, which carries parasympathetic nerve fibers to the gland.

26.2.4 Lingual Nerve and Hypoglossal Nerve

During its course, the lingual nerve loops under the duct running a lateral-to-medial course and travels deep and superior to the SMG; it is most easily identified by reflecting the posterior portion of the mylohyoid muscle [5]. The lingual nerve provides sensory innervation from the anterior two-thirds of the tongue. General sensation fibers for touch, pain, and temperature travel within the mandibular division of the trigeminal nerve (CN-V) as the lingual nerve courses just medial to the inferior alveolar nerve. Special sensation fibers for taste travel with the facial nerve (CN-VII) through the internal acoustic meatus before branching into the chorda tympani nerve, which travels through the middle ear and exits the skull via the petrotympanic fissure into the infratemporal fossa where it joins with the lingual nerve.

Also relevant is the hypoglossal nerve (CN-XII), which lies inferior and medial to the lower third of the gland under the posterior belly of digastric muscle medial to the deep layer of the deep cervical fascia before coursing anteriorly and innervating the extrinsic and intrinsic muscles of the tongue (except for palatoglossus, which is innervated by the pharyngeal branch of the vagus nerve [6].

26.2.5 Investing Fascia and Marginal Mandibular Nerve (MMN)

The SMG is enclosed within a sheath formed by the investing fascia of the neck that is attached superiorly to the mandible. The marginal mandibular nerve (MMN) forms an important external landmark as it passes just superficial to the fascia of the SMG and deep to the plane of the platysma as it courses anteriorly and superiorly toward the ipsilateral corner of the mouth where it innervates the depressor labii inferioris [7]. Thus, surgical dissection within the fascia of the SMG poses the least risk to the MMN.

26.2.6 Vascular Supply

The vascular supply of the SMG is formed by the facial artery and vein. Identification and ligation of these vessels permit complete liberation of the gland in any approach. The facial artery is a branch of the external carotid artery (ECA); it courses through the submandibular space medial and posterior to the digastric muscle and later courses around the muscle and through the submandibular gland and exits into the facial notch of the mandible [5].

26.3 Applied Physiology

26.3.1 Submandibular Gland Function

The submandibular gland is a salivary gland that produces a mixed serous and mucinous salivary output accounting for the majority of baseline salivary production [8]. Saliva produced by the salivary glands provides lubrication to the upper aerodigestive tract, which is crucial for proper taste sensation, deglutition, and speech [9]. Saliva also aids in the preliminary stages of food digestion and serves as a buffer to prevent dental caries and facilitate dental remineralization [10].

26.3.2 Autonomic Innervation

Salivary production by the submandibular gland is mediated by the autonomic nervous system. Parasympathetic innervation originates from the superior salivatory nucleus of the pons. Presynaptic fibers travel with the facial nerve via the chorda tympani, which later is joined with the lingual branch of the mandibular nerve. Fibers synapse at the submandibular ganglion. Postsynaptic fibers act directly on the submandibular gland to induce secretion and vasodilation.

Sympathetic innervation originates from the superior cervical ganglion where fibers synapse. Postsynaptic fibers travel as a plexus within the carotid sheath. Fibers following the facial artery and subsequently submental arteries then enter the gland, where they decrease blood flow to the submandibular gland and decrease salivary production.

26.4 Surgical Pathology

26.4.1 Acute Pathological Disorders

Acute disorders involving the submandibular gland and the ductal system include salivary calculi, strictures, and infectious processes. Unilateral submandibular infectious processes are often bacterial, with *S. aureus*, *S. pyogenes*, *S. viridans*, and *H. influenzae* commonly isolated [10]. These acute bacterial processes are often secondary to duct obstruction or factors that result in salivary stasis, such as dehydration, chronic medical conditions, certain medications, xerostomia, or a history of radiation therapy to the oral cavity. Acute bilateral processes affecting the submandibular glands are often of viral etiology, which may be secondary to the mumps virus, coxsackie, parainfluenza virus, or human immunodeficiency virus (HIV).

26.4.2 Chronic Pathological Disorders

Chronic disorders affecting the submandibular glands include neoplasms of either benign or malignant origin, autoimmune diseases, and infiltrative processes—such as amyloidosis, granulomatous disease, or idiopathic enlargement [10].

26.5 Indications and Contraindications

26.5.1 Indications

26.5.1.1 Chronic Calcular Sialadenitis

The most common indication of submandibular gland excision is salivary calculus (sialolithiasis) with secondary ductal obstruction and sialadenitis. In the setting of an isolated calculus within the submandibular duct, a trans-oral removal of the stone from the duct may be successful. However, most patients with salivary calculus disease have recurrent episodes of obstruction and sialadenitis, which are unlikely to resolve with noninvasive measures alone and are cured by excision of the submandibular gland.

26.5.1.2 Chronic Non-calcular Sialadenitis

Chronic non-calcular sialadenitis is usually considered a "medical disease," with surgical intervention (submandibular sialadenectomy) reserved for intractable symptoms of pain and swelling.

26.5.1.3 Neoplasms

Another indication of submandibular sialadenectomy is the presence of a benign neoplasm within the submandibular gland. Approximately 40–50% of submandibular gland tumors are benign (most commonly pleomorphic adenoma [PA]), and the remaining are malignant (commonly mucoepidermoid carcinoma [MEC], adenoid cystic carcinoma [AdCC], or adenocarcinoma) [11]. Before performing the operation for neoplastic disease, an appropriate preoperative work-up must be completed prior to excision, as a malignant neoplasm should not be managed by a submandibular gland excision alone. In cases of malignancy, a formal neck dissection is often required depending on tumor pathology and stage.

26.5.1.4 Sialorrhea (Chronic Drooling)

Another indication of submandibular gland excision is refractory sialorrhea. When appropriate, this is generally performed bilaterally and may be completed in conjunction with ligation of the parotid ducts. However, sialorrhea may be treated with botulinum toxin injections, which have been shown to be an effective and well-tolerated treatment [12]. Therefore, surgical excision is generally reserved for refractory cases not responsive to conservative treatment.

26.5.2 Contraindications

In the presence of a malignant neoplasm, a submandibular gland excision alone is inappropriate. Comorbid medical conditions may be a contraindication of submandibular gland excision if the patient cannot tolerate the procedure safely. This procedure is performed under general anesthesia in the vast majority of cases, though it has been performed under local anesthesia in selected patients.

26.6 Preoperative Evaluation

26.6.1 Preoperative Evaluation

26.6.1.1 Clinical Evaluation

The work-up of submandibular gland disease should start with complete history-taking and physical examination with attention to symptom onset and course, unilateral or bilateral symptoms, and signs and symptoms of systemic autoimmune, inflammatory, or viral processes. A history of radiation or radioactive iodine treatment should also be obtained. A complete head and neck examination with attention to the oral cavity with bimanual palpation of the floor of the mouth to assess for any palpable calculi, as well as a thorough neck examination to evaluate any masses or lesions, should then be completed. Facial nerve function and symmetry, with close attention to the corners of the mouth, should be assessed.

26.6.1.2 Investigations

Imaging of the submandibular gland is indicated before surgical excision; this includes ultrasonography (US) or computed tomography (CT) scan of the neck to evaluate a neoplastic process and identify the presence of calculi [13]. If any suspicion of a neoplastic process exists on history-taking, physical examination, or imaging, fine-needle aspiration (FNA) of the submandibular gland lesion should be completed and results reviewed prior to surgical excision to rule out a malignant process.

26.7 Approaches to the Submandibular Gland

Submandibular gland (SMG) excision is traditionally performed via a conventional open lateral transcervical approach [1, 2]. Although this approach provides a wide operative field, it sometimes results in an unsatisfactorily accepted scar and does not prevent the occurrence of complications such as injury to the MMN, lingual nerve, hypoglossal nerve, or postoperative infection or bleeding [3].

To avoid visible scarring, some authors have implemented intraoral or trans-oral approaches, which can provide an invisible scar but may cause postoperative complications such as a higher rate of lingual nerve paresis and limitation of tongue movement caused by scar contracture [14]. Other authors described trans-cervical techniques to conceal the scar, using the submental space or hairline (retro-auricular) with or without magnification of the surgical field. Others have used a traditional lateral trans-cervical approach but have reduced the incision size [15] or used a three-port approach to robotic endoscopic resection [16]. These procedures are currently limited in application due to specialized equipment and surgeon experience.

Thus, approaches to submandibular sialadenectomy can be classified as "open" or "endoscopic" approaches as shown in Table 26.1.

26.7.1 Open Techniques (Approaches)

26.7.1.1 External Approaches

As seen in Table 26.1, external approaches include the lateral tans-cervical approach, retro-auricular approach, and submental approach.

26.7.1.2 Lateral Trans-cervical Approach

The lateral trans-cervical approach is the standard and time-tested means of surgical access to the SMG.

26.7.1.3 Indications

Indications for excision via this approach include neoplasm of the SMG, chronic sialadenitis, sialolithiasis, radioactive iodine-induced sialadenitis [17], chronic drooling (sialorrhea), Küttner's tumor, and Kimura's disease [18–20]. Some authors

Table 26.1 Approaches to the submandibular gland

Open techniques	Endoscopic techniques
External approach Lateral trans-cervical Retro-auricular Submental	Endoscopy-assisted Trans-oral Submental Lateral trans-cervical
Trans-oral approach	Completely endoscopic With CO_2 insufflation Robot-assisted

have advocated a partial or total submandibular resection via a trans-cervical approach for facial rejuvenation [21].

26.7.1.4 Anesthesia: General/Local

Lateral trans-cervical submandibular resection is most commonly performed under general anesthesia. However, some authors advocate SMG resection under local anesthesia in a selected patient population.

Criteria for gland excision under local anesthesia include a clinically mobile mass without features of malignancy based on FNA in patients who prefer local anesthesia or are at high risk with general anesthesia. There is no size limitation to the removal of the mass provided, and it can be resected through a 6-cm incision. In the study by Chow et al. (2008), 12 patients (out of 20) with benign submandibular masses underwent sialadenectomy under local anesthesia. They reported that no procedures required conversion to general anesthesia and concluded that SMG excision under local anesthesia is feasible in appropriately selected patients and ultimately can shorten hospital stay and facilitate day surgery [22].

26.7.1.5 Intraoperative Patient Preparation

Generally, antibiotics are not indicated in clean head and neck cases. The patient is positioned supine on the operative table, and a shoulder roll is placed so that the neck is in gentle extension with the head turned away from the operative side. Many surgeons turn the operative table 90° toward the operative side to allow for adequate room for the operative team. Alternatively, some surgeons elect to keep the operative table straight and instead move the table toward the patient's feet. The patient is prepped and draped widely from the nasolabial angle to the clavicles on the operative side. The corner of the mouth is left in view to evaluate for twitching.

26.7.1.6 Steps of the Procedure [18, 19]

The skin incision (4–6 cm) is placed in an upper neck skin crease at least two finger breadths below the angle of the mandible to protect the MMN. This incision provides broad access and a superior cosmetic result. The upper flap consisting of skin, subcutaneous (SC) fat, platysma muscle, deep cervical fascia, and the fascial capsule superficial to the gland is elevated up to the level of the lower border of the mandible in order to avoid injury of the nerve.

The lower border of the gland is grasped and lifted up, the gland is separated from the muscular floor of the submandibular triangle, and the hypoglossal nerve is identified on the hyoglossus muscle. The anterior segment of the gland is released from the mylohyoid muscle. The facial artery is then identified and divided proximal to the gland between strong ligatures. This frees the gland posteriorly.

The gland is retracted downwards in order to divide its superior fascial attachments to the mandible and expose the facial artery and anterior facial vein just below the mandible. These vessels are divided as close to the gland as possible to avoid accidental damage to the MMN. Division of the facial vessels allows caudal retraction of the submandibular gland, providing full exposure of the underlying mylohyoid muscle.

The mylohyoid muscle is retracted forward, thus exposing the deep part of the gland. With traction on the gland still maintained in a downward direction, the lingual nerve is dragged down from its position deep to the mandible, and its attachment to the gland is severed.

Wharton's duct is isolated and divided as close as possible to the floor of the mouth. During this dissection, the hypoglossal nerve is seen in a deeper plane to Wharton's duct and should be carefully protected. If a calculus is present within the submandibular duct, it is important that the duct be ligated distal to the calculus and the calculus (or calculi) removed.

After removal of the surgical specimen, meticulous hemostasis is obtained followed by irrigation with saline solution. A single suction drain is inserted, and the wound is closed in layers as per the surgeon's preference.

26.7.1.7 Postoperative Complications

In general, complications of traditional SMG excision include hematoma formation (2–10%), wound infection (2–9%), fistula formation (1–3%), and neurological complications, which include injury to the MMN (7.7–36%), hypoglossal nerve (0–7%), and lingual nerve (0–22.5%) [17–20, 23, 24].

26.7.1.8 Nerve Injury

The most common complication after submandibular gland excision is injury to the MMN [25]. Temporary injury (temporary paresis) has been reported to range from 1 to 10% of patients [20, 26, 27]. It is highly recommended that the incision should be placed at 3 cm below the angle of the mandible to consistently avoid injury to branches of the facial nerve. Injury to the lingual nerve is uncommon unless a tumor or chronic inflammation presents difficulty in its separation from the gland. Rarer still is injury to the hypoglossal nerve in the course of resection of the contents of the submandibular triangle [26, 27]. Great auricular causalgia and/or the development of neuroma are rather uncommon [28].

26.7.1.9 Other Injuries

Injury to other important structures in the neck may also occur during submandibular sialadenectomy such as the facial artery leading to severe hemorrhage and wall of the pharynx resulting in fistula formation. With careful dissection, these complications are rarely encountered in experienced hands.

26.7.1.10 Surgical Site Complications

The scar that results from cervical incision may be aesthetically unsatisfactory in many patients, particularly those with a slender neck. Avoiding tension of the surgical wound and the use of intradermal sutures can help in preventing an unsightly scar.

26.7.1.11 Submental Approach

The submental approach provides access to the submandibular triangle via a midline horizontal incision just superior to the submental-cervical crease at the level of the hyoid bone. The site of the incision is patient-dependent, determined by pre-existing neck creases, amount of submental fat, and skin texture. The site of the incision is marked preoperatively along the least prominent line of the submental area in the frontal and lateral views of the face and the neck.

The submental approach allows quick access to the gland. The SMG is bluntly dissected free of surrounding fascia in a sub-platysmal plane. The dissection differs from the traditional approach in that the anterior free edge of the gland is first encountered. Following this, the facial vein and artery are ligated, and the gland is separated from the edge of the mylohyoid muscle. The submandibular ganglion is identified and separated from the gland. Finally, the submandibular duct is ligated, and the gland is delivered through the incision. A drain is placed within the incision and is removed on the second or third postoperative day [29].

Roh (2008) compared the submental approach to the traditional lateral trans-cervical approach in a prospective randomized fashion. There were a total of 20 patients with ten patients in each arm of the study. There were no statistically significant differences in the two approaches with respect to incision length, operative time, nerve injuries, and hospital stay. However, the average visual analog scale (VAS) measurements showed a significantly ($p < 0.01$) higher patient satisfaction due to cosmetic concerns in the submental approach group (8.8 versus 5.4) [29].

26.7.1.12 Retro-auricular Approach

Roh (2005) also described a retro-auricular approach to the SMG [30]. Since the initial report in 2005, Roh continued to report on the utility of this approach [31]. The incision is designed in the lower portion of the postauricular sulcus arching toward the middle to upper 1/3 of the sulcus before transitioning across and downward into the hairline; the portion of the incision in the hairline is set to 0.5–1 cm into the hair-bearing area. The main advantage is the improved cosmesis. The main disadvantage is the extent of the skin flap to be raised to access Wharton's duct proximally, which can be 10 cm from the postauricular incision.

The incision is carried downward through the SC tissues and onto the sternocleidomastoid (SCM) muscle at which point the flap is elevated anterior to the SMG. Special attention must be paid to avoid damage to the hair follicles and great auricular nerve (GAN) and its branches during flap elevation in order to avoid postoperative complications.

Once the gland is exposed, extirpation proceeds as in any open approach [30]. Due to the depth of the operative field, endoscopy can enhance the view of the operative field. In his study, comparing this approach to the standard trans-cervical approach, Roh found no significant differences in operative time, scar hypertrophy, and length of hospital stay between the two procedures. In his series, there were no iatrogenic palsies of the MMN with the retro-auricular approach, while there were two such reported complications with the standard lateral trans-cervical approach. The study concluded that the retro-auricular approach is safe and comparable to the standard approach. The overall patient satisfaction with the resultant scar on a VAS was significantly higher with patients from the retro-auricular cohort (8.9 versus 4.2, $p < 0.001$) [31].

26.7.2 Trans-oral Approach

26.7.2.1 Development of the Trans-oral Approach

While first described in modern medical literature in 1960 [32], the trans-oral approach to the SMG did not gain popularity until recently described by Hong et al. in 2000 [33]. Advantages of the trans-oral approach include less risk of iatrogenic injury to the MMN, avoidance of an external scar, minimal risk of postoperative mucocele formation, or inflammation of Wharton's duct [33, 34].

26.7.2.2 Steps of the Trans-oral Procedure

An incision is made in the floor of the mouth from the submandibular papilla to the retromolar trigone. A cuff of mucosa on the gingival side is preserved to allow for tension-free closure and to prevent limitation of tongue mobility due to scar contracture.

The lingual nerve is identified and dissected free of its attachments to the submandibular duct and gland. The submandibular gland is bluntly dissected and delivered into the surgical wound by applying external pressure on the neck. The hypoglossal nerve is identified and preserved. Branches of the facial artery and vein are ligated with care not to disrupt the MMN. The gland is removed, and the wound bed is irrigated and closed in a tension-free manner.

26.7.2.3 Results of the Intraoral Technique

In his series, Hong (2000) reported on 31 patients who underwent a transoral resection of the SMG and later followed this with a retrospective chart review of 77 patients undergoing the same surgery showing similar results. Abnormal tongue sensation was noted in 74% of patients and temporary limitation of tongue movement in 70% of patients [33]. Restriction of tongue movement due to scar contraction was noted in 10% of patients in the first paper, but this was reduced to 2% in the most recent article with these patients being asymptomatic.

In 2007, Weber et al. published their experience with seven patients reporting 43% abnormal tongue sensation, no change in tongue movement, or restriction due to scar contracture. They attributed their lower complication rates to several critical maneuvers such as planning to leave a cuff of gingival mucosa to allow a tension-free closure and prevent tongue tethering. The authors limited the amount of lingual nerve dissection consequently limiting stretch injury to the nerve, which is responsible for abnormal tongue sensation. The authors pointed out that the only patient in their experience where a transoral approach was inadequate to allow excision of the gland had previous surgery and a small oral cavity. These can be considered as relative contraindications to this approach [35].

Hong and Yang later, in 2008, reported excising the SMG with this approach in 12 patients with pleomorphic adenoma. They noted that 50% of patients had anesthesia of the tongue and 40% had limitation of tongue movement, all of which resolved within 2 weeks of surgery [36]. In 2009, Kauffman reported a case series of nine patients with only 22.2% (2/9) of patients having temporary changes in tongue sensation and no patients having lasting complications. This series further validates the safety of trans-oral excision in selected patients [37].

26.7.3 Endoscopic Techniques (Approaches)

With advances in technology and endoscopic procedures, this technology has extended to the excision of the SMG. Endoscopic approaches to the SMG can be classified into "endoscopy-assisted" and "completely endoscopic" approaches.

26.7.3.1 Endoscopic-Assisted Approaches

Endoscopic-assisted approaches to the SMG can be further divided into endoscopic-assisted "transoral," "submental," and "lateral cervical" approaches.

26.7.3.2 Endoscopic-Assisted Trans-oral Approach

Endoscopic-assisted trans-oral excision of the SMG is similar to its open counterpart. The main advantages of this approach (in addition to those of the trans-oral approach, i.e., absence of a cervical scar and lower incidence of facial nerve palsy) are good visualization, magnification, and illumination of the anatomical landmarks and consequently a wider surgical field as compared to the conventional intraoral approach (Figs. 26.1 and 26.2).

Guerrissi and Taborda (2001) described two cases with this technique which were successfully performed for sialadenitis secondary to sialolithiasis [6]. However, Weber et al. did not perceive any difficulties with exposure via the conventional

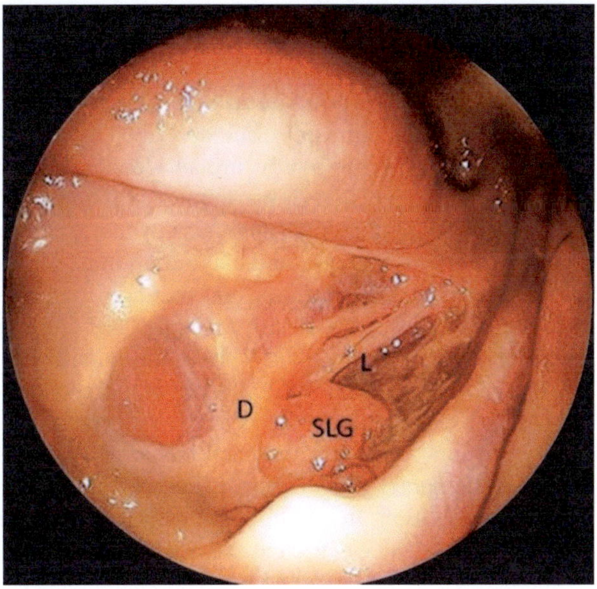

Fig. 26.1 Endoscopic view of trans-oral approach showing the submandibular duct (D), lingual nerve (L), and sublingual gland (SLG)

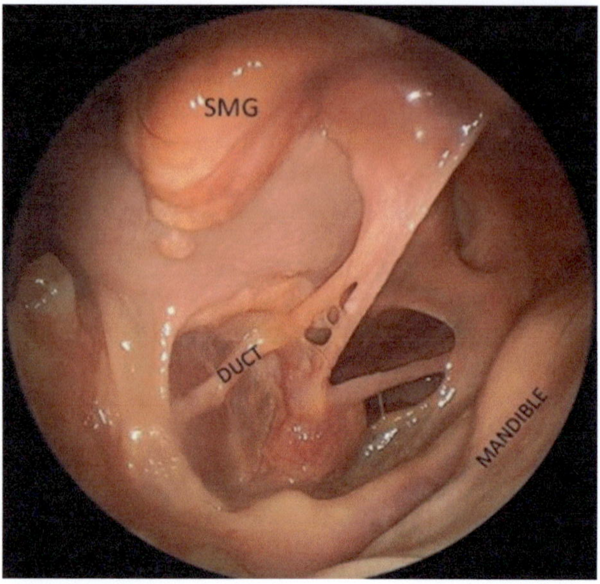

Fig. 26.2 Trans-oral approach. Endoscopic view of the operative field (SMG = submandibular gland)

trans-oral incision. In their series, a single patient required conversion to a trans-cervical approach, which, in their opinion, would not have been preventable even with endoscopic guidance [35].

It must be recognized that the endoscopy-assisted trans-oral approach has several disadvantages, which are common to all endoscopic procedures and include the cost of the endoscopic equipment, the long learning curve associated with the surgeon becoming familiar with the technique, and the increased operative and set-up time as compared to the conventional technique [38].

26.7.3.3 Endoscopic-Assisted Submental Approach

Similar to the submental approach described by Roh et al. (2006) [39], Chen et al. (2006) described a minimally invasive endoscopic resection of the SMG with placement of the incision in the submental area [40]. This procedure differs from the conventional submental approach in that a smaller incision (20–25 mm) is placed over the skin crease in the hyoid midline. Dissection is performed in a sub-platysmal plane. The first assistant maintains an operative view using an endoscope, and the second assistant maintains the working space with two retractors lifting up away from the skin. Vessels are ligated using endoclips, and excision is performed in a standard fashion using an ultrasound-activated scalpel. A drain is then placed for drainage [40].

The advantages of this approach include a smaller incision as compared to the standard submental approach and the previously discussed advantages of endoscopic visualization. In addition, the use of an ultrasound-activated scalpel, which does not transmit an electric current, reduces the risk of thermal injury to the MMN as compared to monopolar and bipolar electrocautery [41]. However, the disadvantages include those that are common to all endoscopic procedures as well as a significant increase in the mean operative time as compared to the conventional submental approach (70 min versus 41 min) [40].

The application of endoscopic approaches in soft tissue surgery has been thwarted by the challenges fundamental to endoscopic neck surgery including the lack of a well-defined sac and the risk of emphysematous dissection [38]. The risk of CO_2 insufflation to create a working space in the neck includes massive SC emphysema, hypercarbia, gas embolization, and some types of arrhythmias [40].

26.7.3.4 Endoscopic-Assisted Trans-cervical Approach

The use of a lateral endoscopic approach was first reported by Komatsuzaki et al. (2003) [15] who performed classic dissection using an ultrasound scalpel and a homemade lifting device in four patients. Meningaud et al. (2006) [42] performed five procedures using video-assisted magnification and classic dissection, and Baek and Jeong (2006) [43] reported using a similar procedure, but with bipolar dissection, in six patients.

In 2009, Hamza and Khalil [44] described a two-step video-assisted technique, using both a harmonic scalpel and an endoscopic monopolar diathermy; they reported 12 procedures for chronic sialoadenitis. While Chen et al. [40] and Komatsuzaki et al. [15] reported no complications, one patient from the series of Baek and Jeong [43] had severe adhesions to adjacent tissue and injury to the lingual nerve, and three patients from the series of Hamza and Khalil had a transient mild deviation of the angle of the mouth [44].

Guyot et al. (2005) [45] described an endoscopic approach for the SMG that does not rely on CO2 insufflation to create an operative pocket. In a cadaveric study carried out on six non-embalmed cadavers, 12 endoscopic submandibular resections were performed. Access to the sub-platysmal plane of dissection was achieved via two 15-mm incisions (one anterior and the other posterior), 10 mm below the submandibular area. A 4-mm-diameter, 30° endoscope provided the surgical view when placed in the posterior incision. The operative pocket was created and maintained using trans-cutaneous sutures. The dissection was otherwise conducted in a usual fashion. Extirpation of the gland was done through one of the incisions. In all cases, gland excision was successful. The operative time decreased with experience from 120 min for the first case to 35 min for the last one.

26.7.3.5 Minimally Invasive Video-Assisted Submandibular Sialadenectomy (MIVASS)

Developed and described by Miccoli et al. in 2000 [46] and 2001 [47], minimally invasive video-assisted thyroidectomy (MIVAT) and parathyroidectomy (MIVAP) are the main gas-free, single-port procedures in the neck. The first MIVASS was performed in 2005. In contrast to thyroid procedures, retraction of the SMG and tissues and the position of the endoscope are limited by the mandibular bone in the working space. Despite this, the resection can be accomplished using the same instruments, and no special instruments need be used as reported by Komatsuzaki [15].

As in other single-port procedures, the edge of the skin suffers pressure and retraction and can be damaged by diathermy or harmonic shears, which may lead to a small but ugly scar. Some authors protect the edges using a rubber cuff [41], but this reduces the working space.

In 2016, Arias et al. [48] reported MIVASS in 15 patients. Indications included proximally located salivary calculus (n = 8), chronic sialoadenitis (n = 3), and benign neoplasm (n = 4). In the cases of neoplasm, US and CT scan revealed that the tumors were completely intraglandular, and FNA revealed benign lesions. Patients with a malignant submandibular tumor, morbid obesity, or long-term sialoadenitis were excluded from MIVASS. Patients were asked at least 6 months after surgery about cosmetic results using a non-standardized scale (poor, fair, good, and excellent). All 15 SMG resections were successfully performed endoscopically. The mean length of the skin incision was 18 mm, and the mean operative time was 84 min (range 45–125 min). The overall complication rate was 13.4%. Bleeding occurred in one patient (6.7%) 1 h after closure, requiring surgical hemostasis. One patient (6.7%) developed an infection with drainage 5 days after surgery, which was successfully treated with antibiotics and local wound care. No nerve palsy was reported.

All operations were performed with the patient under general anesthesia in the supine position. To provide sufficient working space, the neck was rotated to the contralateral side and extended to a smaller degree than with a conventional transcervical approach. A 4-mm-diameter endoscope with 30 and 45° viewing angles and a harmonic scalpel with coagulating shears were utilized. The surgeon was situated on the same side as the operated SMG; the first assistant was on the opposite side, holding the endoscope; and the second assistant was at the top, providing working space by using two retractors to lift the skin up and away from the wound. The mandibular rim and angle, hyoid bone, and facial vein and artery were identified, and a 15–20-mm horizontal incision was created 20 mm below the mandibular rim and centered over the facial artery. The platysma muscle was divided, and the SMG capsule was identified. Using a Miccoli suction dissector (Karl Storz) and Halle-Miccoli elevator (Karl Storz), dissection proceeded between the capsule and the glandular tissue to avoid damage to the MMN. Dissection of the inferior part of the SMG followed to release it from the digastric muscle. The facial artery and vein were then identified at the superior border of the SMG. The facial artery was then ligated using clips (Fig. 26.3).

Following ligation of the facial artery, the SMG was retracted downward, and the mylohyoid muscle was dissected in order to identify the lingual nerve. The lingual nerve branch to the gland was ligated and separated from the gland. Wharton's duct was then identified, and the submandibular gland was pulled out through the surgical wound. Finally, Wharton's duct was suture-ligated and divided at a distal point, and intradermal wound closure was performed.

The main problem with this procedure is that it is more time-consuming than the conventional open method. Few studies report operative time in open submandibular gland excision as a standard variable. However, the comparison of operative time between open and endoscopic methods carries potential bias due to patient selection: Severe inflammatory disease, large tumors, and malignant tumors are more time-consuming and are always treated by an open approach. Chang et al. (2003)

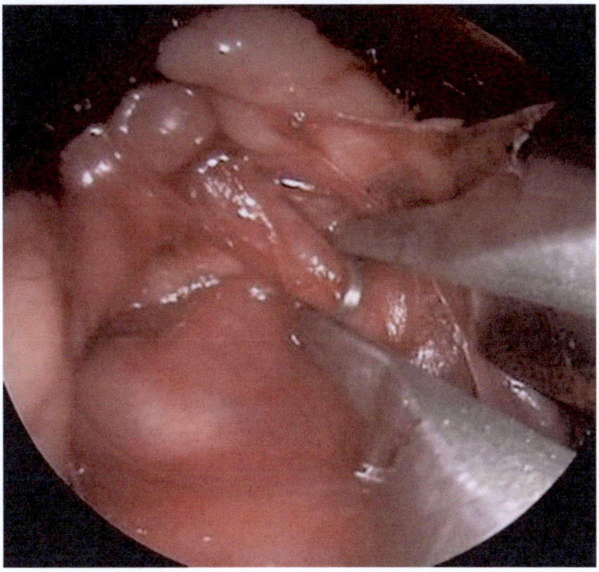

Fig. 26.3 Minimally invasive video-assisted submandibular sialadenectomy (MIVASS): endoscopic ligation of the facial artery using clips

[49] reported a mean of 78 min for a trans-cervical approach, shorter in comparison with an intraoral approach. Roh (2006) [31] reported 38 ± 15 min in a conventional procedure.

The increase in cost due to surgical time can be compensated for by the decrease in hospital stay, which can be more than 4.32 days in an open procedure [49] compared with 1.4 days with the video-assisted approach [44].

26.7.4 Completely Endoscopic Approaches

The "completely endoscopic" approaches can be applied with the use of CO_2 insufflation and may be robot-assisted.

26.7.4.1 Endoscopic SMG Excision Using CO_2 Insufflation

In 2002, Monfared et al. [50] described an endoscopic approach to the SMG in a porcine model using balloon dissection to create an operative pocket, which was constantly maintained with low pressure (not >4 mmHg) CO_2 insufflation. Three incisions were made; the central 14-mm incision accepts the 12-mm trocar, which houses the endoscope, while the two lateral incisions (6–7 mm) were used to place the 5-mm operative trocars. Twelve SMGs were successfully excised endoscopically in seven pigs with no conversion to open surgery. The median operative time was 59 min (range, 42–165 min) [50].

The technique described by Gagner [16] in 1996 (insufflating with CO_2 to create a pocket in the neck and introducing instruments through three ports) was used by Kessler et al. (2006) [51] to investigate submandibular excision in four pigs, four cadavers, and two women. This approach has had only limited use because of the risk of bleeding during puncture, limitation of movement of the instruments, and questionable cosmetic results produced by three scars.

26.7.4.2 Robot-Assisted Excision

Terris et al. (2005) expanded this approach with the addition of the da Vinci robotic system to resect the SMG with a mean operative time of 48 min and with no conversions to open surgery [52].

The main advantage of robotic-enhanced endoscopic surgery includes a virtual three-dimensional vision projection system with an endoscopic arm and two operative arms that can be controlled by the surgeon from a remote console. In addition, the robotic arm permits the use of a full range of articulated instruments, which can reproduce surgical maneuvers in difficult-to-access locations.

The disadvantages of robotic surgery such as high cost and lengthy setup time are great, and further customization of surgical instrumentation for otolaryngology practice remains to be a challenge for the future.

26.8 Complications of Submandibular Sialadenectomy

Particular attention to the MMN should be taken throughout submandibular sialadenectomy. In one series, temporary neuropraxia with full recovery of the MMN following submandibular gland excision occurred in 15.6% of cases, while permanent weakness occurred in 2.2%. Wound healing issues are comparable with other neck surgeries ranging from between 7 and 22% [53]. Injury of the hypoglossal or lingual nerve occurs in less than 2% of cases [54].

Xerostomia is generally believed to be rare in the setting of unilateral submandibular gland excision, though the impact of submandibular gland excision on salivary gland function remains an area of investigation [55]. In the immediate postoperative period, the hematoma formation is also possible. In addition, the facial artery can result in significant bleeding with potential compressive effects on the airway.

References

1. Goh YH, Sethi DS. Submandibular gland excision: a five-year review. J Laryngol Otol. 1998;112:269–73.
2. Winkel R, Overgaard TI, Balle VH, Charabi S. Surgical results of submandibular gland excision. Ugeskr Laeger. 2000;162:5354–7.
3. Hald J, Andreassen UK. Submandibular gland excision: short- and long-term complications. ORL J Otorhinolaryngol Relat Spec. 1994;56:87–91.
4. Cummings C. Otolaryngology and head neck surgery. In: Cummings C, editor. Salivary gland. New York, NY: Mosby; 1998. p. 1201–9.
5. Lalwani A. Current diagnosis and treatment in otolaryngology–head and necksurgery. 2nd ed. New York, NY: McGraw-Hill Medical; 2005.
6. Guerrissi JO, Taborda G. Endoscopic excision of the submandibular gland by an intraoral approach. J Craniofac Surg. 2001;12:299–303.

7. Moore KL, Dalley AF. Clinically oriented anatomy. 4th ed. Philadelphia, PA: Lippincott Williams & Wilkins; 1999. p. 1012–5.
8. Hernandez S, Busso C, Walvekar RR. Parotitis and sialendoscopy of the parotid gland. Otolaryngol Clin N Am. 2016;49(2):381–93.
9. Ogle OE. Excision of sublingual gland. Oral Maxillofac Surg Clin North Am. 2021;33(2):161–8.
10. Porcheri C, Mitsiadis TA. Physiology, pathology and regeneration of salivary glands. Cells. 2019;8(9):976.
11. Mizrachi A, Bachar G, Unger Y, Hilly O, Fliss DM, Shpitzer T. Submandibular salivary gland tumors: clinical course and outcome of a 20-year multicenter study. Ear Nose Throat J. 2017;96(3):E17–20.
12. Jost WH, Friedman A, Michel O, Oehlwein C, Slawek J, Bogucki A, et al. SIAXI: placebo-controlled, randomized, double-blind study of incobotulinumtoxin A for sialorrhea. Neurology. 2019;92(17):e1982–91.
13. Thomas WW, Douglas JE, Rassekh CH. Accuracy of ultrasonography and computed tomography in the evaluation of patients undergoing sialendoscopy for sialolithiasis. Otolaryngol Head Neck Surg. 2017;156(5):834–9.
14. Miloro M. Intraoral submandibular gland excision. Oral Surg Oral Med Oral Pathol Oral Radiol Endod. 1999;88:661–3.
15. Komatsuzaki Y, Ochi K, Sugiura N, Hyodo M, Okamoto A. Video-assisted submandibular sialadenectomy using an ultrasonic scalpel. Auris Nasus Larynx. 2003;30(Suppl):S75–8.
16. Gagner M. Endoscopic subtotal parathyroidectomy in patients with primary hyperparathyroidism. Br J Surg. 1996;83:875.
17. Smith AD, Elahi MM, Kawamoto HK Jr, Lorenz HP, Hedrick MH. Excision of the submandibular gland by an intraoral approach. Plast Reconstr Surg. 2000;105:2092–5.
18. Preuss SF, Klussmann JP, Wittekindt C, Drebber U, Beutner D, Guntinas-Lichius O. Submandibular gland excision: 15 years of experience. J Oral Maxillofac Surg. 2007;65:953–7.
19. Torroni AA, Mustazza MC, Bartoli DD, Iannetti GG. Transcervical submandibular sialoadenectomy. J Craniofac Surg. 2007;18:613–21.
20. Milton CM, Thomas BM, Bickerton RC. Morbidity study of submandibular gland excision. Ann R Coll Surg Engl. 1986;68:148–50.
21. Singer DP, Sullivan PK. Submandibular gland: an anatomic evaluation and surgical approach to submandibular gland resection for facial rejuvenation. Plast Reconstr Surg. 2003;112:1150–4.
22. Chow TL, Chan TT, Choi CY, Lam SH. Submandibular sialoadenectomy with local anesthesia in the era of minimally invasive surgery. Otolaryngol Head Neck Surg. 2008;138:752–5.
23. Berini-Aytes L, Gay-Escoda C. Morbidity associated with removal of the submandibular gland. J Craniomaxillofac Surg. 1992;20:216–9.
24. Smith WP, Peters WJ, Markus AF. Submandibular gland surgery: an audit of clinical findings, pathology and postoperative morbidity. Ann R Coll Surg Engl. 1993;75:164–7.
25. Eisele DW, Johns ME. Complications of surgery of the salivary glands. In: Eisele DW, editor. Complications in head and neck surgery. St Louis, MO: Mosby; 1993. p. 183–200.
26. Kennedy PJ, Poole AG. Excision of the submandibular gland: minimizing the risk of nerve damage. Aust N Z J Surg. 1989;59:411–4.
27. Goh YH, Sethi DS. Submandibular gland excision: a 5 year review. J Laryngol Otol. 1998;112:269–74.
28. Nusair YMH, Dickenson AJ. Great auricular causalgia: an unusual complication of excision of the submandibular gland. Br J Oral Maxillofac Surg. 2003;41:334–5.
29. Roh JL. Removal of the submandibular gland by a submental approach: a prospective, randomized, controlled study. Oral Oncol. 2008;44:295–300.
30. Roh JL. Retroauricular hairline incision for removal of upper neck masses. Laryngoscope. 2005;115:2161–6.
31. Roh JL. Removal of the submandibular gland by a retroauricular approach. Arch Otolaryngol Head Neck Surg. 2006;132:783–7.

32. Downton D, Qvist G. Intra-oral excision of the submandibular gland. Proc R SocMed. 1960;53:543–4.
33. Hong KH, Kim YK. Intraoral removal of the submandibular gland: a new surgical approach. Otolaryngol Head Neck Surg. 2000;122:798–802.
34. Hong KH, Yang YS. Surgical results of the intraoral removal of the submandibular gland. Otolaryngol Head Neck Surg. 2008;139:530–4.
35. Weber SM, Wax MK, Kim JH. Transoral excision of the submandibular gland. Otolaryngol Head Neck Surg. 2007;137:343–5.
36. Hong KH, Yang YS. Intraoral approach for the treatment of submandibular salivary gland mixed tumors. Oral Oncol. 2008;44:491–5.
37. Kauffman RM, Netterville JL, Burkey BB. Transoral excision of the submandibular gland: techniques and results of nine cases. Laryngoscope. 2009;119:502–7.
38. Terris DJ, Amin SH. Robotic and endoscopic surgery in the neck. Oper Tech Otolaryngol. 2008;3:36–41.
39. Roh JL, Yoon YH, Park CI. Removal of nonthyroidal neck masses with improved cosmetic outcomes in skin-lifting surgery. Otolaryngol Head Neck Surg. 2006;135:463–8.
40. Chen MK, Su CC, Tsai YL, Chang CC. Minimally invasive endoscopic resection of the submandibular gland: a new approach. Head Neck. 2006;28:1014–7.
41. Jackson LL, Gourin CG, Thomas DS, Porubsky ES, Klippert FN, Terris DJ. Use of the harmonic scalpel in superficial and total parotidectomy for benign and malignant disease. Laryngoscope. 2005;115:1070–3.
42. Meningaud JP, Pitak-Arnnop P, Bertrand JC. Endoscope-assisted submandibular sialoadenectomy: a pilot study. J Oral Maxillofac Surg. 2006;64:1366–70.
43. Baek CH, Jeong HS. Endoscope-assisted submandibular sialadenectomy: a new minimally invasive approach to the submandibular gland. Am J Otolaryngol. 2006;27:306–9.
44. Hamza Y, Khalil R. Video-assisted submandibular resection: two-step technique. Surg Endosc. 2009;23:2785–9.
45. Guyot L, Duroure F, Richard O, Lebeau J, Passagia JG, Raphael B. Submandibular gland endoscopic resection: a cadaveric study. Int J Oral Maxillofac Surg. 2005;34:407–10.
46. Miccoli P, Berti P, Raffaelli M, Conte M, Materazzi G, Galleri D. Minimally invasive video-assisted thyroidectomy. Am J Surg. 2001;181:567–70.
47. Miccoli P, Berti P, Conte M, Raffaelli M, Materazzi G. Minimally invasive video-assisted parathyroidectomy: lesson learned from 137 cases. J Am Coll Surg. 2000;191:613–8.
48. Arias PL, Mario Fernández MF, Vázquez PV, Muñoz BD. Minimally invasive video-assisted submandibular sialadenectomy: surgical technique and results from two institutions. Surg Endosc. 2016;8:3314–20.
49. Chang YN, Kao CH, Lin YS, Lee JC. Comparison of the intraoral and transcervical approach in submandibular gland excision. Eur Arch Otorrinolaringol. 2013;270:669–74.
50. Monfared A, Saenz Y, Terris DJ. Endoscopic resection of the submandibular gland in a porcine model. Laryngoscope. 2002;112:1089–93.
51. Kessler P, Bloch-Birkholz A, Birkholz T, Neukam FW. Feasibility of an endoscopic approach to the submandibular neck region—experimental and clinical results. Br J Oral Maxillofac Surg. 2006;44:103–6.
52. Terris DJ, Haus BM, Gourin CG, Lilagan PE. Endo-robotic resection of the submandibular gland in a cadaver model. Head Neck. 2005;27:946–51.
53. Chaukar DA, Deshmukh AD, Majeed T, Chaturvedi P, Pai P, D'cruz AK. Factors affecting wound complications in head and neck surgery: a prospective study. Indian J Med Paediatr Oncol. 2013;34(4):247–51.
54. Erbek SS, Köycü A, Topal Ö, Erbek HS, Özlüoğlu LN. Submandibular gland surgery: our clinical experience. Turk Arch Otorhinolaryngol. 2016;54(1):16–20.
55. Jaguar GC, Lima EN, Kowalski LP, Pellizon AC, Carvalho AL, Alves FA. Impact of submandibular gland excision on salivary gland function in head and neck cancer patients. Oral Oncol. 2010;46(5):349–54.

Surgery of the Sublingual Gland

27

27.1 Introduction

The sublingual gland is the smallest of the three major salivary glands [1], which also include the parotid and submandibular glands. The sublingual gland lies between the muscles of the floor of the oral cavity, which include the geniohyoid and hyoglossus muscles medially, and the mylohyoid muscle inferiorly. The mandible borders the sublingual glands laterally [2].

A group of excretory ducts known as the "ducts of Rivinus" drains the sublingual gland. The largest sublingual gland excretory duct called the "sublingual duct of Bartholin" joins Wharton's duct near the sublingual carbuncle, which is a papilla located medial to the sublingual gland and lateral to the lingual frenulum [2]. The sublingual gland contributes about 5% of saliva in the oral cavity [3].

27.2 Embryology

The sublingual gland develops later than the other major salivary glands as it first appears in the eighth week of prenatal development. It originates from epithelial buds surrounding the sublingual folds on the floor of the mouth. These epithelial buds develop into cords, which canalize to form the sublingual ducts and also form the mucous acini. Initially, the sublingual gland develops lateral to the submandibular gland before transitioning to a position anterior and superior to the submandibular gland when development is complete [4].

© The Author(s), under exclusive license to Springer Nature Switzerland AG 2024

M. Sakr, *Surgery of the Salivary Glands*,
https://doi.org/10.1007/978-3-031-82069-4_27

27.3 Surgical Anatomy

27.3.1 Anatomical Position

The sublingual glands lie infero-lateral to the tongue, below the mucosa of the floor of the mouth, and above the mylohyoid muscle. It is separated from the genioglossus muscle medially by Wharton's duct. Sublingual tissue is palpable behind the mandibular canines. The sublingual gland acquires an oval shape when sectioned transversely; however, its shape is longitudinal and lentiform when sectioned parallel to the body of the mandible [2]. The gland is composed of a major sublingual gland and around 8–30 minor sublingual glands [1].

The sublingual gland differs from the other major salivary glands, because it lacks intercalated or striated ducts, so saliva is secreted directly through the ducts of Rivinus. These ducts empty along an elevated ridge called the "plica fimbriate" formed by the sublingual folds, which are oblique to the frenulum linguae bilaterally. The sublingual duct of Bartholin (the largest sublingual gland excretory duct) joins Wharton's duct to form the draining orifice on each side of the lingual frenulum [4]. Sublingual gland hypertrophy may result from congenital absence of the submandibular gland [5].

27.3.2 Blood Supply and Lymphatics

The sublingual glands are supplied primarily by the sublingual and submental arteries, which are branches of the lingual artery and facial artery, which originate from the external carotid artery (ECA). The sublingual vein drains into the lingual vein, which then flows into the internal jugular vein (IJV).

The sublingual glands drain into the submandibular lymph nodes (LNs), which are three to six in number and located in the submandibular triangle, beneath the body of the mandible. The nodes are palpable on the superficial surface of the submandibular gland. Malignant tumors may drain into these regional LNs, requiring more extensive neck dissection for the complete treatment of cancer.

27.3.3 Nerve Supply

The sublingual glands receive their parasympathetic input via the chorda tympani nerve, which is a branch of the facial nerve (CN-VII) via the submandibular ganglion. The nerve functions in a secretomotor capacity. The chorda tympani branches from the motor branch of the facial nerve in the middle ear cavity, which then exits the middle ear through the petrotympanic fissure. The chorda tympani nerve then travels with the lingual nerve to synapse at the submandibular ganglion. The postganglionic fibers reach the sublingual gland and release acetylcholine and substance P. Acetylcholine, the primary neurotransmitter, and the muscarinic receptors work to increase salivation [4].

27.3.4 Surgical Considerations

Sublingual gland excision most commonly involves trans-oral electrocautery and blunt dissection. Structures most at risk of injury during gland excision are the lingual nerve and Wharton's duct. The sublingual tissue can be found in the anterior floor of the mouth and directly deep into Wharton's duct.

A sublingual gland flap can be used to manage major pathologies affecting the mandible and maxilla bones with excellent results [6].

27.4 Applied Physiology

The sublingual salivary gland is predominantly a mucous gland; however, it is considered a mixed serous and mucous gland. It is made up of mainly mucous acini with serous demilunes. It is the only uncapsulated major salivary gland. Sublingual tissue primarily produces a thick mucinous fluid and lubricates the oral cavity, allowing swallowing, initiating digestion, buffering pH, and facilitating dental hygiene [3].

The composition of saliva depends on the salivary flow rate and the overall contribution of each gland. Saliva is comprised of both organic and inorganic components. Inorganic components include electrolytes, urea, and ammonia, while the organic elements contain immunoglobulins, enzymes, and proteins [3]. The primary protein found in mucous saliva is mucin, which functions to lubricate and competitively inhibit bacterial attachment to the salivary duct epithelium. This action allows for antimicrobial protection of the sublingual gland [3].

The use of interferential current stimulation has been investigated for patients who suffer from dry mouth. It may be an approach to stimulate the function of the sublingual and submandibular glands. This therapeutic modality does not create distress or pain for the patient [7].

27.5 Ranula

27.5.1 Definitions

A ranula is a pseudocyst (lacking an epithelial lining) in the floor of the mouth caused by either the extravasation of saliva or the retention of mucous of the sublingual gland [8]. Its name derives from the Latin words rana (frog) and ranula (little frog), due to the typical bluish appearance, similar to a frog's belly [9]. Plunging ranula (also known as cervical ranula) is a pseudocyst that forms following the escape (extravasation) of mucus from the sublingual gland and its subsequent herniation through the mylohyoid muscle into submandibular space and beyond [10, 11]. It is worth mentioning that the term "ranula" has also sometimes been used to refer to other similar swellings of the floor of the mouth such as true salivary duct cysts, dermoid cysts, and cystic hygroma [12].

27.5.2 Classification (Types)

Ranula is anatomically grouped into three different types, namely, (1) superficial ranula (also called "simple," "oral," or "sublingual" ranula), which is confined to the floor of the mouth lying above the mylohyoid muscle; (2) plunging ranula (also called "cervical," "diving," "deep," or "submandibular" ranula) [13], which is an unusual variant found in the neck beneath the mylohyoid muscle; and (3) mixed type, which has both an oral and a cervical component (also called "oral ranula with cervical extension" or "sublingual-submandibular ranula") [12, 14]. While the sublingual type is a simple ranula, the other two appearing in the neck are "plunging" ranulae or "deep cervical ranulae."

27.5.3 Epidemiology

The prevalence of ranula is approximately 0.2 cases per 1000 individuals, accounting for nearly 6% of intraoral cysts of the salivary glands [9]. The age of patients has a wide range between 3 and 61 years, with children and young adults in the second and third decades more affected than others. There is no gender predilection [15].

An ethnic variation in the incidence of plunging ranula has been documented in the literature where it was reported to be more prevalent in people of Asian origin especially the Chinese, natives of New Zealand, and Eskimos. This racial predilection could be attributed to a genetic alteration in people of this race, perhaps predisposing them to either develop areas of deficiencies within the mylohyoid muscle or an anatomically altered variant of the sublingual gland with easy extravasation of mucus following minor trauma [16, 17].

27.5.4 Pathogenesis/Etiology

There are two different concepts for the pathogenesis of ranula: (1) It is a "true cyst" (with an epithelial lining) resulting from ductal obstruction and (2) it is a "pseudocyst" (without an epithelial lining) resulting from injury of the duct and extravasation of mucus [18–20]. Recently, typical ranulae have been considered as an extravasation phenomenon of the sublingual gland [20].

The etiology of plunging ranula can be described by either of two processes. The first is by incomplete blockage of the duct of a sublingual gland, which leads to the development of a true retention cyst lined by epithelium. About 10% of all ranulas develop in this manner [21]. Secondly, the duct or deeper areas of the body of the sublingual gland may become damaged by direct trauma thus initiating mucus to escape into the surrounding area with subsequent formation of a non-epithelial-lined cyst [9, 22, 23]. An obstructed duct secondary to trauma may cause back pressure to build up if severe enough; this will rupture the acini and lead to mucus spillage. In contrast, submandibular and parotid ducts will not usually form ranula from ligation because they only secrete saliva when stimulated, unlike the sublingual that constantly discharges saliva even during the inter-digestive phase [24]. However, ranulae have been reported to also arise from the submandibular duct or the minor salivary gland in the floor of the mouth [25].

Most plunging ranulae usually have also oral components, and several mechanisms have been proposed by which they may arise: (1) Part of the sublingual gland may move through the mylohyoid muscle, or an aberrant sublingual gland may be present below this muscle—this mechanism describes cases without an oral part—(2) the lateral part of the anterior two-thirds of the mylohyoid muscle may have a deficiency (reported in 27–45% of cadavers) through which mucus from the sublingual gland may slip to the submandibular area [13]; (3) the current belief that plunging ranula develops from escape of mucus saliva from the sublingual gland dissecting its way through the mylohyoid muscle [12], with retention of this mucus and its extension into neighboring tissues [23], and rarely extending backwards into the para-pharyngeal space [26]; and (4) finally, the observation that many patients with plunging ranula are young children could point out that perhaps plunging ranula is congenital in origin as reported by Morton et al. (2010) [17], Chin and colleagues (2016) [16], and Olojede et al. (2017) [24].

27.5.5 Clinical Picture

A ranula is usually seen in children and young adults, affecting both sexes equally. The patient usually presents with a painless, slowly growing, submucosal swelling in the floor of the mouth between the symphysis menti and the tongue, just to one side of the frenulum (midline), which helps to distinguish it from a midline dermoid cyst (Fig. 27.1) [12]. The swelling is characteristically translucent and has a bluish tinge. It is spherical in shape (but only the top half is visible) and varies from 1 to 5 cm in size. If it reaches a large size (up to 10 cm), it results in elevation of the tongue and possibly interferes with swallowing causing dysphagia [21]. The edge of

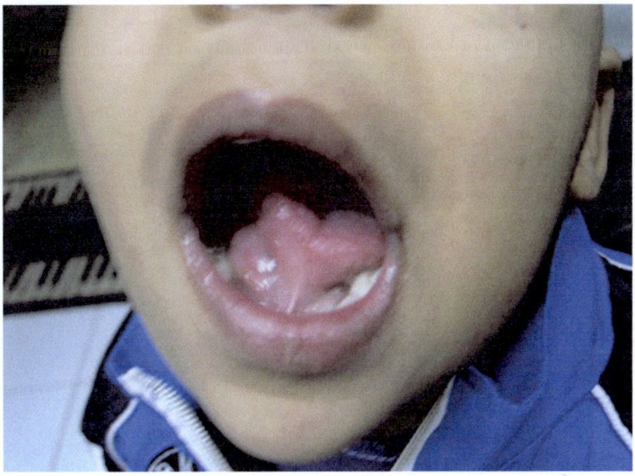

Fig. 27.1 Ranula (oral component) in a child. Swelling in the floor of the mouth to the right side of the tongue. Note the bluish discoloration of the cyst

the swelling is difficult to feel because it is deep and related to the arch of the mandible. The surface is smooth and covered by tortuous veins, and the mucous membrane is mobile over the swelling. The submandibular duct is displaced and stretched over it. A ranula is soft in consistency, usually fluctuant and transilluminates, but cannot be compressed. The fluid within the ranula has the viscous, jelly-like consistency of egg white. A ranula may rupture and refill again.

A ranula is not tender unless it becomes secondarily infected and is not fixed to the overlying mucosa, tongue, or jaw. In the absence of infection, cervical LNs should not be enlarged, and local tissues should be normal [12].

The plunging (cervical) ranula clinically presents as an asymptomatic, progressively expanding swelling in the lateral side of the neck (Fig. 27.2); it may or may not have an intraoral component [27]. When an oral component is present, squeezing the neck mass may increase the size of swelling in the floor of the mouth.

Plunging ranulae have been reported to spread into the submental area, the contralateral side of the neck, the nasopharyngeal region (including the skull base), the retro-pharynx, and sometimes the upper mediastinum [9, 13]. The patient may present with complications of ranula, which in general include infection, repeated trauma, bursting and reformation, and dysphagia (in the case of a large ranula >10 cm in size).

27.5.6 Investigations

27.5.6.1 Imaging Studies

The simple ranula is within the sublingual space above the mylohyoid muscle, but the plunging ranula dives into the submandibular space with a collapsed sublingual portion called the "tail." The key to diagnosing a ranula, especially in cases where they have been dissected some distance away from their origin, is the identification of a connection to the sublingual space, in the form of a thin tail of fluid or a

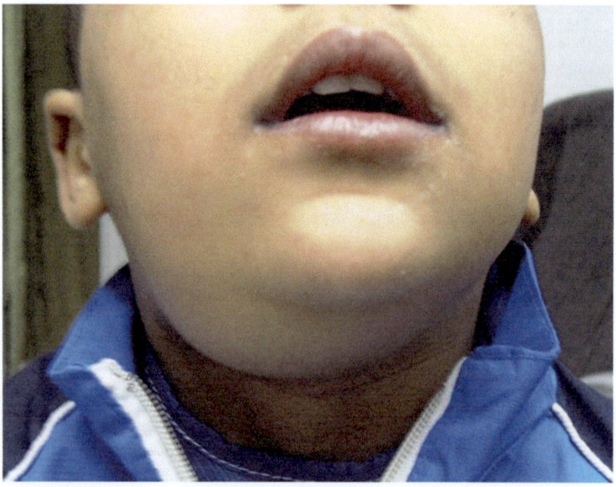

Fig. 27.2 Right plunging ranula (cervical component) bulging into the anterior triangle of the lateral side of the neck (and spreading into the submental triangle)

significant local fluid collection [28]. Imaging studies to investigate plunging ranula include ultrasound (US), computed tomography (CT) scan, and magnetic resonance imaging (MRI) [26].

27.5.6.2 Ultrasonography (US)

High-resolution ultrasound helps to differentiate between a simple or deep ranula as it can confirm the depth above or below the mylohyoid muscle and the overall quality of the lesion. Ultrasound can also identify rupture or herniation of the sublingual gland [24]. It is a noninvasive test with no known biological cost [29]. Uncomplicated ranulas appear as thin-walled cystic lesions and can be imaged both externally from the skin or trans-orally with a small probe.

If infected, the walls are thicker, and the fluid content is more echogenic. The status of the mylohyoid muscle can also be established by this test [13, 15]. This technique will also differentiate plunging ranulae that have plunged behind the posterior border of the mylohyoid into the submental space and the less common ranula that has herniated through a mylohyoid muscle defect into the submental space. The use of US to investigate these lesions has been recommended as the preferred test [27].

27.5.6.3 Computed Tomography (CT) Scan

The classical CT scan finding of plunging ranula is a lesion with a small "tail" that extends into the sublingual space [29]. In the absence of this sign, the diagnosis of a plunging ranula should be made if an identical cyst is seen in the submandibular or para-pharyngeal space with a connection to the sublingual space [13]. An uncomplicated ranula appears as a thin-walled cystic lesion with central fluid attenuation (10–20 HU). If the cyst has been intervened upon previously or has been infected, the content may be increased in attenuation, even occasionally resembling a non-enhancing soft tissue mass. The walls of such lesions are typically thicker. If a superimposed infection is present at the time of imaging, it will be indistinguishable from an abscess, with thicker walls and surrounding fat stranding [28].

27.5.6.4 Magnetic Resonance Imaging (MRI)

Magnetic resonance imaging of the plunging ranula shows a T1 low signal and a T2 high signal. With gadolinium (Gd) contrast (T1 C+), the wall of the lesion may demonstrate some enhancement that is best seen with fat saturation [30].

27.5.6.5 Histopathology

The histological appearance of a ranula is typically that of a pseudocyst without epithelial lining; it consists of a fibrovascular stroma, which contains chronic inflammatory cells including macrophages filled with mucin [21]. Histiocytes or foamy macrophages predominate in the pseudocyst wall, and mucin is also often observed [12] (Fig. 27.3). Occasionally, partial epithelial linings are seen. High amylase and protein are seen in the biochemical analysis of the cystic fluid [9].

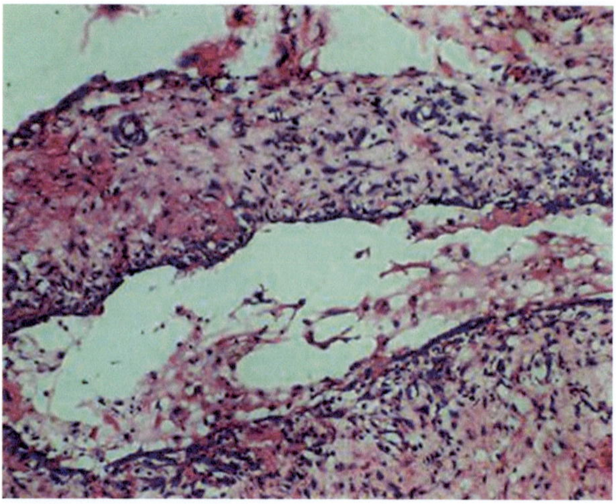

Fig. 27.3 Histology of an excised ranula showing mucin collection in the lumen lined by connective tissue with inflammatory cells. H&E stain ×40

27.5.7 Differential Diagnosis

The differential diagnosis depends on the location of the ranula, intraoral or plunging. In general, a plunging ranula presenting as a cervical swelling should mainly be differentiated from the following [10, 13, 21, 31, 32]:

Dermoid/epidermoid cyst (usually midline)
Cystic hygroma (usually in infants)
Cervical abscess (extensive adjacent fat stranding, usually associated with tooth caries)
Thyroglossal cyst (usually midline)
Second branchial cyst (usually at the anterior border of the SCM muscle)
Lymph node enlargement (cystic/necrotic)
Laryngocele
Thymic cyst
Cysts of endocrine glands of the neck
Benign salivary gland tumors
Some benign mesenchymal tumors

27.5.8 Treatment

Many methods have been used for the treatment of ranulae; these include surgical excision of the lesion, use of cryosurgery, marsupialization, and excision of the oral portion and associated sublingual gland or, rarely, submandibular gland. Other reported procedures include the excision of the sublingual gland through an intraoral approach, drainage of lesions, and excision of the swelling via a cervical approach, sometimes combined with the excision of the sublingual gland [9].

Recurrences have been recorded after these treatments [23]. However, when the sublingual gland together with the associated lesion is excised, a low recurrence rate is recorded [33, 34].

27.5.8.1 Marsupialization of Oral Ranula

Marsupialization is the oldest and most widely used procedure for the treatment of oral ranula; this involves de-roofing the cyst and suturing the edges to surrounding tissues in the floor of the mouth, with the aim of allowing the sublingual gland to re-establish connection with the oral cavity. A high recurrence rate (RR) reaching up to 61–89% was reported within 6 weeks to 12 months of surgery. Early closure of the surgery site due to compression of the tongue on the cyst has been known to increase the RR. Thus, marsupialization and filling (packing) the cavity with gauze for 7–10 days reduced the RR and improved the success rate [24].

Micro-marsupialization involves the placement of a silk suture (Seton) for a minimum of 7 days during which an epithelial tract forms to allow for mucus drainage between the surface and the underlying salivary glandular tissue. This procedure is simple; still, however, recurrence or treatment failure is the primary complication [13].

27.5.8.2 Sublingual Gland Excision and Cyst Drainage

Intraoral excision of the sublingual gland and drainage of the associated cervical content are enough to achieve a cure [23]. With the transcervical approach, total excision of the sublingual gland is challenging because this method requires the pain-staking division of the mylohyoid muscle in the floor of the mouth [13]. However, this method is recommended for recurrent cases and when the plunging ranula is large in size [35]. Cases restricted to the neck are also best treated by the transcervical approach [13].

27.5.8.3 Excision of the Ranula and Sublingual Gland

With the patient under general anesthesia, nasotracheal intubation, and oropharyngeal packing (to prevent aspiration), excision of a ranula can be achieved through the oral cavity, which is opened with a self-retaining mouth retractor. An elliptical incision is then made over the curve of the cystic swelling, and the mucosal flap over the cyst is carefully freed from the ranula, by both blunt and sharp dissection (Fig. 27.4). The cystic swelling is then grasped with serrated forceps and freed from Wharton's duct by blunt dissection and from its connections with the underlying mylohyoid muscle. All small vessels in the field are controlled with bipolar coagulation. After the excision of the ranula together with the sublingual gland, the sound lingual nerve can be seen lying on the floor of the mouth next to Wharton's duct. After careful hemostasis, the wound is irrigated with saline solution, and the mucosa is closed with 3-0 Vicryl sutures. Frequent oral irrigations with oral antiseptic solutions are recommended for optimal oral hygiene, and oral feeding is started with clear liquids and pureed foods.

Yoshimura et al. (1995) [34] compared three methods of ranula treatment in 27 patients and reported a RR of 25% with excision of ranula only, 36% with

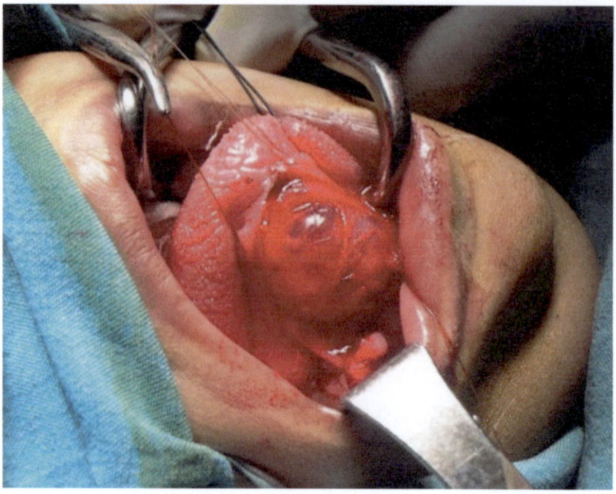

Fig. 27.4 Excision of ranula: intraoperative dissection

marsupialization, and 0% with ranula and ipsilateral sublingual excision. Moreover, the comparative study in children by Crysdale et al. (1988) [36] showed a high RR of 61% with marsupialization and 0% with either excision of ranula only or with ranula and ipsilateral sublingual gland excision.

27.5.8.4 Carbon Dioxide Laser

Carbon dioxide laser has also been used as a treatment option for plunging ranula; this has shown good success with a significant reduction of the RR as reported by Mintz et al. (1994) [37].

27.5.8.5 Radiotherapy (RT)

In very few patients who cannot endure the stress of surgery, a worthwhile alternative would be the use of radiotherapy (RT). Low doses (20–25 Gy) have been known to be effective for the treatment of plunging ranula. The attendant complications of RT especially xerostomia can be circumvented by using low doses and protecting the contralateral parotid gland with a shield. The danger of malignancies developing as a result of treatment with radiation is very low [22].

27.5.8.6 Sclerosing Therapy

Although considered experimental, sclerosing agents have been employed in the treatment of plunging ranula [38]. Woo et al. (2003) reported that Bleomycin and OK-432 have been successfully used to manage plunging ranulae [39]. Rho et al. (2006) reported that OK-432 has been shown to collapse and cause adhesion of the pseudocyst wall of a plunging ranula [38]. In a study of 32 patients with plunging ranula, 31 (97%) achieved a marked decrease in the size of the lesion with an injection of OK-432. While about 50% of all patients experienced local pain or fever, this, however, resolved after some days. Rho et al. thus advocated that sclerotherapy is a safe and potentially curative procedure that may be used as a primary treatment before considering surgery for plunging ranula [38].

Table 27.1 Recurrent rates after treatment of plunging ranula

Procedure	Recurrence rate
Incision and drainage	70%
Marsupialization	53%
Excision of the lesion in the neck	85%
Excision of the lesion in the neck and sublingual gland	3.8%
Intraoral excision of the sublingual gland and drainage of the cyst	0%

27.5.9 Prognosis

27.5.9.1 Outcome

Parekh et al. (1987) reviewed 139 surgeries for plunging ranulae in 89 patients and recorded a RR of over 50% for cases where the sublingual gland was not excised. On the other hand, a RR as low as 3.8% or less was recorded when the sublingual gland was excised, alone or in association with other treatments. They thus advocate that the sublingual gland should at all times be removed to improve the prognosis of this condition [10]. In addition, in the 15 patients treated by Davison et al. (1998) with sublingual gland excision [14], only two cases (13%) recurred after a 2-year follow-up period. This further substantiates the suggestion that the sublingual gland be removed at all times.

Table 27.1 summarizes the RRs observed by Parekh and colleagues (1987) after the different procedures employed for the treatment of plunging ranula [10].

27.5.9.2 Complications

Complications common to intraoral ranula are also associated with plunging ranula with the most common being recurrence of the lesion; lingual nerve injury, which may result in a decrease in tongue sensation; and damage of Wharton's duct. Other complications, which are generally uncommon, are hematoma formation, infection, and dehiscence of the wound. Complications such as marginal mandibular nerve (MMN) paralysis tend also to occur because of the proximity of this nerve to the cyst; proper identification of this nerve can prevent its injury [40].

27.6 Sialolithiasis

27.6.1 Epidemiology

Salivary calculi (sialoliths or stones) obstructing an excretory duct are a common salivary gland disease. The pathophysiology is related mainly to salivary stasis and overall inflammation of the excretory duct. Sialoliths may be single or multiple and occur mainly in the submandibular gland (80–90%) and to a lesser extent in the parotid gland (5–20%). The sublingual gland and the minor salivary glands are rarely affected (1–2%) [3, 41]. The reason for this low incidence remains unknown. From an anatomical viewpoint, the duct of the sublingual gland is shorter and has multiple openings that may drain mucoid saliva more efficiently. Even if a stone develops, it may not cause total obstruction of saliva outflow and subsequent infection. Therefore, most sublingual gland sialolithiasis might be asymptomatic and undetected in clinical practice. Furthermore, because both the ductal systems of the sublingual gland and the submandibular gland duct are located beneath the mucosa of the floor of the mouth, a stone in the sublingual gland duct may be misdiagnosed as submandibular gland sialolithiasis in clinical practice, especially when it is large in size and in close proximity to the gland [42].

27.6.2 Clinical Presentation

Sialolithiasis shows a male preponderance. All ages may be affected, although patients in their third–sixth decade of life represent the majority of cases. Salivary stones may cause swelling of the duct or gland causing colicky peri-prandial pain [43]. On physical examination, calculi are manually palpable when lodged in the salivary duct.

27.6.3 Diagnosis

A stone in the sublingual gland duct may be easily misdiagnosed as being proximally located in Wharton's duct, even using CT, if the index of suspicion is not high. When an accompanying abscess develops, it is easier to identify which gland is involved and where the stone is located by physical examination, because a sublingual gland abscess mainly presents with painful swelling over the unilateral mouth floor, whereas a submandibular gland abscess always presents with painful swelling over the submandibular area of the neck. However, when the abscess becomes larger, with the infection spreading widely into the adjacent tissue, it is somewhat difficult to distinguish between them by physical examination [42].

It is important to preoperatively determine which salivary gland is involved, the sublingual or the submandibular, because they require different surgical approaches. Ultrasound (US) can aid diagnosis along with adjunctive CT scan or MR sialography if the work-up is negative, but suspicion remains high.

27.6.4 Treatment

Initial treatment is conservative, which includes oral hydration and sialagogues. Surgery is only recommended when symptoms persist despite conservative treatment. Hong and Yang (2003) reported multiple sialoliths arising in the sublingual gland. They presented on the right floor of the mouth in a 14-year-old female. The sublingual gland and sialoliths were completely removed with careful preservation of the lingual nerve and Wharton's duct [41]. Liao et al. (2007) reported the case of a 50-year-old gentleman with left sublingual gland sialolithiasis that was successfully treated with excision of the left sublingual gland and the stone via a trans-oral approach, 6 weeks after the infection was controlled [42].

27.7 Sialadenitis

27.7.1 Acute Sialadenitis

Acute sialadenitis of the sublingual salivary gland may be caused by bacterial or viral infection due to an obstructing calculus or hyposecretion. The inflammation may be accompanied by fever, pain, and gland swelling. Conservative treatment includes hydration, warm compresses, massage, pain relief with analgesics, and sialogogues. If the etiology is a bacterial infection, then antibiotics are recommended. Empiric antibiotic therapy starts with amoxicillin/clavulanate or clindamycin. If the formation of an abscess complicates the infection, surgical intervention may be required [3].

27.7.2 Chronic Sialadenitis

Chronic inflammation of the sublingual salivary gland can be related to recurrent infections, duct obstruction, or radiation exposure. If the cause is a calculus, then removal of the obstructing stone or surgical excision of the sublingual gland along with the stone is indicated. The sublingual gland is rarely affected by any of these acute or chronic problems in isolation [3].

27.8 Tumors of the Sublingual Gland

27.8.1 Epidemiology

Neoplastic diseases may affect the sublingual gland as 3–4% of head and neck cancers involve salivary glands. The larger the size of the salivary gland, the higher the possibility of a tumor being benign [3]. Sublingual gland tumors are extremely rare [44]. They are usually malignant (approximately, 75%) and comprise about 1.6% of all salivary gland malignancies. Adenoid cystic carcinoma and mucoepidermoid carcinoma count as the most common sublingual gland malignancies reported, accounting for 80% of all carcinomas arising in this region [45].

27.8.2 Clinical Presentation

Tumors of the sublingual gland usually present as a painless mass under the lateral aspect of the ventral tongue. It may be associated with minimal discomfort, pain, numbness of the tongue, and difficulty with the retention of a dental prosthesis. Most tumors present similarly to benign conditions making diagnosis difficult, and a high degree of suspicion must thus be employed for lesions in this region of the floor of the mouth. These salivary gland tumors can be differentiated from mucosal lesions of the floor of the mouth by their submucosal location. However, it is almost impossible to differentiate primary tumors of the sublingual glands from tumors of minor salivary origin in the floor of the mouth [46, 47].

27.8.3 Treatment of Sublingual Malignant Tumors (MTs)

Since the sublingual gland lies directly beneath the mucosal surface of the anterior floor of the mouth and close to the inner aspect of the mandible, treatment of a sublingual MT usually entails the removal of the gland with a surrounding cuff of normal tissue (floor of the mouth and lateral aspect of the oral tongue). The development of a soft tissue cuff around a MT confined to the sublingual gland without extraglandular extension can be achieved through excision of the mucosa (floor of the mouth and small segment of the tongue), the mylohyoid muscle, and the periosteum of the mandible.

Most salivary gland cancers arising in the floor of the mouth are done in concert with at least level I neck dissection, thus removing the submandibular gland. Treatment of moderately advanced sublingual gland cancer includes ipsilateral neck dissection with resection of the sublingual gland and surrounding tissues (floor of the mouth and lateral aspect of the tongue), usually in association with a marginal resection of the mandible.

More advanced or recurrent cancer of the sublingual gland is likely to require resection of the floor of the mouth along with a partial glossectomy, mandibulectomy, supra-omohyoid structures, and the lingual and hypoglossal nerves. The neck dissection is completed in the usual fashion except for level I, through which the specimen is attached to the primary tumor.

Removal of the sublingual gland is not without potential morbidity, most notably injury to the lingual nerve with subsequent numbness, injury to Wharton's duct with the possibility of obstructive sialadenitis, and ductal laceration causing salivary leakage [48].

27.9 Exciaion of the Sublingual Gland

27.9.1 Positioning and Draping

Under general anesthesia, the patient is placed in a supine position with the neck extended. The skin of the anterior neck and lower face is sterilized. Draping is done in such a way that the mouth and upper neck are exposed. A self-retaining retractor is used to open the mouth. A silk traction suture is passed through the tip of the tongue to better expose the anterior floor of the mouth.

27.9.2 Surgical Approach

The sublingual gland is quite large and is located immediately deep in the mucosa just anterior to the submandibular duct in the anterior floor of the mouth. The sublingual salivary gland is conventionally approached through a simple incision in the floor of the mouth directly over the gland. Using this route, access to dissection is limited, and important related structures are not easy to identify. The use of a flap, proposed by Yates in 1994, greatly improves access and facilitates identification of the submandibular duct and lingual nerve [49].

27.9.3 Important Related Structures

The structures at risk during the dissection of the gland are the duct of the submandibular gland and the lingual nerve. The duct lies superficially in the floor of the mouth medial to the sublingual fold and is crossed inferiorly by the lingual nerve which then enters the tongue. The sublingual artery and vein also lie on the medial aspect of the gland close to the submandibular duct and lingual nerve.

27.9.4 Surgical Technique

Instead of a simple incision, a flap is designed; it is cut squarely at the corners to simplify orientation for repair and in the midline extends between the submandibular duct orifices. A very thin flap is raised to include the submandibular duct. No attempt should be made to produce a more substantial flap as this will cause the operator to enter the gland itself and lose the plane of dissection. Separation of the flap will be most difficult just beneath the sublingual fold where the multiple minor sublingual ducts tether the gland to the mucosa. The submandibular duct is thus raised with the flap, and bearing in mind the anatomical relationship between the duct and the lingual nerve, it leads directly to the latter. In this way, the two key structures at risk in the procedure are identified at a very early stage in the dissection. With this exposure, dissection of the gland from its bed is relatively straightforward, and identification of the sublingual vessels medial and inferior to the submandibular duct and lingual nerve is simplified. The flap is repositioned with resorbable sutures. No drainage is necessary [49].

References

1. Kessler AT, Bhatt AA. Review of the major and minor salivary glands, part 1: anatomy, infectious, and inflammatory processes. J Clin Imaging Sci. 2018;8:47.
2. Bialek EJ, Jakubowski W, Zajkowski P, Szopinski KT, Osmolski A. US of the major salivary glands: anatomy and spatial relationships, pathologic conditions, and pitfalls. Radiographics. 2006;26(3):745–63.

3. Armstrong MA, Turturro MA. Salivary gland emergencies. Emerg Med Clin North Am. 2013;31(2):481–99.
4. Holmberg KV, Hoffman MP. Anatomy, biogenesis and regeneration of salivary glands. Monogr Oral Sci. 2014;24:1–13.
5. Chung J, Lee YW. Functional compensation of a hypertrophied sublingual gland and the absence of the ipsilateral submandibular gland. Br J Oral Maxillofac Surg. 2019;57(8):813–6.
6. Jose A, Rawat A, Singh S, Nagori SA, Roychoudhury A. Management of intraoral surgical defects using sublingual gland flap. J Craniofac Surg. 2020;31(8):e766–7.
7. Hasegawa Y, Sugahara K, Sano S, Sakuramoto A, Kishimoto H, Oku Y. Enhanced salivary secretion by interferential current stimulation in patients with dry mouth: a pilot study. Oral Surg Oral Med Oral Pathol Oral Radiol. 2016;121(5):481–9.
8. Nguyen BN, Malone BN, Sidman JD, Barnett RB. Excision of sublingual gland as treatment for ranulas in pediatric patients. Int J Pediatr Otorhinolaryngol. 2017;97:154–6.
9. Gupta A, Karjodkar FR. Plunging ranula: a case report. ISRN Dent. 2011;2011:806928.
10. Parekh D, Stewart M, Joseph C, Lawson HH. Plunging ranula: a report of three cases and a review of the literature. Br J Surg. 1987;74:307–9.
11. Skouteris CA, Sotereanos GC. Plunging ranula: report of a case. J Oral Maxillofac Surg. 1987;45:1068–72.
12. Bouquot BW, Neville DD, Damm CM, Allen JE. Oral & maxillofacial pathology. 2nd ed. Philadelphia, PA: WB Saunders; 2002. p. 391–2.
13. de Visscher JG, van der Wal KG, de Vogel PL. The plunging ranula: pathogenesis, diagnosis and management. J Craniomaxillofac Surg. 1989;17:182–5.
14. Davison MJ, Morton RP, Mclvor NP. Plunging ranula: clinical observations. Head Neck. 1998;20:63–8.
15. Suresh BV, Vora SK. Huge plunging ranula. J Maxillofac Oral Surg. 2012;11:487–90.
16. Chin SJ, Zeng IS, Morton RP. The epidemiology of plunging ranula in South Auckland. Laryngoscope. 2016;126:2739–43.
17. Morton RP, Ahmad Z, Jain P. Plunging ranula: congenital or acquired? Otolaryngol Head Neck Surg. 2010;142:104–7.
18. de Visscher JG, van der Wal KG, de Vogel PL. The plunging ranula. Pathogenesis, diagnosis and management. J Craniomaxillofac Surg. 1989;17(4):182–5.
19. Batsakis GJ. Cyst, pseudocysts, fistulae and sialectsis of the salivary glands. Tumors of the head and neck. 2nd ed. Baltimore, MD: Waverly Press; 1984. p. 116–7.
20. Davison MJ, Morton RP, McIvor NP. Plunging ranula: clinical observations. Head Neck. 1998;20(1):63–8.
21. Langlois NE, Kolhe P. Plunging ranula: a case report and a literature review. Hum Pathol. 1992;23:1306–8.
22. Dietrich EM, Vasilios B, Maria L, Styliani P, Konstantinos A. Sublingual-plunging ranula as a complication of supraomohyoid neck dissection. Int J Surg Case Rep. 2011;2:90–2.
23. Ichimura K, Ohta Y, Tayama N. Surgical management of the plunging ranula: a review of seven cases. J Laryngol Otol. 1996;110:554–6.
24. Olojede ACO, Ogundana OM, Emeka CI, Adewole RA, Emmanuel MM, Gbotolorun OM, et al. Plunging ranula: surgical management of case series and the literature review. Clin Case Rep. 2017;6(1):109–14.
25. Hupp JR, Ellis E, Tucker MR. Contemporary oral and maxillofacial surgery. 5th ed. St Louis, MO: Mosby Elsevier; 2008. p. 410–1.
26. La'Porte SJ, Juttla JK, Lingam RK. Imaging the floor of the mouth and the sublingual space. Radiographics. 2011;31(5):1215–30.
27. Jain P, Jain R, Morton RP, Ahmad Z. Plunging ranulas: high-resolution ultrasound for diagnosis and surgical management. Eur Radiol. 2010;20:1442–9.
28. Coit WE, Harnsberger HR, Osborn AG, Smoker WR, Stevens MH, Lufkin RB. Ranulas and their mimics: CT evaluation. Radiology. 1987;163(1):211–6.
29. Charnoff SK, Carter BL. Plunging ranula: CT diagnosis. Radiology. 1986;158:467–8.

30. Kurabayashi T, Ida M, Yasumoto M, Ohbayashi N, Yoshino N, Tetsumura A, et al. MRI of ranulas. Neuroradiology. 2000;42(12):917–22.
31. Balakrishnan A, Ford GR, Bailey CM. Plunging ranula following bilateral submandibular duct transposition. J Laryngol Otol. 1991;105:667–9.
32. Horiguchi H, Kakuta S, Nagumo M. Bilateral plunging ranula: a case report. Int J Oral Maxillofac Surg. 1995;24:174–5.
33. Harrison JD. Modern management and pathophysiology of ranula: literature review. Head Neck. 2010;32:1310–20.
34. Yoshimura Y, Obara S, Kondoh T, Naitoh SI. A comparison of three methods used for treatment of ranula. J Oral Maxillofac Surg. 1995;53:280–3.
35. Lesperance MM. When do ranulas require a cervical approach? Laryngoscope. 2013;123:1826–7.
36. Crysdale WS, Mendelsohn JD, Conley S. Ranulas—mucoceles of the oral cavity: experience in 26 children. Laryngoscope. 1988;98(3):296–8.
37. Mintz S, Barak S, Horowitz I. Carbon dioxide laser excision and vaporization of nonplunging ranulas: a comparison of two treatment protocols. J Oral Maxillofac Surg. 1994;52:370–2.
38. Rho MH, Kim DW, Kwon JS, Lee SW, Sung YS, Song YK, et al. OK-432 sclerotherapy of plunging ranula in 21 patients: it can be a substitute for surgery. AJNR Am J Neuroradiol. 2006;27:1090–5.
39. Woo JS, Hwang S, Lee HM. Recurrent plunging ranula treated with OK-432. Eur Arch Otorrinolaringol. 2003;260:226–8.
40. Kim PD, Simental A. Management of mucocele and ranula in Myers EN. In: Ferris RL, editor. Salivary gland disorders. 1st ed. Berlin, Heidelberg: Springer-Verlag; 2007. p. 177–84.
41. Hong KH, Yang YS. Sialolithiasis in the sublingual gland. J Laryngol Otol. 2003;117(11):905–7.
42. Liao L-J, Hsiao J-K, Hsu W C, Wang C P. Sublingual gland sialolithiasis: a case report. Kaohsiung J Med Sci. 2007;23(11):590–3.
43. Williams MF. Sialolithiasis. Otolaryngol Clin N Am. 1999;32(5):819–34.
44. de Oliveira FA, Duarte EC, Taveira CT, Máximo AA, de Aquino EC, Alencar Rde C, Vencio EF. Salivary gland tumor: a review of 599 cases in a Brazilian population. Head Neck Pathol. 2009;3(4):271–5.
45. Pownell PH, Brown OE, Pransky SM, Manning SC. Congenital abnormalities of the submandibular duct. Int J Pediatr Otorhinolaryngol. 1992;24(2):161–9.
46. Codjambopoulo P, Ender-Griepekoven I, Broy H. Bilateral duplication of the submandibular gland and the submandibular duct. Rofo. 1992;157(2):185–6.
47. Graamans K, von der Akker HP. History and physical examination. In: Graamans AK, editor. Diagnosis of salivary gland disorders. Dordrecht, Germany: Kluwer Academic Publishers; 1991. p. 1–3.
48. Baurmash HD. Marsupialization for treatment of oral ranula: a second look at the procedure. J Oral Maxillofac Surg. 1992;50(12):1274–9.
49. Yates C. Surgical technique A surgical approach to the sublingual salivary gland. Ann R Coll Surg Engl. 1994;76:108–9.

Surgery of Minor Salivary Glands

28

28.1 Introduction

The salivary glands are exocrine glands that make, modify, and secrete saliva into the oral cavity. They are divided into two main types: the major salivary glands, which include the parotid, submandibular, and sublingual glands, and the minor salivary glands (MSGs), which line the mucosa of the upper aerodigestive tract (i.e., the palate, lip, pharynx, nasopharynx, larynx, and parapharyngeal space) and the overwhelming entirety of the mouth [1].

28.2 Anatomical Location and Function

While the major salivary glands produce 92–95% of saliva, the remainder is made by roughly 600–1000 minor salivary glands. They are dispersed throughout the submucosa of the sino-nasal cavity, oral cavity, pharynx, larynx, trachea, lungs, and middle ear cavity. Although minor salivary gland tissue can be found anywhere along the aerodigestive tract (except for the gingiva and anterior part of the hard palate), it is most concentrated along the buccal mucosa, labial mucosa, lingual mucosa, soft/hard palate, and floor of the mouth [1, 2]. The greatest glandular densities are located within the hard ($n = 250$) and soft ($n = 150$) palates. Each gland has exactly one duct, and although it contains both serous and mucous acini, its secretion is mainly mucous. Unlike the major salivary glands, they are not encapsulated by connective tissue but merely surrounded by it. Von Ebner's glands, a subset of the minor salivary glands, are found surrounding the circumvallate papillae on the dorsal surface of the tongue. They secrete a serous fluid that helps with lipid hydrolysis and also plays a role in taste perception [3].

Minor salivary gland tissue is not normally seen on conventional imaging but can become apparent when replaced by tumor or benign processes, most commonly mucus retention cysts [4]. Unlike the major salivary glands,

© The Author(s), under exclusive license to Springer Nature Switzerland AG 2024

M. Sakr, *Surgery of the Salivary Glands*,
https://doi.org/10.1007/978-3-031-82069-4_28

secretions by the minor salivary glands are not regulated by neuronal control. Instead, they continuously secrete small amounts of saliva, even at night when the major glands are resting, resulting in sustained lubrication of oral surfaces [5].

28.3 Minor Salivary Gland Sialolithiasis

28.3.1 Introduction

The first histopathologically established minor salivary gland sialolithiasis (MSGS) case was published by Lighterman in 1955 [6]. Since then, some solitary MSGS cases have been described as presenting as small, hard, firm, or movable asymptomatic submucosal nodules [7]. In 1971, Holst published the first extensive report of nine cases, including the first reported tongue–located case, as well as the first with nodules in multiple locations in the same patient (two locations in the upper lip) [7]. Pullon and Miller (1972) [8] reported ten cases of MSGS and performed the first MSGS review of a total of 55 cases in the medical literature. The majority of these lesions were located in the buccal mucosa ($n = 24$), followed by the upper lip ($n = 22$). The male-to-female ratio was 2:1. Similar findings were reported in other case series [9–11].

28.3.2 Epidemiology

Sialolithiasis is a common disease of the salivary glands. The majority of the salivary calculi occur in the major salivary glands, the submandibular (80–92%) and parotid (16–19%), while minor salivary glands are rarely affected (2%) [9, 12].

The largest review of 239 MSGS cases was reported by Ben Lagha et al. in 2005 [12]. It confirmed that (1) the most common lesion location is the upper lip (49.2%), followed by the buccal mucosa (37.3%); (2) MSGS affects both males and females (58.3% and 41.7%), with a slight predilection for males; and (3) the mean age of affected patients is 50 years (range, 9–90 years).

28.3.3 Pathogenesis

The development of sialoliths is a multifactorial event. Sialoliths are composed of a central core of organic material, covered by a layered calcified cortex. That calcified cortex consists of complicated salts of calcium, phosphate, and especially hydroxyapatite [13]. Salivary dysfunction or disturbances of secretion may also contribute to the development of sialoliths. Thus, sialolith formation occurs through the gradual calcification of an organic matrix of glycoproteins or of a foreign body.

28.3.4 Clinical Presentation

Sialolithiasis of the minor salivary gland often occurs in the upper lip and buccal mucosa and typically presents with a small, solitary submucosal nodule (Fig. 28.1), which is hard in consistency and, in some cases, can be movable in the surrounding tissue [9, 12]. The lesion (nodule) is usually painless but may become painful when the salivary gland parenchyma or excretory duct becomes infected, with or without pus. In that case, antibiotic medications are recommended. An antibiotic with high diffusion in saliva, such as macrolide, is preferable [12].

Matiakis and Tzermpos (2021) reported a case of minor salivary gland sialolithiasis in a 65-year-old male who presented with a movable asymptomatic submucosal nodule, about 2 cm in diameter, on the left side of the upper lip. The patient had undergone surgical excision of a similar mass in the same location 2 months prior and reported recurrence after a few weeks. The lesion was removed in total under local anesthesia, along with the adjacent minor salivary glands. Histopathology established the diagnosis [14].

In 2022, Huang et al. [15] reported a case of minor salivary gland sialolithiasis of the upper lip of a 58-year-old gentleman who presented with a small solitary nodule in the left upper lip for more than 2 months. The nodule was asymptomatic, hard, and palpable at the submucosal area of the left upper labial mucosa. It measured approximately 0.2 cm in the greatest dimension. The small hard nodule and the surrounding soft tissues were totally excised under local anesthesia and sent for histopathological examination. Microscopically, it showed a round salivary calculus composed of a relatively homogenous core and concentric alternating basophilic and eosinophilic bands at the periphery. Adjacent minor labial glands revealed slightly dilated acini and salivary ducts with mucin retention in the central lumens.

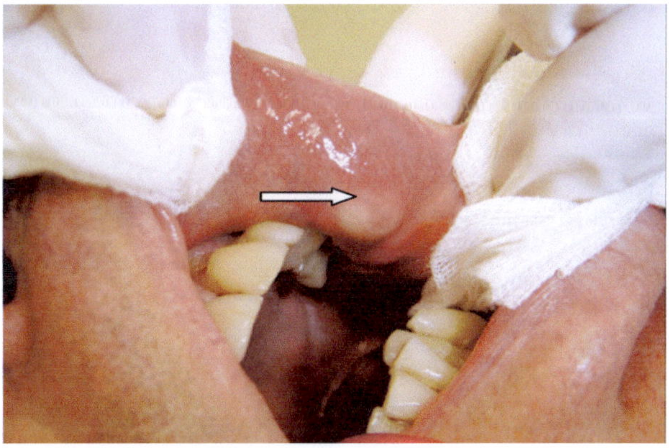

Fig. 28.1 A small minor salivary gland stone presenting as a whitish submucosal nodule, on the left side of the upper lip (arrow)

28.3.5 Investigations

28.3.5.1 Imaging

Sialoliths usually appear as radiopaque masses when the degree of calcification is high enough. Salivary stones in the terminal portion of Wharton's duct can be demonstrated by an occlusal radiograph, and sialoliths of the minor salivary glands of the upper labial or buccal mucosa can be shown by a periapical radiograph [9, 12].

Diagnostic ultrasound (US) may help in establishing the diagnosis and may also contribute to the removal of the calculus or such particles with the use of an ultrasound-guided needle [16]. Nevertheless, the use of US seems to be limited in MSGS diagnosis since there is only one related paper in the literature.

28.3.5.2 Histopathology

Among the histological findings is the presence of a sialolith in the minor salivary gland duct or fragments of sialoliths in different stages of calcification [17, 18]. Stasis of saliva, which accompanies minor salivary gland stones, usually results in minor salivary gland inflammation, with a chronic sialadenitis appearance [18]. Histological examination usually reveals chronic sialadenitis of minor salivary glands, with dilatation of the ducts surrounded by lymphocytes, plasma cells, and eosinophils [13, 18, 19] (Fig. 28.2). Squamous metaplasia and pseudostratified columnar metaplasia in duct epithelium are additional characteristic histological features [19].

28.3.6 Differential Diagnosis

The sialolith of minor salivary glands may be obvious during surgical excision as reported by Matiakis and Tzermpos (2021) [14] or may be absent or fragmented. The differential diagnosis of a nodule in the upper lip includes sialolithiasis, foreign

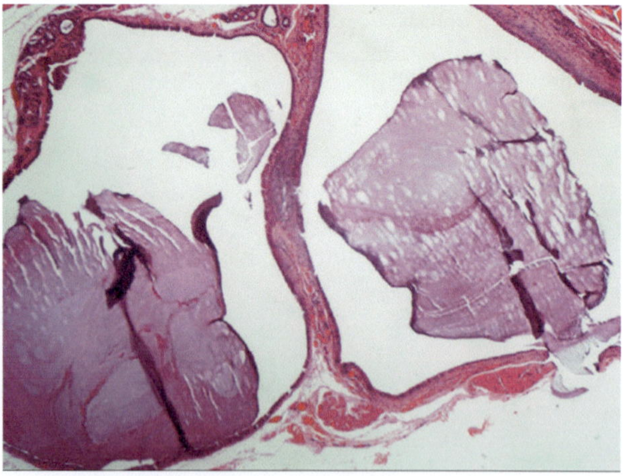

Fig. 28.2 Histopathology showing chronic sialadenitis with lobular atrophy, ductal dilatation, and lymphocytic infiltration in the stroma with lymph follicle formation resulting from a minor salivary gland stone (H&E, ×100)

body, mucocele [10, 20], swelling due to local irritation such as fibroma and diapneusia, chronic abscess of the oral mucosa, benign and malignant salivary neoplasms, and other soft tissue tumors or lesions such as lymphangioma [19, 21]. Sialolith and foreign body may be characterized as a hard nodule. Mucoceles are very common in the lower lip but are rare in the upper lip [9, 12]. Benign and malignant salivary neoplasms are occasionally discovered in the upper lip such as mucoepidermoid carcinoma (MEC) [22], palisaded encapsulated neuroma [23], and Kimura's disease [24]. Histopathological examination is needed to establish the clinical diagnosis of sialolithiasis.

28.3.7 Treatment

Small sialoliths in the excretory ducts of the submandibular and parotid salivary glands may be treated by milking the stones toward the duct orifice. However, larger sialoliths usually need to be removed surgically. Minor salivary gland stones, on the other hand, are best managed by surgical removal. To prevent recurrence, the lesion ought to be excised along with all adjacent minor salivary glands [9, 12]. Lithotripsy, the treatment of choice in sialolithiasis of major salivary glands [25], is not applicable in MSGS [14].

28.4 Subacute Necrotizing Sialadenitis (SANS)

28.4.1 Introduction

Subacute necrotizing sialadenitis (SANS) is generally considered a rare self-limiting, inflammatory condition involving primarily the minor salivary glands of the palatal region [26–28]. It was first described by Werning et al. in 1990 as an erythematous, non-ulcerated, but painful firm swelling of the posterior hard palate [26]. Lombardi et al. (2003) [28] subsequently classified SANS to be a part of the spectrum of the more common, necrotizing sialo-metaplasia (NSM) based on the clinical and histopathological features, while others classified it as a distinct or independent clinical entity with unique clinical and pathological features [29–31].

28.4.2 Epidemiology

Subacute necrotizing sialadenitis (SANS) is rather a rare condition with only 36 cases reported in the literature from 1990 to 2016; 30 cases affecting minor palatal salivary glands and six cases affecting extra-palatal minor salivary glands [29–32]. It occurs more commonly in younger adults and often presents as a painful hard or soft palate nodule with intact mucosa. Unlike NSM, SANS does not ulcerate and heals between 2 and 7 days. On the other hand, NSM often presents in middle-aged adults, and surface ulceration is a prominent feature. Moreover, the average healing time of NSM is between 5 and 6 weeks.

28.4.3 Etiology

The etiology of SANS is still unknown, but clinical and microscopic features have pointed toward a traumatic, infectious, or allergic etiology [30, 33].

28.4.3.1 Trauma

A traumatic etiology of SANS is possible but difficult to prove without patient recollection of trauma or evidence of injury [32].

28.4.3.2 Infection

Clinical features that support an infectious origin of SANS include the prevalence of the disease among young adults living in close quarters as well as the immediate onset, localization, and spontaneous resolution of symptoms [26, 27]. In addition, the cases reported by Werning et al. (1990) [26], as well as Fowler and Brannon (2000) [27], suggested an association with upper respiratory tract infection with a peak incidence in the fall and winter seasons. Viral transmission is likely ruled out as there have not been any viral particles found in samples of the affected glands [28].

28.4.3.3 Allergy

The presence of few eosinophils and the occurrence of spontaneous healing have suggested that SANS is not of allergic origin [27]. Furthermore, all lesions occurred as solitary lesions with no tendency for multi-focality and resolved without the need for topical or systemic medication within 3 weeks duration [29].

28.4.4 Clinical Presentation

Patients with SANS usually present with localized, often erythematous palatal swelling accompanied by an abrupt onset of pain [27]. The mean age of presentation is 27 years (range 15–70). The swelling usually involves the hard or soft palate, but buccal mucosa, upper lip, and ventral tongue are also possible locations. The swelling increases in size in days to weeks but can be gradual in onset. Multifocal presentation is rare. Although the disease usually resolves within 2–7 days, few extra-palatal lesions last longer than 1 week [29].

28.4.5 Pathology

Grossly, these are non-ulcerated, submucosal masses ranging from 0.3 to 2.5 cm. Microscopically, the lesion is characterized by a non-ulcerated nodule

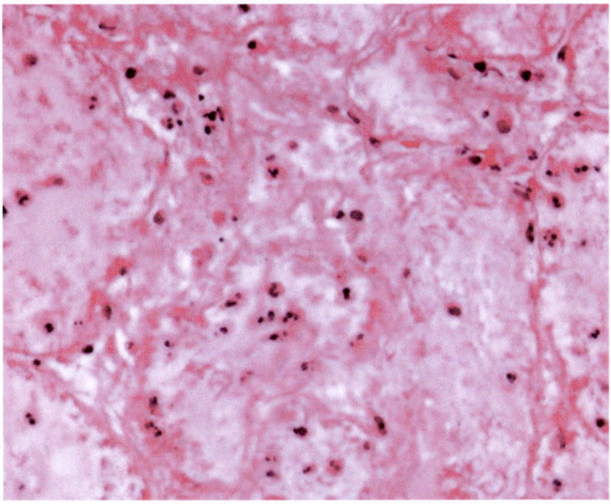

Fig. 28.3 Histopathology of a case of subacute necrotizing sialadenitis (SANS) showing inflammatory infiltrate consisting of neutrophils and eosinophils noted in the necrotic acini (H&E, ×40)

of mucosa in which the underlying salivary glands show subacute inflammation, represented by a mixed infiltrate of lymphocytes, neutrophils, and eosinophils (Fig. 28.3). Most of the ductal structures are lost or atrophic, and the acinar cells are necrotic [27, 28]. No ductal squamous metaplasia or fibrosis is seen [32].

28.4.6 Differential Diagnosis

The differential diagnosis of SANS includes NSM and chronic sialadenitis. Necrotizing sialo-metaplasia (NSM) presents a striking analogy with SANS. Both NSM and SANS share a similar patient profile albeit with involvement at a rather younger age in SANS. They share the same site of distribution on the posterior lateral hard palate, with the exception that NSM can also affect major salivary glands, the nasal cavity, the maxillary sinus, and the larynx. Lastly, they have similar necrosis of mucous acini of minor salivary glands, and both exhibit spontaneous healing [28]. Clinical differences between NSM and SANS are the duration and type of symptoms, the clinical appearance, and the length of the healing time. From the reported cases, the average delay preceding diagnosis is shorter for SANS (~1 week) than for NSM (~3 weeks) [27]. In addition, NSM usually presents as a large ulcer of variable pain, whereas SANS is a smaller, erythematous swelling and is almost always associated with pain [27]. SANS has not been reported as an ulcer. Histologically, the main difference is the prominent squamous metaplasia in the regenerating necrotic acini and ducts seen in NSM. In SANS, microscopy shows ductal loss and atrophy, but squamous metaplasia is normally mild or absent [28].

28.5 Necrotizing Sialo-metaplasia (NSM)

28.5.1 Definition

Necrotizing sialo-metaplasia (NSM) is a reactive nonneoplastic inflammatory process that usually affects the minor salivary glands of the palate; however, it may involve minor salivary glands in any location. It can easily be mistaken for a malignant tumor as it presents with a single, unilateral, painless (or only slightly painful) lesion of the hard palate.

28.5.2 Etiology

Necrotizing sialo-metaplasia is of unclear origin but is thought to result from vascular infarction of salivary gland lobules. Potential causes of diminished blood flow include the following:

Trauma
Local anesthetic injection
Smoking
Diabetes mellitus
Vascular disease
Pressure from dentures

28.5.3 Pathology

Necrotizing sialo-metaplasia is similar in appearance to pseudo-epitheliomatous hyperplasia, which appears as epithelial infiltration into underlying tissue, much like the visualized pattern of a carcinoma. Features distinguishing this condition from a malignant process include the following [34]:

Absence of cellular pleomorphism
Maintenance of salivary lobular morphology
Non-dysplastic appearance of squamous islands or nests
Evidence of residual ductal lumina within the epithelial nests

28.5.4 Clinical Presentation/Treatment

Patients with NSM are usually between the ages of 23 and 66 years. It is two to three times more common in males than in females. Lesions usually appear as large (1–4 cm), painless or painful, deeply ulcerated areas lateral to the palatal midline and near the junction of the hard and soft palates. They are usually unilateral but may be bilateral in some cases. It should be differentiated from other palatal lesions mainly subacute necrotizing sialadenitis (SANS). An excisional biopsy assists in ruling out a malignant process; otherwise, no additional treatment is indicated [34].

28.6 Benign Tumors of Minor Salivary Glands

28.6.1 Epidemiology

Tumors of the major and minor salivary glands account for only 2–4% of head and neck neoplasms. Most (~70%) salivary gland tumors originate in the parotid gland, with the remainder arising in the submandibular gland (~8%) and minor salivary glands (~22%) [35, 36]. Although about 75% of parotid gland tumors are benign, slightly more than 50% of submandibular gland tumors and 60–80% of minor salivary gland tumors are malignant [37]. Benign minor salivary gland tumors thus are relatively uncommon neoplastic entities. Of these, pleomorphic adenoma (PA), cystadenoma, and canalicular adenoma are the most frequently encountered [38].

The minor salivary glands are commonly classified according to their anatomical location—for example, labial glands (upper and lower lips), buccal glands, and so forth. Palatal minor salivary glands are the most common anatomical sub-site affected by minor salivary gland tumors; most series identify a nearly equal distribution between benign and malignant tumors [39].

In a study of 485 cases of minor salivary gland tumors from Northeastern China, PA was found to be the most common type of benign tumor, and adenoid cystic carcinoma (AdCC) was the most common type of malignant tumor [40].

The majority of benign salivary gland tumors (95%) occur in adults, most commonly PAs. Likewise, in children, the most common benign epithelial tumors are Pas, while the most common benign tumors of mesenchymal origin are hemangiomas [41].

28.6.2 Clinical Presentation

Patients with salivary gland lesions require a thorough head and neck evaluation. Cranial nerve function is carefully noted and documented. Careful attention is given to findings that may indicate malignancy, such as rapid growth, fixation to adjacent structures, associated cervical lymphadenopathy, pain, paresthesias, ulceration, and cranial nerve involvement.

Most patients who have benign minor salivary gland tumors present with a painless, progressive, enlarging mass in the affected minor salivary gland or oral cavity mucosal space. These masses can be firm to hard on palpation, mobile if within the salivary gland, and fixed in cases of local invasion [42].

Paranasal sinus minor salivary gland neoplasms may cause obstructive sinusitis, epistaxis, and nasal obstruction. Laryngotracheal salivary gland neoplasms may give rise to hoarseness of voice, dysphagia, odynophonia, and cough. Parapharyngeal space salivary neoplasms often are diagnosed late in their course due to the lack of presenting symptoms until a large tumor size has been attained. Trismus, dysphagia, or dysphonia may be the first indication of a tumor in the parapharyngeal space.

The palate is reported in the literature to be the most common anatomical site for minor salivary gland tumors, of which 42–75% occur in the palatal mucosa. Other sites include the lips (4–21%), the buccal mucosa (5–16%), the tongue or floor of the mouth (4–12%), and the retromolar area (3–7%) [43].

28.6.3 Classification/Histopathology

28.6.3.1 Pleomorphic Adenoma (PA)

Approximately 10% of PAs only occur in the minor salivary glands; the majority (80%) affect the parotid gland. In the oral cavity, the most commonly affected site is the palate, followed by the upper lip and buccal mucosa [44]. These tumors are more frequent in women and may occur in all age groups (mean age, 45 years). The majority of PAs grow slowly and are relatively asymptomatic, but they can become extremely large if neglected. Their gross appearance is that of a round, smooth mass with a thin, delicate, incomplete capsule. Notably, PAs arising in the minor salivary glands usually lack a capsule.

This benign tumor is capable of developing into a metastasizing pleomorphic adenoma (MPA), which is still benign but metastasizes as the name suggests, or into malignant tumors such as carcinoma ex-pleomorphic adenoma (CEPA) and carcinosarcoma. The malignant potential is directly related to the amount of time the tumor in situ (1.5% in the first 5 years, 9.5% after 15 years) [45]. The reported rate of recurrence after surgical excision is 7–15% [45].

Histopathologically, PAs have four components: capsule, epithelial cells, myoepithelial cells, and mesenchymal-stromal elements. Most of these tumors are composed of nearly 50% epithelial-myoepithelial cells and 50% mesenchymal-stromal elements. Tumors in which the percentage of epithelial-myoepithelial cells is 80% or higher are referred to as "cellular Pas," whereas those in which the percentage of mesenchymal-stromal elements is 80% or higher are referred to as "acellular Pas." The epithelial cells are cuboidal to polygonal and appear as small ducts and acini surrounded by a single layer of myoepithelial cells. Tumor cells have eosinophilic-to-amphophilic cytoplasm and central mildly chromatic nuclei with absent or barely discernible nucleoli. Skin adnexal differentiation is frequently observed in palate PA [46]. Myoepithelial cells may appear spindled, plasmacytoid, epithelioid, clear, or oncocytic. The mesenchymal-stromal components range from fibrous to myxoid to chondroid to osseous to lipomatous [47].

28.6.3.2 Basal Cell Adenoma (BCA)

Basal cell adenoma (BCA) accounts for 1–3% of all salivary neoplasms and typically occurs in adults, usually in the fourth to seventh decades of life, with a slight predilection for females [48]. Approximately 75% occur in the parotid gland; the rest involve the submandibular and minor salivary glands, especially the upper lip and buccal mucosa. The tumor typically presents as a slowly enlarging, asymptomatic mass [47], and the risk of malignant transformation is much lower than it is with PA [49].

Histopathologically, BCAs are composed of a mixture of basal, myoepithelial, and ductal cells. Basal cells are morphologically subdivided into (1) small dark cells, with sparse cytoplasm and round hyperchromatic nuclei, forming the periphery of tumor nests and demonstrating peripheral palisading, and (2) larger pale cells that are more polygonal, with basophilic-to-slightly eosinophilic cytoplasm and vesicular nuclei; these cells rest on top of this peripheral layer. Within the center, tumor nests are composed of small ductules lined by cuboidal epithelium [47]. Architecturally, BCAs are divided into six growth pattern subtypes: solid, trabecular, tubular, membranous, cribriform, and myoepithelial-derived stroma-rich [50].

28.6.3.3 Canalicular Adenoma

Canalicular adenoma typically occurs in patients older than 50 years with a slight predilection for women [51]. The majority (80%) affects the upper lip, and the remainder involves the buccal mucosa (10%), palate (3–10%), and parotid gland (<4%) [52]. Canalicular adenoma typically presents as a painless, slowly enlarging submucosal mass covered by intact mucosa that ranges in color from normal to slightly blue, often mimicking a mucocele. It is typically a solitary lesion, but multiple tumors have also been described [53].

Histopathologically, canalicular adenomas may or may not be encapsulated and are composed of cuboidal-to-columnar cells containing dark and often elongated nuclei with light eosinophilic-to-amphophilic cytoplasm. These cells are characteristically arranged in anastomosing cords that are two cells thick; this alternating pattern of abutment and separation has been referred to as "beading" [47].

28.6.3.4 Cystadenoma

Cystadenomas are rare benign cystic neoplasms that predominantly occur in the fifth decade, with a female-to-male ratio of 2:1–3:1 [47], typically found in the parotid and submandibular glands, though they may also be found in the minor salivary tissue of the lips and larynx (oncocytic cystadenoma) [54]. Cystadenomas usually present as fluctuant painless masses. In the oral cavity, they can mimic the clinical presentation of mucoceles.

Histopathologically, cystadenomas may be lined by a variety of epithelial types. Most commonly, the luminal epithelium is cystic to cuboidal with pale eosinophilic cytoplasm, whereas the outer layer is lined by an indistinct layer of basal cells with scant cytoplasm and small ovoid nuclei. A common variant is the "oncocytic cystadenoma," in which the lining is composed of the columnar oncocytic epithelium [47].

28.6.3.5 Ductal Papilloma

Ductal papillomas are divided into intraductal and inverted subtypes. Both are almost always reported in the minor salivary glands and are equally distributed among men and women [49], affecting patients between 50 and 70 years [55, 56].

Histopathologically, the intraductal type is characterized by a papillary network of cell-lined vascular fronds. The papillae partly fill the cystic cavity, and there is no evidence of cytological atypia and mitoses. On the other hand, the inverted type has histological features similar to those of sino-nasal inverted papilloma and is composed of epithelial cells forming a papillary projection. Columnar cells, mucous cells, and microcysts may be seen [49].

28.6.3.6 Lymphadenoma

Only rare cases of lymphadenoma involving the minor salivary glands have been reported in the literature. It usually occurs after the fifth decade of life, with no predilection for either gender [57]. Lymphadenomas typically present as slow-growing painless masses; some degree of cystic change may result in a fluctuant appearance [49].

Histopathologically, lymphadenoma has a prominent lymphoid stroma that does not consist of an oncocytic bilayer, as seen in Warthin's tumor. They are generally subcategorized as either sebaceous or non-sebaceous. Sebaceous lymphadenomas are more common and consist of solid-to-cystic proliferations of squamoid nests with varying degrees of sebaceous differentiation. A unique finding is a granulomatous reaction to keratin and sebum in the surrounding lymphoid stroma. The epithelial component of non-sebaceous lymphadenomas is often basaloid in appearance, ranging from a solid to a tubulo-trabecular growth pattern [49].

28.6.3.7 Myoepithelioma

Myoepitheliomas are rare tumors, comprising 1–2% of all salivary neoplasms. The majority is benign (70–90%), but some are malignant (10–30%). Approximately 75% of all cases occur in the parotid gland and palate. They have been described infrequently in a variety of other minor salivary gland sites, including the sino-nasal tract, oral cavity, and larynx. Unlike the parotid gland, these tumors are uncommon in the submandibular gland. Myoepithelioma affects both sexes equally and most commonly occurs between the ages of 40 and 50 years (range, 9–95 years). The tumor often presents as a mass that enlarges slowly over a period of several months to years [47].

Histopathologically, myoepitheliomas are composed primarily of spindle cells, plasmacytoid (hyaline) cells, or a combination of cells that grow in a solid, nodular, myxoid-mucinous, pseudo-glandular, trabecular, or reticulated pattern. Other cell variants (epithelioid, clear-cell, and oncocytic) are less common. The spindle cells are organized in sheets or swirls and have central oval-to-elongated nuclei with finely dispersed chromatin and blunt tapered ends. The plasmacytoid cells have glassy, dense eosinophilic cytoplasm and eccentric round-to-oval nuclei. In comparison with other subsites, plasmacytoid variants are found more frequently in the palate [47].

28.6.3.8 Oncocytoma

Similar to other oncocytic neoplasms, oncocytoma is a tumor of the elderly, most commonly occurring in the seventh and eighth decades of life, with no predilection for either sex [47]. In nearly 20% of cases, a prior history of irradiation may be present, giving rise to a subpopulation that presents at a younger age [58]. More than

80% of oncocytomas occur in the parotid gland, though they can occur in the submandibular and minor salivary glands as well. These tumors are typically slow-growing painless masses; approximately 7% of patients present with bilateral lesions. Oncocytomas may recur if excision is incomplete [59].

Histopathologically, oncocytomas are composed of polygonal oncocytes that may be arranged in a solid, a trabecular, or occasionally a compressed tubular growth pattern. Nuclei are round and vary from hyperchromatic to slightly vesicular with visible nucleoli. The periphery of tumor nests consists of darker cells with more scant cytoplasm [47].

28.6.3.9 Sebaceous Adenoma

Sebaceous adenomas are extremely rare, accounting for only 0.1% of salivary neoplasms. They are found in the parotid gland 60% of the time; however, when they are located in minor salivary glands, the most common site is the buccal mucosa [60]. Sebaceous adenomas are well-circumscribed encapsulated masses made up of solid nests of sebaceous cells within a fibrous stroma [49].

28.6.3.10 Sialadenoma Papilliferum

Sialadenoma papilliferum makes up 0.4–1.2% of all salivary gland tumors and most commonly occurs on the hard palate (80%) in patients around 60 years of age [61, 62].

Histopathologically, in sialadenoma papilliferum, the salivary duct epithelium demonstrates a biphasic growth pattern into the squamous keratotic epithelium, resulting in papillary epithelial hyperplasia [42, 49].

28.6.3.11 Sialo-lipoma

A sialo-lipoma is a well-circumscribed mass consisting of a salivary gland and mature adipose tissue. It remains unclear whether the salivary tissue within the lesion is neoplastic, hamartomatous, or residual entrapped glandular tissue. Although most commonly seen in the parotid gland, sialo-lipomas can also involve the minor salivary glands, affecting the hard or soft palate. Such lesions should be distinguished from normal fatty replacement of salivary glands, which can occur with the aging process [63].

28.6.4 Imaging Studies

Controversy exists regarding the routine use of imaging for small lesions of the minor salivary glands because radiographic imaging typically does not alter the management of these lesions. Nevertheless, computed tomography (CT) scan, magnetic resonance imaging (MRI), or both may be useful for suspected tumors of the parapharyngeal space. Both MRI and CT scans are also optimal for delineating the complete extent of the tumor and assessing for regional lymphadenopathy. In addition, these imaging modalities are useful for evaluating the possibility of invasion into surrounding tissues and facilitating the planning of definitive surgical resection.

28.6.4.1 Computed Tomography (CT) Scan

When bony erosion is suspected as in palatal minor salivary gland tumors, a CT scan may be required to assess the extent of locoregional involvement, which will play a role in planning for definitive resection and subsequent reconstruction. Similarly, a CT scan is indicated for minor salivary gland tumors involving the paranasal sinuses to delineate the extent of the tumor and differentiate the tumor from obstructive inflammatory changes.

28.6.4.2 Magnetic Resonance Imaging (MRI)

In general, MRI is superior for soft-tissue differentiation and is particularly helpful in assessing tumor extent, marrow infiltration, and perineural spread. It can also detect signal changes and extracapsular spread within regional LNs while simultaneously avoiding exposure to the ionizing radiation of CT. The disadvantages of MRI include its relatively high cost in comparison with CT, its susceptibility to motion artifact, and its poor cortical bone delineation [64].

28.6.4.3 Ultrasonography (US)

Minor salivary gland lesions in the mucosa of the oral cavity, pharynx, and tracheobronchial tree are not easily accessible or visualized via conventional US. Accordingly, ultrasonography is rarely employed in the diagnosis of minor salivary gland lesions.

28.6.5 Cytology/Histopathology

28.6.5.1 Fine-Needle Aspiration Cytology (FNAC)

In general, the histopathology of salivary gland tumors is extremely varied and complex; therefore, correct cytological typing of a primary salivary gland neoplasm can be difficult to perform [65].

The utility of FNA was established by Eneroth et al. (1967), who advocated its routine use and reported accuracy rates of 74–90% [66]. Although the procedure is somewhat operator-dependent, it is generally regarded as safe, simple to perform, and relatively inexpensive. In addition, the risk of seeding the needle tract is negligible (0.003–0.009%) [67].

The Milan System for Reporting Salivary Gland Cytopathology (MSRSGC) (Table 28.1), implemented in 2018, is an evidence-based standardized reporting system for salivary gland FNA that aids in the determination of malignancy risk [37].

28.6.5.2 Core Needle Biopsy (CNB)

Currently, core needle biopsy (CNB) is not as commonly employed in the management of salivary neoplasms, because of the risk of tumor seeding, which ranges between 0 and 22% [68]. The factors implicated in tumor seeding include needle size, use of a single versus coaxial needle, and tumor-related factors. In addition, CNB is unable to evaluate the boundary between the tumor and adjacent tissues and thus is inadequate in distinguishing benign tumors from low-grade malignancies. There may, however, be a role for CNB in cases where prior FNA was nondiagnostic.

Table 28.1 Milan System for Reporting Salivary Gland Cytopathology (MSRSGC)

Grade	Description	Risk of malignancy	Proposed treatment
I	Nondiagnostic	25%	Clinical and radiological correlation/repeat FNAC
II	Nonneoplastic	10%	Clinical follow-up and radiological correlation
III	Atypia of undetermined significance (AUS)	20%	Repeat FNAC or surgery
IV-A	Benign	<5%	Surgery or clinical follow-up
IV-B	Salivary gland neoplasm of uncertain malignant potential (SUMP)	35%	Surgery
V	Suspicious of malignancy	60%	Surgery
VI	Malignant	90%	Surgery

28.6.5.3 Open Biopsy

Open biopsy of minor salivary gland tumors is rarely performed, because of the risk of tumor spillage, associated infection, and tumor recurrence [41].

28.6.5.4 Immunohistochemistry (IHC)

Immunohistochemical diagnostics have specific applications and may facilitate the delineation of different cell components. Various diagnostic markers can be utilized to make an accurate diagnosis such that PLAG1 is specific for PAs and Ki-67 can differentiate between benign BCAs and malignant basal cell adenocarcinomas [69]. PLAG1 and HMGA1 have also been found to be increased in benign tumors and can aid in differentiating benign from malignant neoplasms [70]. Although these markers are helpful for characterizing tumors, they are not essential for diagnosis.

28.6.6 Identification of Genetic Translocations and Fusion Genes

Identification of genetic translocations and fusion genes is another emerging adjunct in the diagnosis of salivary neoplasms. This can be accomplished via fluorescence in situ hybridization (FISH), reverse transcriptase-polymerase chain reaction (RT-PCR), or, more recently, targeted RNA sequencing (RNA-seq) [71], which is capable of identifying fusion genes with rearrangement of PLAG1 and HMGA2 in PAs, for example.

28.6.7 Differential Diagnoses

Differential diagnosis of benign tumors of minor salivary glands includes the following:

Amyloidosis
Cheilitis glandularis
Mucocele and ranula

Mumps
Necrotizing sialo-metaplasia (NSM)
Sarcoidosis
Sjögren's syndrome

28.6.8 Treatment

28.6.8.1 Approach Considerations

The general consensus is that definitive surgical therapy is indicated for most benign tumors of the minor salivary glands. Notable exceptions would be certain tumor-like conditions, such as lymphoepithelial cysts associated with acute immunodeficiency syndrome (AIDS) and small asymptomatic hemangiomas. Historically, physicians have advocated surgery without imaging or FNAC; however, current recommendations include preoperative assessment with these diagnostic tools to assess for locoregional extent and concomitant lymphadenopathy. The primary contraindication of surgical treatment of benign salivary gland tumors is the presence of associated medical comorbidities that preclude general anesthesia.

28.6.8.2 Medical Therapy

Appropriate medical and supportive treatment is warranted for inflammatory or infectious salivary lesions such as acute bacterial sialadenitis or mycobacterial infection. Salivary gland excision is sometimes indicated when chronic, symptomatic, recurrent sialadenitis proves refractory to conservative therapies. If lymphoma is diagnosed, appropriate treatment for the stage and subtype of lymphoma is indicated through consultation with a medical oncologist.

28.6.8.3 Surgical Treatment

Management of benign salivary gland tumors includes complete removal with an adequate margin of peripheral tissue to avoid locoregional recurrence. Excision is performed with the patient under general anesthesia without paralysis. The endotracheal tube is usually positioned in the corner of the mouth opposite the proposed surgical field.

28.6.8.4 Intraoral Minor Salivary Gland Resection

Surgical treatment of minor salivary gland tumors depends on the site of origin and the extent of locoregional disease. For tumors of the lip or palate, this may simply involve wide local excision with primary closure. Benign minor salivary gland tumors of the upper lip and buccal mucosa are often managed with a mucosa-sparing wide local excision that sacrifices the etiologic minor salivary gland tissue with an intact tumor pseudo-capsule [39].

For more extensive palatal lesions, the recommendation is to perform a bone-sparing, periosteal-sacrificing, wide local excision incorporating 5- to 10-mm linear margins within the palatal mucosa, with careful preservation of the tumor pseudo-capsule. The periosteum and tumor pseudo-capsule represent anatomical barrier margins on the deep surface of the tumor. In long-standing cases of benign palatal salivary gland tumors, the thin remaining bone is sacrificed on the deep surface of the tumor specimen; retention of thinned bone often is not technically possible or anatomically meaningful. Immediate soft-tissue reconstruction of the resultant defect is possible and desirable; primary closure with adjunct locoregional flap reconstruction may be used if clinically indicated.

28.6.8.5 Transcervical Approach

Larger tumors of the parapharyngeal space may necessitate a more complex surgical approach; intraoral resection typically is not recommended in such cases. The main options for external approaches to the parapharyngeal space are the cervical-parotid approach and the cervical-parotid approach with mandibulectomy.

Although this procedure does not require a full facial nerve dissection, the inferior divisions must be located and preserved. By retracting the sternocleidomastoid (SCM) muscle laterally, the internal jugular vein, the carotid artery, and the lower cranial nerves (IX-XII) are identified. To improve access to this space, the posterior belly of the digastric and stylohyoid muscles are divided, followed by the external carotid artery (ECA) and the stylomandibular ligament. In addition, the styloid process may be resected for better visualization and delivery of larger tumors. In patients with tumors located in the superior aspect of the parapharyngeal space that approaches the Eustachian tube and skull base, a mandibulectomy may be necessary in order to provide optimal surgical access [72].

28.6.8.6 Trans-oral Robotic Surgery

Recently, applications of minimally invasive trans-oral robotic surgery (TORS) to head and neck surgery have increased. It affords access to the parapharyngeal space and allows precise tumor dissection, avoiding the need for an external approach and thereby improving cosmetic outcomes for patients.

The risk of tumor capsule fragmentation and subsequent cellular spilling with TORS has been found to be low. However, depending on the location of the tumor, a change in approach to a trans-oral blunt instrument dissection may be necessary to avoid damage to the ECA and ensure patient safety [73]. Although TORS can be attempted for tumors medial to the ECA, a transcervical approach is generally recommended for tumors located lateral to the vessels [74].

28.6.9 Prognosis

28.6.9.1 Outcome

With appropriate treatment of benign salivary gland tumors, the outcome is excellent, and the recurrence rate (RR) is very low. In general, PA has the highest risk of malignant transformation and recurrence of all benign salivary gland tumors. Basal cell adenomas (BCAs) also carry a risk of malignant transformation, albeit a much smaller one, whereas the other types virtually never undergo malignant transformation. Recurrence is unlikely for oncocytoma, canalicular adenoma, myoepithelioma, and BCA (membranous subtype). Recurrence is extremely rare for lymphadenoma, cystadenoma, and BCA (solid, trabecular, and tubular subtypes) [49].

28.6.9.2 Complications

Age greater than 60 years and a larger extent of surgical resection are significant predictors of complications. Complications associated with definitive excision and reconstruction of palatal minor salivary gland benign and malignant tumors include Eustachian tube dysfunction, flap loss, trismus, velopharyngeal insufficiency, and wound dehiscence [75]. Complications associated with definitive transcervical excision of parapharyngeal minor salivary gland tumors include facial nerve paralysis, first-bite syndrome, Frey's syndrome, hemorrhage, and infection [76]. Complications associated with TORS include bleeding, dysphagia, infections related to aspiration, and local pain [77].

28.7 Malignant Tumors of Minor Salivary Glands

28.7.1 Epidemiology

Malignant tumors of minor salivary glands are a group of rare cancers with significant heterogeneity in histological types and ultimate clinical behavior. The incidence of salivary gland malignancy is estimated to be 4–135 cases/106/year [78] with only 10–15% arising in the minor salivary glands [79]. The annual incidence of minor salivary gland malignancies has been estimated to be 0.16–0.4/100,000 population [80].

Salivary gland carcinomas demonstrate an unparalleled histological diversity when compared to any other organ system [81]. The two most common histological types reported in the literature are adenoid cystic carcinoma (AdCC) and mucoepidermoid carcinoma (MEC) [82–94]. Clinical series have often shown an increased incidence in females [43, 82, 83, 88, 91, 95–97]. However, a SEER report in 2016 found the incidence to be equal between males and females, 49.9% versus 50.1%, respectively [98]. Hay et al. (2019) reported that malignant tumors of minor salivary glands are mostly encountered in patients in their middle age (around 60 years) (~56%), less commonly in old age (around 80 years) (~6%), and least in the young (<20 years) (~2%) [96]. Similarly, several authors reported that, typically, the most common ages to present with minor salivary carcinoma are the sixth and seventh decades [43, 85, 93–95, 98]. Different peaks of age, depending on the histological type analyzed, have been reported in the literature [88, 92, 98].

A number of recent studies have reported on patients following postoperative radiation and had a lower incidence of early-stage tumors, 20% had T1 tumors in the study by Cianchetti et al. (2009) [99], and 23.4% were T1 in a paper by Salgado et al. [100].

28.7.2 Anatomical Location

Hay et al. (2019) explored the incidence, pathology, clinical behavior, and the factors predictive of outcome in a large cohort of patients ($n = 450$) with minor salivary gland malignancies treated at Memorial Sloan Kettering Cancer Center (MSK) over a 30-year period (1985–2015). They determined the anatomical site of minor salivary gland malignancies using clinical examination and imaging [96]. Accordingly, tumor locations were categorized into the oral cavity, nasal cavity, paranasal sinuses, oropharynx, larynx, and trachea. The oral cavity consisted of the subsites buccal mucosa, floor of the mouth, hard palate, mandible, lip, retromolar trigone, tongue, and upper gum. The oropharynx included the subsites of the base of the tongue, soft palate, and tonsil, while the nasal cavity included the subsites maxillary sinus, nasal cavity, nasal septum, and nasopharynx.

The most frequent site for minor salivary carcinoma was the oral cavity, accounting for 68% of the tumors, and then the oropharynx representing 21% of the tumors [96]. This has also been reported in the SEER data report (2006), with 58.7% in the oral cavity and 21.2% in the pharynx [98].

28.7.3 Pathology

The histopathology of minor salivary glands is complex with multiple different histopathological types. Usually, the WHO Classification of Head and Neck Tumors is used for histological classification and for definitions of grade within pathological groups [95]. Tumors are categorized into low-, intermediate-, and high-risk histology groups to allow for analysis because of the large number of histological types.

Tumors categorized as "high-risk" are salivary duct carcinoma, high-grade MEC, high-grade carcinoma ex-pleomorphic adenoma (CEPA), high-grade adenocarcinoma, high-grade myoepithelial carcinoma, high-grade adenoid cystic carcinoma (AdCC), and high-grade acinic cell carcinoma (ACC). "Intermediate-risk" tumors include AdCC and intermediate-grade MEC, while tumors classified as "low-risk" include low-grade ACC, low-grade MEC, low-grade adenocarcinoma, low-grade CEPA, low-grade myoepithelial carcinoma, and all polymorphous adenocarcinoma and epithelial-myoepithelial carcinomas.

28.7.4 Clinical Presentation

Sarmento et al. (2016) [94] evaluated the clinicopathological profile of patients with minor salivary gland neoplasms over a period of 15 years. This retrospective study included 37 patients with benign and malignant tumors of the minor salivary glands. Malignant neoplasms represented 70.3% of cases. The MEC was the most common neoplasm (45.9%), followed by PA (24.4%). Most patients were female (70.3%), aged between 71 and 80 years. The palate (67.6%) and the retromolar region (10.8%) were the most affected sites. The time of progression was shorter, and the mean size of lesions of benign tumors was smaller than for malignant neoplasms. Signs and symptoms can be related to tumor size and may vary according to the tumor site. Malignant tumors with a late diagnosis can be related to metastasis, especially AdCC [101].

Jansisyanont et al. (2002) [89] observed that 27.95% of malignant tumors were present for >1 year and 13.1% were asymptomatic. Thus, all suspected tumors of minor salivary glands require biopsy to avoid delays and errors in diagnosis. Clinically, it is not possible to differentiate between malignant and benign tumors of minor salivary glands. Swelling (mass) is the most common clinical presentation of malignant minor salivary gland tumors. Ulceration, ill-fitting dentures, difficult speech, and pain are other presentations. It is not clear if pain is a common symptom in malignant neoplasms of minor salivary glands [43, 85, 88, 102–104]. In the series reported by Sarmento et al. in 2016, no case exhibited lymphadenopathy, and only one case showed metastasis [94].

28.7.5 Investigations

Computed tomography (CT) scan and magnetic resonance imaging (MRI) are useful in determining the extension of the disease and the possibility of adequate resection. These investigations are also valuable in the demarcation of metastatic neck lymph nodes (LNs).

Ultrasound (US) evaluation, especially combined with ultrasound-guided fine-needle aspiration cytology (US-FNAC), has been proposed as a means of increasing preoperative accuracy in staging [105]. However, it is generally accepted that pathological staging is the most decisive parameter for further management. In addition, micrometastasis may not be diagnosed but only cured with a neck dissection.

Minor salivary gland carcinomas (MSGCs) can be divided radiologically into "localized" and "invasive" subtypes on the basis of the clinical utility of such categorization. Characteristic invasion patterns of the invasive type include deep submucosal extension, bone marrow infiltration, and perineural spread, which are difficult to assess clinically. MSGCs easily invade adjacent structures because of their submucosal location and may spread along the muscles, nerves, periosteum, and dura mater. Moreover, the tumor may spread into the bone marrow without obvious bone destruction.

28.7.5.1 Localized Type

The localized type manifests as a well-demarcated mass and could cause pressure erosion of the adjacent bone, which corresponds to a low-grade tumor. The tumor may show polypoid growth [106–108]. In clinical settings, the localized type exhibits clinical and radiological features similar to those of benign tumors with slow growth over several years [106]. Painless swelling is the most common symptom of the localized type [109]. Fine-needle aspiration cytology (FNAC) or biopsy is useful in reaching an accurate diagnosis. However, pathologists may find it difficult to differentiate between benign and malignant tumors without assessing the invasion of the interface between the tumor and adjacent normal tissue [110]. Regarding the localized type, malignancy should be suspected on the basis of slight findings associated with malignancy, including irregular shape, ill-defined margins, or absence of a capsule [111]. Localized types are usually treated by surgical resection with a wide safety margin [109, 110].

28.7.5.2 Invasive Type

The invasive type invades surrounding structures and can cause pain, ulceration (that should be differentiated from squamous cell carcinoma), bleeding, or nerve palsy due to neural invasion [110, 112]. At imaging, the invasive type shows an ill-defined border with an obvious invasion of adjacent structures, which corresponds to high-grade tumors. Since MSGCs occur in the submucosa, the tumor may easily invade underlying structures. The characteristic invasion patterns of the invasive type are classified as deep submucosal extension [113–115], bone marrow infiltration with minimal bone cortex destruction (best depicted by MRI), and spread along the nerve sheath [116].

28.7.6 Treatment

The clinical behavior of MSG tumors of the same entities seems to differ significantly depending on clinical staging, histopathological and biological features such as differentiation grade, tumor localization, and different signaling pathways [117–123]. All these factors are important in deciding the best modality of treatment and determining prognosis.

28.7.6.1 Treatment of the Tumor

In general, radical surgical excision is the therapeutic intervention of choice for malignant neoplasms of minor salivary glands (MSGs) followed by adjuvant radiotherapy (RT) [82, 83, 87, 89, 91, 119, 124–132]. Primary radiotherapy (RT) is indicated in cases of irresectable tumors [110].

28.7.6.2 Management of the Neck

The treatment of the clinically negative neck (cN0) remains controversial, as data on cervical metastases are rare and often vary significantly between different publications and tumor entities [132, 133]. The rate of cervical metastases, however, is crucial for treatment planning and patients' outcome, as they have been identified as highly relevant prognostic factors in various head and neck tumors [130, 133, 134].

Many factors usually dictate selective neck dissection, such as the site and size (T) of the tumor, the histological grade, and the age of the patient. Parsons et al. (1996) have classified MSG tumor sites according to the incidence of node positivity [131]. According to this classification, low incidence (<10%) is observed in MSG tumors of the hard palate, nasal cavity, paranasal sinuses, lip, and buccal mucosa. The intermediate risk of positive neck at presentation should be expected in MSG tumors of the floor of the mouth and tongue. The higher risk of LN metastases lies with MSG tumors of the pharynx and larynx. However, other authors advocate significantly lower LN infiltration than hematogenous metastases for MSG tumors [135]. Papadogeorgakis et al. (2011) [136] analyzed the data of 22 patients with malignant tumors of the minor salivary glands, surgically treated over a 10-year period. They recommended modified radical neck dissection (MRND) for clinical, radiological, or frozen section evidence of metastasis. Selective supra-omohyoid neck dissection is reserved for patients with tumors of high-grade or advanced stage (III-IV). Site is not estimated as important for the decision of neck dissection nor is the patient's age [136].

28.7.6.3 Adjuvant Therapy

Papadogeorgakis et al. (2011) recommended adjuvant radiotherapy (RT) for high-grade, tumor-positive LNs and residual disease [136]. Adjuvant RT is also supported as a further means of achieving locoregional control of the disease by several authors [132, 137]. A combination of radiotherapy (RT) and chemotherapy (cisplatin with or without docetaxel) was offered to patients with positive or close margins and advanced stage of the disease at presentation in one study [136]. Other authors reserve such therapy for patients with distant metastases [138, 139] or as palliative treatment [135, 137]. Combination therapy appears to improve the prognosis of patients with MSG tumors. As 10-year survival is poor among such patients [137–139], an effective chemotherapeutic agent may inhibit and prevent late hematogenous metastases.

28.7.6.4 Follow-Up

For patients with malignant MSG tumors, a follow-up of over 10 years is absolutely necessary, with review monthly for the first year, every 3 months for the next 5 years, and every 6 months thereafter. All patients under review should be examined locally and for neck metastases. Physical examination, as well as a yearly MRI, is necessary for follow-up [136].

28.7.7 Prognosis

28.7.7.1 Overall Survival

In 2019, Hay et al. [96] reported 5-year and 10-year overall survival rates of 86% and 69%, respectively, for minor salivary gland malignancies. This is similar to previous reports; Spiro et al. (1991) reported a 5-year survival rate of 75% [140], Vander Poorten et al. (2000) reported 68% [109], and Loh et al. (2009) reported 73.8% [141]. As reported by Hay et al., factors predictive of failure in overall survival on univariate analysis were age greater or equal to 60 years, male gender, tobacco consumption, history of serious comorbidity, perineural invasion (PNI), lymphovascular invasion (LVI), close/positive margins, histological risk group, postoperative radiation, pathological T and N stage, and AJCC oncological overall stage.

On multivariable analysis, age 60 or greater was associated with a 3.62 increased risk of death ($p < 0.001$). Female gender was associated with a lower risk of death ($p = 0.003$). Compared to tumors in the oral cavity site, tumors of the larynx/trachea sites had a decreased risk of death. The high-risk histology group had a 2.40 ($p < 0.001$) increased risk of death compared to the low-risk histology group [96]. Univariate analysis of margins showed that positive/close margins were associated with an increased risk of death compared to a negative margin ($p = 0.042$). Overall stage was an important predictor in the multivariable model. AJCC stage II tumors had a 1.60 increased risk compared to stage I. Stages III and IV had an increased risk of 6.01 and 4.73, respectively, compared to stage I.

28.7.7.2 Disease-Specific Survival (DSS)

According to Hay et al. (2019), the DSS at 5 years and 10 years was 94% and 82%, respectively. Factors predictive of DSS on univariate analysis were male gender, history of tobacco, PNI, LVI, positive margins, histological risk group, postoperative radiation, pathological T and N stage, and AJCC oncological overall stage [96].

On univariate analysis, tumors of the sino-nasal site had a higher risk of disease-related death compared to the oral cavity site. Oropharynx tumors also had a 1.91 times higher rate of disease-specific death. Multivariable analysis showed that gender, high-risk pathology group, and AJCC stage remained significant predictors of disease-related death. However, the tumor sites predictive on univariate analysis and postoperative radiation were no longer significant [96].

28.7.7.3 Recurrence Free Survival (RFS)

Hay et al. (2019) reported that the estimated 5-year and 10-year recurrence-free survival (RFS) was 79% and 69%, respectively. The factors that were significant in univariate analysis were gender, tumor site, PNI, LVI, margin status, pathology risk group, pT stage, pN stage, AJCC stage, and postoperative radiation. Age, alcohol, tobacco, and comorbidities were not significant predictors of recurrence. On multivariable analysis, the factors that remained statistically significant predictors of recurrence were the pathological risk group and AJCC stage. Tumor site and margin status were not significant factors. Compared to the low-risk histology group, intermediate- and high-risk pathologies had an increased risk of recurrence. Higher AJCC stage was also associated with increased risk of recurrence [96].

28.7.8 Analysis of Predictors of Survival/Recurrence

28.7.8.1 Age of the Patient

Several studies have shown that age was important for overall survival but had no effect on the other survival or recurrence outcomes in multivariable analysis [96, 128, 142, 143]. Thus, age should not impact the optimal treatment plan [79], although it may affect the practical considerations in choosing appropriate therapy.

28.7.8.2 Site of the Tumor

Disease site has been shown in the literature to be an important prognostic factor in univariate analysis with sino-nasal tumors having a worse outcome [141, 144]. However, when tumor stage and grade were controlled for multivariable analysis, the site was no longer significant [141]. In the cohort study by Hay et al. (2019) [96], patients with oral cavity tumors had a worse overall survival when age, gender, margin, pathology, stage, and adjuvant radiation were controlled. Further multivariable analysis did not show tumor site had a statistically significant effect on DSS or RFS.

28.7.8.3 Resection Margin

In 2010, Iyer et al. reported that a negative resection margin is correlated with better outcomes [145]. Local and regional control is usually good in most tumors with the long-term mortality attributed to distant failure [79]. In 2019, Hay et al. found that although patients with a positive or close margin had a 56% increased chance of death, there was no statistically significant effect on RFS.

28.7.8.4 Histology of the Tumor

Histology of the tumor has also been reported by several authors to be an important predictor of outcome for salivary malignancy [128, 146–149]. The pathology of the carcinoma, incorporating histological type and high-risk factors, is a major driver of the outcome of this disease. PNI and LVI are both significant predictors on univariate analysis.

28.7.8.5 Stage of the Disease

The stage of the tumor, including the T or N stage or combining these into the AJCC overall stage, has been shown in the literature to have important prognostic significance [140]. The AJCC stage is a statistically significant predictor for all survival and all recurrence outcomes [96].

28.7.8.6 Radiotherapy

Radiation is not considered a curative primary treatment for salivary malignancy, but it has been used extensively as an adjuvant treatment. The indications for postoperative radiotherapy (PORT) are usually high-grade and high-stage salivary gland tumors. Margin status, tumor location, neck disease, and the presence of extra-nodal extension (ENE) have also been considered indications [149, 150]. Local control and survival benefits have been reported with adjuvant radiotherapy in retrospective cohorts [151]. In Hay et al.'s study, univariate analysis showed that patients receiving PORT had worse outcomes, but when other variables were controlled for multivariable analyses, PORT was associated with improved overall survival, DSS, and RFS but was not statistically significant [96].

References

1. Som PM, Brandwin-Gensler MS. Anatomy and pathology of the salivary glands. In: Som PM, Curtin HD, editors. Head and neck imaging. 5th ed. St. Louis, MO: Mosby; 2011. p. 2449–602.
2. Hoang JK. Extramucosal diseases of the head and neck. In: Grossman RI, Yousem DM, editors. Neuroradiology: the requisites. 3rd ed. St. Louis, MO: Mosby; 2010. p. 476–514.
3. Kessler AT, Bhatt AA. Review of the major and Minor salivary glands, part 1: anatomy, infectious, and inflammatory processes. J Clin Imaging Sci. 2018;8:47.

4. Senthikumar B, Nazargi MM. Mucocele: an unusual presentation of the minor salivary gland lesion. J Pharm Bioallied Sci. 2012;4:180–2.
5. du Toit DF, Nortjé C. Salivary glands: applied anatomy and clinical correlates. SADJ. 2004;59(2):65–74.
6. Lighterman I. Sialolithiasis of a minor salivary gland. Oral Surg Oral Med Oral Pathol. 1955;8(2):143–5.
7. Holst E. The clinical entity of sialolithiasis of the minor salivary glands. Acta Odontol Scand. 1971;29:75–84.
8. Pullon PA, Miller AS. Sialolithiasis of accessory salivary glands: review of 55 cases. J Oral Surg. 1972;30:832–4.
9. Anneroth G, Hansen LS. Minor salivary gland calculi. A clinical and histopathological study of 49 cases. Int J Oral Surg. 1983;12:80–9.
10. Brazao-Silva MT, Prosdocimi FC, Lemos-Junior CA, de Sousa SO. Clinicopathological aspects of 25 cases of sialolithiasis of minor salivary glands. Gen Dent. 2015;63:e22–6.
11. Wang WC, Chen CY, Hsu HJ, Kuo JH, Lin LM, Chen YK. Sialolithiasis of minor salivary glands: a review of 17 cases. J Dent Sci. 2016;11:152–5.
12. Ben Lagha N, Alantar A, Samson J, Chapireau D, Maman L. Lithiasis of minor salivary glands: current data. Oral Surg Oral Med Oral Pathol Oral Radiol Endod. 2005;100:345–8.
13. Lee LT, Wong YK. Pathogenesis and diverse histologic findings of sialolithiasis in minor salivary glands. J Oral Maxillofac Surg. 2010;68:465–70.
14. Matiakis A, Tzermpos F. Sialolithiasis of minor salivary gland: a challenging diagnostic dilemma. J Korean Assoc Oral Maxillofac Surg. 2021;47(2):145–8.
15. Huang C-H, Hwang M-J, Lang M-J, Chiang C-P. Minor salivary gland sialolithiasis of the upper lip. J Dent Sci. 2022;17(2):1050–2.
16. Ng SY, Pinto P. Ultrasound-guided retrieval of labial minor salivary gland sialoliths. Dentomaxillofac Radiol. 2000;29:319–22.
17. Barnett ML. Sialolithiasis of a labial gland. Oral Surg Oral Med Oral Pathol. 1971;32:22–8.
18. Ho V, Currie WJ, Walker A. Sialolithiasis of minor salivary glands. Br J Oral Maxillofac Surg. 1992;30:273–5.
19. Boyd AS. Sialolith of a minor salivary gland. J Cutan Pathol. 2013;40:695–8.
20. Okada H, Yokokawa M, Komiya M, Akimoto Y, Kaneda T, Yamamoto H. A rare case of sialolithiasis of the lower lip simulating a mucocele and review of the literature. Quintessence Int. 2011;42:589–94.
21. Suh DW, Lee EJ, Lew BL, Sim WY. Minor salivary gland sialolithiasis of the upper lip. Ann Dermatol. 2013;25:502–4.
22. Lin HP, Cheng CY, Sun A, Chiang CP. Mucoepidermoid carcinoma of the upper lip. J Formos Med Assoc. 2016;115:1015–6.
23. Jin YT, Chang JYF, Hwang MJ, Chiang CP. Palisaded encapsulated neuroma of the upper labial mucosa—case report. J Dent Sci. 2021;16:1041–3.
24. Hwang MJ, Chang JYF, Sun A, Chiang CP. Kimura disease of the upper lip: case report. J Dent Sci. 2021;16:1325–7.
25. Su CH, Lee KS, Tseng TM, Hung SH. Endoscopic holmium:YAG laser-assisted lithotripsy: a preliminary report. B-ENT. 2015;11:57–61.
26. Werning JT, Waterhouse JP, Mooney JW. Subacute necrotizing sialadenitis. Oral Surg Oral Med Oral Pathol. 1990;70:756–9.
27. Fowler CB, Brannon RB. Subacute necrotizing sialadenitis: report of 7 cases and a review of the literature. Oral Surg Oral Med Oral Pathol Oral Radiol Endodontol. 2000;89:600–9.
28. Lombardi T, Samson J, Kuffer R. Subacute necrotizing sialadenitis: a form of necrotizing sialometaplasia? Arch Otolaryngol Head Neck Surg. 2003;129:972–5.
29. Suresh L, Aguirre A. Subacute necrotizing sialadenitis: a clinicopathological study. Oral Surg Oral Med Oral Pathol Oral Radiol Endodontol. 2007;104:385–90.
30. Maloth SGK, Latha S, Pai A, Komali B. Subacute necrotizing sialadenitis—a case report. J Indian Acad Oral Med Radiol. 2007;19:345.
31. Eyibilen AON, Aladağ I, Ozkan F, Kaya Z, Köseoğlu D. An unusual giant subacute necrotizing sialadenitis as an emergency case of otolaryngology. J Ear Nose Throat. 2008;19:216–9.

32. Ko YC, Philipone E, Florin W, Heinz MJ, Rosenberg S, Yudell R. Subacute necrotizing Sialadenitis: a series of three cases and literature review. Head Neck Pathol. 2016;10(4):425–8.
33. Castro WH, Drummond SN, Gomez RS. Subacute necrotizing sialadenitis in the buccal mucosa. J Oral Maxillofac Surg. 2002;60:1494–6.
34. Miloro M, Kolokythas A. Diagnosis and management of salivary gland disorders. In: Hupp JR, Ellis III E, Tucker MR, editors. Contemporary oral and maxillofacial surgery. 7th ed. Philadelphia, PA: Elsevier; 2019. p. 423–49.
35. Spuntarelli G, Santecchia L, Urbani U, Zama M. Minor salivary gland neoplasm in children. J Craniofac Surg. 2013;24(2):664–7.
36. Eveson JW, Cawson RA. Salivary gland tumours. A review of 2410 cases with particular reference to histological types, site, age and sex distribution. J Pathol. 1985;146(1):51–8.
37. Ritwik P, Brannon RB. A clinical analysis of nine new pediatric and adolescent cases of benign minor salivary gland neoplasms and a review of the literature. J Med Case Rep. 2012;6:287.
38. Bradley PJ. Frequency and histopathology by site, major pathologies, symptoms and signs of salivary gland neoplasms. Adv Otorhinolaryngo. 2016;78:9–16.
39. Carlson ER, Schimmele SR. The management of minor salivary gland tumors of the oral cavity. Atlas Oral Maxillofac Surg Clin North Am. 1998;6(1):75–98.
40. Wang XD, Meng LJ, Hou TT, Zheng C, Huang SH. Frequency and distribution pattern of minor salivary gland tumors in a northeastern Chinese population: a retrospective study of 485 patients. J Oral Maxillofac Surg. 2015;73(1):81–91.
41. Califano J, Eisele DW. Benign salivary gland neoplasms. Otolaryngol Clin N Am. 1999;32(5):861–73.
42. Nag D, Biswas PK, Mandal PK, Bhattacharyya NK, Gautam D, Mukhopadhyay S. Tumours of minor salivary glands—a clinicopathologic study. J Indian Med Assoc. 2012;110(8):567–77.
43. Pires FR, Pringle GA, de Almeida OP, Chen SY. Intra-oral minor salivary gland tumors: a clinico-pathological study of 546 cases. Oral Oncol. 2007;43(5):463–70.
44. Pinkston JA, Cole P. Incidence rates of salivary gland tumors: results from a population-based study. Otolaryngol Head Neck Surg. 1999;120(6):834–40.
45. Bokhari MR, Greene J. Pleomorphic adenoma. Treasure Island, FL: StatPearls; 2023.
46. Schmidt LA, Olsen SH, McHugh JB. Cutaneous adnexal differentiation and stromal metaplasia in palate pleomorphic adenomas: a potential diagnostic pitfall that may be mistaken for malignancy. Am J Surg Pathol. 2010;34(8):1205–10.
47. Seethala RR, Barnes EL. Rare malignant and benign salivary gland epithelial tumors. Surg Pathol Clin. 2011;4(4):1217–72.
48. Li J, Fonseca I. Basal cell adenoma. In: El-Naggar AK, JKC C, Grandis JR, Takata T, Slootweg PJ, editors. WHO classification of head and neck tumours, vol. 9. 4th ed. Lyon, France: International Agency for Research on Cancer (IARC); 2017. p. 187–8.
49. Hellquist H, Paiva-Correia A, Vander Poorten V, Quer M, Hernandez-Prera JC, Andreasen S, et al. Analysis of the clinical relevance of histological classification of benign epithelial salivary gland tumours. Adv Ther. 2019;36(8):1950–74.
50. Dardick I, Daley TD, van Nostrand AW. Basal cell adenoma with myoepithelial cell-derived "stroma": a new major salivary gland tumor entity. Head Neck Surg. 1986;8(4):257–67.
51. Nelson JF, Jacoway JR. Monomorphic adenoma (canalicular type). Report of 29 cases. Cancer. 1973;31(6):1511–3.
52. Daley TD, Gardner DG, Smout MS. Canalicular adenoma: not a basal cell adenoma. Oral Surg Oral Med Oral Pathol. 1984;57(2):181–8.
53. Rousseau A, Mock D, Dover DG, Jordan RC. Multiple canalicular adenomas: a case report and review of the literature. Oral Surg Oral Med Oral Pathol Oral Radiol Endod. 1999;87(3):346–50.
54. Brandwein M, Huvos A. Laryngeal oncocytic cystadenomas. Eight cases and a literature review. Arch Otolaryngol Head Neck Surg. 1995;121(11):1302–5.
55. White DK, Miller AS, McDaniel RK, Rothman BN. Inverted ductal papilloma: a distinctive lesion of minor salivary gland. Cancer. 1982;49(3):519–24.

56. Sun S, Wang P, Wang Y, Su W, Wang F, Yang H. Intraductal papilloma arising from the accessory parotid gland: a case report and literature review. Medicine (Baltimore). 2018;97(20):e10761.
57. Ma J, Chan JK, Chow CW, Orell SR. Lymphadenoma: a report of three cases of an uncommon salivary gland neoplasm. Histopathology. 2002;41(4):342–50.
58. Brandwein MS, Huvos AG. Oncocytic tumors of major salivary glands. A study of 68 cases with follow-up of 44 patients. Am J Surg Pathol. 1991;15(6):514–28.
59. Buxton RW, Maxwell JH, French AJ. Surgical treatment of epithelial tumors of the parotid gland. Surg Gynecol Obstet. 1953;97(4):401–16.
60. Gnepp DR. Sebaceous neoplasms of salivary gland origin: a review. Pathol Annu. 1983;1:71–102.
61. Fowler CB, Damm DD. Sialadenoma papilliferum: analysis of seven new cases and review of the literature. Head Neck Pathol. 2018;12(2):193–201.
62. Bobos M, Hytiroglou P, Karkavelas G, Papakonstantinou C, Papadimitriou CS. Sialadenoma papilliferum of bronchus. Virchows Arch. 2003;443(5):695–9.
63. Nagao T, Sugano I, Ishida Y, Asoh A, Munakata S, Yamazaki K, et al. Sialolipoma: a report of seven cases of a new variant of salivary gland lipoma. Histopathology. 2001;38(1):30–6.
64. Lee YY, Wong KT, King AD, Ahuja AT. Imaging of salivary gland tumours. Eur J Radiol. 2008;66(3):419–36.
65. Jayaram G, Verma AK, Sood N, Khurana N. Fine needle aspiration cytology of salivary gland lesions. J Oral Pathol Med. 1994;23(6):256–61.
66. Eneroth CM, Franzén S, Zajicek J. Aspiration biopsy of salivary gland tumors. A critical review of 910 biopsies. Acta Cytol. 1967;11(6):470–2.
67. Guidelines of the Papanicolaou Society of Cytopathology for fine-needle aspiration procedure and reporting. The Papanicolaou Society of Cytopathology Task Force on Standards of Practice. Diagn Cytopathol. 1997;17(4):239–47.
68. Robertson EG, Baxter G. Tumour seeding following percutaneous needle biopsy: the real story! Clin Radiol. 2011;66(11):1007–14.
69. Meyer MT, Watermann C, Dreyer T, Ergün S, Karnati S. Update on diagnostic markers and translocation in salivary gland tumors. Int J Mol Sci. 2021;22(13):6771.
70. Barca I, Mignogna C, Donato G, Cristofaro MG. Expression of PLAG1, HMGA1 and HMGA2 in minor salivary glands tumours. Gland Surg. 2021;10(5):1609–17.
71. Bubola J, MacMillan CM, Demicco EG, Chami RA, Chung CT, Leong I, et al. Targeted RNA sequencing in the routine clinical detection of fusion genes in salivary gland tumors. Genes Chromosomes Cancer. 2021;60(10):695–708.
72. Scianna JM, Petruzzelli GJ. Contemporary management of tumors of the salivary glands. Curr Oncol Rep. 2007;9(2):134–8.
73. Maglione MG, Guida A, Pavone E, Longo F, Aversa C, Villano S, et al. Transoral robotic surgery of parapharyngeal space tumours: a series of four cases. Int J Oral Maxillofac Surg. 2018;47(8):971–5.
74. Bulut OC, Giger R, Alwagdani A, Aldabal N, Stenzinger A, Heimgartner S, et al. Primary neoplasms of the parapharyngeal space: diagnostic and therapeutic pearls and pitfalls. Eur Arch Otorrinolaringol. 2021;278(12):4933–41.
75. Moore BA, Burkey BB, Netterville JL, Butcher RB 2nd, Amedee RG. Surgical management of minor salivary gland neoplasms of the palate. Ochsner J. 2008;8(4):172–80.
76. Horowitz G, Ben-Ari O, Wasserzug O, Weizman N, Yehuda M, Fliss DM. The transcervical approach for parapharyngeal space pleomorphic adenomas: indications and technique. PLoS One. 2014;9(2):e90210.
77. Hay A, Migliacci J, Karassawa Zanoni D, Boyle JO, Singh B, Wong RJ, et al. Complications following transoral robotic surgery (TORS): a detailed institutional review of complications. Oral Oncol. 2017;67:160–6.
78. Albeck H, Nielsen NH, Hansen HE, Bentzen J, Ockelmann HH, Bretlau P, et al. Epidemiology of nasopharyngeal and salivary gland carcinoma in Greenland. Arctic Med Res. 1992;51(4):189–95.

79. Vander Poorten V, Hunt J, Bradley PJ, Haigentz M Jr, Rinaldo A, Mendenhall WM, et al. Recent trends in the management of minor salivary gland carcinoma. Head Neck. 2014;36(3):444–55.
80. Bradley PJ, McGurk M. Incidence of salivary gland neoplasms in a defined UK population. Br J Oral Maxillofac Surg. 2013;51(5):399–403.
81. Seethala RR, Stenman G. Update from the 4th edition of the World Health Organization classification of head and neck Tumours: tumors of the salivary gland. Head Neck Pathol. 2017;11(1):55–67.
82. Oliveira FA, Duarte EC, Taveira CT, Máximo AA, Aquino EC, Alencar Rde C, et al. Salivary gland tumor: a review of 599 cases in a Brazilian population. Head Neck Pathol. 2009;3(4):271–5.
83. Dhanuthai K, Boonadulyarat M, Jaengjongdee T, Jiruedee K. A clinico-pathologic study of 311intra-oralsalivaryglandtumors in Thais. J Oral Pathol Med. 2009;38(6):495–500.
84. Tian Z, Li L, Wang L, Hu Y, Li J. Salivary gland neoplasms in oral and maxillofacial regions: a 23-year retrospective study of 6982 cases in an eastern Chinese population. Int J Oral Maxillofac Surg. 2010;39(3):235–42.
85. Wang D, Li Y, He H, Liu L, Wu L, He Z. Intraoral minor salivary gland tumors in a Chinese population: a retrospective study on 737 cases. Oral Surg Oral Med Oral Pathol Oral Radiol Endod. 2007;104(1):94–100.
86. Shishegar M, Ashraf MJ, Azarpira N, Khademi B, Hashemi B, Ashrafi A. Salivary gland tumors in maxillofacial region: a retrospective study of 130 cases in a southern Iranian population. Pathol Res Int. 2011;2011:934350.
87. Ito FA, Ito K, Vargas PA, Almeida OP, Lopes MA. Salivary gland tumors in a Brazilian population: a retrospective study of 496 cases. Int J Oral Maxillofac Surg. 2005;34(5):533–6.
88. Jaber MA. Intraoral minor salivary gland tumors: a review of 75 cases in a Libyan population. Int J Oral Maxillofac Surg. 2006;35(2):150–4. Review
89. Jansisyanont P, Blanchaert RH Jr, Ord RA. Intraoral minor salivary gland neoplasm: a single institution experience of 80 cases. Int J Oral Maxillofac Surg. 2002;31(3):257–61.
90. Vargas PA, Gerhard R, Araújo VJ, Filho CIV. Salivary gland tumors in a Brazilian population: a retrospective study of 124 cases. Rev Hosp Clin Fac Med Sao Paulo. 2002;57(6):271–6.
91. Venkata V, Irulandy P. The frequency and distribution pattern of minor salivary gland tumors in a government dental teaching hospital, Chennai, India. Oral Surg Oral Med Oral Pathol Oral Radiol Endod. 2011;111(1):e32–9.
92. Tilakaratne WM, Jayasooriya PR, Tennakoon TM, Saku T. Epithelial salivary tumors in Sri Lanka: a retrospective study of 713 cases. Oral Surg Oral Med Oral Pathol Oral Radiol Endod. 2009;108(1):90–8.
93. Ramesh M, Krishnan R, Paul G. Intraoral minor salivary gland tumours: a retrospective study from a dental and maxillofacial surgery centre in Salem, Tamil Nadu. J Maxillofac Oral Surg. 2014;13(2):104–8.
94. Sarmento DJ, Morais ML, Costa AL, Silveira ÉJ. Minor intraoral salivary gland tumors: a clinical-pathological study. Einstein (Sao Paulo). 2016;14(4):508–12.
95. Barnes L, International Academy of P. University Hospital ZDoP. World Health Organization Classification of tumours: pathology and genetics of head and neck tumours. Lyon, France: IARC Press; 2005. p. 430.
96. Hay AJ, Migliacci J, Karassawa Zanoni D, McGill M, Patel S, Ganly I. Minor salivary gland tumors of the head and neck-Memorial Sloan Kettering experience: incidence and outcomes by site and histological type. Cancer. 2019;125(19):3354–66.
97. Buchner A, Merrell PW, Carpenter WM. Relative frequency of intra-oral minor salivary gland tumors: a study of 380 cases from northern California and comparison to reports from other parts of the world. J Oral Pathol Med. 2007;36(4):207–14.
98. Baddour HM Jr, Fedewa SA, Chen AY. Five- and 10-year cause-specific survival rates in carcinoma of the minor salivary gland. JAMA Otolaryngol Head Neck Surg. 2016;1 42(1):67–73.
99. Cianchetti M, Sandow PS, Scarborough LD, Morris CG, Kirwan J, Werning JW, et al. Radiation therapy for minor salivary gland carcinoma. Laryngoscope. 2009;119(7):1334–8.

100. Salgado LR, Spratt DE, Riaz N, Romesser PB, Wolden S, Rao S, et al. Radiation therapy in the treatment of minor salivary gland tumors. Am J Clin Oncol. 2014;37(5):492–7.
101. Guzzo M, Locati LD, Prott FJ, Gatta G, McGurk M, Licitra L. Major and minor salivary gland tumors. Crit Rev Oncol Hematol. 2010;74(2):134–48.
102. Al-Khateeb TH, Ababneh KT. Salivary tumors in north Jordanians: a descriptive study. Oral Surg Oral Med Oral Pathol Oral Radiol Endod. 2007;103(5):e53–9.
103. Speight PM, Barrett AW. Salivary gland tumours. Oral Dis. 2002;8(5):229–40.
104. Pires FR, Almeida OP, Pringle G, Chen SY. Differences on clinicopathological profile from intraoral minor salivary gland tumors around the world. Oral Surg Oral Med Oral Pathol Oral Radiol Endod. 2008;105(2):136–8.
105. Atula TS, Varpula MJ, Kurki TJI, Klemi PJ, Grénman R. Assessment of cervical lymph node status in head and neck cancer patients: palpation, computed tomography and low field magnetic resonance imaging compared with ultrasound-guided fine-needle aspiration cytology. Eur J Radiol. 1997;25:152–61.
106. Kwak SH, Lee KS, Chung MJ, Jeong YJ, Kim GY, Kwon OJ. Adenoid cystic carcinoma of the airways: helical CT and histopathologic correlation. AJR Am J Roentgenol. 2004;183(2):277–81.
107. Kato H, Kanematsu M, Sakurai K, Mizuta K, Aoki M, Hirose Y, et al. Adenoid cystic carcinoma of the maxillary sinus: CT and MR imaging findings. Jpn J Radiol. 2013;31(11):744–9.
108. Krishnamurthy A. Clear cell mypepithelial carcinoma of the base tongue managed by the mandible preserving pull-through oropharyngectomy approach. Indian J Surg Oncol. 2015;6(3):263–6.
109. Vander Poorten VL, Balm AJ, Hilgers FJ, Tan IB, Keus RB, Hart AA. Stage as major long term outcome predictor in minor salivary gland carcinoma. Cancer. 2000;89(6):1195–204.
110. Vander Poorten V, Hunt J, Bradley PJ, et al. Recent trends in the management of minor salivary gland carcinoma. Head Neck. 2014;36(3):444–55.
111. Zheng Y, Xiao Z, Zhang H, She D, Lin X, Lin Y, et al. Differentiation between benign and malignant palatal tumors using conventional MRI: a retrospective analysis of 130 cases. Oral Surg Oral Med Oral Pathol Oral Radiol. 2018;125(4):343–50.
112. Abdel Razek AAK, Mukherji SK. Imaging of minor salivary glands. Neuroimaging Clin N Am. 2018;28(2):295–302.
113. Hasan Z, Tan D, Buchanan M, Palme C, Riffat F. Buccal space tumours. Auris Nasus Larynx. 2019;46(2):160–6.
114. Zvrko E, Golubović M. Laryngeal adenoid cystic carcinoma. Acta Otorhinolaryngol Ital. 2009;29(5):279–82.
115. Ganly I, Patel SG, Coleman M, Ghossein R, Carlson D, Shah JP. Malignant minor salivary gland tumors of the larynx. Arch Otolaryngol Head Neck Surg. 2006;132(7):767–70.
116. Panizza B, Warren T. Perineural invasion of head and neck skin cancer: diagnostic and therapeutic implications. Curr Oncol Rep. 2013;15(2):128–33.
117. Lombardi D, McGurk M, Vander Poorten V, Guzzo M, Accorona R, Rampinelli V, et al. Surgical treatment of salivary malignant tumors. Oral Oncol. 2017;65:102–13.
118. Klussmann JP, Ponert T, Mueller RP, Dienes HP, Guntinas-Lichius O. Patterns of lymph node spread and its influence on outcome in resectable parotid cancer. Eur J Surg Oncol. 2008;34:932–7.
119. Carrillo JF, Maldonado F, Carrillo LC, Ramirez-Ortega MC, Pizano JG, Melo C, et al. Prognostic factors in patients with minor salivary gland carcinoma of the oral cavity and oropharynx. Head Neck. 2011;33:1406–12.
120. Jang S, Patel PN, Kimple RJ, McCulloch TM. Clinical outcomes and prognostic factors of adenoid cystic carcinoma of the head and neck. Anticancer Res. 2017;37:3045–52.
121. Ferrarotto R, Mitani Y, McGrail DJ, Li K, Karpinets TV, Bell D, et al. Proteogenomic analysis of salivary adenoid cystic carcinomas defines molecular subtypes and identifies therapeutic targets. Clin Cancer Res. 2021;27:852–64.
122. Feeney L, Hapuarachi B, Adderley H, Rack S, Morgan D, Walker R, et al. Clinical disease course and survival outcomes following disease recurrence in adenoid cystic carcinoma with and without NOTCH signaling pathway activation. Oral Oncol. 2022;133:106028.

123. Yan K, Yesensky J, Hasina R, Agrawal N. Genomics of mucoepidermoid and adenoid cystic carcinomas. Laryngoscope Investig Otolaryngol. 2018;3:56–61.
124. Geiger JL, Ismaila N, Beadle B, Caudell JJ, Chau N, Deschler D, et al. Management of Salivary Gland Malignancy: ASCO guideline. J Clin Oncol. 2021;39:1909–41.
125. Terhaard CH, Lubsen H, Van der Tweel I, Hilgers FJ, Eijkenboom WM, Marres HA, et al. Salivary gland carcinoma: independent prognostic factors for locoregional control, distant metastases, and overall survival: results of the Dutch head and neck oncology cooperative group. Head Neck. 2004;26:681–92.
126. Zeidan YH, Pekelis L, An Y, Holsinger FC, Kong CS, Chang DT, et al. Survival benefit for adjuvant radiation therapy in minor salivary gland cancers. Oral Oncol. 2015;51:438–45.
127. Wang X, Luo Y, Li M, Yan H, Sun M, Fan T. Management of salivary gland carcinomas—a review. Oncotarget. 2017;8:3946–56.
128. Lopes MA, Santos GC, Kowalski LP. Multivariate survival analysis of 128 cases of oral cavity minor salivary gland carcinomas. Head Neck. 1998;20:699–706.
129. Shi X, Huang NS, Shi RL, Wei WJ, Wang YL, Ji QH. Prognostic value of primary tumor surgery in minor salivary-gland carcinoma patients with distant metastases at diagnosis: first evidence from a SEER-based study. Cancer Manag Res. 2018;10:2163–72.
130. Moratin J, Horn D, Semmelmayer K, Ristow O, Engel M, Hoffmann J, et al. Surgical treatment of carcinomas of the oral minor salivary glands-oncological outcome in dependence of tumor entity and therapeutic strategies. Cancers (Basel). 2023;15(15):3895.
131. Parsons JT, Mendenhall WM, Stringer SP, Cassisi NJ, Million RR. Management of minor salivary gland carcinomas. Int J Radiat Oncol Biol Phys. 1996;35:443–54.
132. Bell RB, Dierks EJ, Homer L, Potter BE. Management and outcome of patients with malignant salivary gland tumors. J Oral Maxillofac Surg. 2005;63:917–28.
133. Moratin J, Ledermann A, Schulz AD, Metzger K, Ristow O, Hofele C, et al. Neck involvement and disease recurrence in adenoid cystic carcinoma of the minor salivary glands: the role of surgery in primary and progressive disease. Int J Oral Maxillofac Surg. 2020;10:1663.
134. Moratin J, Metzger K, Kansy K, Ristow O, Engel M, Hoffmann J, et al. The prognostic significance of the lymph node ratio in oral cancer differs for anatomical subsites. Int J Oral Maxillofac Surg. 2020;49:558–63.
135. Licitra L, Grandi C, Prott FJ, Schornagel JH, Bruzzi P, Molinari R. Major and minor salivary glands tumours. Crit Rev Oncol Hematol. 2003;45:215–25.
136. Papadogeorgakis N, Parara E, Petsinis V, Pappa E, Nikolaidis A, Alexandridis K. A retrospective review of malignant minor salivary gland tumors and a proposed protocol for future care. Craniomaxillofac Trauma Reconstr. 2011;4(1):1–10.
137. Kokemueller H, Swennen G, Brueggemann N, Brachvogel P, Eckardt A, Hausamen J-E. Epithelial malignancies of the salivary glands: clinical experience of a single institution—a review. Int J Oral Maxillofac Surg. 2004;33:423–32.
138. Strick MJ, Kelly C, Soames JV, McLean NR. Malignant tumours of the minor salivary glands—a 20-year review. Br J Plast Surg. 2004;57:624–31.
139. Stannard CE, Hering E, Hough J, Knowles R, Munro R, Hille J. Post-operative treatment of malignant salivary gland tumours of the palate with iodine-125 brachytherapy. Radiother Oncol. 2004;73:307–11.
140. Spiro RH, Thaler HT, Hicks WF, Kher UA, Huvos AH, Strong EW. The importance of clinical staging of minor salivary gland carcinoma. Am J Surg. 1991;162(4):330–6.
141. Loh KS, Barker E, Bruch G, O'Sullivan B, Brown DH, Goldstein DP, et al. Prognostic factors in malignancy of the minor salivary glands. Head Neck. 2009;31(1):58–63.
142. Anderson JN Jr, Beenken SW, Crowe R, Soong SJ, Peters G, Maddox WA, et al. Prognostic factors in minor salivary gland cancer. Head Neck. 1995;17(6):480–6.
143. Kakarala K, Bhattacharyya N. Survival in oral cavity minor salivary gland carcinoma. Otolaryngol Head Neck Surg. 2010;143(1):122–6.
144. Spiro RH. Salivary neoplasms: overview of a 35-year experience with 2,807 patients. Head Neck Surg. 1986;8(3):177–84.

145. Iyer NG, Kim L, Nixon IJ, Palmer F, Kraus D, Shaha AR, et al. Factors predicting outcome in malignant minor salivary gland tumors of the oropharynx. Arch Otolaryngol Head Neck Surg. 2010;136(12):1240–7.
146. Auclair PL, Goode RK, Ellis GL. Mucoepidermoid carcinoma of intraoral salivary glands. Evaluation and application of grading criteria in 143 cases. Cancer. 1992;69(8):2021–30.
147. Li Q, Zhang XR, Liu XK, Liu ZM, Liu WW, Li H, et al. Long-term treatment outcome of minor salivary gland carcinoma of the hard palate. Oral Oncol. 2012;48(5):456–62.
148. Spiro RH, Koss LG, Hajdu SI, Strong EW. Tumors of minor salivary origin. A clinicopathologic study of 492 cases. Cancer. 1973;31(1):117–29.
149. van der Wal JE, Snow GB, van der Waal I. Histological reclassification of 101 intraoral salivary gland tumours (new WHO classification). J Clin Pathol. 1992;45(9):834–5.
150. Lloyd S, Yu JB, Ross DA, Wilson LD, Decker RH. A prognostic index for predicting lymph node metastasis in minor salivary gland cancer. Int J Radiat Oncol Biol Phys. 2010;76(1):169–75.
151. Terhaard CH, Lubsen H, Rasch CR, Levendag PC, Kaanders HH, Tjho-Heslinga RE, et al. The role of radiotherapy in the treatment of malignant salivary gland tumors. Int J Radiat Oncol Biol Phys. 2005;61(1):103–11.

MIX
Papier aus verantwortungsvollen Quellen
Paper from responsible sources
FSC® C105338

If you have any concerns about our products,
you can contact us on
ProductSafety@springernature.com

In case Publisher is established outside the EU,
the EU authorized representative is:
Springer Nature Customer Service Center GmbH
Europaplatz 3, 69115 Heidelberg, Germany

Printed by Libri Plureos GmbH
in Hamburg, Germany